WM 70 DUD

2012

Mental Health and Human Rights

vision, praxis, and courage

Mental Health and Human Rights

vision, praxis, and courage

Edited by

Michael Dudley

Derrick Silove

and

Fran Gale

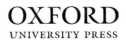

OXFORD

UNIVERSITY PRESS

OXFORD
UNIVERSITY PRESS

Great Clarendon Street, Oxford ox2 6dp
United Kingdom

Oxford University Press is a department of the University of Oxford.
It furthers the University's objective of excellence in research, scholarship,
and education by publishing worldwide. Oxford is a registered trade mark of
Oxford University Press in the UK and in certain other countries

British Library Cataloguing in Publication Data
Data available

Library of Congress Cataloging-in-Publication Data
Data available

ISBN 978–0–19–921396–2

Printed and bound by
CPI Group (UK) Ltd,
Croydon, CR0 4YY

Dedication

For all who live with mental health challenges, users and survivors of mental health services, and all who care.

In Memoriam

In memory of Gene Brody (1921–2010) and Alan Flisher (1957–2010), champions of mental health and human rights.

Foreword

This important volume tells, from different but authoritative perspectives, the story of the very last human right to be recognized—that of the mentally disabled, to participate fully in human society. The 'right to independent living' in Article 19 of the 2006 *Convention on Rights of Persons with Disabilities* insists that these persons shall not be demeaned or discriminated against in choosing their place of residence and where and with whom they live, and should have equal access to community services and facilities. It is, of course, a long process between the crystallization of a right in a Convention and its acceptance in a world where fifty countries still have no laws at all about mental health. Still, a way forward has been found, from the welfare model embodied in the Poor Law (which formally removed social rejects from the community and diminished the quality of their life by unnecessary institutionalization) to a rights-based approach which enables those wrongfully detained or excluded or discriminated against on grounds of mental handicap to use the law as a weapon for redress.

Why have the rights of the mentally disabled been so belatedly and so reluctantly recognized? Way back in 1948, the destruction in part of a race or ethnic group was outlawed by the Convention on the Prevention and Punishment of the Crime of Genocide, which made no reference to groups that had been exterminated as 'useless eaters' by the Nazis, or discarded as 'feeble-minded' by the eugenics movement in the US and the UK or had been the potential victims of sterilization programmes with the slogan 'three generations of imbeciles are enough', or actual victims of 'breeding out' programmes, like the 'stolen generation' of Australian aborigines? The public intellectuals who made eugenic euthanasia fashionable in the 1920s were, of course, still in the grip of the nineteenth century rationalist fallacy, that rights should only belong to those capable of logical thought—a principle that in the Victorian age excluded 'women, dogs, and lunatics' from the professions, the universities and the franchise. Even supporters of female emancipation drew the line at votes for 'lunatics' (although John Stuart Mills' passionate defence of the eccentric proved the community benefit from the right to be different).

It did not help that rights in this period were commonly assumed to come from nature or from God: it was not until 1939 that H.G. Wells pointed out that rights were possessed by individuals 'because a man comes into this world through no fault of his own' and that all governments had a duty to protect the minimum dignity of the most vulnerable.[1] That was the moral imperative which inspired the *Universal Declaration of Human Rights* in 1948 and then its offspring which soon gave protection to women, to children, and to the victims of torture, landmines and racism. But not, until 2006, to those with mental disabilities.

The common law has long afforded them a few basic protections, ever since Chief Justice Edward Coke, back in 1606, declared the unlawfulness of hanging a mentally disabled murderer: "that should be a miserable spectacle, both against law and of extreme inhumanity and cruelty, and can be no example to others".[2] A fine principle, but the problem always lay in the diagnosis.

---

[1] See G Robertson, *Crimes Against Humanity—The Struggle for Global Justice*, (Penguin, 3rd edn 2006) p27.

[2] See G Robertson, *Freedom The Individual and The Law*, (Penguin, 7th edn) p 433.

Daniel McNaughton was 'not at all mad' declared Queen Victoria, on hearing that the young schizophrenic who had tried to assassinate the Prime Minister had Chartist sympathies. Even today, Gary Mackinnon—the hacker with Aspergers who is resisting extradition to America—is regarded by judges as mentally composed because he left a protest about Guantanamo on the U.S army computers he hacked into—as if holding political views means that you cannot have a mental illness! Every expert declared that 'Yorkshire Ripper' Peter Sutcliffe suffered from paranoid schizophrenia, but the Judge, an embodiment of public prejudice, refused to let the Attorney-General accept his plea of diminished responsibility and encouraged the jury to come to an obviously wrongful verdict of 'guilty of murder'. (It was so obviously wrongful to put Sutcliffe in an ordinary prison that within a few months he was moved to Broadmoor).

I found Kiranjit Ahluwhalia languishing in prison with a life sentence for murder, despite her mental condition arising from the fact that the husband she killed had beaten her every day of their ten-year marriage. By the 1990's, it was possible to obtain her release by persuading the Court of Appeal to recognize that post-traumatic stress disorder has diminished her responsibility.[3] By this time the *Confait* Inquiry had demonstrated the extreme vulnerability and suggestibility of children with learning difficulties when interviewed aggressively in police custody (they had confessed to a murder they did not commit) and henceforth they had to be accompanied by a parent or social worker. I handled the successful appeal of David Mackenzie, convicted as a serial killer, but who turned out to be a serial confessor. The Court of Appeal established an important rule that uncorroborated confessions by mentally disordered persons could not henceforth be the basis for a 'guilty' verdict.[4] But these developments, gradually integrating the insights of psychiatry with the mercy of the law, had their limits: the case of *W v Egdell* showed that mental patients had no right of confidentiality to stop professional advisers, without their consent, sending subjective assessments of their 'dangerousness' to the authorities.[5] In many mental hospitals there was still a culture of brutality and repression: the law was limited to occasional police action when an abuse became public. Without management practices and ethical standards based on a human rights code, mental patients continued to be treated as if they are a sub-human species.

This position gradually changed as the *European Convention on Human Rights* took hold, through decisions of its court in Strasbourg. In Britain, for example, the problem for mentally disordered offenders was that any kind of liberty—release, recall, discharge—depended not on a review tribunal (its decisions were no more than recommendations) but on the politician—easily deterred by fear of adverse publicity—who happened to occupy the office of Home Secretary. Human Rights law requires decisions about restoration of liberty to be a matter of independent judgement rather than political discretion, and Article 5(4) of the Convention gives all detainees the right to have the lawfulness of their confinement decided by a court. The Strasbourg judges ruled that the Review Tribunal was not a 'court', because it had no power to do other than make recommendations to the Minister. The law in the UK had to be changed, so that it was henceforth for the Minister to make recommendations to the Review Tribunal.[6] This was an example of a significant contribution by human rights law to ensuring fairness for mentally disordered offenders, by insisting that decisions about their liberty are made independently and impartially. I can whole-heartedly endorse the point made in the introduction to this book, namely that the European Court of Human Rights has generated a remarkable body of case law which has obliged

---

[3] *R v Ahluwalia* (1992) 4 All ER 889.
[4] *R v Mackenzie* (1992) 96 Cr AppR 98.
[5] *W v Egdell* (1990) 2 WLR 471.
[6] *X v United Kingdom* (1981) 4 EHRR 188.

its forty-seven member states to modify their national laws to address the civil rights issues of their citizens with mental disabilities.

There is, of course, much more to be done, and this book provides very helpful guidance to the rights, so recently recognized, that need to be effectuated and enforced. At present, the international reporting system which covers all state parties to human rights Conventions, still fails to include 'mental health' as a matter on which these states must report. This must change, and urgently. In 'advanced' countries massive ignorance remains, often fanned by sensational stories in the media, about 'dangerousness': after having educated judges, mental health campaigners must now educate journalists, and through them the wider public.

The true test of a nation is how it treats its most vulnerable citizens, and mentally disabled people still have their lives made miserable—sometimes too miserable to bear—by being bullied, scapegoated, and taunted. Persecuting people on account of or by reference to their mental capacity should be made a specific criminal offence. Laws and practices, that have the effect of excluding the mentally disabled from community experiences and duties—jury service, for example—must be reconsidered. There are insights provided throughout the chapters of this book which will greatly help in promoting the happiness of those who, through no fault of their own, have minds less adjusted to a world which should value them nonetheless, and especially.

Geoffrey Robertson Q.C.
Doughty Street Chambers
8th March 2012

Foreword

This is a very big book—in size, in scope, and in the range of perspectives it contains. Both mental health and human rights are such vast and overlapping concepts that we lack a consensus on how humans should preserve or restore them. For instance, some people defend the right to treatment, even when people don't want it; while others claim treatment without consent is a violation of human rights. International human rights agencies have rightly objected to the psychiatric incarceration of political dissidents in some countries while turning a blind eye to the compulsory regimes imposed upon ordinary citizens diagnosed with mental illness in other countries. Some experts lament the global inequities that have stalled the development of western style mental health systems in low income countries, while others warn that the introduction of these systems will deliver more profits for multi-national drug companies but worse outcomes for the people who receive them. This book acknowledges the varieties of discrimination against people with a diagnosis of mental illness in many countries and cultures, including the contribution made by even the most benign intentions within psychiatry and the law.

I view all these debates through the lens of someone who has experienced madness and has been part of the international user/survivor movement for nearly three decades. In a word this movement advocates self-determination for people who are diagnosed with mental illness—in our treatment, in the services we use, and in the lives we lead. Although there have been some small gains since the movement began in the 1970s, mad people throughout the world are routinely subjected to compulsory interventions, and a large majority of people who use mental health services in the west do not work, have partners or bring up children, and they die up to 25 years younger than average. The reasons for this are complex but a strong pattern of inequality and human rights breaches are woven into these sobering outcomes.

Why do society and its mental health and human rights institutions allow this situation to continue and even promote some of the practices that remove our self-determination? Perhaps this question I often ask myself comes down to people's deepest beliefs about the nature of madness. These beliefs are sometimes explicit but more often implicit, and they drive people's reasoning about madness as well as their responses to it. Some who work in the busy, chaotic intersection between mental health and human rights still view mad people as 'other'—a compromised class of human beings who are helpless victims of a pathology that robs us of our full humanity. This view ensures that human rights violations against mad people will continue because it invites a justification for inaction, coercion, or exclusion. It would be wrong to minimize or romanticize madness but we need to see it as a full human experience. Imagine if humans viewed this set of experiences as crises of being which stretches people's personal resources to the limit and which takes heroic strength to overcome. Imagine if we could all see that value and meaning can be derived from these experiences, not just for the person themselves but the rest of the community. This would do more to protect our human rights than anything else I can think of.

A major development in mental health and human rights in recent years is the United Nations Convention on the Rights of Persons with Disabilities, adopted by the United Nations General Assembly in 2006. This convention reaffirms the human rights of people with disabilities, including those with 'psychiatric disabilities'. The Convention prohibits discrimination against people with disabilities in civil, political, social, cultural, and economic life and it breaks new ground by stating in Article 14 on liberty and security of the person, that 'the existence of a disability shall in no way justify a deprivation of liberty'. This article may be early sign that the tide is turning on compulsory regimes in mental health across the world.

I hope that this book guides the flow of ideas at the intersection between human rights and mental health into a more unified direction—a direction that moves us all towards a consensus on genuine self-determination for people who experience madness.

Mary O'Hagan
Former Chair, World Network of Users and Survivors of Psychiatry, and
International consultant, writer, and speaker

Contents

Contributors

Gunilla Backman
Health Policy Advisor,
Swedish International Development
Cooperation Agency (SIDA),
Stockholm, Sweden

Catherine R. Bateman Steel
School of Public Health and
Community Medicine,
University of New South Wales,
New South Wales, Australia

Professor Myron L. Belfer
Department of Psychiatry
Children's Hospital Boston
Harvard Medical School
Boston, MA, USA

Professor Dinesh Bhugra
President-Elect of the World Psychiatric
Association
Professor of Mental Health and Cultural
Diversity
Institute of Psychiatry,
King's College London,
London, UK

Professor Michaeline Bresnahan
Assistant Professor of Clinical Epidemiology,
Mailman School of Public Health,
New York State Psychiatric Institute,
New York City, NY, USA

Professor Henry Brodaty
Director,
Primary Dementia Collaborative Research
Centre, School of Psychiatry,
University of New South Wales,
Sydney, New South Wales, Australia

Professor Eugene Brody
[deceased]

Dr Elaine Brohan
Health Service and Population Research
Department, Institute of Psychiatry,
King's College London, London, UK

Professor Ngiare Brown
Associate Professor and Director
Bullana, the Poche Centre for Indigenous
Health, University of Sydney,
New South Wales, Australia

Professor Richard A. Bryant
Scientia Professor,
School of Psychology,
University of New South Wales,
New South Wales, Australia

Judith Bueno de Mesquita
School of Law, University of Essex,
Colchester, UK

Dr Tom Calma
Immediate Past Aboriginal and
Torres Strait Islander Social Justice
Commissioner; and National Coordinator,
Tackling Indigenous Smoking,
Australian Government, Canberra, Australia

Dr Adrian Carter
NHMRC Postdoctoral Fellow in Public Health,
University of Queensland Centre for Clinical
Research, University of Queensland,
QLD, Australia

Associate Professor Dilek Cindoğlu
Associate Professor of Sociology,
Department of Political Science,
Bilkent University, Ankara, Turkey

Professor Peter J. Cooper
Co-Director of the Winnicott Research
Centre and Research Director, Berkshire
Child Anxiety Clinic,
Winnicott Research Unit,
School of Psychology,
University of Reading, Reading, UK

Professor John Copeland
Emeritus Professor of Psychiatry,
University of Liverpool, UK;
Past President, World Federation for
Mental Health, Washington DC, USA

Professor François Crépeau
Professor of International Public Law
Faculty of Law, McGill University,
Montréal, Québec, Canada

Professor Amita Dhanda
Professor and Head,
Centre for Disability Studies,
NALSAR University of Law,
Hyderabad, India

Dr Michael Dudley
Psychiatrist, Sydney Children's and
Prince of Wales Hospitals,
Senior Conjoint Lecturer, School of
Psychiatry, University of New South Wales,
Sydney, Australia

Dr Catherine Esposito
General Manager, International
Programs ActionAid Australia
New South Wales, Australia

Professor Alan Flisher
[deceased]

Tony Fowke
President of the World Federation for Mental
Health, Karrinyup, Australia

Dr Fran Gale
Lecturer, Community and Social Work,
University of Western Sydney,
New South Wales, Australia

Preston J. Garrison
World Federation for Mental Health,
Springfield, USA

Anne-Claire Gayet,
Agent of Domain Justice,
Quebec Metropolis Centre of Immigration
and Metropoles
Montréal, Québec, Canada

Semyon Gluzman
President of the Ukrainian Psychiatric
Association, Director of the International
Medical Rehabilitation Center for the Victims
of War and Totalitarian Regimes, Kiev, Ukraine

Dr Ian Hall
Consultant Psychiatrist for people with
Learning Disability,
East London Foundation NHS Trust,

Community Learning Disability Service,
London, UK

Professor Wayne Hall
NHMRC Australia Fellow and Deputy
Director (Policy),
University of Queensland Centre for Clinical
Research and the Queensland Brain Institute,
University of Queensland,
QLD, Australia

Lillian Craig Harris
Director, Together for Sudan,
Arlington, Virginia, USA

Winton Higgins
Transforming Cultures Research Centre,
Faculty of Arts and Social Sciences,
University of Technology,
Sydney, New South Wales, Australia

Professor Ernest Hunter
Regional Psychiatrist: Queensland Health,
Adjunct Professor: University of
Queensland, Cairns
School of Population Health,
University of Queensland
Cairns, QLD, Australia

Jennifer Jacobs
School of Medicine,
University of Western Sydney,
New South Wales, Australia

Professor Jon Jureidini
Head, Department of Psychological Medicine,
Women's and Children's Hospital,
Adelaide, Australia

Professor Dr. Thomas W. Kallert
Head of the Department of Psychiatry,
Psychosomatic Medicine and Psychotherapy,
Park Hospital Leipzig;
Medical Director, Soteria Hospital
Leipzig; and
Faculty of Medicine,
Dresden University of Technology,
Germany

Aliya Kassam
Health Service & Population Research
Department, Institute of Psychiatry, King's
College London,
London, UK

Professor Laurence J. Kirmayer
James McGill Professor and Director,
Division of Social and Transcultural
Psychiatry, McGill University,
Montréal, Québec, Canada

Professor Arthur Kleinman
Esther and Sidney Rabb Professor of
Anthropology,
Department of Anthropology,
Harvard University,
and Professor of Medical Anthropology and
Professor of Psychiatry,
Harvard Medical School, Boston, USA

Professor Martin Knapp
Professor of Social Policy, Director of the
Personal Social Services Research Unit, and
Director of the NIHR School for Social Care
Research, London School of Economics
and Political Science, and King's
College London,
London, UK

Dr Mireille Landman
Department of Psychology,
Stellenbosch University,
Stellenbosch, South Africa

Oliver Lewis
Executive Director
Mental Disability Advocacy Center
(MDAC) Budapest, Hungary

Elanor Lewis-Holmes
Health Service and Population Research
Department, Institute Of Psychiatry,
King's College London, London, UK

Associate Professor Crick Lund
Director,
Centre for Public Mental Health,
Dept of Psychiatry and Mental Health,
University of Cape Town,
Cape Town, South Africa

David McDaid
Senior Research Fellow in Health Policy and
Health Economics,
LSE Health and Social Care and European
Observatory on Health Systems and Policies,
London School of Economics and Political
Science, London, UK

Professor AC McFarlane
Professor of Psychiatry,
Head CMVH University of
Adelaide Node,
The Centre for Military and Veterans' Health,
The University of Adelaide,
Adelaide, SA, Australia

Dr Tristan McGeorge
Central and North West London NHS
Foundation Trust
London, UK

Professor Patrick McGorry
University of Melbourne,
Executive Director,
Orygen Research Centre, Director of
Clinical Services, Orygen Youth Health,
Parkville, Victoria, Australia

Kathleen Maltzahn
Founder
Project Respect,
Collingwood, VIC, Australia

Dr Roshni Mangalore
Research Associate
Department of Social Policy,
London School of Economics and
Political Science, London, UK

Dr Sarah Mares
Infant, Child and Family Psychiatrist,
Redbank House, Western Sydney, New South
Wales; and Senior Visiting Clinical Fellow,
Menzies School of Health Research,
NT, Australia

Jonathan H. Marks
Associate Professor of Bioethics,
Humanities and Law
Director, Bioethics Program
The Pennsylvania State University
University Park, PA, USA

Janet Meagher
Divisional Manager (Inclusion),
Psychiatric Rehabilitation Australia
Redfern, New South Wales, Australia

Dr Nisha Mehta
Health Service and Population Research
Department, Institute of Psychiatry,
London, UK

Professor Helen Milroy
Director/Winthrop Professor
Centre for Aboriginal Medical and
Dental Health (CAMDH),
University of Western Australia,
Crawley, WA, Australia

Scientia Professor Philip Mitchell
Head, School of Psychiatry,
University of New South Wales,
Sydney, Australia

Professor Paul E. Mullen
Community Forensic Mental Health Service
Forensicare,
Melbourne, Australia

Dr Nell Munro
Faculty of Social Sciences,
University of Nottingham,
Nottingham, UK

Professor Carol Cooperman Nadelson
Brigham and Women's Hospital, and Office
for Women's Careers,
Harvard Medical School, USA

Professor Louise Newman
Director,
Monash Center for Developmental
Psychiatry and Psychology,
Monash University,
Clayton, Victoria, Australia

David W. Oaks
Executive Director,
MindFreedom International,
Eugene, Oregon, USA

Professor Nick O'Neill
Professorial Visiting Fellow,
Faculty of Law,
University of New South Wales,
Sydney, New South Wales, Australia

Professor Vikram Patel
Professor of International Mental Health &
Wellcome Trust Senior Research Fellow in
Clinical Science,
London School of Hygiene & Tropical
Medicine, London, UK
and Sangath, Goa, India

Associate Professor Carmelle Peisah
School of Psychiatry,
University of New South Wales,
Sydney, New South Wales, Australia

Professor Michael L Perlin
Director, International Mental Disability
Law Reform Project,
Director, Online Mental Disability
Law Program,
New York Law School,
New York, USA

Dr Jennifer Randall
Institute of Psychiatry,
Department of Health Service and Population
Research, King's College London,
London, UK

Professor Beverley Raphael
School of Medicine,
University of Western Sydney
New South Wales, Australia

Dr Susan Rees
QE-11 Senior Research Fellow, Australian
Research Council
Psychiatry Research and Teaching Unit
School of Psychiatry
University of New South Wales
Liverpool, New South Wales, Australia

Professor Alan Rosen
Senior Consultant Psychiatrist,
Centre for Rural & Remote Mental Health,
University of Newcastle, and
Greater Western Area Health Service,
Professorial Fellow,
School of Public Health, Faculty of Health &
Behavioural Sciences,
University of Wollongong,
Clinical Associate Professor, Brain & Mind
Research Institute,
Faculty of Medicine/Sydney Medical School,
University of Sydney, Australia

Tully Rosen
Policy & Research Officer,
Mental Health Coordinating Council,
New South Wales, Australia

Diana Samarasan
Director, Disability Rights Fund,
Boston, MA, USA

Professor Benedetto Saraceno
Associate Professor of Social Psychiatry,
Department of Psychiatry,
University of Geneva, Switzerland

Professor Norman Sartorius
President, Association for the Improvement
of Mental Health Programmes,
Geneva, Switzerland

Associate Professor Ufuk Sezgin
Associate Professor of Clinical Psychology,
Istanbul University,
Istanbul, Turkey

Julia Shearsby
Bankstown Mental Health Service,
Bankstown, New South Wales, Australia

Professor Derrick Silove
Director,
Psychiatry Research and Teaching Unit,
Liverpool Hospital,
Liverpool, New South Wales, Australia

Professor Meg Smith
Head of Program Social Sciences Bankstown,
School of Social Sciences,
University of Western Sydney,
New South Wales, Australia

Associate Professor Zachary Steel
Center for Population Mental Health
Research, Sydney South West Area Health
Service, and the Psychiatry Research and
Teaching Unit, School of Psychiatry,
University New South Wales,
Liverpool Hospital,
Liverpool, New South Wales, Australia

Professor Dan J. Stein
Professor and Chair of the Dept of Psychiatry
and Mental Health,
Department of Psychiatry and Mental Health,
University of Cape Town
Groote Schuur Hospital J-2,
South Africa.

Dr Danny Sullivan
Assistant Clinical Director,
Victorian Institute of Forensic Mental Health;
Adjunct Senior Lecturer,
School of Psychology and Psychiatry,
Monash University,
Melbourne, Australia

Professor Ezra Susser
Professor of Epidemiology and Psychiatry
Mailman School of Public Health
Columbia University and New York State
Psychiatric Institute
New York, USA

Dr Tom Sutcliffe
Chairperson,
Mental Health Review Board
of the Western Cape,
Cape Town, South Africa

Professor Leslie Swartz
Department of Psychology,
Stellenbosch University,
Stellenbosch, South Africa

Professor Éva Szeli
Adjunct Professor of Law at New York
Law School;
Senior Lecturer at
Arizona State University,
USA

Professor Daniel Tarantola
Visiting Professorial Fellow,
School of Public Health and Community
Medicine, Faculty of Medicine,
University of New South Wales,
Sydney, New South Wales, Australia

Dr Melanie Taylor
School of Medicine, University of Western
Sydney, New South Wales, Australia

Professor Graham Thornicroft
Professor of Community Psychiatry,
Health Service and Population
Research Department,
Institute of Psychiatry,
King's College London,
London, UK

Professor Mark Tomlinson
Department of Psychology,
Stellenbosch University,
Stellenbosch, South Africa

Professor Robert van Voren
Chief Executive,
Global Initiative on Psychiatry
Kaunas Vytautas Magnus
University, Lithuania
Ilia State University,
Tbilisi, Georgia

Dr Lakshmi Vijayakumar
Head, Department of Psychiatry,
Voluntary Health Services, Adyar,
Chennai, India
Founder, SNEHA, Suicide prevention centre,
Chennai, India

Louella Villadiego
Legal Advisor,
Ing Makababaying Aksyon (IMA)
(Action for Women) Foundation,
Angeles City, Philippines

Peter Walker
Kiloh Centre, Prince of Wales Hospital,
South Eastern Sydney
and Illawarra Area Health Service,
New South Wales, Australia

Dr Charles Watters
Director,
European Centre for the Study of Migration
and Social Care,
University of Kent, Canterbury, Kent, UK

James Welsh
Researcher/Advisor, Special
Thematic Projects,
Amnesty International,
International Secretariat,
London, UK

Dr Evan Yacoub
Consultant Psychiatrist,
Specialist Secure Service for People with
Learning Disability,
John Howard Centre,
London, UK

Professor Dr Sahika Yüksel
Department of Psychiatry,
Istanbul Medical Faculty,
Istanbul University,
Istanbul, Turkey

Tables, Boxes, and Figures

A Personal Testament

Semyon Gluzman

During the Second World War my Mum's sister, an average school teacher and an ethnic Jew, managed to escape from the Nazi occupation in Ukraine. With her little daughter she arrived to the Urals in the East of Russia.

It goes without saying that the municipalities of the Ural cities couldn't provide dwellings to many thousands of refugees, thus they settled these poor people into the flats and houses of local citizens without asking any consent of any parties. So my aunt became one of the many dwellers. Her husband had been arrested and executed in 1937 as a 'Romanian spy' (he could be accused of espionage in favour of Guadeloupe, Ceylon, or even Antarctica). The woman that hosted my aunt and her child knew nothing about the details of their biography. The hostess was mentally ill and was repeatedly admitted to the local psychiatric hospital because of acute delirious impairment. However, the condition didn't prevent her from being a secret agent of the Soviet political police—the NKVD. On a regular basis she revealed more and more new 'foreign spies' among the city population. These people had disappeared in the NKVD prisons and camps, and had been shot by executioners, and my aunt's hostess brought home some belongings of her victims, and sold them to buy food products. And, quite sincerely, she shared the food with her lodgers—a wife and a daughter of a 'people's enemy'. Such a surreal story, strange and eerie.

I believe the Stalinists' investigators were well aware of the fact that their agent suffered from a severe mental disorder. However, this didn't stop them. I assume that the local psychiatrists also knew about the specific activity of their patient. But none of them was bold enough to come to the NKVD and to shed some light on the insane and delirious basis of the information produced by the woman. That sort of initiative can't be expected in the totalitarian country. . .

This terrifying case from the past needs comprehension, a psychiatric comprehension. Even after Stalin's death, and the obvious softening of the political and totalitarian monster, psychiatric abuse in the USSR didn't become a thing of the past.

Under the conditions of dictatorship and total human rights abuse the psychiatrist can't be saved from possible involvement in professional misuse. This misuse may take any form—from tough or inhuman dealings with a patient suffering from mental disease, to admitting a healthy person to a psychiatric hospital only because he/she had expressed 'wrong' political ideas. As a rule, any dictator has beside him a chief psychiatric advisor to sanction illegality and oppression in psychiatric practice by means of handy professional and ideological dictums. Here is a quotation from a scientific work of the last years of the USSR: 'The concept of mental disease should be applied to all disorders relating to the psychiatrist's competence' (Snezhnevsky 1983). Since the statement was declared and written by a psychiatrist who received the highest official recognition, it became a symbol and the matrix for professional conduct. That's why psychiatrists in such countries ascribe criticism of 'the only truthful doctrine by Lenin' (Fidel Castro, Kim-Ir-Sen, etc), interest in the 'reactionary' painting of abstract and surrealist artists, and a desire to leave because of 'worship of the West', to unhealthy mental symptoms.

How many were there of them, the victims of psychiatric abuse in my country? No one knows. Retired executioners do not write their memoirs. I only know about one 'slip of the tongue' made by a competent official of Gorbachev's epoch, when freedom was awakening: 'It shouldn't be pretended that the Serbsky Institute only deals with dissidents, this is not correct: they only make 2% of all our patients' (Dmitrieva 1991). This is a huge number, taking into consideration that the Serbsky Institute was simply the country's main institution where forensic psychiatric examinations were performed. In the meantime, a great number of mentally sane people were exposed to psychiatric treatment without legal proceedings having been instituted, so to speak 'by administrative order'.

Nor can we rely on the personal courage and professional dignity of a psychiatrist. A well-known Russian doctor, VM Morozov, a survivor of the Nazi concentration camp, by the end of his professional and human life turned out to have participated in the psychiatric stigmatizing of several outstanding dissidents. After his verdict, these people found themselves in the most severe conditions of specialized psychiatric clinics for mentally ill criminals.

Now the situation in the former USSR countries is different. In particular, my country, Ukraine is a member of the ICD-10 diagnostic club. Our doctors have long ceased to make a diagnosis of continuous sluggish schizophrenia (which, unfortunately, is still practiced in Russia). Legal procedures and guarantees define the special psychiatric laws, which are slightly different in various post-Soviet countries. Offices of the Ombudsman (never heard of in the USSR) are currently established in every country. However the reality is not that good.

In 2007 my Swedish colleague attended the Kiev psychiatric hospital. 'Unlike my clinic in Stockholm the acute ward here is quiet and calm' was his first feedback. And again I felt ashamed. The calmness and quietness of the post-Soviet hospitals is a result of neuroleptic administration. The big doses of archaic aminazine (chlorpromazine) and trifluoperazine stun our patients without doing them any good. In my country (as well as in the majority of other former USSR countries) no rehabilitation programmes have been developed, no social work schemes, no social psychiatry services. . .

Yes, we should appreciate the fact that there are no cases of psychiatric abuse with a view of political interests. But this is not the victory of psychiatrists. The KGB disappeared and instead of dissidents there is a legal political opposition. However even now, under the circumstances of political freedom, it's a real misfortune to become a psychiatric patient in my country.

Within the last 18 years on a regular basis I receive letters from European and US lawyers dealing with the cases of my compatriots illegally residing in other countries and receiving their psychiatric treatment there. The lawyers ask me very practical questions (always the same): can Mr X or Mrs Y receive the psychiatric treatment in Ukraine adequate to that provided in the country they are staying in now (or in the country whose citizenship they seek)? These are dramatic questions, as I realize that my reply will influence the decision made in the court or in an immigration office about the case of Mr X or Mrs Y. Formally the right for adequate psychiatric treatment exists in the former Soviet countries, but it greatly differs from our everyday life.

According to the current legislation, compulsory admission is only possible in well defined cases. But. . . even today almost all patients who are hospitalized in Kiev, the capital of Ukraine, give their consent to admission and treatment 'on their free will', this is—without any court decision. Do you guess—why?

The right to know your own diagnosis. It is simple—you apply to the doctor, you receive the treatment, but. . . they refuse to tell you your diagnosis.

The right for basic privacy. You stay in the hospital, and here you have some necessary things: a tooth-brush, a handkerchief, a book. . . but you have nowhere to place these. Because you have neither shelf, nor locker, nor bedside table.

The right for social support. The disease is a new social situation for you and your family. Your doctor has prescribed you the medicines and you do feel better, your family are not as scared with your behaviour as they have been before. However your social ties and labels are broken, and you, as an alive and suffering human being, need the support of some competent professional. No use in seeking support—it doesn't exist in this country, because there is no professional institute of social workers.

These, as well as many other things, form the notion of 'human rights observance in psychiatry'—not just the right to have a correct diagnosis and to receive adequate treatment. There are also some small and, at first sight, obvious rights like a right to visit a toilet according to one's need rather than according to a 'Schedule of Patients' Toilet Visits' worked out by staff. A strange limitation, isn't it? Nevertheless it exists in the countries which have signed all necessary international liabilities to observe human rights. The national ombudsmen learn about the cases from mass media or from the reports of international human rights inspectors.

In 1838 in France the first law on humanizing the arrangements of dealing with the mentally sick was adopted. Before that, by the end of the 18th century, the French doctor, Pierre Jean Cabanis, declared: 'If a person is mentally sane, or when some meaningless changes in his/her mental activity do not threaten neither his/her own or someone else's security and do not shatter peace and quiet in the community, nobody, even the whole of the society, may infringe upon his/her freedom' (Cabanis 1994).

Of course, there may be a somewhat different approach to the issue. Michel Foucault had expressed it in the most clear and tough form (Foucault 1972). Later this trend of thought and activity was called 'anti-psychiatry'. The philosophical and methodological maximalism in psychiatry, without any doubt, played an important role in humanization of psychiatry in the 20th century. However, it was preceded by active dehumanization of psychiatry in Nazi Germany with its total killing of mental patients. The anti-psychiatric movement in Western Europe and in Northern America helped psychiatry to see itself in the mirror and the image was far from being nice and attractive. However any maximalism, any revolution, can destroy a building, but also prevent the bricks of a new construction. There are the realities: a disease, often unrecognized by its carrier, the danger presented by the patients to themselves and to the surrounding people. This is a truism, banality. And in this point we see the crash of the arguments adduced by the knights of anti-psychiatry, of the splendid parapsychiatric philosophy.

The compulsory knowledge offered by our university curricula belongs to the sphere of demonstrative, conclusive medicine. This is because the doctor in fact has no right to make mistakes. Our mistake is someone's blasted destiny. Or death. In these cases the judges interfere in our work. This is the law. But there are also the instances when any of us, a member of the psychiatric profession, must recognize this small, meaningless seeming, trifle, which hasn't become a zone of justicial competence yet. In the Soviet political camp, where I've spent seven years of my life, once I ran across a medical journal. An author of one of the articles quoted a well-known Swiss psychiatrist, Bleuler junior. These words sparkled in my grey world of a prisoner, convicted by his own country for his attempt to call the naked king 'a naked king'. And I still remember the words: 'The duty, the responsibility and the art of clinical psychiatry is to serve the ideas of freedom and humanism, but not to destroy them.'

January 2009, Kiev

References

Snezhnevsky A.V. *Manual on psychiatry*, Moscow Medicine, 1983., vol. 1., p.12

Dmitrieva T.B. Newspaper Youth of Estonia November 11, 1991

Cannabih Y. *History of psychiatry*, Moscow ZTR MGPVC, 1994

Michel Foucault (1972) *L'Histoire de la folie à l'âge classique*. Paris Gallimard, 1972

Mental Health, Human Rights, and their Relationship: An Introduction

In recent decades, mental health and human rights have emerged as converging fields of research and practice, as recognition grows that the two domains intersect in multiple and complex ways. By including human rights outcomes within their proposed agendas, initiatives in global mental health have acknowledged this close link (Lancet Global Mental Health Group 2007; Patel and Prince 2010). One key element of this shared concern involves addressing the enormous burden of adverse mental health outcomes following war and other conflicts (Steel et al. 2009) endeavouring to guarantee that the mental health component is integral to humanitarian programmes. Another is to engage cultural considerations at the forefront of thought and practice in both human rights and mental health, thereby ensuring that mental health initiatives do not undermine the traditional healing and recovery processes of indigenous peoples (Steel et al. 2009). Given the intricate relationship between the mental health and human rights communities, there is a pressing need to increase the level of dialogue and strengthen the in-depth analysis of this important relationship.

The present volume, which includes contributors from a variety of perspectives, aims to begin to redress this gap. The increasing salience of mental health and the needs of people with mental disorders[1] is a cause for optimism, but internationally, statements of intent and aspiration often

---

[1] A definition of mental health is given in the main body of text. This book is written for, about and (crucially) with users, potential users and survivors of mental health services; however, there is currently no uniformly acceptable usage in relation to those who suffer mental health problems. We accept that terminology is of political significance because it may act as a means of reproducing stigma, or it may promote social inclusion and establish a human-rights reformative agenda in mental health. In relation to those who suffer these problems, our contributors have used terms such as 'people with mental disorders' as well as 'users [or survivors] of psychiatric services' or 'people with [psychosocial] disabilities' or even 'sufferers'. The intent here is to signify the personhood of those who are affected, while also acknowledging differences (including recognized medical terminology) in describing their experiences of illness. As with other terms in this volume, we have elected to accept some divergence of usage.

Many service users object to the medical overtones of the term 'mental illness', so we therefore generally avoid the term except when it is formally used in the context of the operation of mental health acts (legislation), or in the widespread phrase 'Severe and Persistent Mental Illness', which refers to chronic, highly disabling mental disorders. This reflects the incomplete resolution of the intellectual and political debate regarding the role and place of biological factors and medical approaches in the illnesses, recoveries and well-being of survivors, and potentially, the biomedical domain overshadowing other contributions. Again in this volume we have elected to accept some divergence of usage.

We frequently adopt the international usage of the term 'disorder' by the Classification of Mental and Behavioural Disorders: Clinical Descriptions and Guidelines (ICD-10) (WHO 1992), and the Diagnostic and Statistical Manual of Mental Disorders (DSM-IV) of the American Psychiatric Association (1994).

overshadow real action. There is great variation in the commitment to resourcing, skills development, programme implementation, and standardization of prevention and care that promotes mental health while safeguarding human rights.

This introduction is intended as a reference for all those interested in global mental health, in the international human rights project, and the relationship between them. While it alludes to the different chapters at relevant points, the divisions between the book's sections contain more extended chapter summaries.

We briefly survey the current global situation in mental health and chart the fundamental concepts of human rights, as a prelude to considering the relationship between the two domains. We aim to summarize their common ground, their distinguishing features, their shared histories and potential reciprocity. We consider the prospect of advancing both mental health and human rights by way of legislation. We attend to the challenges of redressing mental health inequity in a globalized yet culturally diverse world. We raise the issue of abuses by examining the controversy surrounding the coercion of those with mental disorders, while noting the contrary, connected problem of neglect and potential abandonment of those with mental disorder in dire need. We extend our focus on abuses to the actions taken by states and non-state actors in perpetrating or providing protection against such abuses. These reflections guide discussions about possible future directions of global mental health and human rights, as potential partners in a joint endeavour. We make reference to the relevant chapters in this volume that address these issues.

Certain key observations emerge. In international relations, human rights currently occupy a pivotal position, mental health does not. This may be because efforts over the last two centuries to advance the cause of human rights culminated in an international benchmark, the Universal Declaration of Human Rights (UDHR), against which all nations are now judged. Advocacy for mental health has not assembled such a broad, influential international constituency, nor have efforts been as sustained. Notably, mental health is absent from international agendas in a way that physical health is not. Nevertheless, mental health is an inescapable necessity for health and well-being and increasingly acknowledged as such. The prerequisite conditions for mental health and psychosocial well-being are precisely those that underpin the promotion of human dignity, and therefore the essence of human rights. Mental disorders are ubiquitous in all societies and produce especially dire impacts in low- and middle-income countries, where they commonly co-exist and interact with problems such as poverty, mass trauma, and social disruption. Yet, mental health remains the 'missing partner' in many global health initiatives, for example, from the Millennium Development Goals, a key omission that must be identified and addressed. To date, the goal of providing universal support to promote the capabilities of those with mental disorders and including those who have been socially excluded because of severe mental illness remains a distant ideal.

Within mental health services, the core agenda must be to move from paternalistic, controlling responses towards emancipatory ones, to recognize the validity of the lived experience of sufferers, and to tackle discrimination, exclusion, and social inequalities that afflict the lives of

---

'Disorder' has the notion of a clinically recognizable set of symptoms and/or behaviours that are associated with distress and impaired functioning, and is not accounted for by social deviance or conflict alone. A disadvantage of the term 'disorder' is its medical connotation and the overtone of a socially prescribed notion of how things are supposed to be ('order'), from which the sufferer presumably deviates. However, it has the advantage of being the internationally accepted term of WHO and international classifications as well as professional bodies.

We recognize that this will not be satisfactory to some, but we hope that this approach will not be taken as a lack of commitment to the emancipatory agenda that this volume represents.

affected persons. Progressive mental health and anti-discrimination legislation may further the well-being of people with mental disorders, assisted by wider societal contact with sufferers, the building of equal partnerships, the promotion of public education, leadership that offers unambiguous advocacy, and the use of protest where practices or policies clearly transgress basic principles. In addressing human rights in mental health, redressing inequities and abuses are both essential components. Building integrated mental health and human rights frameworks that develop and promote rights-based practices in (mental) health, obtaining evidence of the effectiveness of interventions both in clinical and human rights terms, and creating a research agenda and monitoring standards, are all pertinent.

Scope and definitional issues

Footnotes concerning terminology are found immediately above and below. Regarding our basic terms, however, we take 'mental health' to refer to diverse activities directly or indirectly related to the mental well-being component of the World Health Organization (WHO)'s definition of health: 'A state of complete physical, mental and social well-being, and not merely the absence of disease'. While recognizing that common and historical usage tends to equate 'mental health' with professionals and services associated with the diagnosis, treatment and rehabilitation of people affected by mental disorders, mental health also encompasses the promotion of well-being, the prevention of mental disorders (WHO 2010), and the right to the highest attainable standard of physical and mental health.

In this wider perspective, mental health incorporates all the dimensions of human experience: biological, psychological, socio-cultural, developmental, political, ecological, and spiritual. Mental health, while a subject of scientific investigation and empirical study, is also a social construct insofar as different cultures and social groups shape how it is understood and how mental health disturbances arise and are remedied (Weare 2000). Thus this volume allows for both specificity and breadth in usage of the term 'mental health'.

Rights in general, or 'human rights' as a sub-class, may be regarded as special normative entities and strong entitlements but also sets of social practices (Donnelly 2003) which apply to everyone, by virtue of their dignity as humans. While rights have moral, political, and legal functions, they are pre-legal, pre-political, and peremptory in nature. Rights are primarily concerned with human capacities to flourish and develop without arbitrary impediment; they signify the incalculable worth and potential of all humanity. Protecting morally valid, fundamental human interests, human rights especially apply to disadvantaged and marginalized groups for whom realizing rights is imperative to achieving full potential. Rights are inalienable, interrelated, interdependent, and indivisible (UN 1993), and therefore need to be grounded on or at least strive for universal consensus. Expressed and guaranteed by international conventions and treaties and by national laws, they concern systemic, power-related issues that influence well-being, particularly, the individual's relationship to the state. The state remains the principal violator of human rights as well as their most powerful potential protector (Donnelly 2003:35). Hence, state-based human rights standards and laws need to be legitimized by international monitoring and where necessary remediation (a principle that applies equally to provisions governing mental health). Rights provide fundamental protections without qualification or exception (Freeman 2002; Gavison 2003:26; Ife 2001; UN Office of the High Commissioner for Human Rights 2010). Analogous to the task of promoting mental health, human rights rest on social and political foundations, and require a priori commitments to treat rights as if their legitimacy is inviolable, and to make the social changes required to realize the underlying moral vision of human dignity (Donnelly 2003:15, 21).

Global mental health: a snapshot

Some years ago the World Development Report (1993), the Global Burden of Disease report (Murray and Lopez 1996), and other major commentaries (e.g. Desjarlais et al. 1995; WHO 2001) surprised the international health community by documenting the enormous health burden of mental disorders, not just in high income countries but in low- and middle-income countries.

A decade later, in a special issue of the journal, *The Lancet*, the implications of this burden were explored further, particularly regarding the means and barriers to mounting an effective mental health service response in the least resourced developing[2] countries (Prince et al. 2007; Saxena et al. 2007; Patel et al. 2007a; Jacob et al. 2007; Saraceno et al. 2007, Lancet Global Mental Health Group 2007, and others). Asserting that global mental health has come of age, the series initiated a Movement for Global Mental Health, under the WHO banner, proclaiming that there is 'no health without mental health'.

Disability is now recognizably a major global issue: an estimated 978 million people worldwide, 15 per cent of the world's population, and at least 93 billion children under 15 years, have moderate to severe disabilities (WHO and World Bank, 2011, pp xi, 29). Yet mental disorders now comprise five of the ten top causes of years lost to disability[3] worldwide (Demyttenaere et al. 2004). The international mental health burden caused by HIV/AIDS, war, trauma, dislocation, and poverty, and the impact of colonialism on indigenous peoples, is increasingly well documented. Universal forms of abuse, such as gender-based violence, considerably raise the prevalence of mental disorder and disability (Rees et al. 2011). There is growing evidence concerning the substantial incidence and prevalence of severe and persistent mental disorders, such as schizophrenia, bipolar, depressive and related disorders, and also of substance misuse, dementia, and intellectual disabilities,[4] not only in high- and medium- but in low-income countries with diverse

---

[2] The Human Development Index of the UN Development Programme inclusively describes the root causes of inequity between countries. Although these are broader than income, consistency with a widespread usage has led us sometimes to refer to countries as having low-, middle-, and high-incomes, rather than low, middle and high human development. Similarly, references to countries as developed or developing for some may have obsolete overtones of progress in which some countries have 'arrived' and others are aspirational: nevertheless sometimes we also frequently adopt this usage given its ubiquity. Other usages, such as 'North and South', or 'First and Third World' are avoided because of various inaccuracies in their assumptions (Sartorius, 2002).

[3] At times we use the term 'disability' or specifically, 'psychosocial disability'. Following international usage, it is used to describe the condition whereby physical and/or social barriers prevent a person with an impairment from taking part in the normal life of the community on an equal footing with others (UNICEF Innocenti Digest #13). Disabilities may be physical, intellectual, mental, psychosocial, or multiple in nature. The use of the term 'psychosocial disabilities' in UN discussions and recent conventions, signals a recent change in relation to this issue. Whatever the type, the growing use of the term 'disability' signifies the overriding importance of social context in sufferers' lives. We have used it for example where the intention is to signify this context. Again, throughout the volume, there is some variation in usage.

[4] People with intellectual disabilities (a term which supersedes the terms 'mental retardation' and 'learning disability' (the latter when it is used as a synonym for intellectual disability)) may suffer from mental and physical illnesses which may in part have biological origins, yet by no means are necessarily 'sick'. We note that like those with mental disorders, those with intellectual disability share experiences of social exclusion and require the protection of legislation, and that though they may also have mental disorders, they also may differ in important respects to those with mental disorders, for example their capacity to consent over time. Legislation will need to allow for differentiation of these groups. However, sometimes also we have used the term 'mental disability', consistent with the meaning of this term, where the authors' intentions are to signify the negative interactions of the individual with his environmental context.

cultures (Silove et al. 2008). Adults and children with intellectual impairments and mental health problems have more risks and disadvantages of all kinds than those with physical and sensory disabilities; not only like others with disabilities do they face degradation, stigmatization, and discrimination, but they are also routinely confined against their will in institutions, and deprived of freedom, dignity, and basic rights (WHO and World Bank 2011, p36). People with mental disorders also suffer a higher risk of unintentional injury and exposure to violence; and are also much less often employed, a status that arises from misconceptions about their disability and as a consequence of discrimination against them (WHO and World Bank 2011).

Mental disorders not only produce an enormous impact in their own right but through their interaction with physical health conditions (e.g. communicable and non-communicable diseases and accidental and non-accidental injuries), resulting in complex patterns of reciprocal causality. Whatever pathways lead to the concentration of disorders, it is clear that co-morbidity, that is the accumulation of physical and mental health problems over the lifespan, compounds disability and greatly affects the sufferer's quality of life. These patterns massively impact on the quality and effectiveness of services from help-seeking to follow-up, and on levels of mortality and disability (Prince et al. 2007). Those with long-term mental health problems commonly experience 'diagnostic overshadowing' (their physical health problems go undiagnosed), they have more chronic health problems occurring at an earlier age, are at greater risk of poverty, and die earlier (Disability Rights Commission 2006). People with mental disorders are also much less often employed, a status that arises from misconceptions about their disability and as a consequence of discrimination against them: hence, to fulfill their capabilities, they may need access to supported employment (WHO and World Bank 2011).

Moreover, those in greatest need, living in extreme poverty, commonly endure the worst mental health. This is especially true for women, children and young people, who have particular trouble accessing and engaging with services. In general, the burden of mental disability outstrips the funding allocated to this area compared with the resources available for physical disorders (McGorry et al. 2007; Patel et al. 2007b). In low- and middle-income countries (LAMICs), where most children live, and access to mental health care is limited, the gradient of disadvantage is especially steep. Mental health is worse for those living in rural areas and belonging to minority ethnic and religious groups. Thus the most disadvantaged are at greatest risk. Globally, 450 million people with mental, neurological, or behavioural problems are among the world's most vulnerable persons from a social and economic perspective (WHO 2005a).

As confirmed in the photo-essay by Patel and colleagues, observations worldwide attest that persons with mental disabilities often live in the most parlous circumstances: starving, naked, destitute, and denied proper hygiene and sanitation. Frequently shackled, chained, caged, or imprisoned without charge, they may be hidden away or, alternatively, exposed to public view and to ridicule (Silove et al. 2000). Such arbitrary confinement and restriction sometimes lasts for years, even for life. Those suffering psychosis may be forced to have electroconvulsive therapy, sometimes without anaesthetic. With resources and hope cut off, and overwhelmed by shame, families may abandon loved ones to institutions. These establishments, especially in LAMICs, are not infrequently characterized by sexual and physical abuse, neglect (for example of health care), exploitation (for example through forced labour), injury owing to neglect or abuse, discrimination, and rejection. Contrary to popular perception, those with mental disorders far more often endure violence than perpetrate it. Due processes and review of conditions of confinement are lacking, as are opportunities to exercise rights and freedoms. Neither are services, communities, and health and mental health professionals exempt from collusion in these practices. Active exclusion, dehumanization, and social death afflicts many with severe and persistent mental disorders in LAMICs (Kleinman, 2009, Patel and Prince 2010; Patel and colleagues, this volume; WHO 2005a:1–5).

Kleinman (2009) aptly has referred to a 'failure of humanity': 'individuals with mental illness exist under the worst of moral conditions' (p. 603). These accounts provide repetitive evidence of breaches of the fundamental rights that are necessary to promote and preserve mental health: equality, non-discrimination, information and participation, privacy and autonomy, least restrictive treatment, and freedom from inhuman and degrading treatment (WHO 2005a:3; Saxena et al. 2007). Eyewitness professionals detail gross abuses and gross inequities. The worldwide plight of people with mental disorders is an affront, and the task of addressing their needs is not only daunting but morally undeniable. The development of human rights protections may therefore be particularly significant, given their unique limitations and deprivations (Perlin and Szeli, this volume).

The WHO has adopted the mh-GAP programme as its flagship programme in mental health, committing to scaling up care on mental, neurological, and substance use disorders and producing evidence-based guidelines for non-specialist health care workers (Patel and Prince 2010). Likewise, the World Federation for Mental Health (WFMH), and its constituent organizations and user groups, has put forward a global campaign 'The Great Push for Mental Health' in strategic alliance with the Movement to raise mental health up the agenda of governments. The WHO Resource Book on Mental Health, Human Rights and Legislation (2005a) has mapped the roles to be played by progressive mental health legislation.

Yet despite compelling arguments to advance mental health, broader definitions of health, and greater awareness of health's social determinants, mental health is frequently absent from health and social policy-making and research. As mentioned, targets like the Millenium Development Goals (including women's empowerment, maternal and child health, and addressing communicable diseases) omit mental health, despite it being crucial to their realization (Prince et al. 2007).

Resources for mental health—such as beds, staffing, finance—are not only scarce, but inequitably distributed and inefficiently employed. This is especially true of LAMICs, which are home to more than 80 per cent of the world's people, but enjoy less than 20 per cent of its mental health resources (Saxena et al. 2007).

Psychiatric beds in LAMICs are scarce overall, but also are over-concentrated in mental hospitals. Thus only about 50 per cent of LAMICs provide community-based mental health care outside hospitals; and 80 per cent of beds in middle- (neither high- nor low-) income countries are in mental hospitals. This reflects a dearth of available treatments, distancing of service users from their communities, and legacies of institutionalization, including prolonged seclusion and restraint. Such conditions constitute or potentially contribute to rights violations. Ideally, a balance of hospital and community services maximizes population mental health care, but only a few high-income countries have developed programmes that approximate this model (Thornicroft and Tansella 2004).

Mental health professionals are 200 times more available per capita in high-income compared to low-income countries. In low-income countries, the scarcity of professionals, aggravated by the 'brain drain' to well-resourced countries, not only severely limits psychiatric care but may impede transformation of systems and necessitate out-of-state or international solutions to these countries' overall mental health resource problems (Saxena et al. 2007). Thus, these countries can only provide care to one-quarter of those affected by serious mental illnesses, with much of this care being inadequate (Patel and Prince 2010). The worldwide prevalence of mental disorders greatly exceeds service usage. Sufferers not only have less access to health facilities but to health promotion activities (Disability Rights Commission 2006). The unmet need for services also has a major impact on carers, including family members who must provide intensive care and support, often under extreme socio-economic duress (WHO and World Bank 2011:141).

Funding in almost all countries does not match the needs of those with mental disability: the resources allocated relate more closely to general healthcare resources and Gross Domestic Product than to neuropsychiatric burden (Jacob et al. 2007). In most LAMICs, mental health ranks well behind communicable diseases and maternal and child health in resourcing, and in wealthy countries, behind non-communicable diseases that cause early death—heart disease and cancer (Prince et al. 2007). In LAMICs, mental disorders attract under 2 per cent (and in the poorest countries, often under 1 per cent) of the health budget, while 31 per cent of countries report that they do not have a mental health budget, an impediment to accountability (Saxena et al. 2007, Jacob et al. 2007; Kleinman 2009). Also in poor countries, out-of-pocket payments tend to predominate, rather than pre-payment mechanisms which redistribute wealth to the least advantaged for (mental) health care, e.g. taxation, social insurance, and voluntary insurance (Saxena et al. 2007).

Legislation seldom adequately protects those with mental disabilities. Nearly 25 per cent of countries internationally have no mental health legislation, while the legislation of many more nations does not reflect currently accepted mental health practices, offers only poor protection for rights, or worse, blatantly transgresses rights. These matters are discussed below.

Given this extreme picture, it is striking that examples of (cost-) effective mental health interventions are frequently described in LAMIC settings (Patel et al. 2007a; Tennant and Silove 2005). Such promising programmes exist for schizophrenia, depression (a major cause of disease burden in LAMICs), alcohol misuse, and for children and young people, for example with ADHD. Prevention also demonstrably works for anxiety and depression in school students; for various causes of childhood disabilities; for infants at risk (Patel et al. 2007a), and for suicide prevention (Fleischmann et al. 2008). Optimal mental health responses following mass conflict and disasters still require better definition (Silove et al. 2008; Tol et al. 2011). In Iran, nursing students participating in educational counselling over one semester reduced their anxiety in the long-term (Sharif and Armitage 2004)—this has potential relevance for the well-being of the health workforce in LAMICs. However, though these interventions appear cost-effective, the overall process and effectiveness of scaling up mental health interventions awaits adequate assessment (Patel et al. 2007a).

Why does global mental health receive such a low priority? International experts suggest that practitioners and advocates fail to endorse clear, unified messages and indicators concerning mental health needs, evidence-based interventions and cost-effectiveness; service users and their families lack influence and/or are marginalized; and communities may lack awareness and informed knowledge. Ignorance breeds stigma, thereby generating a vicious cycle of neglect (Saraceno et al. 2007).

Stigma against mentally ill people is ubiquitous and has persisted throughout history. Its components, ignorance, prejudice, and discrimination, manifest in multiple forms: stereotyping, fear, embarrassment, anger, cruelty, rejection, ostracism, and avoidance. Service users and survivors highlight risks inherent in the term stigma itself, particularly in locating attributing the phenomenon to individuals rather than depicting it as a dynamic interchange between societal values and practices, group reactions, and the target of the negative appraisal. Anti-stigma campaigns may encourage help-seeking, assuming and assuring the sufferer that services will promote autonomy and act beneficently. Service users however may encounter stigmatizing attitudes and practices that are neither safe nor respectful. Armed with these experiences and a wider critique of practices and institutions, some service users and survivors have challenged the core claims of psychiatry as a beneficent enterprise, citing its medical affinities as an additional problem (Chamberlin 2007): these tensions remain unresolved. Stigma appears in families, neighbourhoods, personal relationships, employment settings, civil and social life, leisure, health care, mental health and social care (including amongst professionals in these fields), health insurance, housing, access to services, and the media. It triggers attributions about the threat of violence posed by mentally ill people and may evince responses of psychological, sexual, or physical abuse. Stigma attaches not just to sufferers, but to families, professionals, institutions, services, and communities (WHO 2005a; Thornicroft 2006; Thornicroft et al. 2007), and may also affect will to allocate health funding (Sartorius and Schulze 2005; Saxena et al. 2007). Randall and colleagues explore the issue of stigma more fully in their chapter.

The first person voices of sufferers are crucial to increasing understanding and effective prevention, and to promoting broad educational and advocacy campaigns about mental disorders. To hear these voices requires tackling the roots of social exclusion of individuals and communities, investing in the human capital of all people, and genuinely re-claiming and endorsing what one scholar has called 'experiential rights' (Cresswell 2009). As Dhanda, Smith, Oaks, Lewis and Munro, and various other authors argue cogently in their contributions to this volume, the participation of people with mental disabilities in legal and policy reforms relating to their lives is critical to the goal of empowerment and to realizing the full range of rights, but also communicates a message of inclusiveness and equity to the wider society. This entitlement, embedded in General Comment No. 14 of the Committee for Economic, Social and Cultural Rights, is confirmed in the shift from welfare to rights in the Convention on the Rights of Persons with Disabilities but remains to be widely implemented in practice.

Human rights: a brief, selective overview

Along with world peace, environmental sustainability and gender equality, human rights constitutes a headline moral project for modernity in its current phase. The predicament of people with mental disorders naturally fits into this project. Moreover, making the link between human rights and mental health provision offers sufferers and their carers considerable leverage in their struggle to overcome the prejudice and neglect of those decision-makers who are capable, should they show the will, to commit resources and introduce better policies in the future.

The literature on human rights and international relations (and related issues), like that for mental health, is vast, and the treatment that follows cannot claim to be representative, let alone comprehensive. The material here and throughout the book is necessarily synoptic and selective, and does not provide any detailed account of the principal UN organs, UN subsidiary bodies, or treaty bodies, nor does it systematically address international humanitarian law, criminal justice, and foreign policy developments. The reader is referred to other sources for more general accounts: excellent coverage and extensive bibliographies are found in Donnelly (2003), Forsythe (2006), Freeman (2002), Griffin (2008), Landman (2005), and Nickel (2009) among many others (see the References for further citations). Allowing for both the specificity and the breadth of the term 'mental health', the material presented here is chosen because it provides a necessary context for understanding or illuminating issues to do with mental health and its relationship with human rights.

Provenance and establishment of standards

The debate about the existence of universal human rights that can be traced throughout history (Freeman 2002; Ishay 2008) is not explored here. Human rights as articulated in the modern era are generally regarded as originating in the West, that is Western Europe, North America, and Australasia (Donnelly 2003). Donnelly (2003:71) contends that while all major cultures have had duty systems that underwrite their acknowledgment of human dignity, these systems arguably are alternatives to, not synonymous with, human rights. Yet while recognition of human rights has not been universally evident across cultures, some hold that non-Western cultures have at times adopted concepts and practices akin to modern precepts of rights (Sen 1999, 2009; Lauren 1998). However this essentially historical debate does not affect the universal applicability, appropriateness, or value of human rights concepts and practices either in or outside the West (Donnelly 2003:69).

Rights in the West have roots in documents such as Magna Carta, notions of natural rights, and an emerging valorization of autonomy. They find their modern enshrinement in sources such as the 1689 English Bill of Rights, the French Declaration on the Rights of Man and Citizen (1789), and the US Declaration of Independence (1776) and Constitution and Bill of Rights (1791). Between the American and French Revolutions and the Second World War, apart from isolated causes such as anti-slavery or workers' rights, the notion of natural rights declined and utilitarianism or scientific positivism as applied to society provided the theoretical basis for political reform (Freeman 2002). Early 19th century nationalists envisaged their movement as leading universal crusades for oppressed peoples, though later in that century, nationalism adopted a more xenophobic character: historical and biological explanations in the form of 'race science' were adopted to justify policies of social exclusion. Socialists and communists questioned whether political rights that ignored economic rights were enough, and whether the right to protect private property could be reconciled with society's fostering the well-being of less fortunate members.

In the West, human rights regained momentum in the mid-20th century—in part propelled by the vivid images depicted in photographs at the liberation of the Nazi death camps, and the subsequent Nuremberg trials, which shockingly demonstrated the consequences of racist and nationalist ideologies. In addition, smaller states and many civic organizations lobbied for the inclusion of strong human rights principles in the United Nations Charter; its new Human Rights Commission decided forthwith to draft a bill of rights (Glendon 2001; Hunt 2007:176–208).

The Universal Declaration of Human Rights (UDHR) (1948) is the cornerstone of the modern human rights movement. As the first inter-governmental statement in world history to approve a set of basic principles on human rights, it has profoundly altered the international landscape, heralding a new age of universal human rights, which has entered common parlance, law and the moral imagination (Freeman 2002; Gruskin and Tarantola 2005; Forsythe 2006). Despite its non-binding character, and the reality that national interests perennially lead to trade-offs with human rights claims and values (Forsythe 2006), the UDHR has 'scattered. . .human rights protocols, conventions, treaties, and derivative declarations of all kinds' (Morsink 1999:x). Hence, particularly in recent decades, there is not a single nation, culture, or people that is not in one way or another enmeshed within human rights regimes. In that sense, the UDHR has provided an overlapping consensus on standards of political legitimacy for nation states (Donnelly 2003:43).

Through the UDHR, the United Nations revived human rights, restoring the natural civil rights tradition, while also beginning to address issues of economic and social justice (Freeman 2002). These precepts are enshrined in the International Covenant on Civil and Political Rights (ICCPR), and the International Covenant on Economic, Social and Cultural Rights (ICESCR) respectively.

Civil and political rights are sometimes known as *negative rights*, entailing freedoms from oppressive or repressive state interventions (Marshall 1965; Berlin 1969:122–131). They include freedom from slavery; from cruel, inhuman and degrading treatment and torture; from arbitrary arrest and detention and intimidation and harassment; the right to fair trial, equality before law and to privacy; and to freedom of speech, assembly, movement, religion, voting, and citizenship. They relate to autonomy and freedom of choice that usually stem from liberal notions of the individual that developed in the West from the late 17th century onwards and are guaranteed through various legal mechanisms (bills, conventions etc). These rights are generally regarded as justiciable (i.e. capable of being decided by a court). Governments are generally obliged to respect (not violate) and protect (prevent non-state actors violating) these rights.

Economic and socio-cultural rights are '*positive rights*' to do something which the individual might be unable to do without state intervention (Marshall 1965; Berlin 1969:131–134). They include the right to education, housing, health, social security, employment, food, clothing, and the benefits of scientific progress and its applications, among others. The underlying principles are those of participation, inclusion, and opportunity, and are based on notions of social democracy, socialism and collectivism, as broadly articulated since the 19th century, although some enjoy ancient provenance (for example, a number of them can be found in the Hebrew scriptures). According to the UDHR, governments need to help fulfill economic and socio-cultural rights by creating supportive living conditions (Ife 2001; Gruskin and Tarantola 2005); nevertheless, positive rights are generally seen as malleable and whether they are justiciable is a moot point. For some, their realization was seen to endanger rather than strengthen the state (Weller 2009).

Together with the UDHR, these treaties comprise what is informally known as the International Bill of Rights. The historical division into the two treaties has been interpreted as referring to the tension between the position of liberal states founded on civil and political rights on the one hand, and on the other, that of socialist, communist and/or welfare states founded on the principles of solidarity and the government's obligation to meet basic economic and social needs (Annas, 2005; Forsythe 2006; Weller 2009).

There have been critiques of this bifurcation. People's lives—and the rights they need for dignity—do not fit neatly into such separate spheres. For example, the right to work is a right to economic participation akin to political participation; and cultural rights are closely related to civil liberties such as freedoms of speech, religion, and mass media. Equally, civil and political rights are violated to protect economic privilege, and poverty can be seen as explicitly arising out of political actions and policies. As noted below, the duties of governments in relation to these categories are not as clear-cut. Feminist thought, in questioning the public–private split, also questions the artificial division between international law protecting public civil–political rights, traditionally exercised by men and defendable in courts on the one hand, and on the other the rights associated with the work of women in the home, in subsistence economies, health care, and family education—rights which law traditionally has not protected (Weller 2009). The actual interdependence of these domains is illustrated by the outcomes of famines in developing countries, where civil and political rights (democratization, freedom of speech and protest) have been integral to securing vital socio-economic rights, commencing with the right to food (Sen 1982). Dichotomous thinking regarding positive and negative human rights (as elsewhere) can perpetuate violations (Donnelly 2003:32–33) which, as the section on so-called 'Asian values' below indicates, can also have consequences for mental health.

Preceding or building on these treaties, other rights treaties focus on specific populations—for example, the Convention on Refugees (1951), the International Convention on the Elimination of All Forms of Racial Discrimination (ICERD) (1965), the Convention on the Elimination of all Forms of Discrimination against Women (CEDAW) (1979), the Convention on the Rights of the Child (CRC) (1989), and the Convention on the Rights of Persons with Disabilities (CRPD) (2008)—or on specific issues, for example, the Convention on Genocide (1948), the Supplementary Convention on the Abolition of Slavery (1956), the Convention against Apartheid (1973), the Convention against Torture and Other Cruel, Inhuman or Degrading Treatment or Punishment (CAT) (1984), and the Framework Convention on Climate Change (1992). Regional agreements, notably in Europe and the Western Hemisphere, have complemented these international instruments. A series of international conferences have aimed to give content to the rights enshrined in many of these treaties (Gruskin and Tarantola 2005).

In addition, collective or solidarity rights (Vasak 1977) have been formulated including such examples as the benefits of economic growth and development, peace, a healthy environment, and self-determination. Based as they are on community development principles, their codification is in the early stages, and their status of rights is debated (Ife 2001). This is further discussed below, under minority rights.

In sum, the political struggles of the last two centuries have gradually expanded the purview of human rights to those who were previously disadvantaged or excluded. Thus for example, working men, colonized peoples, religious dissenters, women, and ethnic minorities have come under the rights umbrella (Marshall 1965; Donnelly 2003:60; Hunt 2007). Furthermore, the International Human Rights Covenants have now extended rights to everyone. In step with this, nation states increasingly have been regarded as being founded on political rights and the rule of law, rather than simply being an expression of shared culture, history, or blood ties; and their citizens, as deriving their rights from being human beings rather than from any other criterion (Donnelly 2003:64). This broad (if uneven and inconstant) shift from ethnic towards civic nationalism (Higgins, 2006) therefore has heralded an advance in the scope of rights. Despite this advance, nation states often fail to encompass those who fall outside their concern—non-citizens, for example asylum-seekers—whose rights remain precarious (Kymlicka 2002:254–255). Mares and Jureidini and Steel and colleagues address their needs and exclusion from the social contract, Moreover, in political struggles for inclusion, those with mental and psychosocial disabilities remain socially marginalized, experience wide-ranging human rights violations and are frequently poorly served by their governments (Drew et al. 2011).

Administration and accountability

Various objections to the concept of human rights are assessed below. However, one frequent criticism considered here is that the human rights project in whole or in part (e.g. the notions of economic and socio-cultural rights) is impractical, involving 'paper victories' that don't translate into hard realities (noted by Perlin and Szeli, this volume). Some go further, saying that in some quarters of the developing world, human rights are seen as an unaffordable luxury, reflecting Western privilege, disconnected from the struggle on the ground (Farmer 2005). Frameworks of administration are dealt with here, and questions about the effectiveness of existing regimes below.

The human rights cause has been driven by a highly politicized process within and outside the UN framework. The process now engages all governments as well as being a principal focus of many international and local non-governmental organizations (NGOs) (including those working in health and mental health). The chief organs of the UN global human rights regime have been the Commission on Human Rights, the prime forum for developing human rights norms which had limited monitoring functions through its resolutions, working groups and special rapporteurs till its dissolution in 2006; the Human Rights Council which has succeeded it; the Human Rights Committee and the Committee on Economic, Social and Cultural Rights, which report on the ICCPR and the ICESCR respectively; and the UN High Commissioner for Human Rights. Various regional rights regimes and single issue regimes—concerning workers' conditions, race discrimination, torture, women's rights, children, genocide, and minorities—complement these arrangements.

Within this global matrix, however, the UN is decentralized and states remain autonomous. In global human rights law, decision-making is also decentralized. No single body (e.g. the UN Security Council, international courts) assumes direct responsibility for human rights *in toto*, so that direct protection and enforcement are rare. Thus the international human rights regime is relatively strong in promoting rights, but generally weaker in implementation and rarely capable of enforcing the regime. However, while national sovereignty remains ascendant, states are more constrained by human rights norms and engage in more indirect implementation than has been the case previously (Donnelly 2003; Freeman 2002; Landman 2005; Forsythe 2006).

The international human rights regime has a coherent set of norms across various categories of rights. Governments ratifying the relevant treaties report periodically to the treaty body which monitors government actions under that treaty. Experts examine and comment on periodic reports from member states. Various UN agencies (e.g. UNICEF, UNAIDS, WHO, the International Labour Organization (ILO), the United Nations Development Programme (UNDP), and the United Nations Population Fund (UNPF) provide the treaty bodies with information based on their evaluation of government compliance. Agency input is often uncoordinated, and different agencies have different levels of country coverage, resulting in somewhat patchy regimes of accountability (Freeman 2002). NGOs have a crucial role, though the dearth of formal reporting mechanisms to treaty bodies, and liaison amongst each other, impairs the effectiveness of the monitoring process. Government reports are the subject of formal dialogue with the treaty body, which prepares the concluding comments and observations. Guidelines for governments reporting to treaty monitoring bodies do not, in the main, specifically refer to mental health. The absence of mental health NGOs in some countries leaves the sole responsibility of review to mainstream rights organizations such as Amnesty International and Human Rights Watch, which do not always have a primary focus on health or mental health (Gruskin and Tarantola 2005).

In recent years, the UN has made progress in mainstreaming human rights: it has made human rights integral to the design, implementation, monitoring and evaluation of policies and programmes in the political, economic, and social spheres. This has led to restructuring of processes within agencies such as UNICEF and WHO (UN 1997). Treaty bodies have also formulated General Comments and Recommendations relating to health, which influence various parties reporting on this issue (Gruskin and Tarantola 2005).

Conceptualizing human rights: a sample of key debates

The emphasis and prominence given to human rights have not inhibited spirited debates about their conceptualization (Griffin 2008; Freeman 2002). In the West, the core idea prevails that humans are unique. For Jews, Christians, and Muslims, this means all humans are created in God's image, and thus are creators too: of ourselves and part of the world around us, for which we account as moral agents (Griffin 2008:26). The breakdown of theistic foundations for natural rights in the West means that the basic idea, that they cover everyone just by being human, has often been seen as insufficiently persuasive. This is notwithstanding good reasons that buttress human rights, including the respect for human dignity (Donnelly 2003), the foundations of moral action (Gewirth 1982), the demands of human sympathy (Glover 1999; Rorty 1993) and the conditions necessary for human flourishing (Nussbaum 2006; Freeman 2002). The moral force of rights, residing in the humanity of the rights-holder, constitutes the great source of their appeal as well as their potential weakness (Gavison 2003:26). Ultimately, as noted above, human rights regardless of their contentious foundations and their loose association with various moral theories, rest on a social and political resolve to recognize rights as valid. They are both the ideal and the practice for implementing that ideal (Donnelly 2003:15, 21).

A range of philosophical frameworks can inform discussions of rights: classically and centrally, liberalism, and social contract theory (Donnelly 2003:35), but also utilitarianism (consequentialism), libertarianism, Marxism, communitarianism, citizenship theories, multiculturalism, and feminisms, among others (Kymlicka 2002). Though reference is made to some of these frameworks, it is impossible to systematically assay them here. However, Donnelly (2003:47–49) notes that liberalism can be associated both with rights-based (Lockean) and goods-based (Benthamite

or utilitarian) social theories, and with thick or thin accounts of the range of rights. Social democracy and libertarianism denote the end points of the 'thick-thin' continuum. Social democracy,
conjoined with strong egalitarianism, an extensive system of economic and social rights, and
robust democratic political control, upholds the UDHR and advances the mental health and well-
being of people with mental disorders. Strong libertarianism—especially in its microeconomic,
utilitarian 'neoliberal' incarnation with its orientation to efficiency—potentially discourages
concerns for the mentally ill as a disadvantaged group.

Some critiques of human rights examine its scope, especially its relationships with other substantial concerns such as goodness and justice, ethics, needs and capabilities, globalization, and
security and technologies. Other critiques more explicitly query the legitimacy of rights.
Arguments about the relationship of rights with realpolitik, law, duties and responsibilities, and
cultures and minorities, typify these critiques. These are briefly considered in the sections that
follow, with a special eye on (mental) health.

Scoping human rights

One scoping question is whether human rights encompass the entire domains of goodness or
justice. While all rights are goods, not all goods—whether love, charity, or compassion, or those
grounded in law, justice, utility, self-interest, or beneficence—are rights (Donnelly 2003:12).
Regarding justice, Griffin (2008) argues that rights are specifically intertwined with the concept
and exercise of personal agency, which he conceives as autonomy, liberty, and minimum provision
for people pursuing their conception of a worthwhile life. Although foetuses, very young infants,
and those with advanced dementia or in comatose state undoubtedly require justice, do they, in
view of their potential, modified, or suspended agency, also possess rights (Griffin 2008)? However,
if one concludes they do not, do those with mental disorders, with modified or suspended agency,
also not possess rights? Concepts of agency and rights may need broadening to accommodate
these groups, as the widening franchise of rights over time illustrates (Hunt 2007; Failer 2002).

Can one distinguish human rights from social justice? Definitions matter here. Social justice is
diversely defined but distinguishes itself from laws that operate to control behaviour. As with
human rights, free market proponents and others may deny, implicitly or explicitly, the possibility
of social justice, because it encompasses notions of distributive equality or social equality
(Kymlicka 2002:195–199). Secondly, social justice links to economic, social and cultural rights:

> Social justice is what faces you in the morning. It is awakening in a house with adequate water supply,
> cooking facilities and sanitation. It is the ability to nourish your children and send them to school
> where their education not only equips them for employment but reinforces their knowledge and under-
> standing of their cultural inheritance. It is the prospect of genuine employment and good health: a life
> of choices and opportunity, free from discrimination (Dodson, quoted by Lawrence 2002).

Thirdly, social justice adopts what liberation theologians have called 'a preferential option for the
poor' (Farmer and Gastineau 2005). It focuses on structural inequity and inequality, and prompts
outrage at the suffering of people marginalized by such arrangements, including those with
psychosocial disabilities.

Whether one discriminates human rights from social justice depends on whether human rights
are seen as encompassing all rights, or only civil–political rights. If the latter neo-liberal constraint
pertains, then social justice expands to fulfill economic, social, and cultural rights. If a broader
perspective on human rights applies, then the framework embraces social justice concerns and
redresses inequities with the same passion. Moreover, such frameworks also support social goods
that do not exclusively focus on relieving the suffering of the marginalized and poor. They entail
a set of agreed-upon standards, and a full range of normative prescriptions (Marks 2005).

Similarly, the concept of social inclusion and exclusion, not expounded in detail here, are frameworks that have had significant uptake in certain Western democracies, where they have been deployed inter alia to interpret and respond to the collective drivers of mental disorder and disadvantage (Queensland Alliance 2010; Long 2010; Suicide Prevention Australia 2011). Social inclusion has been criticized for its imprecision, which leaves it open to alignments with social conformity and conventionality. However, more typically, social inclusion has been linked with marginality, minority, and disability, and has been used to supplant welfare with rights agendas. Thus it promotes participation, accountability, non-discrimination, empowerment, and linkages to human rights standards (Szoke 2009). In this guise, the practical applications of social inclusion are evident in relation to the various groups discussed throughout this volume.

Needs are frequently nominated as the foundations of rights. As Mangalore and colleagues (this volume) discuss, needs are basic necessities that link human rights, capabilities, resource allocation, and equity in mental health. Though context and vantage point delineate them (Ife 2001), needs should not be reduced to empirical verification or independent and objective assessment, without engaging philosophical debates (Donnelly 2003:16–17). One defines needs not merely in relation to economic productivity or efficiency, or survival, but in terms of concepts such as dignity (Donnelly 2003). Some models of need, e.g. the ADAPT Model (Adaptation and Development after Persecution and Trauma), straddle empirical and philosophical domains (Silove 1999).

'Capabilities', a closely related term originating in welfare economics (Sen 1985), refers to substantive freedoms, to what people can do and be, opportunities for functioning that the individual chooses to exploit or not in order to create valued outcomes. Capabilities draw on the concept of personal agency and derive from intuitions about a bare minimum of a life worthy of human dignity. Hence they closely relate to, and supplement and clarify, the notion of rights (Nussbaum 2006). They signify that rights are not merely political artefacts, but oblige affirmative action. Poverty is capability-deprivation (Sen 1999). Capabilities result from the interdependence of liberties and socio-economic arrangements. Nussbaum's list of central human capabilities includes life; bodily health; bodily integrity; senses, imagination, and thought; emotions; practical reason; affiliation; other species; play; and control over one's environment, in political and material aspects (see Nussbaum (2006:76–78, 284–291, and *passim*) for the domains encompassed by these items, though Sen (1999, 2009) argues against any list being definitive).

Most significantly for those with psychosocial disabilities, capabilities confront and arguably overcome the limitations of liberalism and social contractarianism that derive from their starting positions of autonomy and rationality as self-interest, which therefore fail to include those with such disabilities. They envisage social cooperation that arises from fellowship (Nussbaum 2006). According to social contractarianism, each accepts a duty to society in exchange for the freedom and security that society provides (Marks 2005:98–99). Yet social contracts also fail to address the needs of marginalized people. Respect and inclusion of those with disabilities matters because it is good to do so, whether it is economically efficient or not, and whether or not they are regarded as idealized rational citizens (Nussbaum 2006:121).

Also central to health and mental health, the capabilities approach figures prominently in the Human Development Index, which underpins the United Nation's Development Project's Human Development Reports (<http://hdr.undp.org/en/humandev/>). This supersedes the World Bank practice of ranking countries by gross per capita income, and denies the presumption of a close link between national economic growth and the expansion of individual human choices.

Some sceptical views and responses

The concept of rights has attracted various objections. Accusations of impracticality, elitism, and luxury are noted above, while questions of implementation are discussed below. Another is that realpolitik is the only factor that governs political life, a process of advancing rational self-interest and bargaining to mutual advantage: 'justice depends on equality of power, the strong do what they can, the weak accept what they must' (Thucydides 1954/1972). This Hobbesian vision repudiates human rights or an inherently human moral status, and also rejects the essentialist notion of justice, which is arguably most relevant in conditions of extreme inequality of power (Kymlicka 2002:128–138).

Another perspective accepts the notion of rights, but asserts that it is identical with that of law. In this view, rights are artefacts of laws and institutions and the only rights are legally enforceable ones (Kymlicka 2002:128–138; Nussbaum 2006). Jeremy Bentham for example (1962 (1792/1843)) famously declared that 'natural rights is . . . nonsense on stilts'. However, if human rights arise from human dignity, they are pre-legal as well as having legal functions. Against Bentham, unrealized rights, that motivate specific legislation, arguably serve as the parent of law rather than its child (Sen 2009). Thus, as noted above, 'human rights' is not fully subsumed under human rights law.

A related but distinct criticism is that discourses about and declarations of rights encourage people to satisfy individual desires and neglect their duties (Hunt 2007:179). This argument is expanded upon here because of the importance of grasping the debate about the relationship between the common good (exemplified by nations, groups, minorities, cultures, etc.—considered below) and individual rights. It takes several forms. However, some observations firstly need to be made.

To affirm that one has human rights simply by being human does not occlude the complex predicated relationship between rights and duties. Rights may entail duties, duties may entail rights, and rights may be independent of duties (for example, rights to have a promise fulfilled or a loan repaid). Rights imply duty bearers (states and others), yet unrealized rights and imperfect obligations exist without readily identified duty-bearers (Sen 2009). Exercising some rights may infringe those of others: thus free speech does not *ipso facto* prohibit inciting hatred. Though the right remains, the law may punish abuses (Donnelly 2003:114–115). Moreover principles of public health and well-being sometimes override individual rights. Although some rights, such as freedom from torture or slavery, the right to a fair trial, and the right to freedom of thought are unqualified (Gruskin and Tarantola 2005), the state may restrict rights such as freedom of movement or speech to achieve a broader public good. For instance, quarantine applies in epidemics (though responses to HIV/AIDS sometimes have unnecessarily violated this principle); and those who threaten others or themselves with violence may be remanded and/or treated against their wishes if they are also mentally ill or disordered. A legitimate object of general interest, strict necessity which excludes alternatives, and the rule of law must govern the emergency suspension of rights, on the so-called Siracusa Principles (Gruskin and Tarantola 2005). Exercising one's rights goes hand in hand with respecting, protecting and possibly satisfying the rights or capabilities of others (to quote Thomas Scanlon (1998), this is 'what we owe to each other').

According to one formulation of the rights–duties relationship, people have rights but not duties. This conceptualizes distinct individuals with separate existences who are not resources for others (Nozick 1974). This model only succeeds if one adopts a libertarian account of rights that emphasizes non-interference: otherwise the contrast between responsibilities and rights collapses (Okin 1990, quoted in Kymlicka 2002:410). Individualists sometimes propose preferences as 'rights', for example, the rights to bear arms, to unlimited private property, to use corporal punishment on one's children. Such imprecise language requires clarification. Overlap with other rights, insufficient generality, infringing the rights of others and/or being unrelated to a situation of oppression or disadvantage, are all grounds to disqualify these latter 'rights' (Ife 2001).

Another formulation is that rights depend on duties. One riposte to Western notions of rights as autonomy or self-government is that they do not capture the interdependence that character-izes other traditions and cultures. An often cited instance is Confucianism, which envisages cosmic and personal harmony: complex, interlocking, hierarchical roles and relations, focused on filial piety, loyalty, deference, accommodation, and self-mastery (Donnelly 2003:114). Similarly, communitarians believe people understand themselves through participating in common life, expressed through common purposes and shared ends, and that they want these arrangements for their own sake, not just instrumentally. Thus they question the political culture of state neutrality which allows people to choose their goals independently of the public good, and to abandon the public good should it outweigh their individual rights (Taylor 1985; Sandel 1996). This echoes the critique of atomistic liberalism noted above, and it is explored further when considering culture and minorities.

Another formulation, much debated, holds that rights and duties divide along gender lines: women purportedly assume caring roles, and engage different modes of moral reasoning to men, favouring a focus on particular relationships and individuals, as against a preferential concern for universals and humanity in general. This description receives observational support (Gilligan 1982), though critics note that offering care may have a general focus whereas concerns for justice may be specific. However, in some cultures women, men, and children may not believe that women have rights. Redress should correct this misconception and allow women to care for themselves and not just for others, and in turn to be cared for (Kymlicka 2002:398–430). These debates potentially influence women's mental health. Three chapters (by Raphael and colleagues, Maltzahn and Villadiego, and Yuksel and colleagues) deal with implica-tions of the different facets of patriarchy and global capitalism for women's mental health and human rights.

Yet another permutation of the rights–responsibilities relationship surfaces in relation to pas-sive versus active accounts of citizenship. The latter perspective argues that citizenship does not equate with legal status, nor with formal (private) rights, nor even with social rights, such as health care and education (Marshall 1965). Citizenship entails active responsibilities and civic virtues: it requires engagement in public discourse. It marshalls critical thinking, questions author-ity, listens and converses, seeks personal benefit without bargaining or threats (Galston 1991; Kymlicka 2002:287–293). Rosen and colleagues take up the question of citizenship for people with severe and persistent mental illness in their chapter.

All such formulations diverge from the original declaration that all humans possess rights that rest on prior moral (and international legal) entitlement, that are inalienable, and that exist before and irrespective of the discharge of social duties (Donnelly 2003:114). The Marquis de Condorcet (quoted in Hunt 1996:119–121) asserted that since rights either belong to none or to all, whoever votes against the rights of another abjures his own. Consequently, even rights violators, capital offenders (as James Welsh's chapter reminds us), and terror suspects detained in the so-called 'war on terror' whose rights to liberty are abridged, retain inviolable legal rights that extend to situations of emergency.

In sum, Western liberal discourse holds that human rights may entail duties, and notes a com-plex relationship between rights and duties. Moreover the vision of rights as interrelated, interde-pendent, and indivisible (UN 1993) does not dispel tensions between rights. This includes and perhaps especially pertains to mental health (as noted below, and for example in the chapters by Rosen et al. and Sullivan and Mullen. They demonstrate this point in considering those with severe and persistent mental illness, and prisoners with mental disorders respectively).

But Western liberal discourse also holds that the standing of rights does not depend on fulfillment of duties.

Selected issues:

Culture, cultural relativism, and minorities One claim that endures is that though human rights discourse aspires to be universal, it originated in the West and is therefore culturally relative. Can a rights framework that reflects Western liberal traditions apply universally, and be universally acceptable and relevant, to all cultures and social contexts? Or do cultures limit rights? Furthermore, do (and should) cultures, groups and/or minorities, as well as individuals, possess rights? Minority rights (or group, or cultural rights) are potentially two-edged, with both edges being relevant to mental health. (Here we interpret minority, group, and culture interchangeably for the purpose of this argument).

On the one hand, minorities (whether based on ethnicity, religion, age, sexual preference, or disability) frequently suffer events or circumstances that jeopardize their mental health. Minority rights, which are a form of group rights, may supplement individual rights by protecting vulnerable groups from external pressures, and protect against occurrences such as discrimination, genocide, and forced expulsion.

On the other hand, culturally relativist arguments and practices are sometimes used in ways that jeopardize mental health. Protection of the rights of illiberal minorities may assist them to restrict individual rights of their members (e.g. by suppressing internal dissent), or sometimes to oppress majorities (as in the case of the Third Reich or the Apartheid regime in South Africa). We now briefly explore these two senses, illustrating them with case examples.

Minority, group, and cultural rights

In all senses, culture underpins the lives of people and groups: it helps constitute people's multiple meanings and identities. 'Culture' encompasses cultivation, cultural (often ethnocultural) identity, and the broader sense of culture as ways of life (Kirmayer 2007). Proponents of liberal culturalism (e.g. Kymlicka 2002:339) defend cultural or national character within states. They maintain that individual freedom depends on societal culture, defined by language and history, to which most people have a very strong bond. In this view, liberal justice acknowledges cultural membership and requires minority cultural rights, ensuring equal protection for cultural minorities and majorities. Moreover, as just noted, communitarians support such cultural alignments.

Various grounds in international law accept the needs if not the rights of cultural minorities, enshrined for example in the ICCPR. Article 27 of the ICCPR recognizes that group members hold rights to participate in their culture, religion and language. However, it confines this to states where minorities exist (increasing the likelihood states will deny this), to individuals not groups to which they belong, and mandates toleration rather than duties to assist (Freeman 2002:114; Griffin 2008).

Various specific examples of the value of minority or cultural rights for mental health may be briefly noted. One example concerns indigenous people. In 1992, the UN General Assembly adopted the Declaration on the Rights of Persons belonging to National, or Ethnic, Religious and Linguistic Minorities. The Working Group on Minorities and Indigenous Peoples of the UN Sub-Commission has promoted this area in recent years (Donnelly 2003:151). These groups experience unique threats to their mental health, as Hunter and colleagues note in their chapter.

Similarly, the enactment of legislation against hate crimes internationally aims to protect minorities and to enable nations and communities to restrain and correct racism and negative discrimination through legal action. The chapter by McGeorge and Bhugra, with particular reference to the UK, examines racism and class as they affect mental health.

Sexual minorities provide another example of those still to benefit from the progressive extension of rights that has characterized the last two centuries. They suffer significantly higher rates of self-harm, suicide attempts, and possibly suicide than the general population (Suicide Prevention Australia 2009). These afflictions arise from the intolerance they experience in almost all societies. Numerous countries prohibit and criminalize same-sex sexual relations, while sexual orientation constitutes grounds for discrimination in employment, housing, access to public facilities and social services, civil status, inheritance, adoption, parenting, and social insurance. Violence is commonplace and sometimes quasi-official (Donnelly 2003). This is despite the facts that the ICESCR proscribes sex as a ground for discrimination (Article 2.2); that the ICCPR (Article 17) mandates the right to privacy; that the European Court of Human Rights finds laws that criminalize homosexual behaviour violate human rights (Finnemore and Sikkink 1998); and that Amnesty International opposes persecution of or discrimination against same-sex attracted people (Gruskin 2000). In international relations, sexual orientation is becoming a faultline between Western countries that seek to protect sexual diversity, and states that assert that sexual minorities undermine culture, tradition, and religion. For example, some Asian states, under the guise of 'Asian values', have portrayed homosexuality as a distinctly Western form of degeneracy (see discussion below). The Ugandan government attracted widespread international condemnation when it attempted to legislate to make homosexuality a crime punishable by death in May 2011.

Noting that persecution of sexual minorities remains widespread internationally, Newman (this volume) tracks how psychiatry in particular perpetuates such discrimination. She promotes social reform encompassing increasing tolerance of gender diversity, culturally competent health services, and inclusive medicine that aids understanding and insight for self-determination. Strategies for inclusion also include incorporation into international human rights law, and into national legislation (Donnelly 2003).

Limits to minority, group, and cultural rights

Arguments against strong cultural relativism (Kirmayer, this volume) note that despite its formative influence, culture is not destiny (Donnelly 2003:88), nor are cultures essential or immutable. Rather, they are often complex, open, contested, conflicted and in the 'global village', cultures inevitably permeate each other. Moral intuitions based on our common humanity allow us to see the other's 'equivalent centre of self' (as George Eliot put it in 'Middlemarch'), bridging cultures to infer the needs of others. Liberalism often denies moral worth or human rights to groups, while assuming that people will exercise rights as group members. States may promote non-discrimination through toleration of groups or perhaps equal protection, rather than fully-fledged multiculturalism. They may intervene against activities that infringe or violate human rights, and remedy systematic discrimination through promoting freedom of association and economic, political, and socio-cultural participation (Donnelly 2003:205). Rather than individual cultures being irreducible units that cannot be aggregated, negotiations and cross-cultural dialogue as well as interlocking systems of international law can realize universal human rights as expressed in the UDHR model (Donnelly 2003:71; Prasad 2004).

Thus cultures do not represent the final moral arbiter. Precepts concerning the equality of human beings and the protection of innocents or the vulnerable, apply to practices as divergent as the Taliban stoning allegedly adulterous women in Afghanistan, and capital punishment (sometimes with mass jubilation) in parts of the United States (Sen 2005).

Moreover, arguments from strong cultural relativism have magnified alleged differences between Western and non-Western societies over the value assigned to civil–political rights or economic and socio-cultural rights (Cassese 1999; Shue 2003; Inoue 2003; Donnelly 2003), and have been problematic for mental health.

As noted, Western and socialist states diverge in their emphasis on rights. Some Asian political leaders in the 1990s also promoted 'Asian values', emphasizing social harmony, socio-economic rights, and collectivism, asserting the pre-eminence of state interests over individual rights and the dependence of rights on fulfillment of duties. These principles were invoked to resist the West's cultural domination, the alleged neo-colonial imposition of liberal democracy and human rights, and to justify rapid economic development and authoritarian regimes (Donnelly 2003:109). Such rhetoric for example neglected the importance of civil and political rights in accommodating religious and cultural tensions in many Asian countries; and the fact that the tension between communitarianism and individualism runs not between East and West, but through both of them (Inoue 2003). Asian societies may still implement the universal norms of human rights in distinctive ways that do not follow Western models, but human rights may prompt the re-evaluation of local traditions in both West and East (Donnelly 2003).

Conversely, particularly at times in the US, civil and political rights have been elevated, and sometimes equated with state non-interference (Nussbaum 2006:286). Economic and socio-cultural rights by contrast have at times been identified with 'development', requiring redistribution. Governments may view them as more costly to implement and more complex for courts to adjudicate and enforce, than most aspects of civil and political rights (Ife 2001; Gavison 2003). These assumptions have been questioned. The supposed problems of implementing economic and social rights do not support the moral priority of civil and political rights (Donnelly 2003). But just as not all civil and political rights are negative rights—some entail positive actions (and costs), for example the right to property, or educating populations to de-legitimate torture–so social and economic rights are not necessarily all costly, for example, guaranteeing the right to privacy for those on welfare. All human rights require positive action and restraint on the part of the state (Donnelly 2003:30).

However, to emphasize civil and political rights and diminish economic and socio-cultural rights is to align with liberal individualism, which typically views people abstractly, as self-made, self-contained individuals, alone, pitted against the collective, and not reliant on the state. Human rights law and discourse has been criticized for heavily relying on an essentially patriarchal conception, maintaining dominant hierarchies of gender, race and class, and a distinction between public and private spheres, the former regulated by the state, the latter not (Freedman 1999; Nussbaum 2006:290). This perspective in turn narrows the focus of health and mental health, magnifying the significance of individual risks and minimizing psycho-social causal processes. Basic socio-economic rights should also be part of 'the rules of the game'—should, for example, be embedded in constitutions. A person struggling to subsist does not have freedom to pursue any goals (Gavison 2003).

This point pre-eminently applies to those suffering from severe and persistent mental illness in the community, people who are deemed to be at liberty to 'enjoy' their 'anti-rights' on the fringes of society (Arboleda-Flórez, 2008), or 'die with their rights on' (Treffert et al. 1973, quoted by Rosen et al, this volume). If a culture's preoccupation with privileging civil and political rights while diminishing or dismissing socio-economic rights means that some are free to pursue their goals only because others live a life from which this freedom is absent, then the original formulation is problematic. The relationship of these two forms of rights therefore raises one of the core political questions: about the relationship between individual autonomy and mutual social responsibility (Gavison, 2003).

Although at times arguments have been made about the primacy of either 'Eastern' or 'Western' cultures or grouping of rights, no fundamental reasons for recognizing human rights give one cluster of rights primacy over the other. As noted, human lives do not fit into such categories. The authorship of the Universal Declaration of Human Rights was truly international, not merely Western (Glendon 2001). Sen's work on the outcomes of famines and feminist critiques has been discussed above. Civil and political rights, and social and economic rights, are equally required for human dignity and for mental health and well-being. They reinforce each other (Gavison 2003).

Further implications of the conjunction of culture and human rights for mental health are discussed below, and Kirmayer, Rosen, and colleagues also do so in their chapters.

Globalization Globalization has been defined as the shrinking of space and time, and the disappearance of borders (United Nations Development Programme 1999). The international movement of money, trade, culture, people, and information is both centuries-old and contemporary. Its common elements through time include the spread of capitalism and integrated markets, socio-political changes, improved technology and communication, and the sharing of norms and values (Arat 2005).

For mental health and human rights, the consequences of globalization and global economics, especially aid, trade, and commerce, are mixed. Globalization enhances health through information- and resource-sharing, and debatably through competition to provide more widely available, higher quality services. Through global trade and monetary organizations, transnational corporations (TNCs) advance inter-state cooperation and assist poorer countries to develop their economies.

However, since the market does not prioritize equity, it can contribute to widening resource inequalities. For example, informed by neo-liberal free market doctrine, the IMF and the World Bank adopted structural adjustment policies that imposed crippling burdens of debt on poor states, which have especially impacted on women and children (Senarclens 2003; Shue 2003). Foreign aid recently has been labelled an 'unmitigated political, economic and humanitarian disaster' (Moyo 2009), though this has been strongly contested. Globalization can also spread lifestyles and behaviours (such as substance abuse) that jeopardize mental health (Gruskin and Tarantola 2005).

TNCs and other non-state actors that influence health and well-being (such as research institutions, foundations, insurance companies, care providers, and health management organizations) need regulation. However, no formal process for this exists (Gruskin and Tarantola 2005). By design or neglect, TNCs have violated human rights in many countries when they partner authoritarian regimes to exploit domestic labour. Negotiated agreements, independent monitoring, public reporting, and consumer boycotts may prevent such violations. Governments may be persuaded to ensure that TNCs comply with human rights and to avoid complicity in abuses that governmental or corporate partners perpetrate. Organizations like the World Trade Organization (WTO) need to meet their express aims of helping workers and the poor, and assisting the environment. Through preventing access by developing countries to available pharmaceuticals, WTO's Trade-Related Aspects of Intellectual Property Rights (TRIPS) jeopardizes health, mental health, and the right to share in the benefits of scientific progress (see below). Pursuit of the Millennium Development Goals requires raising levels of aid, and reforming the conduits—aid agencies, and as indicated, development organizations such as the IMF and the World Bank. Raising the profile of mental health in all of these activities is paramount (Forsythe 2006:218–248; Kinley 2009). In the case of transgressive nation states, 'principled engagement' may be a middle strategy that avoids the twin poles of ostracism and normal engagement ('business as usual') (Kinley 2009).

Complex clashes occur between globalist economics and human rights over environmental management. This book does not address the particular challenges of international globalization and climate change for mental health and human rights. However these developments have important consequences for communities. Mental health promotion in rural and remote areas should respond to the felt effects of climate change (McEwan et al. 2009).

The globalization of information technology, the media, and social networking similarly poses major questions concerning state's and TNC's respect for human rights, and for the advance of social resilience (Bolzan and Gale 2011a&b), which have only begun to be explored.

Despite some conservative commentary that seeks to disconnect human rights and global economics, considerable evidence suggests that human rights are not only ends but means for global economies to achieve their goals, and a strong albeit complex link between economic well-being and human rights protection. Human rights advocates may need to better appreciate the global economy's role when pursuing human rights standards (Kinley 2009; Kinley and Stewart 2009). Although mental health does not have the same profile as human rights, it should be equally important to the pursuit of aid, trade and commerce: the potential reciprocal relationship between mental health, aid, and business should be highlighted and more strongly asserted.

Challenges to implementation

Just as human rights abuses and neglects contribute to mental disorders, so the ongoing struggle for socially inclusive, civil societies nurtures the right to (mental) health. The rule of law, viable national and international institutions, human rights regimes and social movements, all mediate this struggle. Cross-cultural applicability, as well as education, language, resources and infrastructure, and impacts of globalization, all affect the prospects of implementing and enforcing rights where appropriate (Freeman 2002; Nussbaum 2006).

Acute moral and practical problems complicate international human rights activities. For example, the UN failed to tackle mass murder in Rwanda and the former Yugoslavia. Despite a zero tolerance policy, sexual abuse of children by UN peacekeepers still occurs, a problem that has also reportedly affected NGOs (Associated Press 2007; Pflanz 2008). The International Committee of the Red Cross has had to justify its stance about preserving confidentiality when it perceives human rights violations (Robertson 2006:211–212, 600; Robertson 2007; Daccord 2007). International NGOs have joined nation states in using human rights language, sometimes from UN platforms (such as the UN Human Rights Commission), to issue controversial unilateral condemnations in morally contested situations. These include, but are not confined to, the Arab-Israeli conflict (NGO Monitor 2008, Commonwealth Human Rights Initiative 2011). Chapters by Rees and Silove, Tomlinson and colleagues, and Gale and Dudley, show how researchers in post-conflict and humanitarian situations act to empower or disempower local societies, depending on their assumptions and practices. The question of the effectiveness of the international rights machinery is discussed here.

A notable upswing in human rights activities has occurred since the Cold War. The increasing development and monitoring of human rights conventions and the proliferation in the number and work of international human rights NGOs have sought to restrain and address human rights neglects and abuses.

As private, not-for-profit organizations, international NGOs analyse information for accuracy, disseminate and publish it, energetically lobby public authorities to adopt new human rights standards or to apply existing ones, and sometimes provide direct services to victims of human rights violations. It is hard to determine their success, given the difficulty with evaluating impacts and causal pathways to particular outcomes. Movements like these, however utopian they may seem, nevertheless create a climate of opinion in international relations that is sympathetic to human rights, and may manage to change policies and situations, sometimes over long periods. Historical examples include the anti-slavery movement and the extensive work of the International Red Cross (regarding humanitarian law and human rights in armed conflict). At times repressive governments have tried to restrict NGO access to UN forums, a move that bears witness to the effectiveness of the NGOs in question. NGOs also sustain relief and development efforts, including mental health and psychosocial programmes that reflect human rights principles in their implementation (Forsythe 2006:188–217).

How effective are the periodic formal reporting processes that oblige signatory governments to report to human rights treaty bodies, and the associated communications (complaint) procedures? Reporting is based on self-criticism and good faith efforts, and while allowing periodic review, it lacks a strong system of international monitoring: this is unlikely to tackle severe, systematic violations. Complaints procedures are optional: states engaging in questionable procedures usually exempt themselves (Donnelly 2003:173–175). UN Human Rights Commission and Human Rights Committee reviews of particular countries, or petitioning mechanisms regarding human rights violations have been highly selective, potentially politicized, and slow to reach conclusions. They impact little on the prevalence of human rights violations. However, the reporting regime has motivated legislative change, contributed to advancement of rights through discussion and advice, and sometimes has benefited individual complainants (Freeman 2002). Crepeau and Gayet (this volume) show, with specific reference to Canada, how this happens with mental health at various levels.

Arising from international conventions, treaties, and trans-national institutions, human rights law has vastly proliferated. Changes in law and international human rights institutions have assisted the prosecution of those accused of crimes against humanity (Robertson 2006). The comprehensive violation of human rights in the so-called 'war on terror' (Wilson 2005; Marks, this volume) has expanded litigation on arbitrary detention, torture and ill-treatment, extraordinary 'rendition', extraterritorial application of human rights norms, and the creeping reach of the 'terrorism' label. These cases in turn illuminate how the 'war on terror' affects human rights (Duffy 2008). Human rights law informs cases as diverse as the law of military occupation (Campanelli 2008; Vite 2008), the admissible killing and internment of fighters in non-international armed conflicts (Sassoli and Olson 2008), and international detainee transfers and the practice of non-refoulement (a matter of considerable significance for refugee mental health) (Droege 2008b). The interrelation, applicability, and limits of international humanitarian law and human rights law is being explored (Droege 2008a). Many other strategies hold governments accountable for rights abuses: diplomacy, boycotts, ostracism, etc.

Some regions (for instance, Europe and the Americas) are significantly stronger than others. For example the European Court of Human Rights, as an international court interpreting the European Convention on Human Rights, uniquely provides for enforcement. It hears individual petitions and makes decisions to which the signatory states agree to be bound, by modifying their national laws (Sumption 2011). The result is a considerable body of case law, including that related to mental health (see below). Africa, Asia, and the Middle East do not have such human rights regimes.

Some empirical research regarding the effectiveness of international rights machinery suggests that international law on human rights has had an enduring if limited effect on state practices, after controlling for a number of variables: the level of democracy, wealth, international interdependence, intra- and interstate conflict, size, and regional differentiation (Landman 2005). Not surprisingly, democracies probably ratify instruments that comprise the international human rights regime, and better protect human rights than non-democracies; and internal conflict underpins non-protection. New democracies ratify more frequently but protect more weakly than old ones. The gap between ratification and protection narrowed in recent years, suggesting alignment between international law and state practice. The activities of NGOs are strongly related to human rights treaty ratification and inter-governmental organizations (IGOs) to greater protection of human rights. Overall, promoting democracy, economic development, international institutionalization, and conflict resolution can collectively enhance human rights, and reduce violations (Landman 2005).

Mental health and human rights

Commonalities, differences, reciprocity

What then do mental health and human rights share in common, and what challenges reside in their relationship? Both focus on the broad social, political, and related (cultural) factors that impinge on human health and well-being. They therefore reveal a common humanistic and humanitarian framework. Both tend to employ a progressive political perspective, concerned with social justice and social responsibility, which at times have provoked opposition from more 'conservative' political sectors or representatives of traditional medical science. Their convergence has implications for practitioners trying to integrate the two fields into a coherent set of principles and practices.

Various sources (e.g. WHO 2002, 2003; Gruskin and Tarantola 2005; Gruskin et al. 2007) trace reciprocal relationships between health and human rights, identifying:

♦ The effect of human rights neglect, denial, or abuse (for example including professionals or services participating in abuses and discrimination), on (mental) health

♦ The effect of health on the delivery of human rights, and the impact of (mental) health laws, policies, programmes and practices (or their absence) on human rights

(for example the risk of imposing what are considered to be universal mental health practices on local populations, which may undermine indigenous conceptualizations of mental health and traditional healing processes).

One paradigmatic structure emerges from practical experience in the case of HIV, where public health programmes first explicitly engaged human rights concerns (Gruskin et al. 2007; see Esposito and Tarantola, this volume). It grants the importance of both negative and positive rights in mental health. People with mental health problems suffer both gross abuses and neglects, and gross inequities. The ensuing sections review these key domains.

The connection between mental health and human rights does not annul differences in their priorities, methodologies, and their understanding of their respective missions. One contrast turns on the difference between rights and ethics. Human rights law largely deals with the responsibility of the state to its citizens (often on a case-by-case basis), whereas clinical psychiatry focuses on the well-being of individuals suffering from mental disorders. Mirroring this, clinical professional ethics as traditionally conceived has concentrated on client encounters and environments rather than on social issues impinging on professionals and their clients (Bloch and Pargiter 2009). In the US and various Western countries, medical law has enlarged in recent decades, with an accent on more regulation, litigation, and avoiding legal liability, while interest in medical ethics conceived as the search for good conduct has diminished (Annas 2005). In contrast to the content or emphasis of codes of ethics, human rights frameworks address the systemic or power-related issues relevant to mental health or suicide prevention as well as problems such as dual loyalty. Also in contrast to ethical decision-making which attaches to the worker, human rights perspectives hinge on empowerment, allowing the client to be an active participant in decision-making (Ife 2001).

The two approaches—mental health and human rights—sometimes pursue differing priorities. For example, in truth and reconciliation processes, the human rights impetus may be to record the entire truth relating to past atrocities, whereas mental health professionals may be troubled that the process of truth-telling could re-traumatize survivors. Also, human rights and mental health personnel have sometimes been on opposite sides of the argument about the right to treatment or to refuse treatment for severe mental illness. Debate persists, for example, about the possible intrusion of the legal process (and attendant bureaucracy) into settings that some practitioners may argue are best handled within the medical domain.

Yet the extent of the shared framework is substantial. It covers the domains of education, practice, monitoring and measurement, evaluation, and research.

The right to health

The WHO definition of health covers mental health and has profound human rights implications. In the early post-Second World War era, the health and human rights communities frequently worked in parallel, rarely connecting. Yet there have been clear indicators of a growing rapprochement between the two domains in recent decades. Various factors influenced this process of convergence.

As economic, social, and cultural rights have risen in prominence, so also has the right of everyone to enjoy the highest attainable standard of physical and mental health (the 'right to the highest attainable standard of health' or the 'right to health'). The idea of health care as a human right is closely allied with a primary health care philosophy, espoused by statements such as the Alma Ata Declaration (1978) which helped to entrench this conviction (Hall and Taylor 2003; Gillam 2008; Sartorius, 2002), and the Ottawa Charter of Health Promotion (1986). The Global Programme on AIDS under WHO in the late 1980s became the first world public health programme to explicitly employ human rights language (Gruskin et al. 2007), though it was some time until the comparable connection was made to mental health (see Esposito and Tarantola, this volume).

Health organizations and experts, including those in the field of mental health care, increasingly recognize this right (Backman and Mesquita, this volume), though in recent times of economic recession, the notion that health is a right and that which holds health care as a commodity, have been in active tension (Aggarwal et al. 2010).

In the modern era, the right to health was first proclaimed during the Enlightenment and institutionalized during the French Revolution (as noted by Susser and Bresnahan, and also Backman and Mesquita in this volume). In the 20th century, this principle is stipulated in Article 12 of the International Covenant on Economic, Social and Cultural Rights (ICESCR) (1966), and the UN conventions on the Elimination of Racial Discrimination (1965), the Elimination of Discrimination against Women (1979), the Rights of the Child (1989), and the Rights of Persons with Disabilities (2008). It also appears in several regional charters (for example the African Charter of Human and People's Rights (1981), the Additional Protocol to the American Convention on Human Rights in the Area of Economic, Social and Political Rights (1988), and the European Social Charter (1996)).

Governments must respect (refrain from interfering in), protect (prevent third parties from interfering), and satisfy (facilitate, provide, and promote) the right to health (General Comment 14 on Article 12 of the ICESCR by the Committee on Economic, Social and Cultural Rights (CESCR) (WHO 2005a:10)). This requirement covers the gamut of both negative and positive rights. Human development presupposes such a commitment to such rights in the domains of health outcomes, health systems, and societal and environmental preconditions (Gruskin and Tarantola 2005). General Comment 14 specifies entitlements to autonomy regarding one's health and body, to freedoms from interference, and endorses the interrelated elements of service availability, accessibility, acceptability, and quality. Interrelated rights essential to health and mental health include non-discrimination, the right to enjoy the benefits of scientific progress (this is relevant to inequities regarding access to antiretroviral therapies (Gruskin and Tarantola 2005:11–12) and psychotropics), and the right to participation.

Shared histories of mental health and human rights

Defining histories of mental health and human rights, and their interrelationships have not yet been mapped. A general outline is given here. The specific issue of mental health legislation is noted in the next section.

Throughout history, those with mental disorders have suffered abuses in most if not all societies. Patel and colleagues (this volume) remind us particularly of the scope of these abuses today in developing countries, but rightly note that they occur in all countries.

The Western sources of liberalism, for example, the writings of Locke, Kant, and Mill, exclude those suffering from mental disorders from persons qualifying for rights, though they do not offer justifications for such exclusions. Each assumes rather than explicates sufferers' incapacity for reason, proposing that rationality is necessary for the exercise of all rights, instead of noting that this principle may be true for some rights but not others. Further, collectively, these philosophers do not make clear how those who fail the standards for becoming rights-holders should be treated. Liberalism in general prescribes different treatments for those with mental illnesses. Although it seeks to protect individuals deemed incapable of legitimately asserting rights from themselves, and likewise seeks to shield society from them, it excludes them from the putative civil compact, and thereby forecloses on their rights as against public authorities (Failer 2002).

In the 18th century, subtle social shifts supported the emergence of new social and political concepts of human rights (Higgins, this volume). Such changes may have shaped responses such as Pinel's unchaining of patients in a Paris asylum (noted by Patel and colleagues); and have connected with the emergence of asylums and to more humane 'moral treatments' for mental illness during the 19th century (Rakfeldt 2008). From the mid-19th century, however, a further shift towards a somatic approach promoted the view that 'mental disease is brain disease'. Public health and eugenics converged on mental health to justify the institutionalization of those with mental disorders, sometimes subjecting them to sterilization. In Germany, this notion of mental illness justified involuntary 'euthanasia', through intentional mass starvation of inmates in mental asylums in the First World War and then even more systematic extermination under Nazism. The latter practice foreshadowed the Holocaust (Berg and Cocks 1997; Friedlander 1995; Dudley and Gale 2002). Chapters by Susser and Bresnahan, and Dudley and Gale (this volume) discuss some of this history.

While not directly mentioning mental health, the international foundations of human rights, its conventions, treaties, and institutions, frequently signal its importance. Copeland and colleagues (this volume) discuss the development of the World Federation for Mental Health (WFMH) which championed the relationship of mental health and human rights from the early post-war years. The WHO definition of health has been noted. WHO accepted a mandate for mental health early, though it took another 50 years to introduce mental health into public health programmes in the agency (Sartorius 2002:128–139; Brody, this volume). The move for 'general' hospitals to establish psychiatric units over the last 40 years reflected the intention that psychiatry departments should have the same status as other specialties and avoid the stigmatization of ghettoized care (Wright 2010).

However, it may not have been till the late 1970s to the 1990s that the notion that mental health and human rights had a special relationship began to gain traction. A series of emerging historical factors gave increasing prominence to this relationship.

In this period, various inquiries targeted mental health care. Civil and political rights abuses, including torture and unlawful deprivation of liberty in psychiatric institutions, attracted attention (Perlin and Szeli, this volume; Backman and Mesquita, this volume; Hunt 2005). In 1977, the UN Commission for Human Rights formed a sub-commission charged with determining whether adequate grounds existed for detaining persons on the grounds of mental ill-health, and to formulate guidelines to prevent potentially injurious forms of detention and/or treatment. The UN Principles for the Protection of Persons with Mental Illness and for the Improvement of Mental Health Care (1991) eventually resulted from this inquiry (see also Perlin and Szeli, this volume). From 1979, the European Court of Human Rights (ECtHR) heard cases dealing with mental disability. This has resulted in a remarkable body of case law, which has obliged signatory countries to modify their laws to address civil rights issues such as admission to and discharge from psychiatric and related institutions, institutional standards and controls, medical treatment, life and death, legal capacity, guardianship, and supported decision-making (Bartlett et al. 2007; Perlin and Szeli, this volume).

Various treaties also canvass mental health issues. For example, the CRC addresses mental health via its concerns for children with disabilities having a full and decent life (Article 23), a standard of living adequate for the child's physical, mental, spiritual, moral, and social development (Article 27), periodic reviews of the treatment of children in institutions (Article 25), and their protection from labour that is hazardous, jeopardizes their education, or harms their health and development (Article 32). The CAT requires contracting states to prevent torture and related acts, thus prohibiting a potent source of mental disorder in the form of traumatic stress. In their chapter, Lund and colleagues note where the international human rights instruments address mental health. They remark on their relevance in addressing rights violations, to developing legislation and policy, and in monitoring progress towards appropriate, accessible, and affordable mental health service provision.

The ECtHR has also addressed the question of social participation by people with mental disabilities, and implicitly, the barriers that arise from stereotypes about them: that they cannot make rational choices, are dangerous and unpredictable, are uneducable, should not reproduce, cannot be adequate parents, cannot participate in political life, and need looking after rather than making their own decisions. According to Bartlett et al. (2007:177, 203), in a study of the ECtHR, the heart of the matter is whether or not people with mental disabilities are understood as full members of their societies. Are they to remain marginalized, merely ensuring they are not actively harmed, or do they have a legitimate place in an inclusive society? Decisions concerning the rights to community integration, education, property, marriage, parenthood and family life, voting, association, and work, confront traditional social structures as they pursue the possibility of lasting social change. However, legal judgments are only one path to achieving this.

The assertion and articulation of the rights of black people, women, and other civic groups foreshadowed disability rights, which entered legal, political, and global rights discourse only in 1990s. There has been some explicit overlap between mental health and disability reform. Disability activists, legislators, mental health professionals, and human rights leaders formulated the Declaration of Caracas (1990), which was adopted by the Pan American Health Organization and WHO, and which supported legislation that guards the rights of those with mental disorders, and services that safeguarded these rights while providing appropriate treatment. It opposed exclusive treatment in inpatient psychiatric units, while supporting the remoulding of psychiatric care towards community-based and -integrated mental health services. This reform promoted the policy of ensuring that patients are treated in their natural environments and communities (WHO 2005a:15). The Standard Rules on the Equalisation of Opportunities for Persons with Disabilities (1993) established citizen participation by people with disabilities as an internationally recognized human right (WHO 2005a:14). The user-survivor movement decisively shaped the ensuing Convention on the Rights of Persons with Disabilities (CRPD), which not only upholds a full complement of rights (including highest attainable health and well-being) for those with disabilities, but unlike previous treaties, institutes national and international frameworks of coordination and monitoring to enable its implementation. The CRPD, which is arguably the dawn of a new era in rights (Lewis and Bartlett 2011), is extensively discussed throughout the book. For more information visit <http://www.un.org/disabilities/default.asp?id=150>.

International health and psychiatric organizations have also established connections between mental health and human rights. Following from the development of ethical standards in health (such as the Declaration of Helsinki (1964 and subsequent versions)), the World Psychiatric Association (WPA) adopted the Declaration of Madrid (1996), whose standards of professional behaviour and practice depend on partnerships with people with mental disorders, enforcing involuntary treatment only under exceptional circumstances, and the social responsibility of psychiatrists and mental health professionals. Political misuses of psychiatry in the former Soviet Union were crucial to the development of the latter. Van Voren's chapter discusses this history. The codes of ethics of bodies such as the Royal Australian and New Zealand College of Psychiatrists reproduce these standards (Bloch and Pargiter 2009).

The advent of population mental health has also played its part. While the concerns of epidemiology and human rights both converge and contrast and may operate at different levels, there are considerable synergies (Venkatapuram et al. 2010). Susser and Bresnahan (this volume) also explore this relationship with particular reference to mental health. As noted previously, the World Development Report of the World Bank (1993) and the Global Burden of Disease report (Murray and Lopez 1996) among others, promoted awareness of the magnitude of mental health on a global scale, especially in LAMICs. Continuing research into the scope of mental health worldwide has confirmed and extended the relevant findings. As noted, journals such as *The Lancet* and the *Journal of the American Medical Association* have given a special focus to publishing series linking health and more recently mental health with human rights. Internationally, academic programmes on health and human rights include (among others) the Francois-Xavier Bagnoud Center of Health and Human Rights at the Harvard School of Public Health, the Mailman School of Public Health at Columbia University, the Netherlands Centre of Human Rights, and the Health and Human Rights Programme of the School of Public Health and Family Medicine at the University of Cape Town (Gruskin and Tarantola 2005). WHO has recently established an International Diploma on Mental Health Law and Human Rights with the ILS Law College in Pune, India; and also supports a Masters in Mental Health Policy and Services through the New University of Lisbon, and various courses through the Centre for Public Mental Health, a joint initiative of the Department of Psychiatry and Mental Health at the University of Cape Town and the Department of Psychology at Stellenbosch University in South Africa (WHO 2012).

Professional bodies such as WPA and WFMH—but also other international non-government organizations—have provided leadership to accomplish positive outcomes. The relevant international NGOs include those which have had general human rights agendas, such as the World Medical Association, Amnesty International, Human Rights Watch, Physicians for Human Rights, and those specific to mental health, such as Disability Rights International, Mental Disability Advocacy Centre, Mind Freedom International, and Global Initiative on Psychiatry, as well as national organizations. The achievements of these advocacy organizations throughout the world should not be underestimated. In some countries, including Australia, national and regional inquiries have galvanized momentum towards human rights reforms of mental health systems and practices.

The increasing range of disciplines and audiences now interested in these domains enhances the 'special connection' between mental health and human rights. A non-exhaustive list would include lawyers, mental health and helping professionals, mental health consumers, philosophers, human rights workers and their organizations, the UN and other international agencies, social scientists (not least political scientists, anthropologists, sociologists, and international relations experts), religious professionals and their associations, representatives of government, teachers, researchers, drafters of legislation, and practitioners. There are compelling reasons why helping professionals should be concerned about human rights, a topic is addressed in several chapters. This volume addresses all these groups.

Advancing the mission of mental health through legislation

Charges of irrelevance concerning the human rights movement, such as those mentioned above, cannot be laid against the need for international reform in mental health legislation, and action on human rights violations (Drew et al. 2011). As noted, legislation is currently conspicuous by its absence in nearly 25 per cent of countries worldwide; while in other countries, obsolete laws that aim primarily to safeguard the public mandate long periods of custodial care. The latter practice frequently violates the rights of those suffering mental illness. In some countries public authorities discriminate against those with mental disabilities, for example by excluding them from disability payments or restricting access to medical insurance (WHO 2005a; Saxena et al. 2007), or by failing to ensure adequate support, for example by not providing appropriate conditions to prevent relapse. Poor legislation may translate into abuse and neglect in practice, by mental health workers, lawyers, and judges. The WHO (2005a) report, examined below, discusses potential remedies.

The UN Principles for the Protection of Persons with Mental Illness and for the Improvement of Mental Health Care (1991) established minimum human rights standards in mental health. The Principles are not legally binding, and have not met with universal agreement: the World Network of Users and Survivors of Psychiatry have criticized some provisions (specifically Principles 11 and 16) that are perceived to weaken the criteria governing informed consent. Nevertheless, international oversight bodies have sometimes considered that the Principles are authoritative in interpreting the requirements of conventions such as the ICESCR (WHO 2005a:8). Thus they have provided a framework for mental health legislation in many countries.

To help interpret the Principles and evaluate institutional conditions, WHO developed Guidelines for the Promotion of Human Rights of Persons with Mental Disorders; Mental Health Care Law: Ten Basic Principles (WHO 1996); and the WHO's Resource Book on Mental Health, Human Rights and Legislation (2005a) as guides to countries developing mental health laws. These include the Principles enunciated in Tables 16.1 and 16.2 (pp316–317) (WHO 1996).

As the WHO's Resource Book on Mental Health, Human Rights and Legislation (2005a) makes clear, mental health legislation must protect, promote and improve the lives, well being and rights of citizens suffering from mental disorders, people who are thereby vulnerable to abuse and also stigma. Ideally, legislation shapes good policy by providing for fair, equal, and least restrictive treatment, protection from discrimination, affirmative obligations, and standards and accreditation. Progressive legislation and policy also reinforce each other throughout the intervention spectrum: access to mental health treatment and care, rehabilitation, aftercare, community integration, and mental health promotion in the wider society, as well as developing and maintaining community-based services and integrating these with primary care.

Legislation should also support those with mental disorders in their interaction with the health and housing systems, and employment (including fair remuneration, protection from exploitation, and 'reasonable accommodation' with flexible hours to enable attendance at mental health treatment). Legislation may improve financial resources for access to mental health care by stipulating the need for equality with funding for physical health, redirecting funding, allocating additional funding, or funding statutory bodies. It is also possible to legislate to introduce mental health interventions into primary care, and to enforce non-discriminatory approaches to insurance (WHO 2005a: 27–28).

Elaboration of a number of specific areas for reform and provision falls outside the ambit of this volume, but are discussed in the Resource Book (WHO 2005a). These areas include international best approaches to legislation concerning rights of service users, including confidentiality, access to information, and rights and conditions in mental health facilities; the rights of families and carers; questions of capacity, competence, and guardianship; voluntary and involuntary admission and treatment (including proxy consent), community-based involuntary care, and emergencies; staff skills and qualifications for determining mental disorder; special treatments such as ECT, psychosurgery, and major medical and surgical procedures; seclusion and restraint; research; review processes and bodies; police responsibilities; and mentally ill offenders. However, we return to the generic question of coercion below.

Numerous examples exist of how legal standards have been applied to the delivery of health programmes and interventions for HIV (Gruskin et al. 2007). Similarly, Perlin and Szeli, and Crepeau and Gayet (this volume) do likewise for the application of legal standards to mental health in various jurisdictions.

Crucially, complementary models for legislation and policy require the backing of political will, adequate resources, functioning institutions, community support services, and well-trained personnel (WHO 2005a:1–3). For example, India passed mental health legislation in the 1980s and early 1990s which was not implemented because of a failure to estimate the cost and provide the necessary budgetary support. The situation has somewhat changed with an inquiry into the conduct of mental hospitals after a devastating fire in 2001, along with increased funding and a reinvigorated comprehensive strategy reaching down to the district level. However, recent commentary indicates the massive gaps in treatment and accompanying violations in human rights laws within mental health services, requiring a range of remedies (Ghanashyam and Nagarathinam 2010; Saraceno et al. 2007). Similarly, the policy decision to integrate mental health into primary care in Nigeria failed because of the absence of a clear structured link between primary care and mental health professionals, and the poor funding of mental health, with most monies still being directed at mental hospitals (Saraceno et al. 2007). Drew et al. (2011) and Crepeau and Gayet (this volume) provide examples of successful legal action in relation to rights in mental health. Taking four African countries as examples, Stein and colleagues (this volume) describe innovative theoretical or moral interpretive frameworks that might better guide legislation, policy, and practice in these key areas.

Redressing global inequity for mental health: markets and cultural caveats

As health care workers and those living with mental disorders can attest, the Western mindset did not invent the problem of mental disorder in LAMICs (Patel and Prince 2010). Moreover, while sufferers often experience inequitable care compared to people with physical illnesses, the burden of mental health problems is also inequitably borne by those living in LAMICs, who suffer dire socio-economic circumstances that are made worse by their mental disorders.

What principles should guide those who address the quantitative disparities between regions and countries?

One corollary of following the liberal principle, enunciated by John Rawls (1971), of maximizing the well-being of the least well-off, is to disseminate skills and resources, including technology. In the era of globalization and electronic access to information, the reach of psychiatry and mental health is likely to grow, with governments and societies turning to these disciplines to help grapple with large-scale determinants of mental health and adverse psychosocial consequences of events such as war and disasters. As indicated above, Patel et al. (2007) found numerous efficacious interventions usually originating in the West which were trialled successfully in developing-world settings, but which are seldom deployed in the latter. According to the principles of distributive justice, they should be made generally available. While desirable, achievement of this aim is not straightforward, as two examples will illustrate.

Firstly, as noted above, global capitalism and market mechanisms ignore questions of equity. The behaviour of pharmaceutical companies and the maldistribution of psychotropic drugs in the developing world exemplify this lacuna. Psychotropic drugs may be misused, or given without appropriate psychosocial interventions, but nevertheless they are fundamental to treating many mental disorders and potentially enable everyone, including the most disadvantaged, to share the benefits of scientific progress. Basic first generation antipsychotics and generic antidepressants are essential, whereas newer atypical antipsychotics and antidepressants may have less side-effects, but are only marginally more effective and are certainly more expensive (Saxena et al. 2007; Lancet Global Mental Health Group 2007). However, even the essential drugs are often not available and/or families bear the out-of-pocket expense for these treatments (Patel et al. 2007). Appropriate access would depend on several considerations including the rational selection of medicines, affordability, sustainable financing, and available, reliable health and supply systems, as well as effective mental health policies and legislation. Maintenance and improvement of access to care also require ongoing assessment and monitoring (WHO 2005b).

However, intellectual property rights law and TRIPS (see p20) frequently collide with human rights law and the right to health (Cullet 2005). Because TRIPS provides for a minimum 20 years for patent protection, it precludes populations accessing low-cost generic medicines, even if TRIPS legal safeguards allow some public health exceptions. Governments therefore can and should legislate to allow parallel imports for medicines of public health significance and compulsory licensing of their use. Philip Mitchell (this volume) specifically examines the challenge to the reputation of psychiatry arising from its aberrant relationship with pharmaceutical companies (WHO 2005b).

The second example concerns philosophical and socio-cultural caveats in transferring dominant paradigms of psychiatric knowledge to developing countries. The field of transcultural psychiatry reveals enormous cultural differences in conceptualizing mental disorder and in approaches to healing across diverse settings in the developing world. Western psychiatry however has increasingly focused on neurobiology, the definition of diagnostic criteria, the development of structured diagnostic instruments, and the matching of these procedures to psychopharmacology and packaged psychological treatments. Can such a scientific, evidence-based approach complement rights-based and social science-based frameworks, recognizing that science per se does not address issues of equity or cultural appropriateness?

Western agencies have been accused of exporting interventions to post-conflict societies with different cultural and epistemic traditions, purportedly imposing disorders (such as 'post-traumatic stress disorder' (PTSD) and models of trauma debriefing that may ignore local meanings and priorities, the risk being of uncritically framing participants as victims, and potentially trivializing wider political and socio-cultural questions. As yet, such theoretical criticisms have not been supported by strong evidence; for example, PTSD has been identified across a multiplicity of societies (Silove 2000; Silove et al. 2007; Steel et al. 2009) and ample evidence exists that it is a cause of disability worldwide. Nevertheless, there is growing evidence that a failure to recognize culturally-specific modalities for expressing distress can lead to an under-enumeration of mental disorders in transcultural settings. The risk is that assumptions will be made about a lower level of need in precisely those countries with the least access to mental health resources, a double jeopardy for those in need (Steel et al. 2009). It is vital therefore to acknowledge fully the relevance of culture in shaping mental illness, its understanding, expression, and impact and in setting the context for meaningful interventions is a topic that requires much more extensive attention. There are risks of imposing Western methods of treatment without careful consideration of culture and context, failing to empower populations at the grass roots level, and destroying traditional approaches to dealing with these problems. To ignore these key issues, or to pay only lip service to them, could lead to inadvertent transgressions of human rights in the pursuit of a monolithic global mental health agenda. By contrast, matching external approaches with indigenous cultures in order to achieve some form of hybrid model is a challenge that requires deep respect and understanding for the local culture and history of the recipient population.

Thus in complex emergencies and disasters, psychosocial recovery must embrace an expanded perspective that is rooted in the history, culture, and social structures of the society. A general emergency relief plan that enables communities to re-create a cohesive and secure society will understand acute traumatic stress as a normative response to the threat of death, which tends to subside once conditions of safety are established. The ADAPT Model (see p14) acknowledges identifies the key threats posed to such societies in relation to security, interpersonal bonds, systems of justice, roles, and identities, and institutions that promote meaning and coherence (Silove and Steel 2006). The repair of these systems requires a convergence in planning and implementation that draws centrally on the principles of human rights, development, and culture. Within that broad recovery context, clinical mental health services can focus on the residual minority whose wider mental health needs are inhibiting sufferers from participating in the recovery and development process; even then, this specific activity needs to be culturally and contextually congruent with the social conditions in which it operates, maintaining an eye on the future in shaping mental health policy.

In this volume, Steel and colleagues highlight these debates about how well Western-based trauma models account for and address cultural and indigenous mental health issues and rights, and how these explanatory approaches may work together in research and practice. Similarly, Rees and Silove contemplate how balancing the context-specific, lived experience of diverse communities against the 'objective' findings of science, research, and an evidence-based approach, can help tackle inequity. Mark Tomlinson and colleagues report searching human rights-based reflections on a research collaboration that was designed to investigate a mother-infant intervention in South Africa.

Refreshingly, locally effective interventions in LAMICs may also achieve cross-cultural translation in reverse, before becoming generalizable. An example is Eastern forms of meditation, which have underpinned Western mindfulness therapies. The latter, now developed and evaluated, may be re-packaged and deployed globally.

Cognitive-behavioural therapy (CBT) has also been re-packaged to deliver culturally appropriate interventions to those with medically unexplained symptoms, a common presentation of depression and anxiety especially in some LAMICs (Patel et al. 2007; Sumathipala et al. 2000), though how successfully it is translated in LAMICs will substantially depend on resources and settings (Naeem et al. 2010). Various studies successfully have integrated spiritual content into CBT for depressed patients of different religious persuasions (e.g. Propst et al. 1992; Azhar et al. 1994; d'Sousa and Rodrigo 2004). Interestingly, the efficacy of group psychological interventions in LAMICs may be related to the influence of traditional social supports and collective action.

As noted, evidence must be strengthened if clinical trials in prevention and early intervention are to meet the needs of regional and national populations in a culturally sensitive manner. In Chile, a 'stepped care' intervention for treating depressed women in primary care has launched a national programme (Patel et al. 2007). Kirmayer's essay in this volume highlights the importance of having a robust framework of cultural understanding when approaching all these issues.

Abuse and neglect: coercion and abandonment as twin dilemmas

As suggested by the eyewitness accounts mentioned at the beginning of this introduction, practices of coercion combined with social exclusion and ostracism are commonplace globally in managing mental illnesses and disorders. However, as Kallert, Oaks, Smith, Rosen, and colleagues, as well as others discuss in this volume, duress associated with treatment—even when it is not overtly accompanied by social exclusion and ostracism—remains controversial. Despite many countries tightening standards and procedures for involuntary treatment (Szmukler and Applebaum 2011), in some Western countries, mental health policy imperatives have moved towards increasing pressures to treat within a climate of fear about risk to public safety posed by service users. In various jurisdictions, including the UK, controversial new mental health legislation extends the compulsion powers of services operating outside of hospital-based care (Department of Health (UK) 2007; Lewis 2009). While some want to get out of the mental health system, others want or need access to it: they need treatment to restore their autonomy, because it has already been breached by mental illness (Large et al. 2008b). Moreover, pressure in treatment is not homogeneous. Assertive community treatment (ACT) for example includes assertive engagement, interpersonal leverage, inducements, and a 'no-drop out' policy, yet is not particularly associated with actual or perceived coercion (Szmukler and Applebaum 2011; Killaspy and Rosen 2011). These issues which are of enduring interest (Kallert et al. 2011), are briefly discussed here.

The recently promulgated Convention on the Rights of Persons with Disabilities (CRPD) represents a seismic shift in the treatment of people with disabilities. In signalling the shift from welfare to rights and acknowledging the centrality of disability in human experience, the CRPD challenges coercion. This is notwithstanding the WHO Mental Health Legislation book (WHO 2005a) which has addressed international codes and essential operational and regulatory requirements surrounding involuntary treatment; and WHO and network members offering technical advice and assistance to several countries.

Treatment pressure occurs in relation to admission and discharge, seclusion and restraint, inpatient and outpatient treatment (the latter including community treatment orders (CTOs)), and chemical and other somatic treatments, such as psychosurgery and electroconvulsive therapy (ECT). Despite being ubiquitous (with rare notable exceptions), systematic international information is lacking on trends and practices relating to coercion and other forms of treatment pressure. For example, it is mandated that ECT requires informed consent (WHO 2005), but the frequency of adherence to this injunction is unknown. WHO has proposed a ban on direct (unmodified) ECT (i.e. ECT without anaesthetic) but the practice is still used in a number of countries (see, for instance, James et al. 2009). How often involuntary ECT is used as an emergency medical procedure or for other reasons is also unclear. Potentially chronic iatrogenic effects from anti-psychotic and other psychotropic drugs (e.g. Moncrieff and Leo 2010; Correll et al. 2009) are of significant concern, especially for people with severe, persistent mental illness treated involuntarily. These long-term adverse outcomes of treatments that compound disability and that may be given involuntarily should occasion extra caution and consultation. Various responses to duress in practice demonstrate how tension can arise between different rights and how international standards can differ in spite of apparent universal agreement on principles.

Mental health laws that allow for involuntary admission and/or treatment (typically to administer psychotropic drugs against someone's will) are traditionally justified on several grounds. These include risk to life (of self or others) putatively due to mental illness or disorders, the potential for profound impact on physical and mental health, including personal reputation, the duty of society to those who cannot care for themselves and their right to this care, the likelihood that treatment may avert these outcomes, and no less restrictive alternative being available.

Risk to life in particular is a vexed issue. Although clinicians must constantly make judgements about risk to life, predicting suicide or homicide is impossible (Large et al. 2008b). Though mental disorders as a whole somewhat increase the risk for violence, the vast majority of people suffering from mental disorders are not violent or dangerous, and a great proportion of violence is not so much associated with mental disorder as it is with specific factors such as substance misuse, paranoid symptoms, and non-adherence to treatment (Swanson et al. 1994). Given that incidents of serious violence are rare, and predicting rare events is inherently inaccurate, constraining large numbers of people deemed at risk is both impractical and unethical. Similar observations are true for suicide, except that the association between mental disorders and self-directed violence is much stronger (Goldney 2008).

It is a moot point whether involuntary admission and treatment per se save lives. Analysing international legislation, Large et al. (2008a) reported that where legislation decrees that danger (i.e. threat to the patient's life or that of others) rather than assessed need is the criterion for involuntary treatment, duration of untreated psychosis (DUP) is significantly prolonged. Citing studies connecting DUP to worsening prognosis including suicide and homicide, these authors argue that ethically, dangerousness criteria unfairly discriminate against people with mental disorders. They represent an unreasonable barrier to treatment without consent, and they spread the burden of risk that any mentally ill person might become violent across large numbers of mentally ill people who will never become violent. They conclude by supporting removing such criteria for involuntary admission and treatment.

Conversely, organizations representing users and survivors of psychiatry (e.g. World Network of Users and Survivors of Psychiatry, Mind Freedom International), oppose coercion (Declaration of Dresden 2007). Citing scientific and first-person accounts of the traumatic, disabling, or personality-altering effects of psychotropic medications and ECT, their sometime use for non-therapeutic purposes, and related psychiatric abuses, they contend that coercion breaches the CAT and the CRPD, and they regard all legislation authorizing imposed psychiatric interventions as illegitimate (Minkowitz 2007). This countermands previous landmark decisions: for example, the European Court of Human Rights rejected claims that nonconsensual psychiatric interventions amount to torture, inhuman or degrading treatment, or punishment, in so doing articulating a standard of therapeutic necessity that permits force to be used 'to preserve the physical and mental health of patients who are entirely incapable of deciding for themselves and for whom [the medical authorities] are therefore responsible' (*Herczegfalvy v Austria*, App. No. 10533/83, 15 Eur. H.R. Rep. 437,1 82 (1992), quoted in Minkowitz 2007). McSherry (2008) alternatively suggests that Article 17 of CRPD, which enshrines the right to respect for physical and mental integrity on an equal basis with others, is more correctly viewed as a limitation on practices of restraint and seclusion, and as providing protection from both unbeneficial treatment and overly intrusive treatment. Both writers, however, invite a re-evaluation of the 'taken for granted' practices in mental health care that may infringe Article 17, including non-therapeutic practices imposed for administrative purposes, convenience, or punishment (Weller 2009).

In this vein, some service users and survivors have asserted 'experiential rights', deriving from the 'madness-experience'. For them, institutional systemic trauma is superimposed on interpersonal trauma. Cresswell (2009) argues that this is a ('third generation') solidarity right which revalorizes a formerly devalued experience. What may be needed is an alternative non-medical perspective on this 'madness-experience'—based upon solidarities forged between 'critical practitioners' and psychiatric survivors (Spandler and Calton 2009). Controversy also surrounds the question of how to acknowledge and respond to impaired capacity among those with mental disorders, especially when incapacity is profound or complete. The premise in some mental health legislation that patients cannot make key decisions (e.g. regarding treatment, finances), comes up against the CRPD's Article 12, on the legal capacity of those with psychosocial disabilities and their need for support in exercising it. The CRPD's Article 25—on the right to health, defined by accessible, appropriate services, non-discrimination, and free informed consent—informs this whole discussion. In her chapter, Dhanda traces the struggle between the proponents of supported and of substituted decision-making for people with disabilities.

The value of CTOs is undecided. While some evidence supports the view that CTOs may avert hospitalization (Segal and Burgess 2009), and are effective where there is intensive support and longer durations (e.g. more than six months), randomized control trials have not demonstrated consistent benefits. Objections arise regarding the inadequacy of services supporting such measures, effects on the therapeutic relationship, potential workable alternatives such as proxy consent and advance directives, treatment refusal for medication side-effects, and other valid reasons. Overall, CTOs remain controversial (Swartz and Swanson 2004; Chaimowitz, 2004; O'Reilly, 2004).

Other psychiatric and legal scholars note that people with mental disorders vary in their legal capacity. While mental illnesses are often associated with denial of disorder and of the need for care (Szmukler and Applebaum, 2011), these scholars oppose the discriminatory assumption that mental disorders *ipso facto* incapacitate sufferers in making key decisions. They detect unjustified legal discrimination against mentally disordered persons compared with persons with physical disorders, and recommend amalgamating capacity and mental health laws to bring psychiatric practice into line with other health interventions. Thus they designate the patient's decision-making (in)capacity as the central criterion for involuntary treatment in all medical contexts (Dawson and Szmukler 2006). This approach allows autonomy to trump paternalism and the claim of public protection. The considerable literature on mental capacity (e.g. Candia and Barba 2011) is not reviewed here. The Declaration of Madrid (WPA 2005) states that where involuntary treatment is unavoidable, the psychiatrist should consult the patient's family and lawyers to ensure protection of the patient's rights. Although coercion may interfere with therapeutic engagement, and therefore with treatment, objective and subjective 'coercion' may not coincide. Perceptions of fairness in treatment and motives of decision-makers may weigh more heavily than actual legal status (Szmukler and Applebaum 2011). It is sometimes claimed that attitudes to treatment improve as treatment leads to clinical improvement and insight (Surguladze and David 1999; Kane et al. 1983).

The CRPD's implications for mental health require active exploration, and the dearth of relevant current evidence is of concern. The CRPD clearly favours autonomy, but other standards note that when mental illness undermines mental capacity and autonomy, beneficial interventions must aim to promote and where possible restore these capabilities. Thus autonomy, beneficence, and non-maleficence all undergird service users' rights, and beneficence in particular requires support for autonomy rather than opposing it. Treatment pressures may be reduced by making services as acceptable and attractive as possible and enhance patients' involvement in planning their own care (Szmukler and Applebaum 2011).

One undesired outcome of coercion or its failure is abandonment. Unfortunately, deinstitutionalization and 'community care' are empty alternatives to coercion if there is not governmental, institutional, and community support for the full participation of those living in society. Surveying this area, Arboleda-Flórez (2008) contends that the challenges facing those with mental disabilities in many countries are not individual abuses of freedom and autonomy, but structural and systematic neglect of sufferers as an unprotected social underclass. He notes how those suffering mental disorders are no longer in asylums but in prisons, which have become veritable mental hospitals, ones that in turn reinforce prejudice against those with mental disorder. He cites the factors contributing to this 'underclass' attribution: the effects of stigma against those with severe and persistent mental disorders; the often chronic, incapacitating nature of their illnesses, which can result in their virtual social annihilation; but also anti-rights policies and practices. In a parody of liberty, deinstitutionalized sufferers drift without protection or connection to the fringes of society, homeless and destitute. This trend represents systemic, structural violence. Their powerlessness is a consequence of poverty, political disenfranchisement, extreme disability, and championlessness (Arboleda-Flórez, 2008).

State-directed abuses

Abuses of psychiatry, especially by sovereign states, continue to afflict mental health professionals and service users in many countries. Historical examples (see the chapters by Dudley and Gale, and van Voren) can inform thinking about contemporary conundrums. These contributors along with Marks, and Mares and Jureidini explore formulations that strike a balance between systemic determinants of abuse and individual/professional responsibility and culpability, especially where practitioners are caught up in the abuse of psychiatry in settings such as prisons, detention centres, and the military. In Australia, harsh policies of deterrence and indefinite mandatory detention towards asylum-seekers wilfully expose adults and children to abuse and neglect and materially contribute to negative developmental and mental health outcomes. These policies continue at the time of writing, with Australia attempting to expel unauthorized boat arrivals, including children, to Malaysia—a nation that has not signed the Convention Relating to the Status of Refugees—in the face of the UNHCR's criticism. Mares and Jureidini, and Steel and colleagues, examine the human rights implications of Australia's policy, with the former authors conducting an analysis of the consequentialist arguments advanced in this case. Also in Australia, the well-being of indigenous communities is jeopardized by the continuation of the Federal Government's paternalistic, non-consultative 'Intervention' policy in the Northern Territory, which suspended the Racial Discrimination Act and compulsorily acquired Aboriginal lands (Hunter and colleagues, this volume). The UN Human Rights Commissioner (2011) has criticized this intervention.

A vital question that requires a fresh assessment is how psychiatry as a profession and other mental health professions can defend and promote human rights where institutional or political factors threaten the capacity of the profession to maintain its integrity. Whereas previously, writers mostly focused on abuses occurring under autocratic regimes (Nazi Germany, the Soviet Union, and the Japanese empire up to the end of the Second World War), new circumstances have embroiled Western countries that traditionally champion human rights, as the Australian case exemplifies.

Mental health professionals from Western countries have been accused of complicity in the abuse of political prisoners. Silove and colleagues ponder how the absolute prohibition against torture incorporated in several international and regional human rights instruments is being undermined, and critically re-analyse whether and why leading politicians and some philosophers have shifted ground on this key issue. Marks, and Dudley and Gale contemplate what can be done where professionals wear two or more hats (for example, as clinicians and as advisors to governments), or where they have dual loyalties such as when working in the military in the so-called 'war on terror'. How can human rights and mental health mount an inter-disciplinary coalition with the capacity to withstand and respond to these new geopolitical forces? The group Global Lawyers and Physicians exemplifies one such response to this challenge. GLP was formed on the fiftieth anniversary of the Nuremberg trials to reinvigorate the collaboration of the legal and medical/public health professions to protect the human rights and dignity of all persons. GLP has taken up such disparate causes as campaigning against the continuing force-feeding of Guantanamo hunger-striking prisoners, documenting rape of women as a war strategy in Darfur and Chad, and treating traumatized Tibetan monks with strategies other than meditation (which may for some worsen ruminations over bad memories and guilt). Can further inter-disciplinary partnerships be galvanized to safeguard and promote a rights-based approach?

Vulnerable groups

The present monograph cannot cover in depth all vulnerable groups. In particular, we elected not to cover diagnostic groups per se; as with the potential proliferation of potential candidate diagnoses, this would have been impossible. The groups chosen, however, include local and particular groups, such as indigenous people and refugees; we also include cultures that may constitute 'ways of life', such as sexual minorities and those with problems with addiction. Many groups are discriminated against, persecuted, or victimized because of their gender, social, or cultural backgrounds, or their political, religious, or other beliefs, with consequences for their mental health.

This volume considers a range of such vulnerable groups, including people with serious and persistent mental illness (Rosen and colleagues, Smith, Oaks, Walker and colleagues), those who are tortured (Silove and colleagues) or under sentence of death (Welsh), detainees in the 'war on terror' (Marks), those with mental disorders who are coerced (Kallert, Smith, Oaks), people with mental disorders in developing countries (Patel and colleagues), prisoners and those in custody with mental disorders (Sullivan and Mullen), refugees and asylum seekers (Mares and Jureidini; Steel and colleagues), women (Raphael and colleagues; Yüksel and colleagues), victims of trafficking (Maltzahn and Villadiego), particular racial and ethnic groups (Bhugra and McGeorge), indigenous people (Hunter and colleagues), people with intellectual disabilities (Hall and Yacoub), children and adolescents with disabilities (Belfer and Samarasan), disabled, marginalized, and mentally ill older people (Peisah, Brodaty, and O'Neil), people with diverse sexual identities and orientations (Newman), individuals treated for drug addiction (Carter and Hall), and those who die or are affected by suicide (Vijayakumar and Harris). Contributors reflect on what differences occur in the impact and manifestations of distress experienced by these groups, and what principles and practices guide mental health professions in undertaking prevention, service development, and advocacy.

Future directions

A consensus implicit in this volume is that 'there is no health without mental health.' Perhaps the most crucial element therefore for the progression of human rights in mental health is naming mental health as a key international social issue: combating stigma, bringing the invisible to light. Mental health awareness should transfigure all health and social policy, planning, and delivery (Prince et al. 2007). Global human rights violations experienced by those with psychosocial disabilities should spearhead this call to action (Drew et al. 2011; Patel and colleagues, this volume).

Indeed, massive upscaling of global health initiatives will miss its mark if mental health continues to be neglected (Patel and Prince 2010). Exemplifying this, Susser and Bresnahan note in this volume how training public health professionals to recognize that 'there is no health without mental health' can enable them to raise the profile of mental health within public health. This means not merely reducing inequalities in health and wealth across the general population, but being committed to excluded social groups such as those with severe mental disorders, and raising issues such as the status of mental health in LAMICs. Public health and mental health may exchange skills through establishing training opportunities and public mental health courses.

The lived experience of those with mental disorders and their contact with mental health services should sculpt this transformation of health and social policy. The CRPD champions this approach, having brought those with lived experience together with other stakeholders to produce a document that emphasizes autonomy and control: 'nothing about us without us'. It demands a major shift in vision and praxis: from welfare to rights, towards autonomy with support and equality, thus granting both the same and different to persons with disabilities; and most importantly, acknowledging disability as a part of the human experience (Dhanda and Narayan 2007; Dhanda 2008). Key steps to recognizing and supporting the role of those with lived experience entail moving from paternalistic and controlling service responses to emancipatory ones, from misrecognizing service users' experience and denying their full humanity to respecting that experience, and appreciating how social inequalities frame discrimination and exclusion that affect service experiences (Lewis 2009). Addressing stigma necessitates legislation, public education, contact and partnerships, coalitions and protest, and clear unambiguous political leadership. The same set of principles need to be extended to whole societies, particularly in the move to a Global Mental Health strategy. It is not sufficient to transplant knowledge, systems and interventions from dominant societies to LAMICs. The process requires a careful and equitable approach to engagement, the formation of partnerships and the empowering of local structures to ensure that mental health developments are firmly rooted in the traditions, way of life, and world views of the indigenous populations.

There are cogent reasons to add this set of principles to the otherwise valuable five primary indicators of progress promulgated by the Lancet Global Mental Health Group (2007): national and regional health plans which sufficiently attend to mental health; increased funding (with monies earmarked, even quarantined, for this purpose (Jacob et al. 2007)); increased numbers of trained mental health care staff; available basic pharmacological treatments; and increasing the treatment coverage of people with schizophrenia. Its secondary indicators included: balancing expenditure in hospital and community services; providing adequate basic medical and nursing training in mental health; distributing staff equitably between urban and rural areas; ensuring least restrictive practice; protecting the human rights of people with mental disorder; and lowering the suicide rate. Collectively, these dynamically address planning, investment, workforce, human rights and outcomes. Research priorities also have been caucused and refined. However, it is of note that rights of people with mental illness are listed as a secondary outcome. Adding all the major rights groupings together (civil–political, economic and socio-cultural, spiritual and collective) would encompass all the goals and actions just listed, and make human rights the overarching outcome for these two lists (Lancet Global Mental Health Group 2007).

Discussing health and human rights, Gruskin et al. (2007) suggest creating a health and human rights research agenda, building evidence of the effects of applying health and human rights frameworks to health practice, and the development of monitoring standards. The latter, not further examined here, is illuminated in recent discussions concerning the Human Development Index (United Nations Development Programme 2011; see also Mokhiber 2005; Raworth 2005). Mental health and human rights requires a similar agenda at various levels. Cooper et al's (2010) examination of Uganda's mental health system offers one recent example of standards application. As observed by Jonathan Marks in his chapter, and also by Gale and Dudley, human rights need to pervade social and institutional frameworks, policy guidelines, health systems and workforce, education and mentorship, and structural reforms. These recommendations apply to both state and non-state actors: the latter is particularly significant in an era of government deregulation.

Since the psychosocial determinants of health often fall outside the health sector and health care, a multiplicity of sectors need to be involved in a 'whole of community, whole of government' approach to effective primary health and mental health care. Just as psychosocial factors contribute to so many health problems, so psychosocial assessments ought to be integral to all (mental) health care.

At the other end of the spectrum, only briefly addressed by this volume but of enormous potential relevance, are developments in biological knowledge in mental health that have direct and sometimes alarming human rights implications. McFarlane and Bryant, and also (in part) Gale and Dudley, ponder this cross-cutting issue, where so much more work is required.

A primary health care philosophy, as exemplified by the Alma Ata Declaration and the Ottawa Charter of Health Promotion, is best suited for whole populations and for remedying disadvantage, rather than one based on market forces and the economic benefits of health (Hall and Taylor 2003; Gillam 2008). Alma Ata proclaimed that 'governments have a responsibility for the health of their people which can be fulfilled only by the provision of adequate health and social measures . . . made universally accessible to individuals and families in the community' (1978 Alma Ata WHO/UNICEF declaration). Alma Ata emphasized scientific soundness regarding treatment and prevention, social acceptability (despite the complex moving nature of this target), universal accessibility, population involvement, and affordability (Sartorius 2002), and also helped to entrench the importance of essential health care as a human right.

Yet if mental health services are to be sustained in primary care, they crucially depend also on the prior or simultaneous development of community mental health services, allowing for training, supervision, and continuous support for primary care workers, and the reallocation of tasks. For some health challenges, such as HIV/AIDS, chronic diseases, and maternal and child health, pragmatism and efficiency suggest the value of integrating mental health care into existing primary care programmes. Such settings may not suit all needs. For example, severe, disabling, and persistent conditions such as intellectual disabilities, schizophrenia, and dementia urgently require decentralization, deinstitutionalization, and the provision of acute and continuing mental health services closer to communities where those affected live (Saraceno et al. 2007; Patel and Prince 2010). Basic psychotropic drugs and psychotherapeutic interventions need to be available at all levels (Saraceno et al. 2007; Patel and Prince 2010).

For many countries, improving equity depends on moving from reliance on mental hospitals to a population health model. 'The solution is not to virtually imprison affected people in costly and largely ineffective psychiatric hospitals, where human rights abuses are often rampant. Evidence tells us that service delivery in a primary care setting is far more cost-effective, equitable, efficient, and humane' (Chan 2008). Many factors may impede this transfer, and need to be overcome. However, there are remarkable examples where the move out of mental hospitals to community (including primary) care has been achieved, such as in Brazil. The two tasks (scaling-down and scaling up) intertwine, and may require extra funding in the transitional phase (Saxena et al. 2007; Sartorius 2002; Jacob et al. 2007; Saraceno et al. 2007).

As we have seen, state and other jurisdictions need to enact legislation consistent with international human rights standards, establishing mechanisms for its implementation (such as review boards), and linking them to service provision and resource allocation (see Lund et al's chapter). The need to combine effective legislation and policy-making has already been noted (WHO 2005a:27–28).

LAMICs may be unwilling to seize control of their own budgets, rather than relying on external programme funding from donor countries. Yet providing a core mental health care package has been costed at $US2 per person per year in low-income countries and $US3–4 in lower- and middle-income countries—a modest impost when compared with scaling up services for other major contributors to the global health burden (Lancet Global Mental Health Group 2007).

Professional bodies such as the WPA and the WFMH, human rights organizations, WHO and other other international and UN agencies, governments, and local professional groupings each make a key contribution to the mental health and human rights agenda. Working in concert, they are relevant to early detection and intervention, policy formulation, advocacy, education, and most importantly, direct practice in relation to assisting persons at risk or those who have suffered human rights violations. One challenge for health and rights practitioners is how to avoid the charge that one can study rights abuses independently. Everyone is implicated in unjust social structures, but one's actions either help the sufferers or the system (Farmer and Gastineau 2005; Rees and Silove, this volume). The bodies and organizations mentioned are central to reflecting on, developing, and promoting a rights-based practice in mental health provision and intervention. Special aspects of practice concern survivor groups and individuals: how to engage such groups, how to ensure that the services provided promote dignity and protect them from further abuses, and the extent to which standard psychiatric practices support or potentially obstruct these endeavours. Empirical research and intervention in this area is just beginning (Drew et al. 2011; Rees and Silove, this volume). Critical psychiatry and mental health practice may have much to offer in this latter respect (Gale and Dudley, this volume; and see further below).

In sum, mental health firstly and finally needs to be placed on international agendas. Too long it has been absent from those agendas, in a way that human rights and also physical health have not. It is time to recognize that the quest to overcome stigma attached to psychosocial disabilities is an international one. At the time of writing, the WFMH and the Movement for Global Mental Health are campaigning to have mental health, mental illness and neuropsychiatric disorders put on the agenda of the United Nations Special Session on Non-communicable Diseases (September 2011). To make policy, legislative and structural changes that add up to substantive mental health reform, political will is a crucial element. Achieving it requires clear, unified, coordinated advocacy targeting decision-makers: politicians, donors, and government and non-government agencies. Such leadership and advocacy may be improved using participatory action methods common in community development (Saraceno et al. 2007; Lancet Global Mental Health Group 2007).

Mental health encompasses all dimensions of the human experience. The complex web of mental health problems that impede the exercise of rights, and the rights that oblige recognition from professionals and services, require affirmation rather than being seen as impediments. Creating and maintaining the link between mental health and human rights is a task that requires the vision, praxis and courage referred to in this collection's sub-title. For professionals and for those with lived experience of such disabilities, being engaged in this quest goes to the heart of their citizenship and humanity.

Limitations

This volume is necessarily incomplete. The knowledge of the editors (two of whom are psychiatrists, one a political scientist and social worker, all three Australian) of all the relevant domains and geographical trends is, despite our best efforts, partial. There are authorities on the issues addressed whose points of view are not represented. Had the editors been, for example, lawyers coming from the vantage point of human rights, different judgments may have come to light.

Some areas have not been included. The landscape has changed rapidly in the course of assembling the book: for example, as mentioned the human rights and mental health challenges posed by climate change, and the new technologies. We have already noted the importance of biological developments in relation to mental health and their human rights implications. Critical psychiatry and anti-psychiatry has evolved as an area in its own right, with a continuous flow of informative articles and books in recent years (see <http://www.mentalhealth.freeuk. com/article.htm>), and its treatment in relation to human rights will have to wait for another volume. We left untouched the domain of specific treatments, such as the human rights and state-related implications of electroconvulsive therapy and deep brain stimulation (Loo et al. 2010); we have decided, at least at this point, that these domains have been well considered elsewhere, for example in books on psychiatric ethics (Bloch and Green, 2009). We have focused little on positive mental health or protective factors in general or specifically, for example, including little on the topic of religion or spirituality and their link to mental health disorder and human rights. Continuing work will also need to focus on specific vulnerable groups, such as the rights of foetuses and infants, or those with physical impairments who may also have coincident psychosocial disabilities, such as those with chronic illnesses or specific sensory impairments. The issue of disseminating psychotropic drugs internationally also requires further work. A future instalment or sequel to this volume will also need to consider resources required for intensifying human rights activities in mental health at all levels. Attentive readers will doubtless find other gaps.

In such a vast terrain, there is still much linkage work to be done. It should be taken as a point of departure to stimulate discussion and further research, rather than a definitive work.

Acknowledgements

All chapters have been peer-reviewed. As well as thanking the contributors for their patience with the process, and their uncomplaining willingness to contribute to the internal review process (often on multiple occasions), we wish to thank the following (often indefatigable) reviewers:

Peter van Arsdale, Eileen Baldry, Peter Bartlett, José Manoel Bertolote, Sid Bloch, Vaughan Carr, Edmond Chiu, Erminia Colucci, Adele Cox, Jackie Curtis, Richard Day, Pat Deegan, Kate Diesfeld, Eric Emerson, Karen Engle, Michael Fairley, Anne Gallagher, Michael Grodin, Sofia Gruskin, Dusan Hadzi-Pavlovic, Abraham Halpern, Angela Hassiotis, Edvard Hauff, John Highfield, Barbara Hocking, Tony Holland, Frank Hume, Vanessa Johnston, Archibald Kaiser, Judith Klein, Gerald Koocher, Ryan McGlaughlin, Vijaya Manicavasagar, John Mendoza, Atari Metcalf, Jakob Mertz, Steven Miles, Anne Mitchell, Robin Munro, Srinivasa Murthy, Robert Parker, Sasha Pavkovic, Jill Peay, Gordon Parker, Campbell Paul, Nicholas Procter, Gerard Quinn, Hans Reinders, JS Reinders, Konya Roy, Leonard Rubenstein, Perminder Sachdev, Richard Shweder, Vikki Sinnott, Christopher Slobogin, John Snowden, Nirmala Srinivasan, Michael Stein, Jill Straker, David Stephens, Nora Sveaass, Colin Tatz, R Thara, Samantha Thomas, Bruce Tonge, Carol Ping Tsao, Harvey Whiteford, Sallie Yea.

As well as authoring his chapter, we are profoundly grateful to Winton Higgins, who has done an outstanding job with critical mentoring and stylistic suggestions. We thank all members of the mental health, suicide prevention, and refugee advocacy networks in Australia, especially the sustaining inspiration and mentorship of the Asylum-Seekers and Mental Health Interest Group, the Board and team at Suicide Prevention Australia, and our families and friends: Caroline Aebersold, Peter and Ros Bennett, Isobel and Jim Bishop, Natalie Bolzan, Vaughan Bowie, Lena Bruselid, Michaela Byers, Stephen Blanks, Lyn Bender, Pat Cleary, Ian Colley, Diego De Leo, Suzana Dekanovic, David Dudley, Patricia Dunn, Nicole Emdur, Paula Farrugia, Di Fitzjames, Michael Fitzjames, Kerry Graham, Martin Harris, Keith Hawton, Ian Hickie, John and Trish Highfield, Adele Horin and Paul Ireland, Jon Jureidini, Trish Langford, David and Isla Lonie, Ryan McGlaughlin, Pat McGorry, Sarah Mares, Louise Newman, Jon Nicholas, Lesley O'Connor, Dawn O'Neil, Margot O'Neill, Chris Paulin, Tania Perich, Ian Rintoul, the Miller-Rosen family (Alan Rosen, Viv Miller, Zacha Rosen and Pilar Angon Urquiza Rosen, and Tully Rosen), Michael Robertson, Lionel and Dawn Robson, Seb Rosenberg, Ngareta Rossell, Hazel Schollar, Alan and Lois Staines, Rodney Smith and Liz Hill, Zac Steel, Freddy Steen, Darryl Taylor and Anne-Marie Codrington, Colin and Sandra Tatz, Ross and Susie Tzannes, Michael Wearing, and Mark Williams. David Webb has persistently challenged Michael Dudley to push the boundaries of the medical model, and think through the issues for users and survivors. We also thank the tireless and dedicated staff at OUP—Martin Baum, Carol Maxwell, Charlotte Green, Abigail Stanley, Simon Witter, and Vimal Stephen at Cenveo Publisher Services— for their commitment to quality and their patience with our many requests. Many others have been important on this journey, and our thanks to you all. Special thanks are due to our inspirational workplace colleagues and our students. The assistance of those with lived experience has been the life-blood of this project.

References

Aggarwal, NK, Rowe, M, and Sernyak MA (2010) 'Is health care a right or a commodity? Implementing mental health reform in a recession', *Psychiatric Services*, 61(11), 1144–5.

Annas, G (2005) 'Human rights and health: the Universal Declaration of Human Rights at 50', in S Gruskin, M Grodin, G Annas, and S Marks (eds) *Perspectives on health and human rights*. New York and London: Routledge, Chapter 3, 63–70.

Arat, Z (2005) 'Human rights and globalisation: is the shrinking world expanding rights?' *Human Rights and Human Welfare*, 5, 137–46. Available at <http://www.du.edu/korbel/hrhw/volumes/2005/arat-2005.pdf>, accessed 27 June 2011.

Arboleda-Flórez, J (2008) 'Mental illness and human rights: editorial review', *Current Opinion in Psychiatry*, 21, 479–84.

Associated Press (2007) 'UN probes over 300 for sexual abuse: official says more needs to be done, spotlight on peacekeepers in Sudan'. Available at <http://www.msnbc.msn.com/id/16495713>, accessed 18 May 2011.

Azhar, MZ, Varma, SL, and Dharap, AS (1994) 'Religious psychotherapy in anxiety disorder patients', *Acta Psychiatrica Scandinavica*, 90, 1–3.

Bartlett, P, Lewis, O, and Thorold, O (2007) *Mental disability and the European Convention on Human Rights*. Leiden/Boston: Martinus Nijhoff.

Bentham, J (1962) 'Anarchical fallacies', in *The Works of Jeremy Bentham*. 11 vols. (John Bowring (ed) Edinburgh: William Tait, 1838–1843). Limited edn. Reprinted New York: Russell & Russell. Vol 2.

Berg, M, and Cocks, G (eds) (1997) *Medicine and modernity: public health and medical care in nineteenth and twentieth-century Germany*. Washington DC: German Historical Institute and Cambridge University Press.

Berlin, I (1969) *Four essays on liberty*. London: Oxford University Press.

Bloch, S, and Green, S (eds) (2009) *Psychiatric ethics*. 4th edn. Oxford: Oxford University Press.

Bloch, S, and Pargiter, R (2009) 'Codes of ethics', in S Bloch, S Green (eds) *Psychiatric ethics*. 4th edn. Oxford: Oxford University Press, 151–73.

Bolzan, N, and Gale, F (2011a) 'Expect the Unexpected', *Child Indicators Research*, 4(2), 269–81.

Bolzan, N and Gale, F (2011b) 'Using an interrupted space to explore social resilience with young people', *Qualitative Social Work*. Published online 24 June 2011, http://qsw.sagepub.com/content/early/2011/05/24/1473325011403959

Campanelli, D (2008) 'The law of military occupation put to the test of human rights law', *International Review of the Red Cross*, 90(871), 653–68.

Candia, PC and Barba, AC (2011) 'Mental capacity and consent to treatment in psychiatric patients: the state of the research', *Current Opinion in Psychiatry*, 24, 442–46.

Cassese, A (1999) 'Are human rights truly universal?', in Savic O (ed) *The politics of human rights*. New York: Verso, 149–65.

Chaimowitz, GA (2004) 'Community Treatment Orders: An Uncertain Step', *Canadian Journal of Psychiatry*, 49(9), 577–78.

Chamberlin, J (2007) 'Foreword', in G Thornicroft, *Shunned: Discrimination against People with Mental Illness*. Oxford: Oxford University Press, xi–xiv.

Chan, Dr Margaret (Director-General of the World Health Organization) (2008) *Address at the launch of the WHO Mental Health GAP Action programme*, Geneva, Switzerland, 9 October 2008. Available at <http://www.who.int/global_health_histories/seminars/presentation40a.pdf>, accessed 7 August 2011.

Commonwealth Human Rights Initiative (2011) *Easier said than done*. Available at <http://www.humanrightsinitiative.org/publications/hradvocacy/ESTD_2010/Full_report_with_Annexure_III.pdf>, accessed 18 May 2011.

Cooper, S, Ssebunnya, J, Kigozi, F, Lund, C, Flisher, A, and The Mhapp Research Programme Consortium (2010) 'Viewing Uganda's Mental Health System through a Human Rights Lens', *International Review of Psychiatry*, December, 22(6), 578–88.

Correll, CU, Manu, P, Olshanskiy, V, Napolitano, B, Kane, JM, and Malhotra, AK (2009) 'Cardio-metabolic risk of second generation antipsychotic medications during first-time use in children and adolescents', *JAMA*, Oct 28, 302(16), 1765–73.

Cresswell, M (2009) 'Psychiatric Survivors and Experiential Rights', *Social Policy & Society*, 8(2), 231–43.

Cullet, P (2005) 'Patents and medicines: the relationship between TRIPS and the right to health', in S Gruskin, MA Grodin, G Annas, and SP Marks (eds) *Perspectives on Health and Human Rights*. New York and London: Routledge, 179–202.

Daccord, Y (2007) 'ICRC and confidentiality', *The Lancet*, 370(9590), 823–2.

Dawson, J and Szmukler, G. Fusion of mental health and incapacity legislation (2006) *The British Journal of Psychiatry*, 188, 504–509.

Declaration of Dresden against Coerced Psychiatric Treatment, 2 June 2007. Available at <http://www.mindfreedom.org/kb/mental-health-global/wpa-dresden/declaration/>, accessed 14 April 2011.

Demyttenaere, K, Bruffaerts, R, Posada-Villa, J, et al. (2004) 'WHOWorld Mental Health Survey Consortium. Prevalence, severity, and unmet need for treatment of mental disorders in the World Health Organization, World Mental Health Surveys', *JAMA*, 291(21), 2581–90.

Department of Health (UK) (2007) *2007 Mental Health Act—overview*. Available at <http://www.dh.gov.uk/en/Policyandguidance/Healthandsocialcaretopics/Mentalhealth/DH_078743>, accessed 6 June 2011.

Desjarlais, R, Eisenberg, L, Good, B, and Kleinman, A (1995) *World Mental Health: Problems and Priorities in Low-Income Countries*. New York/Oxford: Oxford University Press.

Dhanda, A (2008) 'Constructing a new human rights lexicon: Convention on the Rights of Persons with Disabilities', *Sur International Journal on Human Rights* (English edition), 5(8), 43–59. Available at http://www.surjournal.org/eng/conteudos/pdf/8/dhanda.pdf, accessed 27th March 2011.

Dhanda, A and Narayan, T (2007) 'Mental health and human rights', *The Lancet*, 370(9594), 1197–98.

Disability Rights Commission (2006) *Equality treatment: closing the gap: a formal investigation into the physical health inequalities experiences by people with learning disabilities and/or mental health problems*. London: Disability Rights Commission.

Dodson, M (1993) *Annual Report of the Aboriginal and Torres Strait Islander Social Justice Commissioner*. Available at <http://www.safecom.org.au/social-justice.htm>, accessed 26 June 2011.

Donnelly, J (2003) *Universal Human Rights in Theory and Practice*. 2nd edn. Ithaca, NY and London: Cornell.

Drew N, Funk M, Tang S et al. (2011) Human rights violations of people with mental and psychosocial disabilities: an unresolved global crisis. *Lancet* 378: 1664–1675.

Droege, C (2008a) 'Elective affinities: human rights and humanitarian law', *International Review of the Red Cross*, 90(871), 501–48.

Droege, C (2008b) 'Transfers of detainees: legal framework, non-refoulement, and contemporary challenges', *International Review of the Red Cross*, 90(871), 669–701.

D'Souza, R and Rodrigo, A (2004) 'Spiritually augmented cognitive behavioural therapy', *Australasian Psychiatry*, 12(2), 148–52.

Dudley, M and Gale, F (2002) 'Psychiatrists as a moral community? Psychiatry under the Nazis and its contemporary relevance', *Australian and New Zealand Journal of Psychiatry*, 36(5), 585–94.

Duffy, H (2008) Human rights litigation and the 'War on Terror', *International Review of the Red Cross*, 90(871), 573–97.

Failer, JL (2002) *Who qualifies for rights? Homelessness, mental illness and civil commitment*. Ithaca and London: Cornell.

Farmer, P (2005) *Pathologies of power: health, human rights and the new war on the poor*. (With a new preface by the author). Berkeley and Los Angeles, CA: University of California Press.

Farmer, P and Gastineau, N (2002) 'Rethinking health and human rights: time for a paradigm shift', *Journal of Law and Medical Ethics*, Winter, 30(4), 655–66.

Finnemore, M and Sikkink, K (1998) 'International norm dynamics and political change', *International Organisation*, 52(4), 667–917.

Fleischmann, A, Bertolote, JM, Wasserman, D, de Leo, D, Bolhari, J, Botega, NJ, De Silva, D, Phillips, M, Vijayakumar, L, Värnik A, Schlebusch, L, and Huong, Tran Thi Thanh (2008) 'Effectiveness of brief intervention and contact for suicide attempters: a randomized controlled trial in five countries', *Bulletin of the World Health Organization*, 86, 703–709.

Forsythe, DP (2006) *Human rights in international relations*. 2nd edn. Cambridge, UK: Cambridge University Press.

Freedman, LP (1999) 'Reflections on emerging frameworks of health and human rights', in JM Mann, S Gruskin, MA Grodin, GJ Annas (eds) *Health and human rights: a reader*. New York and London: Routledge, 227–52.

Freeman, M (2002) *Human rights: an interdisciplinary approach*. Cambridge: Polity.

Friedlander, H (1995) *The origins of Nazi genocide: from euthanasia to the Final Solution*. Chapel Hill, NC: University of North Carolina Press.

Galston, W (1991) *Liberal purposes: goods, duties and virtues in the liberal state*. Cambridge: Cambridge University Press.

Gavison, R (2003) 'On the relationships between civil and political rights, and social and economic rights', in JM Coicaud, MW Doyle, and AM Gardner (eds) *The globalization of human rights*. Tokyo and New York: United Nations University, 23–55.

Gewirth, A (1982) *Human rights: essays on justification and applications*. Chicago: University of Chicago Press.

Ghanashyam, B and Nagarathinam, S (2010) 'India is failing the mentally ill as abuses continue', *The Lancet*, 376, November 13, 1633–34.

Gillam, S (2008) 'Is the Alma Ata Declaration still relevant to primary health care?', *British Medical Journal*, 336, 8 March, 536–38.

Gilligan, C (1982) *In a different voice: psychological theory and women's development*. Cambridge, MA: Harvard University Press.

Glendon, MA (2001) *A world made new: Eleanor Roosevelt and the Universal Declaration of Human Rights*. Random House: New York.

Glover, J (1999) *Humanity: a moral history of the twentieth century*. New Haven and London: Yale.

Goldney, RD (2008) *Suicide Prevention*. Oxford: Oxford University Press.

Griffin, J (2008) *On human rights*. Oxford: Oxford University Press.

Gruskin, S (2000) 'The conceptual and practical implications of reproductive and sexual rights: how far have we come?', *Health and human rights*, 4(2), 1–6.

Gruskin, S, Mills, EJ, and Tarantola, D (2007) 'History, principles and practice of health and human rights', *The Lancet*, 370, 449–55.

Gruskin, S and Tarantola, D (2005) 'Health and human rights', in S Gruskin, MA Grodin, G Annas, and SP Marks (eds) *Perspectives on Health and Human Rights*. New York and London: Routledge, 3–58.

Hall, JJ and Taylor, R (2003) 'Health for all beyond 2000: the demise of the Alma-Ata Declaration and primary health care in developing countries', *Medical Journal of Australia*, 178, 17–20.

Higgins, W (2006) 'Could it happen again? The Holocaust and the national question', in C Tatz, P Arnold, and S Tatz (eds) *Genocide Perspectives III*. Blackheath NSW: Brandl & Schlesinger.

Hunt, L (1996) *The French Revolution and human rights: a brief documentary history*. Boston: Bedford/ St Martins Press.

Hunt, L (2007) *Inventing human rights: a history*. New York: WW Norton.

Hunt, P (2005) *Report of the UN Special Rapporteur on the right of everyone to the enjoyment of the highest attainable standard of physical and mental health*, UN doc. E/CN. 4/2005/51.

Ife, J (2001) *Human rights and social work: towards rights-based practice*. Cambridge: Cambridge University Press.

Inoue, T (2003) 'Human rights and Asian values', in JM Coicaud, MW Doyle, and AM Gardner (eds) *The globalization of human rights*. Tokyo and New York: United Nations University Press, 116–36.

Ishay, M (2008) *The history of human rights: from ancient times to the globalization era*. Edition with new preface. Berkeley, Los Angeles, and London: University of California Press.

Jacob, KS, Sharan, P, Mirza, I, Garrido-Cumbrera, M, Seedat, S, Mari, JJ, Sreenivas, V, and Saxena, S (2007) 'Mental health systems in countries: where are we now?', *The Lancet*, 370, 1061–77.

James, BO, Omoaregba, OJ, Igberase, OO, and Olotu, SO. (2009) 'Unmodified electroconvulsive therapy: changes in knowledge and attitudes of Nigerian medical students', *African Health Sciences*, 9(4), 279–83. Available at <http://www.bioline.org.br/pdf?hs09066>, accessed 9 July 2011.

Kallert, T, Mezzich, J, Monahan, J. (2011) *Coercive treatment in psychiatry: clinical, legal and ethical aspects*. Chichester: Wiley.

Kane, JM, Quitkin, F, Rifkin, A, et al. (1983) 'Attitudinal changes of involuntarily committed patients following treatment', *Archives of General Psychiatry*, 40, 374–77.

Killaspy, H, Rosen, A. (2011) Case management and assertive community treatment. In Thornicroft, G, Szmukler, G, Mueser, KT, Drake, RE (eds), *Oxford Textbook of Community Mental Health*, Oxford: Oxford University Press, pp. 142–150.

Kinley, D (2009) *Civilising globalisation: human rights and the global economy*. Cambridge: Cambridge University Press.

Kinley, D and Stewart, D. (2009) *Interview (October 6)*. Available at <http://www.policyinnovations.org/ideas/briefings/data/000145>, accessed 27 June 2011.

Kirmayer, L (2007) 'Cultural psychiatry in historical perspective', in D Bhugra and K Bhui (eds) *Textbook of cultural psychiatry*. Cambridge: Cambridge University Press, 3–19.

Kleinman, A (2009) 'Global mental health: a failure of humanity', *The Lancet*, 374 (Aug 22), 603–604.

Kymlicka, W (2002) *Contemporary political philosophy: an introduction*. 2nd edn. Oxford: Oxford University Press.

Lancet Global Mental Health Group (2007) 'Scale up services for mental disorders: a call for action', *The Lancet*, 370, 1241–52.

Landman, T (2005) *Protecting human rights: a comparative study*. Washington, DC: Georgetown University Press.

Large, MM, Nielssen, O, Ryan, CJ, and Hayes, R (2008a) 'Mental health laws that require dangerousness for involuntary admission may delay the initial treatment of schizophrenia', *Social Psychiatry and Psychiatric Epidemiology*, 43, 251–56.

Large, MM, Ryan, CJ, Nielssen, OB, and Hayes, RA (2008b) 'The danger of dangerousness: why we must remove the dangerousness criterion from our mental health acts', *Journal of Medical Ethics*, 34, 877–81.

Lauren, PG (1998) *The evolution of international human rights: visions seen*. Philadelphia: University of Pennsylvania Press.

Lawrence, C (2002) *What is social justice?* Address given at Curtin University, Western Australia, 23 September. Available at <http://www.safecom.org.au/social-justice.htm>, accessed 26th June 2011.

Lewis, L (2009) 'Introduction: Mental Health and Human Rights: Social Policy and Sociological Perspectives', *Social Policy & Society*, 8(2), 211–214.

Lewis, O and Bartlett, P (2011) International human rights and community mental health. In Thornicroft, G, Szmukler, G, Mueser, KT, Drake, R (eds), *Oxford Textbook of Community Mental Health*. Oxford: Oxford University Press, 230–7.

Long, E (2010) 'The Australian Social Inclusion Agenda: a new approach to social policy? *Australian Journal of Social Issues*, 45(2), 161–82.

Loo, C, Trollor, J, Alonzo, A, Rendina, N, and Kavess, R (2010) 'Mental health legislation and psychiatric treatments in NSW: electroconvulsive therapy and deep brain stimulation', *Australasian Psychiatry*, 18(5), 417–25.

McEwan, A, Bowers, J, and Saal, T. (2009) *Tailoring mental health promotion in rural and remote areas in the context of climate change: an NGO perspective*. Poster. Queensland: Centre for Rural and Remote Mental Health. Available at <http://www.crrmhq.com.au/media/Climate-Change-Poster.pdf>, accessed 27 June 2011.

McGorry, PD, Purcell, R, Hickie, IB, and Jorm, A (2007) 'Investing in youth mental health is a best buy', *Medical Journal of Australia*, 187(7 Suppl), S5–7.

McSherry, B (2008) 'Protecting the integrity of the person: developing limitations on involuntary treatment', in B McSherry (ed) *International Trends in Mental Health Law*, 11–124, 121.

Marks, S (2005) 'Human rights in development: the significance for health', in S Gruskin, M Grodin, G Annas, S Marks (eds) *Perspectives on health and human rights*. New York and London: Routledge, Chapter 5, 95–116.

Marshall, TH (1965) *Class, citizenship and social development*. New York: Anchor.

Minkowitz, T (2007) 'The United Nations Convention on the Rights of Persons with Disabilities and the right to be free from nonconsensual psychiatric interventions', *Syracuse Journal of International Law and Commerce*, 34, 405–28.

Mokhiber, CG (2005) 'Towards a measure of dignity: indicators for rights-based development', in S Gruskin, MA Grodin, G Annas, and SP Marks (eds) *Perspectives on Health and Human Rights*. New York and London: Routledge, 383–92.

Moncrieff, J and Leo, J (2010) 'A systematic review of the effects of antipsychotic drugs on brain volume', *Psychological Medicine*, 40, 1409–22. Published online: 20 January 2010.

Morsink, J (1999) *The Universal Declaration of Human Rights: origins, drafting and intent*. Philadelphia: University of Pennsylvania Press.

Moyo, D (2009) *Dead aid: why aid is not working and how there is a better way for Africa*. New York: Farrar, Straus and Giroux.

Murray, CJL and Lopez, AD (1996) *The Global Burden of Disease*. Geneva: World Health Organization, Harvard School of Public Health, World Bank.

Naeem, F, Gobbi, M, Ayub, M and Kingdon, D (2010) 'Psychologists' experience of cognitive behavior therapy in a developing country: a qualitative study from Pakistan', *International Journal of Mental Health Systems*, 4(2). Available at <http://www.ijmhs.com/content/4/1/2>, accessed 9 July 2011.

Naito, K (2009) *The Necessity of 'Conflict Transformation' in Approaches to Psychosocial Interventions*. Submitted in partial fulfillment of the requirements for the degree of Master of Social Work. Northampton, MA: Smith College School for Social Work. Available at <http://dspace.nitle.org/bitstream/handle/10090/9920/The%20Necessity%20of%20Conflict%20Transformation%20-%20NaitoA09.pdf?sequence=1>, accessed 28 May 2011.

NGO Monitor (2008) *Watching the watchers: the politics and credibility of non-governmental organisations in the Arab-Israeli conflict*. Available at <http://www.ngo-monitor.org/data/images/File/watchingthewatchers-small.pdf>, accessed 18 May 2011.

Nickel, J (2009) *Human rights and globalization*. (From IVR encyclopedie). Available at <http://ivr-enc.info/index.php?title=Human_Rights_and_Globalization>, accessed 26 June 2011.

Nozick, R (1974) *Anarchy, state and utopia*. Basic Books: New York.

Nussbaum, M (2006) *Frontiers of justice: disability, nationality, species membership*. Boston and London: Belknap (Harvard University Press).

Okin, S (1990) 'Thinking like a woman', in D Rhode (ed) *Theoretical perspectives on sexual difference*. New Haven: Yale University Press.

O'Reilly, R (2004) 'Why Are Community Treatment Orders Controversial?', *Canadian Journal of Psychiatry*, 49, 579–84.

Patel, V, Araya, R, Chatterjee, S, Chisholm, D, Cohen, A, De Silva, M, Hosman, C, McGuire, H, Rojas, G, and van Ommeren, M. (2007a) 'Treatment and prevention of mental disorders in low-income and middle-income countries', *The Lancet*, 370, 991–1005.

Patel, V, Fisher, AJ, Hetrick, S, and McGorry, P (2007b) 'Adolescent Health 3—Mental Health of young people: a global public-health challenge', *The Lancet*, 369(9569), 1302–1313.

Patel, V and Prince, M (2010) 'Global mental health: a new global health field comes of age', *JAMA*, 303(19), 1976–77.

Pflanz, M (2008) *Six year olds sexually abused by UN peacekeepers*. Available at <http://www.telegraph.co.uk/news/worldnews/2032996/Six-year-olds-sexually-abused-by-UN-peacekeepershtml>, accessed 18 May 2011.

Prasad, A (2004) 'Review article', Jack Donnelly's *Universal Human Rights in Theory and Practice*. Alternatives: *Turkish Journal of International Relations*, 3(2&3), Summer & Fall. Available at <http://www.alternativesjournal.net/volume3/number2/ajnesh.pdf>, accessed 8 May 2011.

Prince, M, Patel, V, Saxena, S, Maj, M, Maselko, J, Phillips, MR, and Rahman, A (2007) 'No health without mental health', *The Lancet*, 370, 859–77.

Propst, LR, Ostrom, R, Watkins, P, et al. (1992) 'Comparative efficacy of religious and non-religious cognitive-behavioural therapy for the treatment of clinical depression in religious individuals', *Journal of Consulting and Clinical Psychology*, 60, 94–103.

Queensland Alliance (2010) *From discrimination to social inclusion: a review of the literature on anti stigma initiatives in mental health*. Available at <http://www.qldalliance.org.au/discrimination-social-inclusion-research-report>, accessed 6 August 2011.

Rakfeldt, J (2008) 'Book review: Inventing human rights: a history', *Psychiatric Services*, 59, 215, February.

Rawls, J (1971) *A theory of justice*. London: Oxford University Press.

Raworth, K (2005) 'Measuring human rights', in S Gruskin, MA Grodin, G Annas, and SP Marks (eds) *Perspectives on Health and Human Rights*. New York and London: Routledge, 393–411.

Rees, S, Silove, D, Chey, T, Ivancic, L, Steel, Z, Creamer, M, Teesson, M, Bryant, R, McFarlane, AC, Mills, KL, Slade, T, Carragher, N, O'Donnell, M, and Forbes, D (2011) 'Lifetime Prevalence of Gender-Based Violence in Women and the Relationship With Mental Disorders and Psychosocial Function', *JAMA*, 306(5), 513–21.

Robertson, G (2006) *Crimes against humanity: the struggle for global justice*. 3rd edn. Camberwell, Victoria: Penguin (Australia).

Robertson, G (2007) 'Health and human rights series', *The Lancet*, 370, 368–69.

Rorty, R (1993) 'Human rights, rationality, and sentimentality', in S Shute and S Hurley (eds) *On Human Rights: the Oxford Amnesty Lectures 1993*. Basic Books: New York.

Sandel, M (1996) *Democracy's discontent: America in search of a public philosophy*. Cambridge, MA: Harvard University Press.

Saraceno, B, Van Ommeren, M, Batniji, R, Cohen, A, Gureje, O, Mahoney, J, Sridhar, D, and Underhill, C (2007) 'Barriers to improvement of mental health services in low-income and middle-income countries', *The Lancet*, 370, 1164–74.

Sartorius, N (2002) 'The limits of mental health care in general medical services', in N Sartorius, *Fighting for mental health: a personal view*. Cambridge: Cambridge University Press.

Sartorius, N and Schulze, H (2005) *Reducing the stigma of mental illness*. New York: Cambridge University Press.

Sassoli, M and Olson, L (2008) 'The relationship between international humanitarian and human rights law where it matters: admissible killing and internment of fighters in non-international armed conflicts', *International Review of the Red Cross*, 90(871), 599–627.

Saxena, S, Thornicroft, G, Knapp, M and Whiteford, H (2007) 'Resources for mental health: scarcity, inequity, and inefficiency', *The Lancet*, 370, 878–89.

Scanlan, T (1998) *What we owe each other*. Cambridge, MA: Harvard University Press.

Segal, SP and Burgess, P (2009) 'Preventing psychiatric hospitalization and involuntary outpatient commitment', *Social Work in Health Care*, 48(3), 232–42.

Sen A (1982) *Poverty and Famines: An Essay on Entitlements and Deprivation*. Oxford: Clarendon Press.

Sen, A. (1985) *Commodities and Capabilities*. Oxford: Oxford University Press.

Sen, A (1999) *Development As Freedom*. New York: Knopf.

Sen, A (2005) 'Human rights and capabilities', *Journal of Human Development*, 6(2) (July), 151–66.

Sen, A (2009) *The idea of justice*. Harvard: Harvard University Press.

Senarclens, P (2003) 'The politics of human rights', in JM Coicaud, MW Doyle, and AM Gardner (eds) *The globalization of human rights*. Tokyo and New York: United Nations University, 137–59.

Sharif, F and Armitage, P (2004) 'The effect of psychological and educational counselling in reducing anxiety in nursing students', *Journal of Psychiatric Mental Health Nursing*, 11, 386–92.

Shue, H (2003) 'Global accountability: transnational duties towards economic rights', in JM Coicaud, MW Doyle, and AM Gardner (eds) *The globalization of human rights*. Tokyo and New York: United Nations University, 160–77.

Silove, D (1999) 'The psychosocial effects of torture, mass human rights violations, and refugee trauma: toward an integrated conceptual framework', *Journal of Nervous Mental Disorders*, 187, 200–7.

Silove, D (2000) 'Trauma and forced relocation', *Current Opinion in Psychiatry 2000*, 13(2), 231–36.

Silove, D, Ekblad, S, and Mollica, R (2000) 'The rights of the severely mentally ill in post-conflict societies', *The Lancet*, 355(9214), 1548–49.

Silove, D, Steel, Z (2006) 'Understanding community psychosocial needs after disasters: implications for mental health services', *Journal of Postgraduate Medicine*, 52(2), 121–25.

Silove, D, Steel, Z, and Bauman, A (2007) 'Mass psychological trauma and PTSD: epidemic illusion?', in JP Wilson and CS Tang (eds) *Cross-Cultural Assessment of Psychological Trauma and PTSD*. International and Cultural Psychology, Part 3, 319–36.

Silove, D, Bateman, CR, Brooks, RT, Fonseca, CA, Steel, Z, Rodger, J, Soosay, I, Fox, G, Patel, V, and Bauman, A (2008) 'Estimating clinically relevant mental disorders in a rural and an urban setting in postconflict Timor Leste', *Archives of General Psychiatry*, 65(10), 1205–1212.

Spandler, H and Calton, T (2009) 'Psychosis and Human Rights: Conflicts in Mental Health Policy and Practice', *Social Policy & Society*, 8(2), 245–56.

Steel, Z, Bateman-Steel, CR, and Silove, D (2009) 'Human rights and the trauma model: Genuine partners or uneasy allies?', *Journal of Traumatic Stress*, (Sep 9) 22, 358–65.

Steel, Z, Chey, T, Silove, D, Marnane, C, Bryant, RA, and van Ommeren, M (2009) 'Association of torture and other potentially traumatic events with mental health outcomes among populations exposed to mass conflict and displacement: A systematic review and meta-analysis', *JAMA*, 302(5), 537–49.

Suicide Prevention Australia (August 2009) *Suicide and self-harm among Gay, Lesbian, Bisexual and Transgender communities*. Available at <http://www.suicidepreventionaust.org>, accessed 6 November 2010.

Suicide Prevention Australia (September 2011) *Social inclusion and suicide prevention*. (Position statement). Available at <http://www.suicidepreventionaust.org>, forthcoming.

Sumathipala, A, Hewege, S, Hanwella, R, and Mann, H (2000) 'Randomized controlled trial of cognitive behaviour therapy for repeated consultations for medically unexplained complaints: a feasibility study in Sri Lanka', *Psychological Medicine*, 30, 747–57.

Summerfield, D (1999) 'A critique of seven assumptions behind psychological trauma programmes in war-affected areas', *Social Science and Medicine*, 48, 1449–62.

Sumption, J (2010) 'Do the right thing. Review of the Last Utopia: Human Rights in History by Samuel Moyn (Belknap)', *Literary Review*, Dec 2010/Jan 2011, 6–7.

Surguladze, S and David, A (1999) 'Insight in major mental illness', *Advances in Psychiatric Treatment*, 5, 163–70.

Swanson, JW (1994) 'Mental disorder, substance abuse, and community violence: an epidemiologic approach', in J Monahan and HJ Steadman (eds) *Violence and mental disorder: developments in risk assessment*. Chicago: University of Chicago Press, 101–36.

Swartz, MS and Swanson, JW (2004) 'Involuntary Outpatient Commitment, Community Treatment Orders, and Assisted Outpatient Treatment: What's in the Data?', *Canadian Journal of Psychiatry*, 49, 585–91.

Szmukler, G and Applebaum PS (2011) Treatment pressures, coercion and compulsion. In Thornicroft G, Szmukler G, Mueser KT, Drake RE (eds), *Oxford Textbook of Community Mental Health*, Oxford: Oxford University Press, pp 237–44.

Szoke, H (2009) *Social inclusion and human rights—strange bedfellows on the road to an authentically Australian inclusion agenda*. Victorian Equal Opportunity and Human Rights Commission. Available at <http://www.humanrightscommission.vic.gov.au/index.php?option=com_k2&view=item&id=307: social-inclusion-and-human-rights-strange-bedfellows-on-the-road-to-an-authentically-australian-inclusion-agenda&Itemid=514>, accessed 6 August 2011.

Taylor, C (1985) *Philosophy and the Human Sciences: Philosophical Papers 2*, Cambridge: Cambridge University Press.

Tennant, C and Silove, D (2005) 'The development of a mental health service in East Timor: An Australian mental health relief project', *International Psychiatry*, 2(8), 17–19.

Thornicroft, G (2006) *Shunned: Discrimination against People with Mental Illness*. Oxford: Oxford University Press.

Thornicroft, G, Rose, D, and Kassam, A (2007) 'Discrimination in health care against people with mental illness', *International Review of Psychiatry*,19, 113–22. PMID: 17464789.

Thornicroft, G and Tansella, M (2004) 'Components of a modern mental health service: a pragmatic balance of community and hospital care: overview of systematic evidence', *British Journal of Psychiatry*, 185, 283–90.

Thucydides (1972) *History of the Peloponnesian War*. (trans. Rex Warner). Revised edn. London: Penguin Books Ltd. From the Melian Dialogue, v. 86–111.

Tol, WA, Barbui, C, Galappatti, A, et al. (2011) 'Mental Health and Psychosocial Support in Humanitarian Settings: Linking Practice and Research', *The Lancet* 378L 1581–1591. Published online 17 October 2011.

Treffert, D (1973) '"Dying With Their Rights On". Letters to the editor', *American Journal Of Psychiatry*, 130(9), 1041.

United Nations (1993) *United Nations General Assembly: Vienna Declaration and programme of action*. World Conference on Human Rights, Vienna 14–25 June 1993. UN Document A/CONF. 157/23. New York: UN.

United Nations (1997) *United Nations General Assembly: Renewing the United Nations: A Programme for Reform, 14 July 1997*. UN Document A51/950. New York: UN.

United Nations Development Programme (UNDP) (1999) *Human Rights Development Report*. Geneva: UN.

United Nations Development Programme (2011) *Human Development Report 2010*. Available at <http://hdr.undp.org/en/humandev/>, accessed 31 May 2011.

United Nations Office of the High Commissioner for Human Rights (2010). Available at <http://www.ohchr.org/EN/Issues/Pages/WhatareHumanRights.aspx, accessed 16 December 2010.

UN Human Rights Commissioner (2011) *Interviews with Ms Navi Pillay on 29 May 2011*. Available at http://stoptheintervention.org/>, <http://indymedia.org.au/2011/05/29/wgar-news-interview-with-un-human-rights-commissioner-navi-pillay-on-the-nt-intervention>, and <http://caama.com.au/united-nations-high-commissioner-navi-pillay-on-caama-radio>, accessed 6 June 2011.

Vasak, K (1977) 'Human rights: a thirty-year struggle—the sustained efforts to give force of law to the Universal Declaration of Human Rights', *UNESCO Courier*, 30, 11.

Venkatapuram, S, Bell, R, and Marmot, M (2010) 'The right to sutures: social epidemiology, human rights, and social justice', *Health Human Rights*, Dec 15, 12(2), 3–16.

Vite, S (2008) 'The interrelation of the law of occupation and economic, social and cultural rights: the examples of food, health and property', *International Review of the Red Cross*, 90(871), 629–51.

Weare, K (2000) *Promoting mental, emotional and social health: A whole school approach*. London: Routledge Falmer, 12.

Weller, P (2009) 'Human rights and social justice: the Convention on the Rights of Persons with Disabilities and the Quiet Revolution in International Law', *The Journal of Law and Social Justice*, 4, 74–91.

Wilson, RA (ed) (2005) *Human rights in the 'War on Terror'*. Cambridge: Cambridge University Press.

World Health Organization (1992) *The ICD-10 Classification of Mental and Behavioural Disorders: Clinical descriptions and diagnostic guidelines*. Geneva: World Health Organization.

World Health Organization (1996) *Global action for improvement of mental health care: policies and strategies*. Geneva: World Health Organization.

World Health Organization (2001) *The World Health Report 2001. Mental health: new understanding, new hope*. Geneva: World Health Organization.

World Health Organization (2002) *Written submission to the United Nations Sub-Commission on the Promotion and Protection of Human Rights, Fifty-fourth session*. Geneva: World Health Organization.

World Health Organization (2003) *Written submission to the United Nations Sub-Commission on the Promotion and Protection of Human Rights, Fifty-fifth session*. Available at <http://www.who.int/hhr/information/WHO_Written_Submission_to_54th_Session_of_Sub-Commission.pdf>, accessed 13 April 2012.

World Health Organization (2005a) *WHO Resource Book on Mental Health, Human Rights and Legislation*. Geneva: World Health Organization.

World Health Organization (2005b) *Improving access and use of psychotropic medicines*. (Mental Health Policy and Service Guidance Package). Geneva: World Health Organization.

World Health Organization (2010) *Health topics: mental health*. Available at <http://www.who.int/topics/mental_health/en/>, accessed 17 December 2010.

World Health Organization (2012) *Mental Health Policy and Services: Mental Health Improvement for Nations Development: the WHO Mind Project. Training Opportunities*. Available at <http://www.who.int/mental_health/policy/training/en/index.html>, accessed 9th April 2012.

World Health Organization and World Bank (2011) *World Report on Disability*. Geneva: World Health Organization. Available at <http://www.who.int/disabilities/world_report/2011/en/index.htm>, accessed 13 June 2011.

World Psychiatric Association (2005) *Madrid Declaration of Ethical Standards for Psychiatric Practice*. (enhanced version, original version 1996). Available at <http://www.wpanet.org/detail.php?section_id=5&content_id=48>, accessed 9 November 2011.

Wright, D (2010) *Mental health history and the WHO: from Bedlam to Brock Chisholm. Seminar for Global Health Histories*. World Health Organization. Available at <http://www.who.int/global_health_histories/seminars/2010/en/index.html>, accessed 6 June 2011.

Part 1

Overarching Conceptual Issues

This first section introduces wide-ranging issues that are raised by the consideration of the relationship of mental health and human rights. Winton Higgins traces the historical emergence of the idea, culture, and institutional framework of human rights; the gradual spreading of the human rights net under the 'universal' rubric from white males to many other human categories (black people, women, sexual minorities, etc), and eventually to people with mental disorders; and the process whereby abusers lost impunity and rights therefore became meaningful by becoming enforceable. Charles Watters complements this by exploring linkages over time between mental health and illness and ideas of human rights. He highlights the conditions of those both within and outside mental health systems. He notes how the parameters of mental health have expanded, particularly in terms of familial relations and societal contribution, beyond what would formerly have been expected for people with mental disorders. He distinguishes 'bare' survival or 'negative liberty' as freedom from constraint, and the positive liberty of citizens, in which the state facilitates people realizing their goals. Watters illustrates how disorders are historically conditioned, as seen in the history of post-traumatic stress disorder, how entitlement is not true access (highlighted by the case of asylum-seekers), and the limits of social contracts as applied to those with mental illnesses.

Michael Perlin and Eva Szeli consider the relationship between human rights and the law, and specifically, the relatively recent meeting of mental health law and human rights law. They note the neglect of human rights of people with disabilities for decades by international human rights protection agencies. Although recent political, legal, social, and cultural developments have helped shift the environment so as to support a movement that 'extends' rights to this population, these rights are often ignored or granted only on paper. They argue the cause is sanism: an irrational prejudice akin to other prejudices of racism, sexism, homophobia, and ethnic bigotry, that infects jurisprudence and lawyering practices, that is largely invisible and socially acceptable, based predominantly upon stereotype, myth, superstition, and deindividualization, is sustained and perpetuated by 'ordinary common sense' (OCS) and heuristic reasoning in an unconscious response to events in everyday life and in the legal process. They issue the challenge to give life to international human rights for this population.

The connection between culture, context, mental health and human rights is addressed in Laurence Kirmayer's chapter. He addresses three broad questions concerning the cross-cultural applicability of human rights in the domain of psychiatry: (1) Do the theory and practice of psychiatry and other mental health disciplines apply across disparate cultures? (2) Are human rights principles universally applicable? and (3) Are human rights principles applicable to mental health issues across cultures? Kirmayer notes that 'culture' names a process, not a thing, that cultural knowledge and institutions as part of open, fluid, dynamic systems are contested, and that a multiplicity of types of cultures are available in the contemporary world. He notes the twin dangers of endorsing cultural stereotypes and dismissing 'culture' altogether, rather than acknowledging its place in all our lives. Cultural context (whether local, or imported, Western and medical) potentially shapes all aspects of mental disorders and the meaning of and response to symptoms and illnesses. Psychiatry may have a liberating or debilitating role depending on how it is culturally experienced or received, and when used for involuntary treatment, may be empowering or oppressive. Kirmayer examines the meanings of relativism and universality in human rights discourse, and the contrast between Western autonomy and non-Western interdependence. Despite their anchorage in different cultural forms of life, Kirmayer advances arguments for the universality of human rights across and embedded within cultures. He discusses cultural notions of human, humanness, the humane, and dehumanization understood through cultures; comments on the right to culture and community; the potential for engaged dialogue between diverse cultures in a global society; the cultural responsiveness of mental health services; and the globalization of psychiatry as a human rights opportunity and challenge.

Jennifer Randall, Graham Thornicroft, Elaine Brohan, Aliya Kassam, Elanor Lewis-Holmes, and Nisha Mehta consider forms of social exclusion and systematic disadvantage affecting people with mental disorders in all domains of life. They examine stigma as comprising ignorance, prejudice, and discrimination; relevant international human rights conventions; three Articles of a recent human rights convention to illustrate stigma as a critical human rights issue; and give examples of the work of relevant international non-governmental organizations active in this field. They examine the right to health (Article 25 of Convention on the Rights of Persons with Disabilities (CRPD)), the Right to Work and Employment (Article 27 of CRPD), the work of NGOs in the area, the significance of stigma, and particularly how it can be effectively reduced.

Sandy McFarlane and Richard Bryant discuss the relationship of advances in genetics and neurobiology and human rights with particular reference to the case example of traumatic stress. They appraise positive and negative possibilities associated with providing biological information—the latter associated for example with employment and insurance. They place this in the context of the later 19th century preoccupation of the role of heredity in mental illness, and the prejudices, abuses, and atrocities that flowed from this. They review the implications of the impact of traumatic stress on genes and chromosomes, with implications for mental health, and the ethical dilemmas associated with genetic testing for participants (including denial of life opportunities) and families. They examine a range of risk factors for post-traumatic stress disorder (PTSD) which could constitute potential markers, problems with their reliability and predictive capacity, and the ethical problems arising. They also consider genetic screening, the rights of the unborn child, parental rights, and the potential psychosocial consequences and injustices for those children at high genetic risk, who may never express the genetic disorder. Such scenarios have profound, even alarming implications, and need to proceed with due regard to people's rights.

Tristan McGeorge and Dinesh Bhugra tackle the topic of race, class, mental health, and human rights. They ponder differential rates of mental disorders (especially depression and psychosis) among racial and ethnic minorities in the UK, and note negative and adversarial pathways to care for black and minority ethnic patients. They document self-reported racism as a confirmed contributor to common mental disorders and psychosis, and institutional racism in mental health services. They note strategies for improving race equality in mental health, including the role of education in medical schools and psychiatrist training, government organizations, and advocacy groups, and note the role of human rights frameworks in the reform process, including international, regional, and national measures.

Roshni Mangalore, Martin Knapp, and David McDaid contemplate mental health economics, mental health policies, and human rights. How do states and the international community achieve positive mental health outcomes, given their human rights duties and the limits of available resources? Noting that mental health problems and mental health policies and programmes (or lack thereof) can violate human rights and diminish capabilities, they propose introducing fundamental freedoms and human rights into the analysis of economic processes. They adopt the notion of core capabilities, the empirical application of which they discuss in examining individual entitlements, modelling achievement for different groups regarding prevention and interventions, and freedom of choice and opportunity freedom. They introduce the notion of needs, as the basic entity linking human rights, capabilities, resource allocation, and equity in mental health. Further analysing need, especially of the least favoured or worst off, they ask whether applying utilitarian principles of cost-effectiveness in allocating mental health care resources results in denial of human rights (e.g. rationing access to interventions). Resource efficiency, where only economic needs that produce net benefits are met, or where health is regarded as a market commodity, is contrasted with equity approaches. These may sacrifice efficiency gains to focus resources on those socially marginalized and/or suffering severe mental illness, and may include normative need for services, providing good health and equal opportunity for quality living. The authors also consider resource insufficiency (e.g. budgetary allocations, pharmaceuticals), barriers to resource sufficiency (resource inappropriateness, attitudes, financing mechanisms), recognizing value judgments (e.g. re cost-effectiveness) and the importance of economic evaluation in rationing.

Catherine Esposito and Daniel Tarantola trace the important history of how the confrontation with HIV was critical to making the link between health and human rights. They expound on the reciprocal relationships between HIV, health, and human rights, and make suggestions about how this relationship could be improved, through overcoming structural, systemic, and financial obstacles that pre-empt comprehensive, effective responses to co-morbidity. They cite unnecessary hospitalizations of people with serious mental disorders, and in various parts of Asia, compulsory treatment of drug addicts at high risk of HIV in mandatory drug treatment facilities without access to due process. The power to reduce vulnerability is rooted in governments' ability to deliver on their human rights obligations. They argue for supportive policy, legal, and research environments that acknowledge rather than ignore the relationships between HIV, mental health, and human rights, that increase awareness of the advantages of bridging these domains, and adopt strategies in mental health, HIV, primary care, and social services to do so, including making these services economically affordable, high-quality, and non-discriminatory. Mental health literacy campaigns may assist participation for those living with HIV. Accountability processes and reports (e.g. declarations, international treaty monitoring, Millenium Development Goals, national monitoring) need to attend to the issue and impact of HIV/mental health co-morbidity.

Amita Dhanda discusses universal legal capacity as a universal human right. She accepts the enriching value of universalism for human rights discourse, provided (with some postmodern and feminist critiques) it is inclusive and does not privilege the preferences of dominant groups, nor allow hierarchies within groups such as people with disabilities. She contends the CRPD in Article 12 recognises universal legal capacity for people with disabilities, whilst acknowledging differences between them in exercising this, through strategies such as reasonable accommodation and support through co-facilitation or joint decision-making. Universal legal capacity promotes social interaction between all members of society, disabled and non disabled. This inclusive mode of social relationship creates opportunity for developing the capabilities of empathy and social solidarity, and supports self-determination. It challenges the privileging of cognitive faculties, recognizes multiple intelligences potentially affecting decision-making, and confronts the discriminatory denial of legal capacity to those suffering mental disorders compared with physical disorders. It extends general defences for criminal responsibility already available to non-disabled persons, as well as individuated procedures in these cases. The author details the battle, often with states parties, for universal capacity with support against the paradigm of selective capacity with provision for substitution. These arguments are of central significance to mental health law.

In their commentary, Ezra Susser and Michaeline Bresnahan observe the history of public health and its connections to social justice, as illustrated through its outstanding practitioners. Thus Philippe Pinel and colleagues proposed that people with mental illnesses should be treated with respect and dignity, William Farr reported appalling mortality rates in English asylums; Edward Jarvis exposed misleading US Census statistics about freed black people's rates of mental illness; Joseph Goldberger discovered the nutritional origins of pellagra through working in asylums; Edgar Sydenstricker envisioned public health as social justice. Recently, reducing cigarette smoking was a capstone achievement, but the link with mental health (through addictive behaviour, and common mental disorders) has been almost completely missed. The low priority given to mental health by public health, tobacco companies' denials, and public mental health leaders not realizing their central role, have all contributed. Though non-communicable diseases have the largest global mortality, the authors emphasize that, as longevity increases, life quality as well as duration increasingly matters. Mental disorders are leading causes of disability and their neglect constrains the advance of health (including mortality) and wealth globally. The public health community needs to stop neglecting mental health and make it central to its agenda.

We are very fortunate to have Eugene Brody's commentary which offers a personal perspective on technology and human rights. Gene Brody died during the preparation of this book. As someone who worked tirelessly and fruitfully in this field for decades, he reflects on his understanding of human rights in relation to mental health, the challenge of moving to practical application, and the impacts of bio- and communications technologies and globalization. In particular he crystallizes this through his early experience as an eyewitness of Nazi prisoners of the International Military Tribunal, and his personal encounter with and response to one in particular, a military gauleiter. The episode goes to the heart of some of the dilemmas raised by this book.

Chapter 1

Human Rights Development: Provenance, Ambit, and Effect

Winton Higgins

Either no individual in mankind has true rights, or all have the same ones; and whoever votes against the rights of another, whatever be his religion, his colour, or his sex, has from that moment abjured his own rights.

The marquis de Condorcet, July 1790.

Where, after all, do universal human rights begin? In small places, close to home—so close and so small that they cannot be seen on any map of the world. Yet they are the world of the individual person; the neighborhood he lives in; the school or college he attends; the factory, farm or office where he works.

Eleanor Roosevelt, speech to the UN general assembly, 27.3.53.

In mental health reform, as in many other areas of progressive policy, human rights doctrines and institutions inspire a great deal of today's discontent and striving for amelioration. The needs and entitlements of people with mental disorders thus find their place as subsets of more general conceptions of rights attaching to the human person as such. For well over two centuries human rights have been discursively available in the West, and in the latter half of the 20th century they gained a significant degree of global applicability, as well as cultural and institutional purchase. For people with mental disorders and other groups who have traditionally suffered stigmatization, discrimination, and exclusion from effective citizenship, the human rights project enjoys an obvious appeal. Yet the premises on which human rights emerged meant people with mental disorders have counted among the last groups to attract the attention of human rights activists and institutions.

In this chapter I seek to sketch the historical development of human rights so as to illuminate the social and moral assumptions that underpin the concept, and to illustrate its problematic coverage—not least of people with mental disorders—and implementation in key historical moments. In passing I will indicate why human rights pioneers often failed to acknowledge the mentally ill; other contributors to this volume will treat today's amelioration of this problem in greater detail. I will start with an account of the philosophical and cultural rise of human rights doctrine premised on the dignity of the human person understood as a rational and potentially autonomous moral agent. From there I will draw attention to the sweeping implied exclusions built into the formally universal terms in which rights were originally couched, and how these exclusions gradually eroded towards our own time. Thirdly, I will look at attempts since the Second World War to make human rights effective in practice. Finally, I will sketch the contradictory influence that globalization now exercises on the human rights project.

The coming of universal human rights

As we shall see, considerable convergence would later appear between Western and non-Western ideas on human rights. Nonetheless, the Western tradition came to provide the pedigree of today's international human rights project. Western moral philosophers began writing about 'the rights of man' during the European Enlightenment, 'the age of reason', in the 18th century. But they themselves drew on an intellectual heritage that stretched back to the Greek philosophers and their conceptions of 'the good life' (a life worthy of a human being) and moral agency— that is, how individuals shoulder their responsibility to cultivate virtue and make moral choices, including what we today would call 'life choices', ones informed by fundamental moral priorities.

Another venerable Western institution that would come to underpin the development of human rights is the gradual crystallization of the rule of law, which we can trace back to the English Magna Carta of 1215. The rule of law (or *Rechtsstaat* in German) seeks to impose legal rights, protections, duties, and due process on rulers and their subjects alike, including (under the *habeas corpus* doctrine) the subject's immunity from arbitrary arrest and detention. The Magna Carta was conceived as an antidote to 'tyranny', or arbitrary power, which has ever since stood for the counter-pole to the rule of law. However, the Western tradition also erected a major barrier to internationalizing the rule of law by promulgating the principle of national sovereignty, enunciated at the Peace of Westphalia in 1648. To this day, regimes that violate human rights typically appeal to their hallowed national sovereignty to denounce universal human rights as a 'foreign', even 'imperialist' imposition, and in this way to deflect 'interference' in their 'internal' affairs by international rights bodies.

The Enlightenment thinkers also inherited a doctrine of natural rights from medieval theologians and early-modern philosophers. In articulating and then superseding these ideas, not least around the emerging concept of individual autonomy, the Enlightenment triggered a veritable cultural revolution in the late 18th century, one that often turned on empathy for the socially excluded. It ushered in 'the age of revolutions' in which the first declarations of human rights provided rallying cries for mass mobilization, seized the popular imagination, and legitimated new forms of government and citizenship.

Philosophical development

The Romans invented the idea that there are moral and legal principles which bind all human collectivities. As their empire sprawled across the known world, and had dealings with many different cultures, they sought an agreed basis of cross-cultural interaction, a *ius gentium* (law of the peoples—*jus gentium* in medieval Latin) based on 'natural law', that is, principles of good conduct that otherwise disparate cultures upheld in common. Moreover, under the influence of the Greek stoics, Cicero and some other Roman law-makers used this concept to argue successfully, for instance, that the children of slaves should not inherit slave status, but rather be restored to the natural rights of free Roman citizens.

The idea of a natural law would resurface in theological debates in medieval Europe, at a time when Christendom was highly institutionalized, and its institutional imperatives trumped its original ethic. The latter proclaimed an order of love, kindness, forgiveness, and peace, yet actually-existing Christianity presented a tableau of gruesome wars of conquest from the successive crusades in the East to the 'American holocaust' (Stannard 1992) in the West, and soon enough, the widespread bloodshed between Catholic and Protestant powers. Maintaining institutional orthodoxies and power bases also involved the routine use of torture, literal and metaphorical witchhunts, and grisly forms of capital punishment for dissidents. Mainstream theologians reinforced institutional power by proclaiming that a Christian's moral responsibility was to obey God, whose dictates were made known by the reigning ecclesiastical authorities. Inevitably under the circumstances, some thinkers began to wonder what God really expected of mere mortals, and on what basis he did so.

St Thomas Aquinas (1225?–1274) founded what came to be known as the 'intellectualist' school, which presented God and humans as occupying the same moral terrain and consulting the same rational map to navigate it. By deploying their own reasoning faculty, humans could infer what God wanted, because he wanted what we can all deduce to be good. The opposing school, the 'voluntarists' (who included Martin Luther [1483–1546], but later also René Descartes [1596–1650]), held that God was in no way bound by human rationality; he could will whatever he put his mind to, and his will-formation was beyond human ken. Ironically, both sides fell back on a revived notion of natural law—the intellectualists because this represented the ultimate basis of both divine and human morality, the voluntarists because they had in effect disqualified God as a moral codifier, which left humans to fend for themselves.

A nascent third school, the sceptics exemplified by Michel de Montaigne (1533–1592), also colluded in seeking a naturalistic ethic—an artefact of human reason and intuition independent of the (unreadable) will of God. Whereas all the thinkers mentioned were devout Christians who retained God as a guarantor of morality in the last instance, their conclusions set the stage for thoroughly secular moral philosophers, such as David Hume (1711–1776) who sought to ground the principles of a naturalistic ethic in science to the exclusion of religion (Schneewind 1998:354; see also Tuck 1979).

Jerome Schneewind (1998) proposes as his basic thesis that these developments in moral philosophy shifted the whole basis of human moral conduct from obedience to ecclesiastical authority ('God') towards human self-governance. The human shift from cosmic vassalage to independent moral agency imbued the human person with a whole new dignity as a rational self-determining individual. In the new version of natural law, this individual enjoyed *rights* to give effect to the choices he (and eventually she) made. Liberalism's 'father', John Locke (1632–1704), conceived of individuals (by which he meant white, male, property-owning ones endowed with 'Life, Liberty and Estate') as the bearers of *pre-social* rights, that is, natural rights that precede and inform individuals' entry into political community.

Immanuel Kant (1724–1804) clinched this development with 'the invention of *autonomy*' (Schneewind 1998) as the ideal condition of the individual in society. The ideal of individual autonomy furnishes the leitmotif of human rights development from this point on.

In certain polities, these rights were already codified to a degree, such as in the English Bill of Rights of 1689. But it only defined 'the ancient rights and liberties' of Englishmen. The rights proposed in the 18th century to uphold autonomous moral agency were not the birthright of a particular nationality; rather, they purported to be *universal* human rights that naturally attached to human beings as rational, autonomous agents. In theory at least, autonomy and the rights required to underpin it attached to human subjects as such, an idea that implied *equal* entitlement irrespective of social status. Late 18th-century revolutionary movements would germinate this egalitarian seed, and its later fortunes will detain us in the sections of this chapter on 'Imperfect universality' and 'Giving effect to human rights'.

Kant based his account of autonomy on a difficult moral theory that no longer rested on a concept of natural rights. Only partly because of this, the concept began to disappear from leading philosophical discourse (Tuck 1979:1). Another reason for its eclipse was a point made by the prominent natural-law theorist Samuel Pufendorf (1632–1694), and more famously picked up by Jeremy Bentham (1748–1832): if one person has a right, then s/he must be the beneficiary of another's duty, and for analytic purposes it would be better to focus on the duty from which the right derives. We will return to this point in the section of this chapter on 'Giving effect to human rights'. By and large prominent philosophers, not least in the English-speaking world, began to avoid the concept of rights as such, with the glaring exception of the neoliberal ideologue Robert Nozick (1974) in his *Anarchy, state, and utopia*. Nonetheless, later contributors to the human rights project would continue to see the rights in question as ones that naturally attach to humans as rational beings.

In a sense the philosophers had done their work in enunciating a doctrine of rights, and the baton now passed to political commentators and activists. Before we turn to them, we might acknowledge the permanent legacy of the philosophers' ideas that would prove crucial to human rights development from the late 18th century. As Schneewind (1998:5) notes, 'we can only be what we can think and say we are. Philosophical debate in the seventeenth and eighteenth centuries was a major source of new ways of conceptualizing our humanity and of discussing it with one another . . . [W]e came to a distinctively modern way of understanding ourselves as moral agents.'

But the 'new ways of conceptualizing our humanity', which turned so crucially on the individual's putative reason and autonomy, did not augur well for people with mental disorders, who were defined as lacking both these qualities.

Revolutionary rights

In the latter half of the 18th century, new ways of *experiencing* our humanity in Western Europe crystallized dramatically to lend philosophical conceptions of human dignity the power to mobilize for the overthrow of state power in the name of rights. Once again, these new ways had been accumulating less dramatically over the preceding four centuries. Norbert Elias ([1969] 2000) has given a brilliant account of them in his magnum opus, *The civilizing process*.

More and more refined 'manners' gradually diffused from court life to broader social strata, and expressed a growing sense of the individual's bodily and affective integrity. Privacy came to shroud the bodily functions of excreting, urinating, and bathing, for which enclosed spaces were set aside; people no longer shared beds (other than with spouses) so readily; special rooms for beds became normal; people no longer ate with their fingers or shared morsels of food, plates, and cutlery. Displays of aggression and strong emotion in public became taboo. *Social acceptance came to demand self-control.*

These innovations contributed to a wider, thoroughgoing social transformation of the 'psychological habitus known as "civilization"' (Elias 2000:369). As the early modern states emerged in the form of absolutist monarchies, they curbed and monopolized violence, thus opening the way for Western European societies to become more differentiated and functionally complex, Elias argues. The requirements of civility became qualitatively more exacting to ensure that individuals discharged their roles precisely and interacted harmoniously.

What Elias (2000:x–xi) calls 'the threshold of socially instilled displeasure and fear' thus dropped appreciably, and those who transgressed were dismissed as bestial or mad. The failure of many people with mental disorders (and later, indigenous peoples) to comply with the new requirements of *civilité* contributed to the sharper relief in which they were identified and stigmatized. 'It is not polite to drink from the dish,' asserts one medieval German authority on table manners, 'although some who approve of this rude habit insolently pick up the dish and pour it down *as if they were mad*' (quoted in Elias 2000:73; emphasis added). The line between the 'well-adjusted' and the disruptively 'mal-adjusted' hardened, and the custodial segregation of the latter in 'bedlams' or asylums became an increasingly attractive option for the maintenance of the civilized social habitus. To an extent, the concept of mental illness and the whole issue of the human rights of people with mental disorders arose out of the civilizing process itself (see Elias 2000:373–9).

A respect for the privacy and the inner life of the individual accompanied the strengthening sense of bodily integrity. Audiences took to listening to concerts and watching theatre in silence, which activities they now regarded as private, inner experiences akin to the rapidly spreading habit of reading novels and journals in silence and solitude. And as Charles Taylor (1989:11–14) has pointed out, these developments fostered a heightened sensitivity to the inner life and suffering of others, in other words, *empathy* with their subjective experience.

In her important contribution to the history of human rights, the cultural historian Lynn Hunt (2007:82) characterizes these changes as the emergence of 'the self-contained person', the bearer of the 18th-century ethos of individual autonomy. (We may pause to note that the development of human rights on this basis did not augur any better for people with mental disorders than the philosophers' conception of rationalistic, autonomous agency.) She emphasizes two cultural practices that turned the autonomous individual into a revolutionary ideal in the latter half of that century. The first of these consisted of hugely popular epistolary novels which dramatized the trials and suffering of lowly but virtuous individuals attempting to assert their autonomy in the teeth of social injustice.

Hunt highlights Richardson's *Pamela* and *Clarissa*, and Rousseau's *Julie*, all of whose heroines under reigning social arrangements are disbarred from autonomy by their sex; but David Bell (2007) suggests she could have included Montesquieu's *Persian letters* and Voltaire's *Candide*. In this new age of the print media and of a swelling reading public asserting its authority as 'public opinion', these novels channelled widespread discontents, and in turn evinced a startling public reaction—including extravagant outpourings of sympathy for the lot of obscure, imagined individuals. Such was their impact that both Catholic and Protestant authorities excoriated them as threats to public decency and established order, and they quickly found their way onto the Vatican's index of forbidden books (Hunt 2007:45–52).

Routine torture, cruel punishments, and (literally) spectacular ways of putting condemned people to death constitute the second cultural practice that mobilized support for human rights in Hunt's (2007) account. Up until the 1760s, judicial torture to extract confessions and the names of accomplices, and such punishments as public flogging, branding, and mutilation, were part of the routine maintenance of the spiritual and temporal order in Western Europe, as were public executions by burning at the stake, breaking on the wheel, drawing and quartering, and slow hanging, with the corpses gibbeted afterwards. Visiting similar retribution on members of miscreants' families completed the judicial edifice. As Foucault (1977) has explained, these gruesome spectacles offered public entertainment which also had the salutary effect of impressing on the populace the awesome majesty of the sovereign and the church that had suffered affront from the felony, heresy, blasphemy, or apostasy in question.

Opposition to this regime galvanized in 1762 around the case of Jean Calas, an aged Calvinist who found his adult son hanged in his home. In the context of ongoing persecution of the Calvinists in France, the authorities accused Calas of murdering his son to prevent him converting to Catholicism; he underwent judicial torture, and though he never admitted guilt, he was sentenced to death by breaking on the wheel, and his surviving family members faced a similar ordeal. Voltaire led the public outcry, but at first only challenged the religious-persecution aspect of the case. This soon changed, however, and Calas's torture and slow, agonizing death became the subject of Voltaire's furious and sustained attack on the responsible institutions, attacks which likeminded publicists joined.

The new cultural practice of empathy and sense of the individual's bodily inviolability had taken hold. Riots in sympathy with the prisoners now began to break out when public punishments were staged, as spectators empathized with their suffering. The print media teemed with demands for the abolition of cruel punishments, including Cesare Beccaria's *Essays on crimes and punishments* (1764), which went through many editions in several languages. 'Once sacred only in a religious order, in which individual bodies could be mutilated and tortured for the greater good,' Lynn Hunt (2007:82) concludes, 'the body became sacred in its own right in a secular order that rested on the autonomy and inviolability of individuals.'

Penal reform took centre stage in Enlightenment-inspired demands for social and political reform. Eminent theologians entered spirited defences of judicial torture and grisly public punishments, but temporal authorities—including even the *ancien régime* in France—saw the writing on the wall: within two decades judicial torture and cruel punishments had been curtailed in much of Western Europe (Hunt 2007:70–82). But as Foucault (1977) points out, a new technology of power and domination was already emerging out of the proposals for penal reform, one that would find application well beyond the confines of the penal system. This was the power of discipline and regimentation whereby people in all sorts of social settings 'internalized the gaze' of the coordinating authority, such that they were 'drilled' into acting in unison without need of external force. 'Disciplinary society' contributed yet another set of demands for predictable behaviour and precise social conformity, such as punctuality and work discipline, to the modern social and psychological habitus, which in turn made it even harder for people with mental disorders to 'fit in'. In 'the age of reason', many of those who manifested unreason found themselves prisoners in 'vast houses of confinement' which threw together the insane, criminals, and the simply indigent (Foucault 2006:47).

While the American and French Revolutions of 1776 and 1789 respectively responded to socio-economic and political discontents, the *putatively self-evident* 'rights of man' figured prominently in mass mobilization and the solemn declarations in which the Revolutionaries couched their missions. 'We hold these truths to be self-evident,' intoned the American Declaration of Independence of 1776, in words penned mainly by Thomas Jefferson, 'that all men are created equal, that they are endowed by their Creator with certain inalienable Rights, that among these are Life, Liberty and the pursuit of Happiness.' Thirteen years later, in Jefferson's physical presence, the marquis de Lafayette would formulate 'the natural, unalienable, and sacred rights of man' for the Declaration of the Rights of Man and of the Citizen adopted by the French National Assembly in 1789, six weeks after the Bastille fell. 'Men are born and remain free and equal in rights,' the substantive rights begin. 'The aim of all political association is the preservation of the natural and imprescriptible rights of man. These rights are liberty, property, security, and resistance to oppression.'

In form, at least, universal human rights had now been invented, albeit in gender-exclusive terms. Two ironies attended their emergence. Firstly, the universalism of their language hid more exclusions than inclusions—a matter I will take up in the section on 'Imperfect universality'. Secondly, human rights had now been nailed to the mast, but in each case the mast in question graced a nation-state, and the gesture contributed to a radical departure in state formation and a renovation of national identity. The progressive aspect of the latter consisted in the new dignity of individual members of the nation as 'citizens' instead of subjects. From now on, at least in Scandinavia and continental Europe, some important new rights came to attach to citizenship, especially political, economic, social, and industrial rights that organized labour and other progressive movements fought for from the mid-19th century (Marshall 1950).

Mainstream Anglo-American conceptions of rights have tended to confine themselves to individualistic civil and political rights to the exclusion of 'collectivist' social and economic ones. Their critics have long argued that civil and political rights mean little to people denied socio-economic rights and thus subjected to social inequity, relative deprivation, and exclusion from the life chances enjoyed by most of their fellow citizens. Real individual autonomy depends on socio-economic security, which progressive movements now sought to put in place (Higgins and Ramia 1999). This point applies with particular force to people with mental disorders, who typically suffer from extreme social marginalization and socio-economic insecurity. The cleavage between these opposed positions has marked the struggle for human rights to the present time.

With the exception of socio-economic rights in some countries, anti-slavery measures, uneven steps towards Jewish emancipation, and limited reforms in favour of women, the Western rights project stagnated from the end of the Napoleonic wars in 1815 to the end of the Second World War in 1945. Other partial exceptions to this pattern include attempts to ameliorate the savagery of modern warfare (the Geneva and Hague Conventions), and the work of the League of Nations which, however, focused more on collective rights than on human ones. In general, regressive forms of nationalism, as well as colonialism and similar geopolitical schemes, created a hostile environment for the development of human rights.

These preoccupations sundered any sense of 'a common humanity', not least as their apologists biologized differences of race and sex to make ubiquitous patterns of oppression and segregation based on these factors appear natural and inevitable. It was only when the Third Reich (1932–45) gathered, distilled, and acted out all these atavistic elements of Western thought in its 'perfect storm' of unprecedented atrocity that support galvanized around the human rights project once more.

For the first time the project now achieved international status, and rights violators faced real retribution. Amid the rubble of Nazism's symbolic heart, Nuremberg, an international tribunal asserted geographically unbounded jurisdiction to try and sentence human rights offenders, and took the further step of grounding humanity's right to be spared the horrors of aggressive war, which had just claimed 50 million lives. We will return to Nuremberg in the section on 'Giving effect to human rights'. Seven weeks after the Third Reich fell, the United Nations Charter was signed; its preamble declared that the new world organization was intended inter alia 'to reaffirm faith in fundamental human rights, in the dignity and worth of the human person, in the equal rights of men and women and of nations large and small.' Three years later the UN would adopt the Universal Declaration of Human Rights (UDHR), which remains the cornerstone of the human rights project to this day.

In hindsight, the development and adoption of the UDHR was—under the historical circumstances of the beginning of the Cold War and a first peak in the Arab-Israeli conflict—something of a miracle, and certainly an astonishing feat of Eleanor Roosevelt, who chaired the UN Human Rights Commission as the document was hammered out under its aegis. The drafting committee included representatives of the protagonists in both conflicts, not least Charles Malik of the Arab League and René Cassin, a staunch French Zionist, both of whom made major contributions to the document. The prominent contributors also included the Chinese philosopher, diplomat, and playwright Peng-chun Chang; and Hansa Mehta, a Brahmin woman, India's representative on the commission, and a well-known campaigner for women's rights and against colonialism. (Glendon 2001:xx, 35). Their substantial participation put paid to the idea that human rights represented a Western imposition on the rest of the world.

The Commission also received the advice of an international panel of leading philosophers set up under the auspices of the UN Educational, Scientific and Cultural Organization (UNESCO), which also attracted significant non-Western participation. The panel found that the rights the draft declaration listed were endemic to their own diverse traditions: 'Where basic rights are concerned, cultural diversity has been exaggerated,' the panel noted (quoted in Glendon 2001:221). The philosophers identified 15 commonly agreed human rights, some of considerable relevance to people with mental disorders: the rights to life; protection of health; work; social assistance in the case of need; property; education; information; freedom of thought and inquiry; fair procedures; political participation; freedom of speech, assembly and association; freedom of worship and the press; citizenship; to rebel against an unjust regime; and to share in progress (Glendon 2001:73–77). The list does not respect Anglo-American inhibitions towards socio-economic rights. All these rights, along with others, found their way into the UDHR.

Thanks to Hansa Mehta's long struggle on the Commission (against the opposition of its feminist chairwoman, among others), the declaration was finally couched in gender-inclusive terms. Apart from that, its debt to the late 18th-century declarations could hardly be clearer. The preamble treats as self-evident that 'recognition of the inherent dignity and of the equal and inalienable rights of all members of the human family is the foundation of freedom, justice and peace in the world.' And in the first two Articles we find, 'All human beings are born free and equal in dignity and rights. They are endowed with reason and conscience and should act towards one another in a spirit of brotherhood . . . Everyone is entitled to all the rights and freedoms set forth in this Declaration, without distinction of any kind, such as race, colour, sex, language, religion, political or other opinion, national or social origin, property, birth or other status.' The rationalist conception of the human person is still there, and the quoted list of exclusions from rights that the declaration overrules does not include people with mental disorders. While there was little warrant by this time to imply exclusion of people with mental disorders from the 'everyone' whom the UDHR endows with rights, its drafters appear not to have considered the plight of those who languished in the rights-free universe of the asylum.

In December 1948, the UN general assembly adopted the UDHR by a 48–0 vote, with eight abstentions. At the time, UN member countries represented 80 per cent of humanity. In her speech to the assembly, Eleanor Roosevelt commended the declaration for its potential to 'become the international Magna Carta of all men everywhere' (quoted in Glendon 2001:166). Subsequent UN conventions and protocols on human rights have complemented the declaration with provisions dealing with specific categories whose rights are in jeopardy, including racial minorities, women, children, indigenous peoples, migrants and their families, 'the disappeared', and most recently, the disabled. The last is of particular relevance to people with mental disorders, and will receive detailed treatment in other contributions to this book. Other UN human rights conventions deal with specific applications of human rights—to genocide, torture and cruel treatment, capital punishment, child prostitution and pornography, and working life.

Imperfect universality

John Locke who, as we saw, developed the idea of the rights-bearing individual, assiduously promoted the slave trade as secretary to the British Board of Trade and as a major shareholder in the Royal Africa Company; he also advocated the extermination of indigenous peoples who resisted European colonization (Coleman and Higgins 2000:55–58). Thomas Jefferson—like several of his declaration-drafting colleagues who also deemed all men to be equal and endowed with inalienable rights—owned slaves. During the French Revolution, the female antislavery activist and playwright, Olympe de Gouges, was guillotined for publishing the 'counterrevolutionary' and 'unnatural' suggestion that women be made equal in rights to men (Hunt 2007:171). Were the pioneering disquisitions and declarations on human rights mere exercises in hypocrisy by privileged poseurs?

Throughout most of the development reviewed here, implicit (and sometimes explicit) exception clauses attached to formally universal declarations and manifestos. The exceptions flowed consistently from what defined human beings as such, and what was understood to constitute a rational and autonomous individual; and later, from the responsibilities and privileges of citizenship. According to the reigning pre-19th century legal fiction, slaves had bargained away their autonomy; social institutions disbarred women and the property-less from ever achieving autonomy; foreigners and prisoners had no place in the social fabric; and children and the insane enjoyed neither reason nor autonomy. So 'the rights of man' were assumed not to extend to any of these groups.

Strenuous campaigns and social changes gradually eroded some of these exceptions. Between the French Revolution and the American Civil War, slavery gradually disappeared from the metropolitan Western countries. Meaningful inroads into women's subordination and marginalization had to wait well over a century from Mary Wollstonecraft's rejoinder to the French Revolutionaries' patriarchal attitudes in 1792, *A vindication of the rights of woman*. Women's rocky road to amelioration lay primarily through mobilization around claims to citizenship rights in national affairs. Apart from limited property and political rights, women's formal rights only see the light of day internationally, and then only as an also-ran, in the UDHR, and later in the 1979 UN convention on discrimination against women. The property-less became beneficiaries of enacted socio-economic rights, and the universal suffrage that most of the Western world had adopted by the late 1920s. Civil rights campaigns from the 1960s eradicated some racial discrimination in some countries, such as the US.

Until recent years, there has been no comparable mobilization around the human rights of people with mental disorders. By the mid-20th century, few advocates of human rights would have excluded them from the rights-bearing 'everyone' of the UDHR. Thanks to Freud's influence, which peaked in Western countries at that time, 'madness' was no longer an inexplicable black box to the educated and even the general public, but rather a form of irrationality that was now rationally explicable. His ideas had penetrated several branches of the social sciences, as well as the arts and literature; at times—as in Alfred Hitchcock's blockbuster, *Spellbound* (1945) and Anatole Litvak's acclaimed *The snake pit* (1948)—they found a place in popular film culture. This cultural influence brought people with mental disorders in from the cold to some extent, but still did not restore them to 'a common humanity' for the purposes of defending their human rights against the institutions and professionals into whose hands they were committed. The other contributions to this book take up this far more recent enterprise.

Giving effect to human rights

None of the declarations of human rights cited above, from the 1776 American Declaration of Independence on, has enjoyed any constitutional status. Human rights, their declaration, and promotion constitute a cultural practice in the sense in which Lynn Hunt coined the term (see Bonnell and Hunt 1999:11–14). In the first instance their efficacy does not take the form of positive law, but rather that of contributing to an international cultural environment in which denial of the rights in question can lead to condemnation and hostile mobilization. The UDHR 'provided the language of accusatory rhetoric,' Mary Ann Glendon (2001:214) comments; and conversely, governments and institutions might seek legitimacy by enacting rights as positive law or working regulations. The UDHR itself does not legally constrain anyone to do anything, for example, but within a year of its adoption most of its provisions reappeared in the 19 Articles of Part 1 of today's German constitution, first promulgated in 1949, where they clearly enjoy the force of positive law.

The UN proclaimed the UDHR precisely as '*a common standard* of achievement for all peoples and all nations, to the end that every individual and every organ of society, keeping this Declaration constantly in mind, shall strive by teaching and education to promote respect for these rights and freedoms and by progressive measures, national and international, to secure their universal and effective recognition and observance.' In other words, in seeking to promote a culture of human rights, the UN invoked the well-understood mechanism of standardization, whereby standards bodies develop—in representative and transparent mechanisms comparable to the UN's own Human Rights Commission—generic optimal solutions to recurring problems (Higgins and Tamm Hallström 2007:691–5). In the first instance a standard is a voluntary instrument, but it aims to establish a visible benchmark, and is available for adoption by collectivities large and small as an integral part of their governance—at which point the initially voluntary standard becomes mandatory. In terms of the quote from Eleanor Roosevelt that heads this chapter, this is where *effective* human rights *begin*.

Once the standard is set and gains moral authority, failure to comply with it attracts negative consequences. For example, the Chinese dictatorship faced a crisis of legitimacy over its egregious (and increasingly notorious) human rights record as it prepared to host the 2008 Olympic Games—a crisis it appears not to have foreseen or known how to respond to.

As we saw in the first section of this chapter, on 'The coming of universal human rights', some early philosophers argued that rights enjoyed by certain people derive from duties imposed on others, which duties should command our primary attention in any rights discourse. Historically, the revived notion of inalienable, universal human rights and the UDHR itself derive from the 1945–6 proceedings of the International Military Tribunal in Nuremberg, and its successor trials under American auspices in that city throughout 1946–9 (Reginbogin and Safferling 2006:13). Human rights culture gained irreversible momentum from the tribunal's overriding perpetrators' impunity under the 'Westphalian' principle of national sovereignty. The latter had up until then shielded from prosecution those who infringed human rights while discharging the authority of the state, and functionaries acting on their orders, that is, the vast majority of rights violators. Under the principles laid down in the tribunal's enabling London Charter, 'state crimes' now became personal crimes to which the ultimate penalty attached. The charter also announced the new indictable counts of waging aggressive war ('crimes against peace') and crimes against humanity. Here was the solution to Pufendorf and Bentham's problem: all human beings now had rights because those who infringed them could be held accountable for doing so. All individuals in authority now became accountable as autonomous moral and legal agents.

The successor trials in Nuremberg included two directed at gross institutionalized human rights abuse by professionals—lawyers and doctors in Nazi Germany. Both cases involved flagrant violation of long-standing professional ethics which imposed clear duties on the practitioners concerned, and by implication asserted the rights of people over whom they exercised power, authority, and expertise. Notoriously, the German medical establishment had colluded in horrific experiments on concentration-camp inmates during the Nazi period (Harmon 2006), and psychiatrists in particular helped mount the T4 'euthanasia' programme in which ten of thousands of people with mental disorders were murdered (Dudley and Gale 2002). For the latter in particular, making human rights effective obviously requires enforced professional ethics and—in line with Eleanor Roosevelt's dictum heading this chapter—institutional codes that incorporate human rights at the local level.

Several tribunals have been set up since Nuremberg to enforce human rights across state borders and thereby reinforce a global culture of human rights. By far the most important and efficacious has been the European Court of Human Rights set up in Strasbourg under the 1950 European Convention on Human Rights. Both the court and the convention are the work of the

47-state Council of Europe, and thus transcend the membership of the EU. Since the convention enjoys the status of a treaty, it binds the state parties, and in recent times individuals have been empowered to approach the court directly to enforce their rights.

The 1998 Treaty (or 'Statute') of Rome established a more direct successor to the international tribunal in Nuremberg: the International Criminal Court (ICC), which has its seat in the Hague and came into existence in 2002. The treaty binds only state parties (120 states have ratified it at the time of writing), and the court's jurisdiction is confined to 'most serious crimes' (genocide, war crimes, crimes against humanity, and aggression) committed by or on the territory of state parties, or by parties nominated by the UN Security Council. Its jurisdiction complements that of national courts: it should only consider cases that the latter cannot or will not pursue. Though the ICC and its enabling instruments do not address human rights by name, quite clearly the broadly defined crimes listed in Articles 7 (crimes against humanity) and 8 (war crimes) of the statute cover many if not all of the ways in which human rights might conceivably be infringed, including those of people with mental disorders.

The ICC is still very much in its infancy, but the chances are that it will prove a worthy successor to—and a logical progression from—the Nuremberg tribunal (Kaul 2006). Its process against the major war criminal Radovan Karadzic, and indictment of a reigning president (Hassan Al Bashir of the Sudan, for genocide, crimes against humanity, and war crimes) augur well for the court's future effectiveness. It takes its place as part of a developing international human rights regime; as the earlier Pinochet and Milosevic cases attest, the world has become an increasingly hostile place for perpetrator heads of state and government in particular. Robert Harris's (2007) novel *The ghost* builds on the intriguing premise that a recently retired British prime minister, temporarily sojourning in the US (an ICC resistor and thus a haven for perpetrators), faces arrest if he returns home because the ICC has taken up the case of his collusion with the CIA's notorious post-9/11 kidnap and torture programme euphemistically entitled 'extraordinary rendition'.

Human rights under globalization

Thanks mainly to the coordinated aggressive neoliberalism of the Thatcher government in Britain (1979–90) and the Reagan administration in the US (1981–89), major changes in governance unfolded in the developed world. Their socio-economic effects would impact on the world more generally, and by the mid-1990s both sets of changes would be conflated in the term 'globalization' (Higgins and Tamm Hallström 2007). In the initial, destructive phase of neoliberalism—diffused through such international institutions as the International Monetary Fund and the World Bank—welfare provisions, social transfers, and thus socio-economic human rights were undermined by the push to slash public expenditures and to 'deregulate'; market forces trumped democratic choices for national socio-economic development. Market outcomes came to determine—and so polarize—the distribution of wealth, income, and life chances to a far greater extent, both domestically in developed societies, and globally along the north-south divide.

As we have seen, human rights mean little in the absence of social equity and security, and in this sense at least, effective human rights have shrunk in the global era (see George 2003; Chomsky 2003; Shiva 2003). For people with mental disorders, the slashing of social budgets in tandem with a 'freedom' rhetoric has in many cases taken them out of now-defunct closed institutions where they were rightless, and thrown them equally rightlessly onto the street or into the arms of overstretched (usually female) relatives and grossly underfunded outpatient clinics.

Developments in American policy and political culture in particular have boded ill for human rights. After the high tide of the US human rights commitment in the immediate aftermath of the Second World War, that country's enthusiasm waned and narrowed to civil and political rights, before going into reverse across the board in more recent times. As noted above, the US was one of just seven countries (in good company with China, Iraq, Israel, Libya, Qatar, and Yemen) that voted against the 1998 Treaty of Rome and the establishment of the ICC. At the last minute (31 December 2000) the Clinton administration signed it, but predictably, the incoming Bush administration refused to ratify it. The latter and its closest allies showed their contempt for the court and the laws it applies in their unprovoked invasion of Iraq in 2003—a specific crime for which the Nuremberg tribunal sentenced eight individuals to death in 1946, and which now attracts the jurisdiction of the ICC.

Continuing US recalcitrance on human rights includes non-ratification of a host of relevant UN covenants and optional protocols thereto, including ones setting up the UN Human Rights Committee, the abolition of the death penalty, abolition of discrimination against women, against torture, and in defence of the rights of the child and of migrant workers. Post-9/11 the US broke ranks with the rest of the Western world in reintroducing torture as a routine recourse for its military and intelligence services, and its quasi-judicial military commissions in Guantánamo Bay were empowered to admit evidence extracted under torture—a throwback to the pre-1770s judicial torture in Western Europe (Sands 2008). These developments have gone hand in hand with the domestic erosion of rights and the rule of law itself within the US (Wolf 2007). This regressive trajectory of the world's sole 'hyperpower' has a negative demonstration effect on the global culture of human rights as a whole.

Yet globalization also has a more positive aspect for human rights defenders, one based on neoliberalism's penchant—in its second, 'constructive' phase—for reorganizing power and imposing regulation 'at a distance', through 'relays' to semi-autonomous (and sometimes actually autonomous) non-government organizations (NGOs), including international ones (Rose 1996:55–6). Neoliberal deregulation called for the partial dismantling of nation-states' direct, mandatory, 'hard' regulation; a new 'soft' regulation compensates for this, and consists of national, international, and transnational NGOs issuing norms, standards, and regulations. Together with other bodies, they thereafter monitor compliance through audits, reports, and certification processes. In the new 'information society', the norms themselves and transgressions against them attract instant notoriety through the internet, and established standards such as the UDHR thereby gain a new efficacy (Korey 2001). The culture of human rights has taken root sufficiently for most governments and public authorities to fear the odium of an adverse report from a UN compliance committee, Amnesty International, Human Rights Watch, and others—or in the case of people with mental disorders, from the likes of Disability Rights International (formerly Mental Disability Rights International). Closer to home, ombudsman's offices and human rights and equal opportunity commissions also exercise increasing moral suasion. Indeed, many public authorities orient their policy to the prospect of gaining a clean bill of health from watchdogs such as these.

Over the last three decades human rights monitoring has gained great impetus from the 1975 Helsinki Accords, the 'final act' of a diplomatic conference held in Helsinki and attended by representatives of Canada, the US, and virtually all European countries, including the USSR. The conference served the purposes of détente as the Cold War wound down. But the enduring importance of its 'final act', signed by 35 countries, lay in its recommitment to the principles of the UDHR and subsequent international human rights conventions, and its commitment to monitoring compliance. Thus arose the International Helsinki Federation for Human Rights, a peak body of the national human rights committees of state parties to the accords; and Helsinki Watch, an umbrella organization for regional 'watch committees'. In 1988 the latter were restructured into today's Human Rights Watch (HRW), an important research and investigative network.

It complements the work of the older Amnesty International, which was founded in 1961 on the mass-movement model: Amnesty now has 3 million members in 150 countries. It, too, produces regular country-by-country reports. Both HRW and Amnesty have gained in profile and clout through the new dignity that globalized 'soft regulation'—as well as the new information and telecommunication technologies—confer on them.

Globalization is thus proving a mixed blessing for human rights. The neoliberal allocation of resources, wealth, income, and life chances have undermined the socio-economic preconditions to effective human rights by intensifying socio-economic insecurity and relative deprivation, and by depriving public authorities of resources with which to respond to needs and develop long-term strategies. Neoliberal ideologues tout markets and their outcomes as both universal panaceas and irresistible forces of nature, beyond moral and political disputation, thus setting the scene for blame-the-victim dismissals of manifest human distress. In their world view, everything from the malign neglect of people with mental disorders to the widespread return of the slave trade (especially in women and children) are matters of indifference: people are commodities who attract their natural price in the marketplace, not dignified bearers of equal, inalienable rights. And the linchpin of the 'globalized' world, the US, has been leading a retreat from the whole human rights project. The Obama administration shows little interest in restoring the country's post-war commitment to that project.

In spite of all this, in this same globalized world, human rights are an idea whose time has come. When activists in Burma, China, Zimbabwe, and many developing countries mobilize against tyranny today, they do so in the name of their human rights. The old objection that human rights represent a Western, 'imperialist' imposition is now merely risible and heard only from dictators in trouble. At the same time, human-rights culture and supporting institutions enjoy a new dignity and efficacy thanks to globalization's own 'soft regulation', transnational monitoring bodies, and their supporting information and communication technologies.

Those who work to realize the rights of people with mental disorders where they matter—in local institutional arrangements—may have a long way to go, but they have considerable cultural and soft-regulatory resources to call on.

References

Bell, D (2007) 'Un dret egal', *London Review of Books*, November, 14–15.

Bonnell, VE and Hunt, L (1999) 'Introduction', in VE Bonnell and L Hunt (eds) *Beyond the cultural turn: new directions in the study of culture and society*. Berkeley, CA: University of California Press, 1–32.

Chomsky, N (2003) '"Recovering rights": a crooked path', in MJ Gibney, *Globalizing rights: the Oxford Amnesty lectures 1999*. Oxford: Oxford University Press, 45–80.

Coleman, A and Higgins, W (2000) 'Racial and cultural diversity in contemporary citizenship', in A Vandenberg (ed) *Citizenship and democracy in a global era*. London: Macmillan, 51–76.

Dudley, M and Gale, F (2002) 'Psychiatrists as a moral community? Psychiatry under the Nazis and its contemporary relevance', *Australian and New Zealand Journal of Psychiatry*, 36, 585–94.

Elias, N (2000) *The civilizing process: sociogenetic and psychogenetic investigations*. Revised 2nd edn. Oxford: Blackwell.

Foucault, M (1977) *Discipline and punish: the birth of the prison*. New York: Vintage.

Foucault, M ([1961] 2006) *History of madness*. London and New York: Routledge.

George, S (2003). 'Globalizing rights?', in MJ Gibney, *Globalizing rights: the Oxford Amnesty lectures 1999*. Oxford: Oxford University Press, 15–33.

Gibney, MJ (2003) *Globalizing rights: the Oxford Amnesty lectures 1999*. Oxford: Oxford University Press.

Glendon, MA (2001) *A world made new: Eleanor Roosevelt and the Universal Declaration of Human Rights*. New York: Random House.

Harmon, L (2006) 'The doctors' trial at Nuremberg', in HR Reginbogin and CMJ Safferling (eds) *The Nuremberg trials: international criminal law since 1945*. Munich: KG Saur.

Harris, R (2007) *The ghost.* London: Hutchinson.

Higgins, W and Ramia, G (1999) 'Social Policy', in W Hudson and J Kane (eds) *Rethinking Australian citizenship.* Melbourne: Cambridge University Press, 136–149.

Higgins, W and Tamm Hallström, K (2007) 'Standardization, globalization and rationalities of government', *Organization,* 14(5), 685–704.

Hunt, L (2007) *Inventing human rights: a history.* New York: Norton.

Kaul, H-P (2006) 'The international criminal court: key features and current challenges', in HR Reginbogin and CMJ Safferling (eds) *The Nuremberg trials: international criminal law since 1945.* Munich: KG Saur.

Korey, W (2001) *NGOs and the Universal Declaration of Human Rights: 'a curious grapevine'.* New York: Palgrave.

Marshall, TH (1950) *Citizenship and social class and other essays.* Cambridge, UK: Cambridge University Press.

Nozick, R (1974) *Anarchy, state, and utopia.* Oxford: Oxford University Press.

Reginbogin, HR and Safferling CJM (eds) (2006) *The Nuremberg trials: international criminal law since 1945.* Munich: KG Saur.

Rose, N (1996) 'Governing "advanced" liberal democracies', in A Barry et al. (eds) *Foucault and political reason: liberalism, neo-liberalism and rationalities of government.* London: UCL Press, 37–64.

Sands, P (2008) *Torture team: deception, cruelty and the compromise of law.* London: Allen Lane.

Schneewind, JB (1998) *The invention of autonomy: a history of modern moral philosophy.* Cambridge, UK: Cambridge University Press.

Shiva, V (2003) 'Food rights, free trade and fascism', in MJ Gibney, *Globalizing rights: the Oxford Amnesty lectures 1999.* Oxford: Oxford University Press, 87–108.

Stannard, D (1992) *American holocaust: Columbus and conquest of the New World.* New York: Oxford University Press.

Taylor, C (1989) *Sources of the self: the making of modern identity.* Cambridge, MA: Harvard University Press.

Tuck, R (1979) *Natural rights theories: their origin and development.* Cambridge, UK: Cambridge University Press.

Wolf, N (2007) *The end of America: letter of warning to a young patriot.* Melbourne: Scribe.

Chapter 2

Mental Health and Illness as Human Rights Issues

Philosophical, Historical, and Social Perspectives and Controversies

Charles Watters

Introduction

In this chapter various senses in which mental health and illness are linked to ideas of human rights are explored. I argue that the understanding of mental health and illness as human rights issues is necessarily linked to the placement of these concepts in historical context. It is beyond the scope of this chapter to do more than highlight a few examples of the way these concepts have changed and evolved over time. The arguments are largely confined to examination of instances where there are distinctive interrelationships between the two fields. What is suggested is that, through emphasizing the historical contexts, these relationships are revealed as complex and nuanced. Mental illnesses are, to paraphrase one notable commentator, disorders 'in time' and it is a distortion to position them as though they were fixed and immutable entities. Human rights are likewise appropriately seen not as a mere 'given' but operate in distinctive ways within particular political contexts (Chandler 2006). The interplay of these two discourses has developed in distinctive ways in contemporary times and with acute impacts on some of the world's most vulnerable populations.

The parameters of mental health and illness have evolved and changed over time to encompass an ever wider range of disorders. As conceptualizations of mental health and illness have encompassed an ever wider set of conditions, so has the range of treatments available. In one important sense, human rights here relates to a right to appropriate health care for identifiable mental health problems. Thus we speak of members of the public having a right to treatment for conditions such as depression. The rights to treatment may, however, be mitigated by a person's economic status, for example, in countries where the health care system is based on a health insurance model, and where provision for the poor in limited to emergency services. The right to treatment may also be crucially related to one's immigration status, as in the case of asylum seekers in industrialized countries. In these contexts, advocacy for human rights may provide strong challenges to governments that are inclined to limit entitlement to health care to those with rights to remain in the territory.

A second set of rights can be identified as relating to the rights of people who have already been diagnosed as having mental illnesses and are receiving treatment from mental health services. This group is variously identified as 'the mentally ill', or in more recent terminology, 'service users'. Questions arise as to the extent to which service users have a right to full participation in society and how this right may be embodied in and facilitated by policies and procedures. In many countries, concern to address this right has resulted in various policies aimed at ensuring that service users are consulted about the services they are offered. This consultation can take the form of the development of 'patients councils' in hospitals and 'user groups and forums' in the community. There is ongoing debate regarding the extent to which these initiatives offer genuine consultation or are merely 'tokenistic', in that service users rarely actually influence decision making (Pilgrim and Rogers 1997).

An extreme but still widespread issue relating to the human rights of service users is their often forced incarceration and the conditions they experience within psychiatric hospitals. Disability Rights International (formerly Mental Disability Rights International), for example, reports ongoing human rights abuses in every corner of the globe, with recent investigations highlighting the situations in Serbia, Kosovo, Argentina, Mexico, Romania, Turkey, and Hungary (<http://www.disabilityrightsintl.org/>). The often appalling conditions under which people are detained represent gross violations of human rights. The author has personally witnessed situations in Latin America in which patients are routinely tied to beds and maintained in unsanitary conditions. Neglect of basic human rights is not confined to so-called 'developing countries', and instances have been recorded also within the EU and in North America.

While there are specific concerns relating to the treatment of those who have been diagnosed with mental health problems, there are further concerns relating to populations who may be in need of mental health care but are placed outside of mental health systems. Silove and colleagues in Australia have, for example, highlighted the mental health problems among asylum seekers detained in camps while their asylum claims are examined or while facing deportation (Silove et al. 2007). Here widespread mental health problems often have gone undetected and have been systematically neglected. These include the ongoing impact of experiences within asylum seekers' countries of origin that have led to continuing mental health problems in post-migration contexts. Silove and others have shown that adverse experiences in countries of asylum can exacerbate existing mental health problems such as post-traumatic stress disorder and lead to the creation of new mental health problems.

The expanding parameters of mental health

As indicated above, the relation between mental health and human rights should be seen within a historical context. Both are relatively modern concepts that may be seen as developing from principles dating back to antiquity. Mental health encompasses a range of meanings and associations that have undergone significant changes over time. In contemporary times its usage is ubiquitous, with 'mental health' referring to an anticipated standard of psychological well-being, and 'mental illness' often replaced by the arguably less stigmatizing reference to 'mental health problems'. What were previously referred to as psychiatric services are now routinely referred to as mental health services and these encompass the work of professionals from a range of disciplines.

While the use of the term is commonplace, it is often ill defined. This gives rise to questions as to what constitutes a mentally healthy person and in turn wider questions regarding optimal personal characteristics and social conditions. Over the past century or so there has been a significant shift from a conception of mental health as a product of individuals' innate personal characteristics and position within society, to one in which familial and social environments play an ever more significant role. Derek Russell Davis, in a contribution to the *Oxford Companion to the Mind*, argued that for the English middle class at the turn of the 19th century, 'mens sana in corpore sano'—a sound mind in a sound body—would have included 'a disciplined intelligence, a well-stocked memory, qualities of leadership appropriate to a persons' station, a respect for morality and a sense of what life means' (Russell Davis 1987:469). Thus, a 'sound mind' was related both to psychological qualities of intelligence and memory, and additionally to what was deemed an appropriate orientation towards society through moral behaviour and propriety. This appropriate orientation included conducting oneself in accordance with one's position within highly stratified societies. Furthermore, mental health was predicated upon a healthy body, and was thus inconceivable for those with physical disabilities.

In general there is a consensus across most salient disciplines that mental health and illness should not be viewed primarily in a context of inalienable personal characteristics but rather one of familial and societal relations. Pilgrim and Rogers (1999), point out that childhood 'is a time when most of the rules and mores associated with the society and particular class and culture which the child inhabits are learned'. Bowlby has contributed significantly to perspectives offering a link between maternal deprivation and mental health by arguing in oft-cited remarks that an essential condition for the mental health and development of the child is a 'warm, intimate, and continuous relationship with his mother in which both find satisfaction and enjoyment' (1951:1). Where familial relations were disrupted, this would have adverse consequences for children's development and for mental health. Erikson proposed a series of developmental landmarks or 'crises' through which children and adolescents must pass in order to develop into mentally healthy adults. The social training the child receives within their familial environment equips or disables their ability to negotiate these crises successfully (Erikson 1995).

In recent times the parameters of the concept of mental health have widened considerably so that the World Health Organization defines mental health as:

> . . . a state of well-being in which every individual realizes his or her own potential, can cope with the normal stresses of life, can work productively and fruitfully, and is able to make a contribution to her or his community (WHO 2007)

The implications of this capacious definition are considerable and imply that the achievement of mental health in a population can only be gained through the coordinated efforts of a wide range of agencies operating well beyond what are normally viewed as services for people suffering from mental illnesses. The achievement of each individual's potential implies a society in which everyone has full access to the resources necessary to help them achieve the best possible employment commensurate with their capabilities. The ability to cope with the 'normal stresses of life' implies not only personal resources but also access to familial and community networks.

Moreover, the WHO definition suggests potentially a much wider role for mental health services than that normally perceived by those responsible for their development and implementation. This greatly exceeds the role of a mental health team receiving referrals in respect of people suffering neurotic and psychotic disorders, and implies a closer link to conceptions of preventative psychiatry associated, for example, with Caplan and others (Samson, 1995:67).

These definitional issues are important in considering the relationship between mental health and illness and human rights. The relationship can be seen across three axes or trajectories:

- The rights of people to lives that will support their mental health and well-being;
- The rights of people with mental health disorders to appropriate mental health services;
- The rights of people with mental health problems not to be discriminated against in education, employment, and other aspects of economic and social life.

These various rights have distinctive implications for the development and organization of mental health services and of wider society. As such it suggests a wider area of engagement than does a preoccupation with the rights of the mentally ill, as a predefined segment of society. The vision here is of a society that does not merely respond to mental illness but that creates a nurturing and supportive environment for its members that serves to promote and enhance their mental health.

Its rather utopian terms envisage a society that fully supports human rights. How else could a 'state of well-being in which everyone realises their full potential' be achieved?

The third orientation is present in recent formulations on human rights and mental health. Parker, for example, argues that a human rights perspective mental health policy must ensure that people with mental health problems 'can participate in society as equal citizens' (2007:308). There is, in short, a distinctive group of people with mental health problems and the goal of policy makers must be to facilitate their equitable access to social goods. By contrast, the WHO definition has a strongly preventative orientation and implies that people have the right to live in societies where their mental health and well being are supported. It suggests positive action in a range of areas, including housing, community development, education, health care, and employment, to provide an infrastructure that enhances mental health. The process of supporting mental health is thus the province of a range of policy makers and cuts across traditional delineations of government departments.

As such, concern with mental health is closely linked to concern about communities and specifically with the fragmentation of social networks documented in recent research. This association is, of course, hardly new. In Brown and Harris' (Brown and Harris 1978) classic study of depression among women in London, they presented strong evidence that close, confiding relationships could be important factors in mitigating the chance of depression following major life events. Further studies have shown that 'regardless of how much stress an individual is under, people with a higher level of social contacts tend to report better mental health' (Halpern 2005:77). Halpern has noted further that social interaction within neighbourhoods may be of more significance for well being that the quality of residences. Research has also shown a 'group density effect' on well being whereby people from ethnic groups develop 'bonding' social capital in areas with populations from the same group.

This emphasis on the social aspect of mental health may thus be seen as having two possible orientations: an orientation towards prevention in which people are seen as having the right to a society that supports their mental health and well being; and towards social support towards those people who are already deemed to be suffering from mental health problems.

Human rights and bare life

There is a further fundamental issue here concerning the rights enjoyed by people who are deemed to be suffering from mental health problems. An emphasis on human rights can potentially undermine that of a fuller set of rights enjoyed by the citizen. Arguably, by invoking the *human* rights of the mentally ill, attention may shift away from the range of rights and entitlements mentally ill people should enjoy as citizens of a society. This concern is implicit in the work of Hannah Arendt who argues that for the 'survivors of the extermination camps, the inmates of concentration and interment camps…the abstract nakedness of being nothing but human was their greatest danger'. To counter this fear, they 'insisted on their nationality, the last sign of their former citizenship, as their only remaining and recognised tie with humanity' (1976:300). The contemporary philosopher Giorgio Agamben continues in this vein invoking the Aristotelian distinction between bare life—acta vita—and the position of the citizen of the city state. The citizen enjoyed political rights that elevated him or her above those outside the city who existed in a form of bare life.

Arendt's argument suggests that the invocation of human rights for disadvantaged populations may be tantamount to a denial of a population's potential for citizenship. Extending this to the mentally ill suggests that the invocation of human rights may suggest a diminution in the potential for full engagement in society as a citizen of a country. If we return to the image of a patient tied to a bed within a psychiatric hospital, we can see both the power and limitations of an emphasis on human rights. Through invoking human rights legislation and conventions, those who support the rights of the patient may bring national and international pressure to bare on the relevant authorities in an effort to change the systems and the practices within them. Human rights conventions have been a powerful tool used by NGOs such as Human Rights Watch and Amnesty International to bring to light a wide range of abuses undertaken by arms of government in various countries. However, the scope of human rights is often to challenge gross abuses. It may result in the patient being untied but does not ensure her rehabilitation as a citizen, participating fully in her society.

The strengths and limitations of a human rights approach may be usefully explored further in relation to the concepts of positive and negative liberty (Berlin 1969). Put simply, negative liberty implies a freedom from constraint. Conversely it suggests individuals will receive little support from the state to realize their goals. Positive liberty, by contrast, suggests that the state has a fundamental role in creating the environment within which individuals can realize their goals. For the psychiatric patient chained to a bed, negative liberty could be construed as giving the patient freedom from 'cruel, inhuman or degrading treatment' referred to in Article 5 of the Universal Declaration of Human Rights. In practice, this freedom may ensure that the patient has access to no more than a form of 'bare life' referred to by Agamben, for example. However, arguably, for the patient to go beyond bare life requires the introduction of external factors that will facilitate her engagement with wider society; in other words, a form of positive liberty involving intervention by the state to provide a programme of health care and rehabilitation.

This relationship between human rights and the responsibilities of agencies to help individuals realize those rights has been explored by Amartya Sen in what he has termed 'the coherence critique' (Sen 1999:230). It refers to the position that a person's right, 'must be coupled with another agent's duty to provide the first person with that something'. Otherwise the invocation of a person's human rights may be seen as little more than 'loose talk'. While seeing the merits of this view, particularly in legal contexts, Sen nevertheless argues that in 'normative discussions rights are often championed as entitlements or powers or immunities that it would be good for people to have'. Furthermore, he points out that it is surely possible to distinguish between a right that a person has which has not been fulfilled and a right a person does not have.

Entitlement and access

As I have argued elsewhere, it is useful in this respect to distinguish between entitlements and access (Watters 2008). Entitlements here relates to a formal right enshrined in law and policy to receive a certain range of services. An example here would be an entitlement to a full range of health care services. The question of access relates to the extent to which an individual or group is able to realize this entitlement. An example here is the provision of health care for asylum seekers in industrialized countries. In some countries, asylum seekers have entitlement only to a limited range of health provision, in relation, for example to emergency care while in others they may be formally entitled to the full range of health care provided to the general population. This entitlement is important in articulating and forming a legal and policy basis for judging the appropriate practice in services. However, to understand access one must move beyond entitlement and consider the extent to which in practice asylum seekers are able to receive the services to which they are entitled. Investigation may show, for example, that while asylum seekers may be entitled to receive the services of a GP, they may have problems in gaining access to one. Refugee children may be entitled to school places but may have problems in gaining places in local schools because of restrictive admissions policies.

In terms of mental health care, entitlement to a full range of services may be enshrined in law and policy but in practice there is evidence that certain groups have difficulties in gaining access to particular types of services. Research evidence has shown for example that women may have problems in gaining access to services for particular complaints and that ethnic minority groups have particular problems in gaining access to, for example, counselling and psychotherapy (Fernando 1995). These limitations to services may be considered within a context of positive freedom in that they involve the intervention of a collectivity, i.e. the state. However, the idea of entitlements suggests here something more benign than the many concepts of positive liberty. Entitlement does not suggest coercion but rather a set of resources that may be available to a person. I am, for example, feeling ill and am entitled to free treatment by a GP so may choose to go and see one. The question of access relates to possible impediments on the way to realizing my entitlement. In Berlinian terms, access may be construed as a constraint on negative liberty as it affects the realization of choices I have made within a framework of entitlement.

From a historical perspective, the ever widening range of identifiable mental health problems has given rise to a concomitant increase in the range of potential treatments. There is an ongoing and energetic debate about the categories of mental disorders and the effectiveness of treatments. The official recognition of particular conditions as mental illnesses introduces their insertion into formal entitlements for treatment, whether through health insurance policies or a national health system. The introduction of a new disease may have considerable consequences in relation to the economics and the structures of service provision. In other words, it introduces, or in cases where a condition is no longer regarded as a mental health problem may circumscribe, the right to and availability of treatments.

Post-traumatic stress disorder

A notable case here relates to the introduction of post-traumatic stress disorder (PTSD) into the official nosology of the American Psychiatric Association in 1980. According to Allan Young's detailed examination of the origins and development of PTSD, the disorder should not be regarded as an ever present phenomenon that was 'discovered' by science in recent times. Rather, he contends, 'it is glued together by the practices, technologies, and narratives with which it is diagnosed, studied, treated, and represented by the various interests, institutions and moral arguments that mobilised these efforts and resources' (Young 1995:5). He goes on to demonstrate how these elements have evolved historically and, in particular, to show the role of distinctive interests and institutions in the emergence of a diagnostic category. Young's study has wide ranging implications, not least for the philosophy of science. While it is not possible to explore these in depth in the present paper, it is useful for the present purposes to reflect a little on its implications for examining the relationship between mental health and human rights.

Young highlights the role of specific American veterans' organizations in campaigning for official recognition of, and treatment for, veterans who were experiencing traumatic effects from their engagement in the Vietnam War. The formulation of the diagnostic category PTSD had far reaching effects on the funding and shape of professional services for veterans. Specifically, the linkage of the disorder to soldiers' experiences of events in the war provided a legitimate context for the release of significant financial resources. In other words, psychiatric aetiology moved beyond the parameters of scientific endeavour to a hotly contested site for the determination of federal funding and the structuring of service provision. As such, it was inextricably linked to the rights of soldiers to treatment for injuries resulting from war. In the provision and funding of services 'top priority goes to providing health care and benefits for disabilities incurred in the course of active duty, that is, for service connected" disabilities. And there lay the rub, for there was no doubt that PTSD would qualify as service connected" once it entered the official nosology' (Young, 1995:113).

As Young demonstrates, the creation of PTSD is appropriately seen as a historical process in which the role of various interest groups can be identified in its conception and development. That a history of PTSD can be traced in this way is not to dismiss the disorder as somehow lacking reality. Young addresses the issue directly: 'If, as I am claiming, PTSD is a historical product, does this mean that it is not real? …On the contrary, the reality of PTSD is confirmed empirically by its place in people's lives, by their experiences and convictions, and by the personal and collective investments that have been made in it' (1995:5). Indeed, if the development of psychiatric taxonomies is subjected to historical scrutiny then considerable fluctuations can be observed in the emergence and disappearance of a range of disorders over time. For example, in 1973, homosexuality was removed from the Diagnostic and Statistical Manual of Mental Disorders (DSM) by the American Psychiatric Association, to be replaced by the less capacious diagnosis of ego-dystonic homosexuality. The explicit diagnostic reference to homosexuality within DSM was only abandoned fully in 1986. The emergence and disappearance of hysteria, for example, also displays distinctive historical contours.

More generally, enquiries into the origins and development of mental disorders reveal a dialectical relationship between nature and history. The ostensibly fixed and immutable disease entities discovered by science are revealed through historical enquiry to be composite phenomena involving a convergence of various interests and orientations, of which pure scientific enquiry may be only one. The emergence of discourses of rights in these contexts may be inextricably linked to the recognition of a disorder in official nosology. In the case of PTSD, the accordance of official status within DSM had the attendant effect of ensuring that veterans were entitled to treatment and to the costs of that treatment being met.

Asylum seekers and refugees

A concern with the right to treatment also underpins recent research into the health and mental health care of asylum seekers and refugees. Researchers have noted significant levels of mental health problems among refugees and these problems often going unrecognized and untreated (Silove et al. 2000). NGOs such as Physicians for Human Rights have, through their campaign for the 'Right to Health', enshrined a right to appropriate and adequate medical care as a cornerstone of meeting the human rights of disadvantaged populations. This right to treatment also underpins the work of leading researchers and campaigners who highlight the ways in which governmental and corporate interests may operate to cause and to perpetuate health inequalities resulting in some of the most desperate peoples lacking access to basic medications and consequently dying of avoidable diseases (Farmer 2003).

A recent focus for these rights based approaches has been the situation of unaccompanied and asylum seeking children in industrialized countries. In 2009, the plight of 'hidden children' in Scandinavia was highlighted at a major conference organized by the eminent paediatrician and human rights campaigner, Henry Ascher. Save the Children has reported that hundreds of children arrive in Sweden without appropriate papers and live hidden and precarious lives with no access to health care, accommodation, and education. Further concerns have been expressed across industrialized countries at the large numbers of undocumented and asylum seeking children who experience severe problems in accessing health care. Here again a distinction between entitlement and access is important. While many countries sign the relevant conventions, for example the Convention on the Rights of the Child, in practice undocumented children are not given access to basic services and often live in appalling conditions. Recent reports by Human Rights Watch and Amnesty International, for example, have provided detailed accounts of the destitution faced by children in signatory countries such as Greece and Spain (Human Rights Watch 2002; Amnesty International 2005).

In the field of mental health and human rights, the gap between laws and policies and their implementations raises important methodological and practical questions. It implies the necessity for multi-dimensional and multi-disciplinary approaches towards investigating the provision of mental health services, embracing the examination of laws and policies as well as actual practice 'on the ground'. In other words, the investigation of human rights requires more than examination of the formal realm of entitlements, and must encompass investigation into processes through which particular groups and individuals gain, or are excluded from, access to services.

The study of the particular challenges facing asylum seekers and refugees with mental health problems reveals further important dimensions of the relationships between mental health and human rights. Specifically there is evidence that in recent years asylum seekers arriving in industrialized countries are having their claims viewed with increasing scepticism within a predominant 'culture of mistrust' (Knudsen 1995; Bhabha and Finch 2006). This mistrust is linked to increasingly prevalent views that these are not people fleeing from well founded fear of persecution, but are economic migrants seeking better lives in the West. In this context, asylum seeking has been depoliticized and delegitimized and has been contrasted to refugee flows in the 1970s, when those arriving in Western countries were seen as victims and worthy of social and political support. These refugees were often fleeing communist countries or military dictatorships such as Pinochet in Chile. It may be argued that part of the delegitimation in recent years arises from the fact that the refugees arriving in the West are fleeing counties that are embroiled in conflicts involving Western powers, for example, Iraq and Afghanistan. Here, the vision of the enemy 'other' fighting 'our' troops elides into the vision of the other arriving and seeking sanctuary on our shores.

In an analysis of the situation in France, Fassin has noted that while the numbers of asylum seekers being recognized as legitimate refugees has decreased markedly, there has been a concomitant increase in the numbers allowed to stay for humanitarian reasons, with health and mental health reasons prominent (Fassin 2001). Elsewhere, ever increasing emphasis has been placed on the mental health problems of refugees with particular emphasis placed on levels of PTSD. Rutter has argued that no less than 70 per cent of the published papers on refugee children concern mental health issues (Rutter 2006). The centrality of concern for refugees' mental health represents a shift in emphasis from the political body to the sick body (Fassin 2001). It also importantly marks a shift in emphasis from consideration of human rights in general as in the universal right to seek asylum from persecution to an arguably more circumscribed set of rights, the recognition of which hinges on the legitimacy of disease. Within this context, asylum seekers in industrialized countries seek to prove the damaging effects on their mental and physical health caused by exposure to violence. This allows the possibility of achieving legitimacy through what I have referred to elsewhere as the 'avenue of access' offered by sickness (Watters 2001b).

This shift from a depoliticization of asylum seeking towards an emphasis on the sick or suffering body gives rise to a central role of medical evidence in asylum cases. Reports offered, for example, by the London based Medical Foundation for the Care of Victims of Torture may be of crucial significance in determining an individual's right to remain. For asylum seekers whose claims are rejected, the revealing of mental health problems may be a last resort in seeking to circumvent deportation. I have elsewhere identified this as a process of 'strategic categorization' whereby mental health is emphasized by those working with asylum seekers, not to misguide authorities, but to highlight an area of potential legitimacy within a general erosion of political asylum (Watters 2001a).

This shift may be seen in the wider context of global political economy, thus presenting human rights not as a universal and timeless value system but as a discourse embedded in specific political contexts. A historical analysis of the development and positioning of human rights may help reveal the complex interrelationships with mental health. This analysis is not only of theoretical import. By locating the truncated and ever narrowing avenues of access available to vulnerable populations, we can reveal ever more acutely the constraints placed on those seeking a way of life that is merely routine and commonplace to so many in the industrialized world.

Locating human rights and mental health

Let us return to the concerns raised by Arendt, specifically the argument that the location of individuals within a discourse of human rights can be at the expense of a concern with their full participation in society. This has, I argue, resonance also in respect of a preoccupation with issues of entitlement at the expense of concerns about access and, further, with a complex interrelationship between negative and positive liberty. If, as Arendt's work implies, human rights offers only recourse to a most basic level of being in which rights are accorded by virtue of being human rather than as a full member of a society, we can enquire as to what circumstances the rights of the mentally ill can be realized fully as citizens.

An inhibiting factor in the realization of this goal is, according to Nussbaum, the very context in which political liberalism has developed. Specifically, Nussbaum examines the foundations and implications of Rawls' conception of a social contract. According to Rawls, the 'fundamental problem of social justice arises between those who are full and active and morally conscientious participants in society, and directly, or indirectly associated together throughout a complete life' (Rawls 1980:546 cited in Nussbaum 2006:110). A resonance of the idea of participating citizens can be found in 17th and 18th century accounts of the origins of the idea of rights and justice that underpins political liberalism. According to Nussbaum, the central idea of the social contract is underpinned by a 'general image of society as a contract for mutual advantage…among people who are 'free, equal and independent' with the classical theorists assuming that 'their contracting agents were men who were roughly equal in capacity, and capable of productive economic activity' (p. 14).

These formulations presupposed the exclusion of various parties including women, children, and elderly people. Despite these groups being recognized in some subsequent formulations, Nussbaum argues that no social contract doctrine, however, 'includes people with severe and atypical physical and mental impairment in the group of those by whom basic political principles are chosen…people with severe mental impairments in particular were not even educated. They were hidden away in institutions or left to die from neglect, they were never considered part of the public realm' (p. 15).

This implicit exclusion of the mentally ill underpins Rawls' evocation of the principles of a just society. Here, the guiding idea for the principles of justice are 'the principles that free and rational persons concerned to further their own interests would accept in an initial position of equality' (p. 11). Rawls' highly influential work on theory of justice and political liberalism excludes at a foundational level people with disabilities and those with mental impairments. Engaging with the latter is of secondary concern. According to Nussbaum, 'it is clear enough that Rawls believes we can adequately design basic political principles without taking abnormal" impairments, either physical or mental and either temporary or permanent, into account' (Nussbaum 2006:111).

It is beyond the scope of this chapter to explore Nussbaum's extensive critique of Rawls in detail. However, her central argument for what she has termed a 'capabilities approach' offers a potential to resolve some of the problems and complexities highlighted above. A virtue of the capabilities approach is that it offers a balance between the laissez-faire implied in theories of negative liberty and offering a positive role for government in assisting people experiencing disadvantages. Sen, for example, has highlighted a range of 'instrumental freedoms' that may be a prerequisite to people enjoying overall freedom. These include political freedoms, economic facilities, social opportunities, transparency guarantees, and protective security. Social opportunities here refers to 'the arrangements that society makes for education, health care and so on, which influence the individual's substantive freedom to live better' (Sen 1999:39). Throughout the development of capabilities theory, as articulated by Nussbaum and Sen, there is a fundamental interpenetration between entitlement and the social and political actions that may be necessary to realize entitlement in practical form. In proposing a programme of social and political action, the exercise of human agency is seen as interdependent with a set of social obligations.

As such, capabilities theory offers a potential bridge between the expounding of rights and entitlements and the actions necessary to realize them. It is not predicated upon a foundational conception of a contract between physically and mentally healthy people but rather seeks to engage with the totality of humanity. In addressing the relationship between mental health and human rights, it offers a potentially fruitful middle way between entitlement and access, and negative and positive freedoms. It further offers an opportunity to encourage programmes that are not predicated upon a discrete group of people labelled the 'mentally ill', 'service users', or suchlike but views mental health as foundational for the whole of society.

References

Agamben, G (1998) *Homo Sacer: Sovereign Power and Bare Life*. Palo Alto, CA: Stanford University Press.

Amnesty International (2005) *Spain: the Southern border*. London: Amnesty International.

Arendt, H (1976) *The Origins of Totalitarianism*. San Diego, CA: Harcourt.

Berlin, I (1969) *Four Essays on Liberty*. Oxford: Oxford University Press.

Bhabha, J and Finch, N (2006) *Seeking Asylum Alone: Unaccompanied and Separated Children and Refugee Protection in the UK*. London: Macarthur Foundation.

Bowlby, J (1951) *Maternal Care and Mental Health*. Geneva: WHO.

Brown, GW and Harris, TO (1978) *The Social Origins of Depression*. London: Tavistock.

Chandler, D (2006) *From Kosovo to Kabul and Beyond: Human Rights and International Intervention*. London: Pluto Press.

Erikson, E (1995) *Identity: Youth and Crisis*. New York, NY: Norton.

Farmer, P (2003) *Pathologies of Power, Health, Human Rights, and the New War on the Poor*. Berkeley, CA: University of California Press.

Fassin, D (2001) 'The biopolitics of otherness: Undocumented foreigners and racial discrimination in French public debate', *Anthropology Today*, 17(1), 3–7.

Halpern, D (2005) *Social Capital*. Cambridge, UK: Polity Press.

Human Rights Watch (2002) *Nowhere to Turn: State Abuses of Unaccompanied Migrant Children by Spain and Morocco*. New York, NY: Human Rights Watch.

Knapp, M, McDaid, D, Mossialos, E, and Thornicroft, G (eds) (2007) *Mental Health Policy and Practice Across Europe*. European Observatory on Health Systems and Policies Series. Milton Keynes: Open University Press.

Knudsen, J (1995) 'When Trust is on Trial: Negotiating Refugee Narratives', in E Valentine Daniel and J Knudsen (eds) *Mistrusting Refugees*. Berkeley, CA: University of California Press, 13–35.

Nussbaum, M (2006) *Frontiers of Justice: Disability, Nationality, Species Membership*. Cambridge, MA: Harvard University Press.

Parker, C (2007) 'Developing Mental Health Policy: A Human Rights Perspective', in M Knapp, D McDaid, E Mossialos, and G Thornicroft (eds) *Mental Health Policy and Practice Across Europe*. European Observatory on Health Systems and Policies Series. Milton Keynes: Open University Press, 308–335.

Pilgrim, D and Rogers, A (1999) *A Sociology of Mental Health and Illness*. 2nd edn. Milton Keynes: Open University Press.

Russell Davis, D (1987) 'Mental Health', in R Gregory (ed), *Oxford Companion to the Mind*. Oxford: Oxford University Press.

Rutter, J (2006) *Refugee Children in the UK*. Milton Keynes: Open University Press.

Samson, C (1995) 'Madness and Psychiatry', in B Turner (ed), *Medical Power and Social Knowledge*. 2nd edn. London: Sage, 55–83.

Sen, A (1999) *Development as Freedom*. Oxford: Oxford University Press.

Silove, D, Austin, P, and Steel, Z (2007) 'No Refuge from Terror: The Impact of Detention on the Mental Health of Trauma-affected Refugees Seeking Asylum in Australia', *Transcultural Psychiatry*, 44(3), 359–93.

Silove, D, Steel, Z, McGorry, P, and Dobny, J (1999). 'Problems Tamil asylum seekers encounter in accessing health and welfare services in Australia', *Social Science and Medicine*, 49, 951–56.

Silove, D, Steel, Z, and Watters, C. (2000) 'Policies of Deterrence and the Mental Health of Asylum Seekers', *Journal of the American Medical Association*, 284(5), 604–11.

Watters, C (2001a) 'Emerging Paradigms in the Mental Health Care of Refugees', *Social Science and Medicine*, 52, 1709–18.

Watters, C (2001b) 'Avenues of Access and the Moral Economy of Legitimacy', *Anthropology Today*, 17(2), 22–3.

Watters, C (2008) *Refugee Children: Towards the Next Horizon*. London: Routledge.

World Health Organization (2007) *What is mental health?* Online Q&A, 3 September. available at http://www.who.int/features/qa/62/en/index.html, accessed 18th January 2012.

Young, A (1995) *The Harmony of Illusions*. Berkeley, CA: University of California Press.

Chapter 3

Mental Health Law and Human Rights

Evolution and Contemporary Challenges

Michael L. Perlin and Éva Szeli

Introduction

As recently as 19 years ago, disability was not broadly acknowledged as a human rights issue. Although there were prior cases decided in the United States and in Europe that, retrospectively, had been litigated from a human rights perspective[1] the *characterization* of 'disability rights' (especially the rights of persons with *mental* disabilities) was not discussed in a global public, political, or legal debate until the early 1990s. Instead, disability was seen only as a medical problem of the individual requiring a treatment or cure. By contrast, viewing disability as a human rights issue requires us to recognize the inherent equality of all people, regardless of abilities, disabilities, or differences, and obligates society to remove the attitudinal and physical barriers to equality and inclusion of people with disabilities.[2]

In this chapter, we seek to provide a selective overview of some key developments and issues in the mental disability rights area. First, we discuss the path via which disability rights have finally, and tardily, become seen as human rights issues. Next, we look at the newly-ratified UN Convention on the Rights of Persons with Disabilities and consider the expansion of human rights in disability law in an international context. We then turn to the role of sanism, and explain why that must be 'centre stage' in any consideration of these issues. Following that, we discuss how sanism, pretextuality, and international human rights must all be studied together to make sense of this entire subject matter area. We end with some brief conclusions.

---

[1] See e.g. *O'Connor v Donaldson* (1975) 422 US 563 (unconstitutional to confine a non-dangerous person capable of surviving safely in freedom to a mental hospital); *Wyatt v Stickney*, 325 FSupp. 781 (MD Ala 1971); aff'd sub nom *Wyatt v Aderholt*, 503 F2d 1305 (5th Cir 1974) (persons with mental illness have constitutional right to adequate treatment in mental hospital); *Lessard v Schmidt*, 349 FSupp. 1078 (ED Wis 1972) (a statute that fails to provide person alleged to be mentally ill with adequate procedural safeguards is unconstitutional); *Winterwerp v the Netherlands* (1979) 2 EHRR 387 (detention on grounds of unsoundness of mind must be based on objective medical evidence of a true mental disorder, be a proportionate response and be carried out in accordance with a procedure prescribed by law); see generally, 1 & 2 Michael L Perlin (1998) *Mental Disability Law: Civil and Criminal*, 2nd edn. chapters 2 and 3.

[2] The first section of this article is adapted from Michael L Perlin et al. (2006) *International Human Rights and Comparative Mental Disability Law*, 3–7. See generally, Michael L Perlin (2011) *International Human Rights and Mental Disability Law: When the Silenced are Heard*; Michael Perlin and Éva Szeli (2009) 'Mental Health Law and Human Rights: Evolution, Challenges, and the Promise of the New Convention', in Jukka Kumpuvuori and Martin Scheinen (eds) *United Nations Convention on the Rights of Persons with Disabilities: Multidisciplinary Perspectives* 241.

Disability rights have at last been recognized as human rights

Remarkably, the issue of the human rights of people with disabilities, particularly people with mental disabilities,[3] had been ignored for decades by the international agencies vested with the protection of human rights on a global scale. Early developments in global international human rights law following the Second World War—and the various forms of human rights advocacy that emerged in the decades that followed—failed to focus on mental disability rights. As Dr Theresa Degener, a noted disability scholar and activist, has observed:

> [D]rafters of the International Bill of Human Rights did not include disabled persons as a distinct group vulnerable to human rights violations. None of the equality clauses of any of the three instruments of this Bill, the Universal Declaration of Human Rights (1948) (hereinafter UDHR), the International Covenant on Civil and Political Rights (1966) (hereinafter ICCPR), and the International Covenant on Economic, Social and Cultural Rights (1966) (hereinafter ICESCR), mention disability as a protected category.[4]

It was not until the United Nations' declaration of 1981 as the *International Year of Disabled Persons*[5] that there was significant activity on an international level. The United Nations General Assembly subsequently established the *World Programme of Action Concerning Disabled Persons*,[6] and declared 1983 to 1992 to be the *Decade of Disabled Persons*.[7] As part of these efforts, the United Nations Human Rights Commission appointed two special rapporteurs to investigate and report on the human rights of persons with mental disabilities,[8] and in 1991, the General Assembly adopted the Principles for the Protection of Persons with Mental Illness and for the Improvement of Mental Health Care (widely referred to as the 'MI Principles').[9] The MI Principles established the most comprehensive international human rights standards for persons with mental disabilities, and their adoption was a critical global step in recognizing mental disability rights issues within the human rights arena.

---

[3] There is no single, universally-accepted definition of 'mental disabilities.' The terminology varies from country to country, jurisdiction to jurisdiction, and even document to document. In this chapter, we use 'mental disabilities' to encompass both psychiatric disorders and intellectual disabilities.

[4] Theresa Degener (2000) 'International Disability Law—A New Legal Subject on the Rise: The Interregional Experts' Meeting in Hong Kong, December 13–17, 1999', 18 Berkeley J. Intl. L., 18, 180, 187.

[5] GA Res 123, UN GAOR, 31st Session (1976).

[6] GA Res 52, UN GAOR, 37th Session (1982).

[7] GA Res 53, UN GAOR, 37th Session (1982).

[8] United Nations, Economic and Social Council, Commission on Human Rights, Sub-Commission on Prevention of Discrimination and Protection of Minorities: *Human Rights and Disability*, UN Doc. E/CN.4/Sub.2/1991/31 (report by Leandro Despouy), and *Principles, Guidelines, and Guarantees for the Protection of Persons Detained on Grounds of Mental Ill-health or Suffering from Mental Disorder*, UN Doc E/CN.4/Sub.2/1983/17 (report by Erica-Irene Daes).It is sobering that these reports were, for all practical purposes, the first major governmental documents ever published discussing these issues. As we discuss in this chapter, we believe that sanism—manifested here by a refusal to take seriously the issues that affect persons with mental disabilities, especially *institutionalized* persons—is the root cause of this phenomenon.

[9] GA Res 119, UN GAOR, 46th Sess, Supp No 49, Annex at 189, UN Doc A/46/49 (1991). See Eric Rosenthal and Leonard S. Rubenstein (1993) 'International Human Rights Advocacy under the "Principles for the Protection of Persons with Mental Illness"', 16 Int'l J. L. & Psychiatry 257 for a detailed discussion of the development of mental disability rights protections within the United Nations human rights system.

Degener's writings reflect the change that has taken place in disability rights jurisprudence. In 2000, she stated further that 'disability has been reclassified as a human rights issue,' and that 'law reforms in this area are intended to provide equal opportunities for disabled people and to combat their segregation, institutionalization and exclusion as typical forms of disability-based discrimination.'[10]

Yet, historically, mainstream human rights protection systems and advocacy organizations had difficulty acknowledging mental disability rights as part of their mandates. The human rights issues encountered by persons with mental disabilities may have been perceived as too complex or esoteric. This challenge was sometimes articulated in rather unfortunate ways, such as 'We work in human rights, not mental disability rights.'[11] While the oblique suggestion that people with mental disabilities were not 'human' was generally unintended, it may well have reflected deep-seated beliefs that they were somehow less human than the broader population whose human rights merited unquestioned protection.[12] But while human rights are—by definition—universally possessed by *all* humans, the formal recognition of the applicability of these rights in contexts specific to vulnerable populations is critical for their enforcement.

To some extent, this new interest in human rights protections for people with disabilities echoes a larger international movement to protect human rights,[13] and appears to more precisely track C. Raj Kumar's observation that 'the judicial protection of human rights and constitutionalization of human rights may be two important objectives by which the rule of law can be preserved and which may govern future human rights work.'[14]

To be sure, some of the results to date have been modest. Few will quarrel with Douglass Cassel's observation that '[t]he direct impact of international human rights law on practice in most of the world remains weak and inconsistent.' But, as Cassel perceptively noted further:

> Both this incipient body of law, and to a lesser degree its direct and even more its indirect influence on conduct, have grown rapidly in historical terms, and appear to be spreading in ways that cannot be explained by a worldview based solely on state power and rational calculations of self-interest. To appreciate its effectiveness and potential, international human rights law must be understood as part of a broader set of interrelated, mutually reinforcing processes and institutions—interwoven strands in a rope—that together pull human rights forward, and to which international law makes distinctive contributions.

---

[10] Degener, supra n. 4, at 181.

[11] Variations on such a statement have been encountered by the authors and their colleagues in discussions with human rights organizations across the globe, on practically every continent.

[12] See Michael L Perlin, '*When the Winds of Changes Shift': International Teaching For Social Change, or, Why Doing What We Do Keeps Us 'Forever Young'*, (paper presented at Society of American Law Teachers conference, University of California Berkeley Law School, 15 March 2008), manuscript at 9:

> When I have shared with others our vision of [doing mental disability law advocacy work and teaching on-line mental disability law courses] in sub-Saharan East Africa, those others have often scoffed, suggesting that the problems faced in that part of the world are so profound that it is almost frivolous to create the programs we are seeking to launch. As you might expect, I disagree, profoundly.

[13] See BG Ramcharan (1991) 'Strategies for the International Protection of Human Rights in the 1990s', 13 Hum. Rts. Q. 155 (Ramcharan is former Deputy UN High Commissioner for Human Rights).

[14] C. Raj Kumar (2003) 'Moving Beyond Constitutionalization and Judicial Protection of Human Rights—Building on the Hong Kong Experience of Civil Society Empowerment', 26 Loy. L.A. Int'l & Comp. L. Rev. 281, 282.

Thus understood, international law, Cassel concluded, 'can be seen as a useful tool for the protection of human rights, and one which promises to be more useful in the future.'[15]

Within the legal literature, the first time disability rights was directly conceptualized as a human rights issue may have been as recently as 1993. In their groundbreaking article, Eric Rosenthal and Leonard Rubenstein applied international human rights principles to the institutionalization of people with mental disabilities.[16] In the political context, disability as a human rights issue first appears to have been raised in remarks made the next year by former United States Senator Bob Dole: 'As a nation that has been a pioneer in promoting the dignity of its own citizens with disabilities, we have a special obligation to assume leadership in establishing the international human rights of people with disabilities.'[17] Later, in 2004, Senator Tom Harkin introduced the concept of human rights protections for people with disabilities when he successfully won US Congressional approval for an amendment to the foreign assistance act requiring accessibility of government-funded construction overseas.[18]

Meanwhile, regional human rights courts across the globe had begun to exhibit an increasing willingness to address mental disability rights issues.[19] In 1979, over a decade earlier, the European Court of Human Rights had already heard its first mental disability rights case, *Winterwerp v Netherlands*,[20] under the European Convention of Human Rights.[21] Over the following decades, the European Court heard dozens of mental disability rights cases, defining and refining the contours of human rights as applied in mental health contexts under the European Convention.[22]

---

[15] Douglass Cassel (2001) 'Does International Human Rights Law Make a Difference?', 2 Chi. J. Int'l. L. 121, 135.

[16] Rosenthal and Rubenstein, supra n. 9. This article was relied on almost immediately by scholars and activists studying the human rights implications of mental disability laws in nations as diverse as Japan, see Pamela Schwartz Cohen (1995) 'Psychiatric Commitment in Japan: International Concern and Domestic Reform', 14 UCLA Pac. Basin L. J. 28, 35 n. 48, and Uruguay, see Angelika C Moncada (1994) 'Involuntary Commitment and the Use of Seclusion and Restraint in Uruguay: a Comparison with the United Nations Principles for the Protection of Persons with Mental Illness', 25 U. Miami Inter-Am. L. Rev. 589, 591 n. 6.

[17] Bob Dole (1994) 'Promises to People with Disabilities?—Commentary on Blanck', 79 Iowa L. Rev. 925, 931.

[18] Harkin inserted several measures in the Fiscal Year 2004 Omnibus Appropriation Bill, which require the United States government to ensure the inclusion of people with disabilities in post-war Iraq and Afghanistan. Harkin also successfully added disability-related criteria to the Millennium Challenge Account, a new foreign aid initiative which will spent over $5 billion in next five year, and he required that USAID develop access standards to govern all construction overseas. See <http://abilitymagazine.com/Senator_Harken_Views.html>; see also *Foreign Policy and Disability: Legislative Strategies and Civil Rights Protections to Ensure Inclusion of People with Disabilities*, report commissioned by the National Council on Disability (with E. Rosenthal) (9 September 2003). This report resulted in amendments requiring disability accessibility under the Foreign Assistance Act, 23 January 2004; <http://www.ncd.gov/publications/2003/Sept92003> (last visited 5 November 2011).

[19] There is still no regional court in Asia and the Pacific, although it has been recently proposed that a disability rights tribunal for that area be created. See Michael L Perlin and Yoshikazu Ikehara, *Creation of a Disability Rights Tribunal for Asia and the Pacific: Its Impact on China?*, paper presented to the European Chinese Studies Association (Copenhagen, Denmark, June 2010). Available at <http://papers.ssrn.com/sol3/papers.cfm?abstract_id=1744196>; Perlin, supra n. 3, at 169–202.

[20] 33 Eur Ct HR (ser. A), reported at 2 EHRR 387 (1979).

[21] Convention for the Protection of Human Rights and Fundamental Freedoms, ETS No. 5, 213 UNTS 222, opened for signature 4 November 1950, entered into force 3 September 1953.

[22] See Lawrence O Gostin (2000) 'Human Rights of Persons with Mental Disabilities: The European Convention of Human Rights', 23 Int'l J. L. & Psychiatry 125; Oliver Lewis (2002) 'Protecting the Rights of People with Mental Disabilities: The European Convention on Human Rights', 9 Eur. J. Health L. 293.

In the Americas, the Inter-American Commission on Human Rights heard its first mental disabil-ity rights case, *Victor Rosario Congo v Ecuador*,[23] under the American Convention on Human Rights[24] in 1999, breaking new ground in formalizing the use of the MI Principles as a guide for interpreting and applying binding human rights standards. And subsequently, in 2003, the African Commission decided its first mental disability rights case, *Purohit and Moore v The Gambia*, under the African Charter.[25] All of this case law has served to validate the connection between mental health and human rights, providing regional fora for recognizing and enforcing the human rights of individuals labelled with mental disabilities.[26]

However, during the late 20th century, much of the mental disability rights advocacy occurred outside of formal legal settings. Local, regional, and international non-governmental organiza-tions conducted investigations, wrote reports, and brought media attention to egregious human rights abuses suffered by people labeled with mental disabilities.[27] Most significantly, the emer-gence of a 'consumer movement' supported the natural advocacy capacities of stakeholders. By definition, the focal point of the mental disability rights movement is, or certainly should be, individuals who are identified as having mental disabilities. Yet, historically, their voices were often ignored, while others deemed to speak for those who purportedly could not speak for them-selves. Referring to themselves as *consumers, users, ex-users, ex-patients*, or *survivors* of mental health services, individuals who had been labelled with mental disabilities began to organize not only locally, but also regionally and globally.[28] Such self-advocacy groups have since become instrumental in identifying violations of their human rights, and in advocating reform in the policies and systems that directly affect their lives.[29]

---

[23] Case No 11.427 (1999) Inter-Am. C.H.R. 63.

[24] OAS Treaty Series No 36, 1144 UNTS 123, entered into force 18 July 1978.

[25] Comm No 241/2001, 16th activity report of the AfrCHPR (2002–2003). African [Banjul] Charter on Human and Peoples' Rights, OAU doc CAB/LEG/67/3 rev 5, 21 ILM 58 (1982), adopted 27 June 1981, entered into force 21 October 1986.

[26] We cannot fall into the trap of assuming that, simply because a court issued a decision, that conditions in institutions immediately changed or that procedural safeguards were immediately instituted in response to such decisions. The history of mental disability law is all too often the history of 'paper victories,' and even the most rights-protective court decisions may be slow to produce significant real-life changes. See infra n. 43.

[27] See, e.g. Disability Rights International (DRI), Projects: Neuro-Psychiatric Hospital of Paraguay, available at <http://www.disabilityrightsintl.org/work/country-projects/paraguay/> (last visited 5 November 2011); *Mental Disability Rights International, Human Rights and Mental Health: Mexico* (2000); *Mental Disability Rights International, Human Rights & Mental Health: Hungary* (1997); *Mental Disability Rights International, Human Rights & Mental Health: Uruguay* (1995).

DRI's work has continued to gain momentum into the new century, with additional investigations and reports, including *Mental Disability Rights International, Torment Not Treatment: Serbia's Segregation and Abuse of Children and Adults with Disabilities* (2007); *Mental Disability Rights International, Ruined Lives: Segregation from Society in Argentina's Psychiatric Asylums* (2007).

[28] Examples include, but are not limited to, the European Network of (ex-)Users and Survivors of Psychiatry (ENUSP), and the World Network of Users and Survivors of Psychiatry (WNUSP). For discussions of US-based groups, see infra nn. 82–83.

[29] See, e.g. Gabor Gombos et al. (2002) 'Hungary: The Social Care Home Report', 21 N.Y.L. Sch. J. Int'l & Comp. L. 361, describing the results of an extensive nationwide human rights investigation into conditions at long-term residential facilities for persons with mental disabilities, conducted by the Hungarian Mental Health Interest Forum, an organization of users/survivors of psychiatric services.

The Disability Rights Convention

Disability rights as a human rights issue has taken centre stage at the United Nations, and the involve-ment of stakeholders has been critical in the most significant historical development in the recogni-tion of the human rights of persons with mental disabilities: the drafting and adoption of a binding international disability rights convention.[30] In late 2001, the United Nations General Assembly estab-lished an Ad Hoc Committee 'to consider proposals for a comprehensive and integral international convention to promote and protect the rights and dignity of persons with disabilities'.[31] The Ad Hoc Committee drafted a document over the course of five years and eight sessions, and the new Convention on the Rights of Persons with Disabilities (sometimes 'convention' or 'Disability Convention')[32] was adopted in December 2006 and opened for signature in March 2007.[33] It entered into force—thus becoming legally binding on states parties—on 3 May 2008, thirty days after the 20th ratification.[34] One of the hallmarks of the process that led to the publication of the UN Convention was the participation of persons with disabilities and the clarion cry, 'Nothing about us, without us'.[35] This has led commentators to conclude that the convention 'is regarded as having finally empowered the "world's largest minority" to claim their rights, and to participate in international and national affairs on an equal basis with others who have achieved specific treaty recognition and protection.'[36]

The Disability Convention furthers the human rights approach to disability and recognizes the right of people with disabilities to equality in most every aspect of life.[37] It calls for 'respect

---

[30] On the singular role of this convention, see e.g. Frederic Megret, *(2008)* 'The Disabilities Convention: Toward a Holistic Concept of Rights', 12 Int'l J. Hum. Rts. 261; Frederic Megret (2008) 'The Disabilities Convention: Human Rights of Persons with Disabilities or Disability Rights?', 30 Hum. Rights, 2, 494–516.

[31] GA Res 56/168 (2001).

[32] GA Res A/61/611 (2006).

[33] GA Res A/61/106 (2006).

[34] On the 20th ratification, see <http://www.un.org/News/Press/docs/2008/hr4941.doc.htm>. See generally, Tara Melish (Winter 2007) 'The UN Disability Convention: Historic Process, Strong Prospects, and Why the U.S. Should Ratify', 14 Hum. Rts. Brief 37, 44; Michael Ashley Stein and Penelope JS Stein (2007) 'Beyond Disability Civil Rights', 58 Hastings L. J. 1203. As of 24 December 2011, there have been 108 ratifications and 153 signatories. As of the same date, there have been 63 ratifications and 90 signatories of the Optional Protocol to the Convention.

[35] See e.g. Rosemary Kayess and Phillip French (2008) 'Out of Darkness into Light? Introducing the Convention on the Rights of Persons with Disabilities', 8 Hum. Rts. L. Rev. 1, 4 n. 15:

> See, for example, Statement by Hon Ruth Dyson, Minister for Disability Issues, New Zealand Mission to the UN, for Formal Ceremony at the Signing of the Convention on the Rights of Persons with Disability, 30 March 2007: 'Just as the Convention itself is the product of a remarkable partnership between governments and civil society, effective implementation will require a continuation of that partnership.' The negotiating slogan 'Nothing about us without us' was adopted by the International Disability Caucus, available at: <http://www.un.org/esa/socdev/enable/documents/Stat_Conv/nzam.doc> (last accessed 5 November 2011).

[36] Id., n. 17 (See, for example, statements made by the High Commissioner for Human Rights, Louise Arbour, and the Permanent Representative of New Zealand and Chair of the Ad-Hoc Committee on a Comprehensive and Integral International Convention on the Protection and Promotion of the Rights and Dignity of Persons with Disabilities, Ambassador Don Mackay, at a Special Event on the Convention on Rights of Persons with Disabilities, convened by the UN Human Rights Council, 26 March 2007, available at: <http://www.crin.org/resources/infodetail.asp?ID=12917>, accessed 5 November 2011).

[37] See e.g. Aaron Dhir (2005) 'Human Rights Treaty Drafting Through the Lens of Mental Disability: The Proposed International Convention on Protection and Promotion of the Rights and Dignity of Persons with Disabilities', 41 Stan. J. Int'l L. 181.

for inherent dignity'[38] and 'non-discrimination'.[39] Subsequent Articles declare 'freedom from torture or cruel, inhuman or degrading treatment or punishment',[40] 'freedom from exploitation, violence and abuse',[41] and a right to protection of the 'integrity of the person'.[42] However, it is still a *very* open question as to whether or not these will actually be given life, or whether they will remain little more than 'paper victories'.[43] The enforcement of the Disability Convention remains a critical issue.[44]

---

[38] UN Convention, Art. 3(a).

[39] Id., Art. 3(b).

[40] Id., Art. 15.

[41] Id., Art. 16.

[42] Id., Art. 17.

[43] Michael L Perlin (2002) 'What's Good is Bad, What's Bad is Good, You'll Find out When You Reach the Top You're on the Bottom': Are the Americans with Disabilities Act (and *Olmstead v. L.C.*) Anything More Than 'Idiot Wind?' 35 U. Mich. J.L. Reform 235, 246 ('Mental disability law is strewn with examples of "paper victories"), quoting Michael Lottman (1976) 'Paper Victories and Hard Realities', in Valerie J Bradley and Gary J. Clarke (eds) *Paper Victories and Hard Realities: the Implementation of the Legal and Constitutional Rights of the Mentally Disabled* 93.

[44] Many obstacles to the enforcement of UN human rights conventions have been identified in the decades since the entry into force of the ICCPR and the ICESCR. These include concerns that 1) there is limited enforcement machinery; 2) the existing machinery is understaffed, underfunded, and may not have the authority to compel compliance with—or to punish violations of—human rights standards; 3) ultimately, human rights enforcement may be viewed as a State function (the fox guarding the henhouse); and 4) the general lack of accountability that results from some of these issues. See, e.g. *Enforcing Human Rights: The U.N. Machinery*, 30 UN Chron. 93 (Mar. 1993)

Also, note that even with the general human rights instruments (and this may be even more true about the Disability Convention), the lack of universal consensus about the rights to be protected creates a considerable sticking point in enforcement.

Courts in the US have been inconsistent in their enforcement of and adherence to UN Conventions. See generally, Michael L Perlin and Henry A Dlugacz (2009) '"It's Doom Alone That Counts": Can International Human Rights Law Be An Effective Source of Rights in Correctional Conditions Litigation?', 27 Behav. Sci. & L. 675. Compare e.g. *Lareau v Manson*, 507 F Supp 1177, 1187–89 n. 9 (D Conn 1980), aff'd in part & rev'd in part, 651 F 2d 96 (2d Cir 1981) (citing to United Nations Standard Minimum Rules for the Treatment of Prisoners standards in cases involving, the 'double bunking' of inmates), to *Flores v Southern Peru Copper Corp*, 414 F.3d 233, 257, 259 (2d Cir 2003) (United Nations' Convention on the Rights of the Child [CRC] does not convey a private right of action to plaintiffs as a matter of law). In at least one case, however, while noting that the -non-ratified convention was not binding on US courts, the Massachusetts Supreme Judicial Court 'read the entire text of the convention . . . and conclude[d] that the outcome of the proceedings in this case are completely in accord with principles expressed therein': *Adoption of Peggy*, 767 NE 2d 29, 38 (Mass 2002). In *Roper v Simmons* (2005) 543 US 551, 578 in the course of striking down the juvenile death penalty, the Supreme Court (per Justice Kennedy) acknowledged that the United States had not ratified the CRC, but added:

> It is proper that we acknowledge the overwhelming weight of international opinion against the juvenile death penalty, resting in large part on the understanding that the instability and emotional imbalance of young people may often be a factor in the crime. See Brief for Human Rights Committee of the Bar of England and Wales et al. as *Amici Curiae* 10–11. The opinion of the world community, while not controlling our outcome, does provide respected and significant confirmation for our own conclusions.

International attention to disability rights

At least 42 countries have adopted disability anti-discrimination laws.[45] Although some countries rely on the medical model of disability, others have chosen instead to incorporate a human rights perspective in their domestic legislation, thereby guaranteeing the right of people with disabilities to equality and full participation in society. Arguably, at no previous time in history has the confluence of international and domestic efforts with and for people with disabilities challenged policy makers, scholars, and activists to reframe the meaning of equality and inclusion for people with disabilities.

For people with mental disabilities, in particular, the development of human rights protections may be even more significant than for people with other disabilities. Like people with other disabilities, people with mental disabilities face degradation, stigmatization, and discrimination throughout the world today.[46] But disproportionately and more frequently, many people with mental disabilities are routinely confined, against their will, in institutions, and deprived of their freedom, dignity, and basic human rights. People with mental disabilities who are fortunate enough to live outside of institutions often remain imprisoned by the social isolation they experience, often from their own families. They are not included in educational programs, and they face attitudinal barriers to employment because they have not received the education and training needed to obtain employment or because of discrimination based on unsubstantiated fears and prejudice.[47]

Discrimination against people with mental disabilities does not always take the form of hatred or hostility, however. More often, discrimination against people with mental disabilities takes the form of fear, pity, or patronization.[48] Yet only recently have disability discrimination laws and policies in the United States and elsewhere focused on changing such attitudes and promoting the integration of people with disabilities into our schools, neighbourhoods, and workplaces.

Soberingly, a recent survey by Professor Jean Koh Peters found that almost three-quarters of children worldwide live in countries where CRC is not observed or where evidence as to observance is inconclusive, despite CRC's widespread ratification. Jean Koh Peters (2006) 'How Children are Heard in Child Protective Proceedings, in the United States and Around the World in 2005: Survey Findings, Initial Observations, and Areas for Further Study', 6 Nev. L.J. 966, 968–69. On how ratification of a UN Convention has had a salutary impact on domestic law, see Adrian James (2008) Children, the UNCRC, and Family Law in England and Wales, 46 Fam. Ct. Rev. 53.

[45] Arlene S Kanter (2003) 'The Globalization of Disability Rights Law', 30 Syr. J. Int'l L. & Comm. 241, 249, n. 33; Sally Chaffin (2005) 'Challenging The United States Position On A United Nations Convention On Disability', 15 Temp. Pol. & Civ. Rts. L. Rev. 121, 138. An analysis of the effectiveness of these laws is beyond the scope of this chapter. See generally, Yoshikazu Ikehara, *What is DRTAP and its Future?* Paper presented to the International Conference on Disability Rights Tribunal in Asia & the Pacific (Bangkok, Thailand, October 2010), powerpoint slides accessible at <http://tokyo-advocacy.com/drtapeng/conference_bangkok.html>.

[46] See *City of Cleburne v Cleburne Living Center* (1985) 573 US 432, 462 (Marshall, J dissenting in part), arguing that '[T]he mentally retarded have been subject to a "lengthy and tragic history" of segregation and discrimination that can only be called grotesque', and describing a 'regime of state-mandated segregation and degradation . . . that in its virulence and bigotry rivaled, and indeed paralleled, the worst excesses of Jim Crow.'

[47] See e.g. sources cited supra n. 27; Susan Stefan (2001) *Unequal Rights: Discrimination Against People With Mental Disabilities and the Americans With Disabilities Act.*

[48] See generally, Michael L Perlin (2000) *The Hidden Prejudice: Mental Disability on Trial.*

Professor Harold Koh, now Dean of Yale Law School, called attention to the developing inter-national movement with and on behalf of people with mental disabilities[49] when the late Stanley Herr[50] contacted him in 1995 to suggest the convening of a conference:

> Why not bring together at Yale [Stan asked] the leading spokespeople from two of the greatest social movements of the past half-century: the international human rights movement and the disability rights movement? We would talk about disability rights as human rights.[51]

That conference led to the promulgation of what is called the 'Yale Declaration', 'reaffirm[ing] the universality of human rights and [calling] on all nation-states to bring about without delay the full enforcement of the rights of persons with mental retardation.'[52]

It is clear that, within the past decade, there has been nothing short of an explosion of interest in the area of human rights and mental disability law[53]—by academics, practitioners, advocates, and self-advocates.[54] Groups such as Disability Rights International (formerly Mental Disability Rights International)[55] and the Mental Disability Advocacy Center[56] have investigated conditions of institutions for people with mental disabilities and issued scathing reports about the quality of services made available in psychiatric institutions and social care homes in Eastern Europe and Latin America.[57] Organizations such as Amnesty International and the Helsinki Committees have finally, albeit tardily, recognized that violations of persons' mental health rights are violations of human rights.[58]

---

[49] This particular development in mental disability rights was specific to people with intellectual disabilities (i.e. mental retardation). See supra n. 3, regarding terminology.

[50] For a tribute to Stanley Herr's commitment and passionate advocacy in this specific area of the law, see e.g. Karen Rothenberg (2002) 'Eulogy for Stan Herr', 8 Clinical L. Rev. 293, and see Douglas Colbert, Lawrence Gostin, and Harold Hongju Koh (2003) 'Dedication: In Memory of Stanley Sholom Herr, 1945–2001', in Stanley S Herr et al. (eds) *The Human Rights of Persons with Intellectual Disabilities: Different but Equal,* ix (discussing Herr's career and his 'commit[ment] to social justice').

[51] Harold Hongju Koh (2004) 'Different But Equal: The Human Rights of Persons with Intellectual Disabilities', 63 Md. L. Rev. 1, 2.

[52] Id. at 3, citing 'Yale Declaration' in *The Human Rights of Persons with Intellectual Disabilities: Different but Equal,* supra n. 50, at 520–25.

[53] See e.g. Michael L Perlin (2002–03) 'Things Have Changed: Looking at Non-institutional Mental Disability Law Through the Sanism Filter', 46 N.Y.L. Sch. L. Rev. 535, 539, discussing the recent explosion of case law and commentary in this area of the law; see also, Kanter, supra n. 45, at 268 (noting that in recent years the situation has changed dramatically as 'the principle of non-discrimination and equality for people with disabilities has entered center stage in the international arena').

[54] See generally, 1–5. Perlin, supra n. 2; Michael L Perlin (2005) *Mental Disability Law: Cases and Materials.* 2nd edn.

[55] DRI is a Washington, DC-based non-governmental organization dedicated to the recognition and enforce-ment of the human rights of persons with mental disabilities. See <http://www.disabilityrightsintl.org>.

[56] MDAC is an international non-governmental organization based in Budapest that promotes and protects the human rights of people with mental health problems and intellectual disabilities across Central and Eastern Europe and Central Asia. See <http://mdac.info/>.

[57] Excerpts from many of these reports are reprinted in Perlin et al, supra n. 2, at 859–85.

[58] Symposium Transcript, *The Application of International Human Rights Law to Institutional Mental Disability Law,* 21 N.Y.L. Sch. J. Int'l & Comp. L. 387, 391 (2002) (Comments of Eric Rosenthal):

> I began my research . . . by examining the human rights studies of non-governmental organizations such as Human Rights Watch and Amnesty International. I also looked at the U.S. Department of State's Country Reports on Human Rights Practices. What I found is shocking: those human rights organiza-tions and human rights reports criticized governments when political dissidents were put in psychiatric

A challenge remains: fighting 'sanism'

As indicated above, there has always been great ambivalence on the part of the human rights community in its perception of the rights of persons with mental disabilities, and the *value* of those rights. We believe that the explanation for the roots of this ambivalence can be found in what we call 'sanism' and what we call 'pretextuality.' It is critical, we believe, for those seriously interested in this topic to understand these concepts and how their malignancy has distorted all aspects of mental disability law, domestic and international.

'Sanism' is an irrational prejudice of the same quality and character of other irrational prejudices that cause (and are reflected in) prevailing social attitudes of racism, sexism, homophobia, and ethnic bigotry. It permeates all aspects of mental disability law and affects all participants in the mental disability law system: litigants, fact finders, counsel, expert and lay witnesses. Its corrosive effects have warped mental disability law jurisprudence in involuntary civil commitment law, institutional law, tort law, and all aspects of the criminal process (pretrial, trial and sentencing).[59] It reflects what civil rights lawyer Florynce Kennedy has characterized as the 'pathology of oppression'.[60]

'Pretextuality' defines the ways in which courts accept (either implicitly or explicitly) testimonial dishonesty and engage similarly in dishonest (and frequently meretricious) decision-making. It is especially poisonous where witnesses, especially expert witnesses, show a 'high propensity to purposely distort their testimony in order to achieve desired ends.'[61] This pretextuality infects all participants in the judicial system, breeds cynicism and disrespect for the law, demeans participants, and reinforces shoddy lawyering, blasé judging, and, at times, perjurious and/or corrupt testifying.[62]

In previous works, one of us (MLP) has explored the relationships between sanism and pretextuality in matters involving, inter alia, competency to stand trial,[63] sexual autonomy,[64] the right

---

facilities, but they did not speak out about the abuses against other people who may or may not have mental disabilities.

See also Krasimir Kanev (2002) 'State, Human Rights, and Mental Health in Bulgaria', 21 N.Y.L. Sch. J. Int'l & Comp. L. 435, 435 (Amnesty International first involved itself in this issue in Bulgaria in 2001). For commentary on the work done by groups such as DRI and MDAC, see e.g. Alex Geisinger and Michael Ashley Stein (2007) 'A Theory of Expressive International Law', 60 Vand. L. Rev. 77, 107–08; Laura E Hortas (2004) 'Asylum Protection for the Mentally Disabled: How the Evolution of Rights for the Mentally Ill in the United States Created a "Social Group"', 20 Conn. J. Int'l L. 155, 181–82; Lance Gable (2007) 'The Proliferation of Human Rights in Global Health Governance', 35 J. L., Med. & Ethics 534, 540; Arlene S Kanter (2007) 'The Promise and Challenge of the United Nations Convention on the Rights of Persons with Disabilities', 34 Syracuse J. Int'l L. & Com. 287, 316.

[59] See e.g. Michael L Perlin (2003) '"You Have Discussed Lepers and Crooks": Sanism in Clinical Teaching', 9 Clinical L. Rev. 683, 684 (Perlin, *Lepers*). Perlin, supra n. 48, at 21–58.

[60] See e.g. Michael L Perlin (1999) '"Half-Wracked Prejudice Leaped Forth": Sanism, Pretextuality, and Why and How Mental Disability Law Developed As It Did', 10 J. Contemp. Legal Issues 3 (Perlin, *Half-Wracked Prejudice*); Perlin, supra n. 47, at 36–39; Michael L Perlin (1992) 'On "Sanism"', 46 SMU L. Rev. 373.

[61] Michael L Perlin (1991) 'Morality and Pretextuality, Psychiatry and Law: Of 'Ordinary Common Sense,' Heuristic Reasoning, and Cognitive Dissonance', 19 Bull. Am. Acad. Psychiatry & L. 131, 135.

[62] See generally, Perlin, *Half-Wracked Prejudice*, supra n. 60, at 5.

[63] E.g. Michael L Perlin (2004) '"Everything's a Little Upside Down, As a Matter of Fact the Wheels Have Stopped": The Fraudulence of the Incompetency Evaluation Process', 4 Houston J. Health L. & Pol'y 239; Michael L Perlin (1993) 'Pretexts and Mental Disability Law: The Case of Competency', 47 U. Miami L. Rev. 625. (Perlin, *The Case of Competency*).

[64] E.g. Michael L Perlin (1993–94) 'Hospitalized Patients and the Right to Sexual Interaction: Beyond the Last Frontier?' 20 NYU Rev. L. & Soc'l Change 302.

to refuse treatment,[65] 'autonomous decision-making,'[66] the Americans with Disabilities Act,[67] competency to plead guilty or waive counsel,[68] jury decision-making in death penalty cases,[69] and the bar's attitude towards mentally disabled counsel.[70] But, these factors can be even *more* pernicious as they relate to the job that lawyers do when they represent persons with mental disabilities in court proceedings. Writing about this latter topic four years ago, one of us (MLP) alleged:

> Sanism permeates the legal representation process both in cases in which mental capacity is a central issue, and those in which such capacity is a collateral question. Sanist lawyers (1) distrust their mentally disabled clients, (2) trivialize their complaints, (3) fail to forge authentic attorney-client relationships with such clients and reject their clients' potential contributions to case-strategizing, and (4) take less seriously case outcomes that are adverse to their clients.[71]

Sanism, pretextuality, and international human rights

There is now some nascent literature on the relationship between sanism, pretextuality, and international human rights law,[72] especially focusing on circumstances in nations with developing

---

[65] E.g. Michael L Perlin (2005) 'And My Best Friend, My Doctor/Won't Even Say What It Is I've Got: The Role and Significance of Counsel in Right to Refuse Treatment Cases', 42 San Diego L. Rev. 735 (Perlin, *Best Friend)*; Michael L Perlin and Deborah A Dorfman (1996) '"Is It More Than Dodging Lions and Wastin' Time"? Adequacy of Counsel, Questions of Competence, and the Judicial Process in Individual Right to Refuse Treatment Cases', 2 Psychology, Pub. Pol'y & L.114.

[66] E.g. Michael L Perlin (1997) '"Make Promises by the Hour": Sex, Drugs, the ADA, and Psychiatric Hospitalization', 46 DePaul L. Rev. 947.

[67] E.g. Michael L Perlin (1993–94) 'The ADA and Persons with Mental Disabilities: Can Sanist Attitudes Be Undone?' 8 J. L. & Health 15.

[68] E.g. Michael L Perlin (1996) '"Dignity Was the First to Leave": *Godinez v. Moran*, Colin Ferguson, and the Trial of Mentally Disabled Criminal Defendants', 14 Behav. Sci. & L. 61.

[69] E.g. Michael L Perlin (1994) 'The Sanist Lives of Jurors in Death Penalty Cases: The Puzzling Role of Mitigating Mental Disability Evidence', 8 Notre Dame J. L., Ethics & Pub. Pol. 239.

[70] E.g. Michael L Perlin (2008) '"Baby, Look Inside Your Mirror": The Legal Profession's Willful and Sanist Blindness to Lawyers with Mental Disabilities', 69 U. Pitt. L. Rev. 589.

[71] Perlin, *Lepers*, supra n. 59, at 695. On the issues raised when a client may be unable to express a position to an attorney or remains silent, see Perlin, supra n. 1, § 2B-8.1, at 237, and Michael L Perlin and Robert L Sadoff (Summer 1982) 'Ethical Issues in the Representation of Individuals in the Commitment Process', 45 Law & Contemp. Probs. 161, 173 (attorney obligated to question friends, families and others in an attempt to make a collateral determination of the client's views; such an investigation 'should be pursued in every instance').

[72] See e.g. Michael L Perlin (2007) 'International Human Rights Law and Comparative Mental Disability Law: The Universal Factors', 34 Syracuse J. Int'l L. & Commerce 333, 333 (Perlin, *Universal Factors);* Michael L Perlin (2006) 'International Human Rights and Comparative Mental Disability Law: The Role of Institutional Psychiatry in the Suppression of Political Dissent', 39 Israel L. Rev. 69, 89–92; Perlin et al., supra n. 2, at 283–319; Perlin, supra n. 3; Perlin and Szeli, supra n. 3. Other authors have begun to explore the dimensions of the same issue. See e.g. Jennifer Fischer (2005) 'A Comparative Look at the Right to Refuse Treatment for Involuntarily Hospitalized Persons with a Mental Illness', 29 Hastings Int'l & Comp. L. Rev. 153, 161; David Katner (2006) 'The Mental Health Paradigm and the MacArthur Study: Emerging Issues Challenging the Competence of Juveniles in Delinquency Systems', 32 Am. J.L. & Med. 503, 542–43.

economies.[73] For example, an analysis of the European Commission on Human Rights[74] concluded that it has interpreted the European Convention on Human Rights 'very restrictively in psychiatric cases'.[75] The cases included in this analysis, which characterize the handcuffing of patients as 'therapeutically necessary',[76] or sanction the use of seclusion for 'disciplinary' purposes,[77] certainly bespeak pretextuality.[78] It is essential that such pretextuality be identified and answered.[79] This is especially timely in light of the ratification of the new UN Convention. The Convention's focus on questions of empowerment[80] forces us to consider whether the legal system will continue to perpetuate the sort of sanism and pretextuality that has had such a negative impact on the lives of persons with mental disabilities, and will continue to condone teleological judicial behaviour through overreliance on cognitive-simplifying heuristics.[81]

---

[73] See e.g. Michael L Perlin (2008) '"I Might Need a Good Lawyer, Could Be Your Funeral, My Trial": Global Clinical Legal Education and the Right to Counsel in Civil Commitment Cases', 28 Wash. U. J. L & Poly (Perlin, *Global Clinical Education*).

By way of example, residents of nations with developing economies in Central and South Americans nations are no strangers to pretextuality in many other areas of the law and of society. Hernando DeSoto (1989) *The Other Path: The Economic Answer to Terrorism*; Margaret Popkin (2000) *Peace Without Justice: Obstacles to Building the Rule of Law in El Salvador*; Susan Eckstein (ed) (2001) *Power and Popular Protests: Latin American Social Movements*; Eduardo Galeano (1997) *Open Veins of Latin America: Five centuries of the Pillage of a Continent*. On the relationship between this history and the importance of a vigorous mental health advocacy movement, see Michael L Perlin (2007) 'An Internet-based Mental Disability Law Program: Implications for Social Change in Nations with Developing Economies', 40 Fordham Int'l L.J. 435 (Perlin, *Social Change*).

[74] On the ways that the European Commission is, for these purposes, similar to the Inter-American Commission on Human Rights, see e.g. Ann Powers (2002) 'Justice Denied? The Adjudication of Extradition Applications', 37 Tex. Int'l L.J. 272; George William Mugwanya (1999) 'Realizing Universal Human Rights Norms Through Regional Human Rights Mechanisms: Reinvigorating the African System', 10 Ind. Int'l & Comp. L. Rev. 35.

[75] David Hewitt (2001) 'Do Human Rights Impact on Mental Health Law?', 151 New L. J. 1278, 1278.

[76] See id. (discussing *Herczegfalvy v Austria* (1993) 15 Eur Ct HR 437).

[77] See id. (discussing *Dhoest v Belgium* (1987) 12 Eur Ct HR 135).

[78] It should be underscored; there have been *many* decisions about *many* aspects of substantive and procedural civil commitment law in the ECHR and other bodies. These decisions, however, by themselves, have *not* created a robust corpus of international human rights law.

[79] See Michael L Perlin (2008) '"Through the Wild Cathedral Evening": Barriers, Attitudes, Participatory Democracy, Professor ten Broek, and the Rights of Persons with Mental Disabilities', 13 Tex. J. Civ. Libs. & Civ. Rts 413 (discussing the UN Convention in this precise context).

[80] See Kayess and French, supra n. 35, at 17.

[81] See e.g, Michael L Perlin (2009) '"His Brain Has Been Mismanaged with Great Skill": How Will Jurors Respond to Neuroimaging Testimony in Insanity Defense Cases?' 42 Akron L. Rev. 885, 892–93, 902–04, discussing the dominance and the power of the *vividness heuristic,* a cognitive-simplifying device through which a 'single vivid, memorable case overwhelms mountains of abstract, colorless data upon which rational choices should be made,' see Michael L Perlin (1997) '"The Borderline Which Separated You From Me": The Insanity Defense, the Authoritarian Spirit, the Fear of Faking, and the Culture of Punishment', 82 Iowa L. Rev. 1375, 1417.

By *teleological*, we refer to outcome-determinative reasoning; social science that enables judges to satisfy predetermined positions are privileged, while data that would require judges to question such ends are rejected or subordinated. See e.g. Perlin, *The Case of Competency*, supra n. 63.

As discussed above, although there is a robust 'psychiatric survivor' movement both in the United States and elsewhere,[82] this voice is typically ignored.[83] For at least 30 years, formerly-hospitalized individuals and their supporters have formed an important role in the reform of the mental health system and in test case litigation. 'Yet, there is little evidence that these groups are taken seriously either by lawyers or academics.'[84]

In the civil commitment context, any sanism-inspired blunders by lawyers can easily be fatal to the client's chance of success.[85] If a lawyer rejects the notion that his client may be competent (indeed, if s/he engages in the not-atypical 'presumption of incompetency' that is all to often *de rigeur* in these cases),[86] the chances are far slimmer that s/he will advocate for such a client in the

---

[82] See e.g. Peter Margulies (1992) 'The Cognitive Politics of Professional Conflict: Law Reform, Mental Health Treatment Technology, and Citizen Governance', 5 Harv. J.L. & Tech. 25, 57 n. 132; Jennifer Honig and Susan Fendell (2000) 'Meeting The Needs of Female Trauma Survivors: The Effectiveness of The Massachusetts Mental Health Managed Care System', 15 Berkeley Women's L.J. 161, 185; (1997) 'Taking Issue with Taking Issue: Psychiatric Survivors Reconsidered', 48 Psychiatric Services 601–05.

[83] But see, Perlin, *Lepers*, supra n. 59, at 700 n. 90:

One important exception is Shin Imai, A Counter-Pedagogy for Social Justice: Core Skills for Community-based Lawyering, 9 Clin. L. Rev. 195, 199 (2002) (discussing Osgoode Hall Law School's clinic's collaborative work with Parkdale Community Legal Services in representing one such group). See also *Tewksbury v. Dowling*, 169 F. Supp. 2d 103 (E.D.N.Y. 2001), and *Charles W. v. Maul*, 214 F.3d 350 (2d Cir. 2000) (litigants represented by Prof. William Brooks and the Mental Disability Law Clinic of Touro Law School).

[83] Id. at 700 n. 90.Survivors, on the other hand, *were* an important voice in the drafting of the UN Convention. See e.g. *News about the MFI Global Campaign Committee*, available at <http://www.mindfreedom.org/campaign/global/news-about-the-mfi-international-campaign-committee>, accessed 5 November 2011 (discussing role of MindFreedom in enabling 'psychiatric survivors enter the UN to participate in international negotiating sessions about the human rights of people labeled with disabilities'). For an early discussion of the role of such groups in the UN drafting process, see Degener, supra n. 4, at 189 n. 38.

[84] Perlin, *Lepers*, supra n. 59, at 699–700 (footnotes omitted). See also, Perlin, *Social Change*, supra n. 73, at 444 n. 39:

[S]urvivor groups generally have opposed the constitutionality or application of involuntary civil commitment statutes, see, e.g. *Project Release v. Prevost*, 722 F.2d 960 (2d Cir. 1983), or supported the right of patients to refuse the involuntary administration of psychotropic drugs, see *Rennie v. Klein*, 653 F.2d 836, 838 (3d Cir. 1981) (Alliance for the Liberation of Mental Patients, amicus curiae), but also have involved themselves in a far broader range of litigation. See, e.g. *Colorado v. Connelly*, 479 U.S. 157 (1986) (impact of severe mental disability on Miranda waiver; Coalition for the Fundamental Rights and Equality of Ex-patients, amicus). The involvement of such groups in test case litigation—exercising the right of self-determination in an effort to control, to the greatest extent possible, their own destinies, see, e.g. Judi Chamberlin, On Our Own: Patient-Controlled Alternatives to the Mental Health System (197[8])—is a major development that cannot be overlooked by participants in subsequent mental disability litigation.

[85] One of the core factors of comparative mental disability law is the abject lack of counsel made available to persons facing involuntary civil commitment:

Neither counsel nor judicial review is present in most of the world's mental disability law systems. It is rare for even minimal access to counsel to be statutorily (or judicially) mandated, and, even where counsel is legislatively ordered, it is rarely provided. Moreover, the lack of meaningful judicial review makes the commitment hearing system little more than a meretricious pretext.

Perlin, *Universal Factors*, supra n. 72, at 342. See also generally, Perlin, *Global Clinical Education*, supra n. 73.

[86] Michael L Perlin (2003) 'Therapeutic Jurisprudence and Outpatient Commitment: Kendra's Law as Case Study', 9 Psychol. Pub. Pol'y & L. 183, 193 ('In short, the presumption in which courts have regularly

way that lawyers have been taught—or, at the least, *should* be taught—to advocate for their clients. In nations with no traditions of an 'expanded due process model'[87] in cases involving persons subject to commitment to psychiatric institutions or those already institutionalized, sanism in lawyers can be fatal to an individual's chance for release or for a judicial order mandating amelioration of conditions of confinement and/or access to treatment and/or to be free from unwanted treatment interventions.[88]

Conclusion

The legislative and judicial creation of rights, both positive and negative, is illusory unless there is a parallel mandate of counsel that is (1) free and (2) regularized and organized.[89] Without the presence of such counsel, any rights articulated by a court or human rights commission or legislature become merely 'paper victories'.[90] Further, to be authentically effective, counsel needs to be available both for individual cases (in which commitment, initial or extended, of the patient is being sought) and in 'affirmative' cases (that is, cases consciously thought of as 'public interest' or 'law reform' cases in which persons with disabilities file suit as plaintiffs seeking variously to have courts articulate procedural and/or substantive due process rights in the commitment process,[91] or to have courts articulate such rights with regard to conditions of confinement, the latter cohort encompassing both positive rights, e.g. a right to treatment services,[92] and negative rights, e.g. the right to refuse treatment).[93]

An argument can certainly be made that the presence of sanism (a factor that affects lawyers, even those active in the clinical movement,[94] in the same ways that it affects others) and the additional technical complexity of involuntary civil commitment cases (involving, necessarily, expert

---

engaged-that there is both a de facto and de jure presumption of incompetency to be applied to medication decision making appears to be based on an empirical fallacy: psychiatric patients are not necessarily more incompetent than nonmentally ill persons to engage in independent medication decision making') (footnote omitted).

[87] See Perlin, supra n. 66, at 971.

[88] This analysis and critique are not leveled solely at the practice in the United States. See e.g. Perlin, *Global Clinical Education,* supra note 73) (discussing lack of adequate counsel in civil commitment cases in almost all nations), and Perlin, *Universal Factors,* supra note 72 (discussing the significant number of nations in which there is *no* provision of counsel to individuals facing civil commitment).

[89] See generally, Perlin, supra n. 1, Chapter 2B; Perlin, *Global Clinical Education,* supra n. 73.

[90] See sources cited supra n. 43.

[91] E.g. *Lessard v Schmidt*, 349 F Supp 1078 (ED Wis 1972) (a statute that fails to provide person alleged to be mentally ill with adequate procedural safeguards is unconstitutional).

[92] E.g. *Wyatt v Stickney*, 325 F Supp 781 (MD Ala 1971); aff'd sub. nom. *Wyatt v Aderholt*, 503 F 2d 1305 (5th Cir 1974) (mentally ill have constitutional right to adequate treatment in mental hospital).

[93] E.g. *Rennie v Klein*, 653 F 2d 836 (3d Cir 1981) (patients with mental illness committed involuntarily retain their constitutional right to refuse antipsychotic drugs).
On the role of counsel in mental disability/law reform cases in general, see Perlin supra n. 1, Chapter 2B. Without the presence of effective counsel, substantive mental disability law reform recommendations may turn into 'an empty shell.' Perlin, *Best Friend,* supra n. 65, at 748.
Lawyers have significant advocacy roles beyond their work in the courtroom, and the importance of these roles is magnified in areas of law such as this that are so under-litigated (as the body of case law is so thin as to be evanescent in many nations). A fuller discussion of this important issue is beyond the scope of this chapter.

[94] See Perlin, *Lepers,* supra n. 59; Keri K Gould and Michael L Perlin (2000) '"Johnny's in the Basement/ Mixing Up His Medicine": Therapeutic Jurisprudence and Clinical Teaching', 24 Seattle U. L. Rev. 339.

testimony by mental health professionals and subtle predictions about 'future dangerousness')[95] that the gap would be even wider in such cases. In arguing why the United States should ratify the new UN Convention, Tara Melish focused on the 'deeply entrenched attitudes and stereotypes about disability that have rendered many of the most flagrant abuses of the rights of persons with disabilities "invisible" from the mainstream human rights lens.'[96] These stereotypes are the essence of sanism; vigorous, advocacy-focused counsel is needed to answer and rebut them.

Acknowledgements

The authors wish to thank Naomi Weinstein for her excellent research assistance.

---

[95] See generally, Perlin, supra n. 1, Chapter 2A.
[96] Melish, supra n. 34, at 44.

Chapter 4

Culture and Context in Human Rights

Laurence J. Kirmayer

Notwithstanding their European origins, human rights today represent the universal language in which global relations can be normatively regulated. In Asia, Africa, and South America, they constitute the sole language in which the opponents and victims of murderous regimes and civil wars can raise their voices against violence, repression, and persecution, and against violations of their human dignity. But as human rights have won acceptance as a transcultural language, disagreements between cultures over their proper interpretation have also intensified. Insofar as this intercultural discourse on human rights is conducted in a spirit of reciprocal recognition, it can also lead the West to a decentered understanding of a normative construction that is no longer the property of Europeans and may no longer exclusively reflect the particularities of this one culture

Habermas 2006:155

Introduction

Human rights are moral, legal, and political devices for protecting the dignity, well-being, and survival of human beings. As such they are directed against oppressive powers that seek to undermine and attack these same basic human values. Because their intended use is directed against power, human rights must be understood not as abstract and timeless principles but as urgent calls to action in the face of specific threats. The universality of human rights may be justified by ethical arguments and claims about human nature, but these necessarily appeal to particular cultural notions of morality and personhood. In practice, human rights are legitimated by social, political, and legal institutions that are part of an emerging global civil society (Benhabib et al. 2006). Diverse nations and peoples participate in this global system but they retain their own local cultures and social contexts through which they interpret and apply human rights laws and arguments (Nash 2009). Any discussion of the universality of human rights therefore requires careful attention to the diverse contexts of their application.

The respect for individual autonomy at the heart of human rights is intended to speak directly to the forms of power that threaten to silence and efface the vulnerable individual (Turner 2006). This emphasis on protecting individual autonomy has led some to argue that human rights do not apply to cultures or societies that do not embrace the ideology of individualism. Beyond this, some have argued that human rights rhetoric and institutions are themselves agents of Westernization. However, the need to protect individual autonomy against oppression is more basic than any cultural preoccupation with individualism. As Ignatieff has cautioned:

> Relativism is the invariable alibi of tyranny. There is no reason to apologize for the moral individualism at the heart of human rights discourse; it is precisely this that makes it attractive to dependent groups suffering exploitation or oppression (Ignatieff 2001:74–75)

At the same time, many forms of oppression are not targeted at individuals; there have been many systematic attempts to marginalize, exclude, subjugate, or annihilate whole groups or peoples. Other forms of persistent social inequity and injustice arise from economic arrangements that aim to maintain the advantage of some at the cost of many. Human rights language and legislation have been employed to counter these forms of collective oppression and structural violence to seek redress and social change.

This chapter will address three broad questions basic to the cross-cultural applicability of human rights in the domain of psychiatry: (1) Do the theory and practice of psychiatry and other mental health disciplines apply across disparate cultures? (2) Are human rights principles in general universally applicable? and (3) Are human rights principles specifically applicable to mental health issues across cultures?

Culture in a globalizing world

There are four main contexts that raise questions about the cross-cultural applicability of human rights in mental health: (1) *internationally,* that is, across national political or geographic boundaries; (2) within *culturally diverse societies* that contain ethnocultural or other minority groups, whether as a result of migration or the formation of nation states; (3) with respect to *indigenous peoples,* who form relatively homogeneous societies that have been engulfed by colonizers and settlers, and that have faced repeated displacement, marginalization, and forced assimilation; and (4) among *refugees and displaced peoples* who find themselves forced to flee for their lives and who occupy marginal or extra-territorial spaces, in refugee camps or in transition, while they struggle to gain a foothold in a new land. Human rights are crucial to the protection of individuals, communities, and peoples in each of these contexts and, in each case, cultural issues arise in the application of human rights and in the assertion of specific rights claims for vulnerable groups or minorities. However, each context involves different uses of the concept of culture. Of course, diversity has a much broader definition than culture including, for example, differences in age, gender, sexual orientation, and bodily experience (e.g. the disabled or chronically ill, deaf culture). However, all of these distinctions, no matter how deeply rooted they are in biology, are framed in terms of cultural values and concepts.

Within each geographic region or society as well as in the larger contexts of global society, various minorities or distinctive groups are defined in terms of language, ethnicity, religion, race, and other shared or assigned characteristics. These distinctions are based on a particular history that gives rise to a set of social categories and institutional practices through which individuals identify themselves, form communities, or are grouped together by others. While this cultural-historical basis is obvious for ethnicity, language, and religion it applies as well to race and to other forms of social categorization. For example, some of the distinct ethnic or cultural groups in Africa and other regions owe their current boundaries and definition in part to European colonial powers that imposed distinctions based on racialized categories. Race is a culturally constructed category (though it may use biologically influenced variations in appearance as social markers) because the choice of categories, the ways of assigning people to these categories, and the uses of this distinction are all determined by cultural practices. The meaning of these categories changes with social context, but racial categories have usually been imposed by a group or society to justify its domination, exploitation, or annihilation of another group (Fredrickson 2002). Challenging such discriminatory practices is a basic function of human rights.

Until recently, discussions of culture in the mainstream literature on human rights tended to work with a view of cultures as closed, static, homogenous systems, which produce individuals who are culture-bearers and whose behaviour is largely determined by shared cultural models, values, and perspectives (Eriksen 2001). This approach has been thoroughly critiqued on the grounds that it reifies and essentializes cultures and stereotypes individuals while exaggerating the homogeneity of culture (Freeman 2002; Preis 1996; Wilson 1997). Contemporary anthropological approaches insist that 'culture' names a process, not a thing, and that cultural knowledge and institutions are part of open, fluid, dynamic systems with much internal variation, conflict and contestation (Kuper 1999). Individuals draw from culture to construct their identities and, in the process, they may challenge and reshape cultural practices. Increasingly, there is intermixing of cultural systems giving rise to new hybrid forms of identity; this process has been accelerated by globalization (Kraidy 2005).

Theorists of multiculturalism have recognized this dynamic view of culture; however, in many cases they still identify culture with a more or less localized community. For example, Kymlicka offers this definition of culture: 'The sort of culture that I will focus on is a societal culture—that is, a culture which provides its members with meaningful ways of life across the full range of human activities, including social, educational, religious, recreational, and economic life, encompassing both public and private spheres. These cultures tend to be territorially concentrated, and based on a shared language' (Kymlicka 1995:76). In this view, culture is synonymous with a society or a people, but the contemporary world offers many compelling hybrid cultures, subcultures, or delocalized cultures maintained through transnational or virtual networks.

Although the notion of culture is an abstraction that describes a complex dynamic system, there is a strong tendency in human perception to reduce culture to ethnic stereotypes. Cultural stereotypes can have the same invidious effects as racial stereotypes. The conceptual difficulties with notions of culture and their history of abuse, have led many to argue that it would be best to dispense with the idea of culture entirely (Phillips 2007). However, this is problematic for scientific, moral, and political reasons. Scientifically, it is clear that we are cultural beings, requiring culture to achieve our full functioning. The human brain is essentially an organ of culture, and the ways in which we become ill reflect culture as much as biology (Kirmayer 2006; Wexler 2006). Morally, since culture is the source of our individual values and the means by which we organize communities, recognizing culture is essential to recognizing and respecting each other's commitments and concerns. Finally, every political system, no matter how much it strives for equity privileges some groups while ignoring or disadvantaging others. Acknowledging the domain of culture and recognizing specific ethnocultural groups are essential to identifying and correcting these biases and inequities.

Psychiatry across cultures

The first question concerns the extent to which mental health principles and practices are applicable across cultures. Our ability to answer this question is limited by the available research, which is generally framed in ways that minimize the possibility of identifying salient cultural differences. In much international psychiatric research, culture is conflated with geographic region or nation. Thus, the World Health Organization has coordinated studies on schizophrenia, depression, and common mental disorders in primary care based at centres in several countries and, despite the absence of measures of cultural identity or practices, this is sometimes presented as information about cultural diversity. In the US, membership in large, heterogeneous, 'ethnoracial blocs' defined by the census (i.e. African American, Asian American and Pacific Islander, Hispanic, American Indian and Alaska Native, White), is often taken as a proxy for culture (Hollinger 1995). While it may serve the political purposes of identifying health service needs among socially demarcated groups, this type of research does not engage with cultural variation at a level where specific mediators can be identified. A more fine-grained understanding of culture is required to unpack the elements relevant to any specific mental health problem. Without this contextualized understanding of human strengths and vulnerability, we are left with a 'one-size-fits-all' approach that is a form of one-sided cultural proselytization or imperialism that silences dialogue and exchange (Alegria, Atkins, Farmer, Slaton and Stelk 2010; Gone and Kirmayer 2010).

Nevertheless, there is evidence both for universal aspects of mental health and illness and culture-specific dimensions that require adaptation of conventional models and practices developed in Euro-American contexts. Clinical, epidemiological, and ethnographic research has provided evidence of significant variation in the causes, course, symptoms, treatment, and outcome of mental disorders across cultures (Kirmayer 1989; Kleinman 1988; López and Guarnaccia 2000). While the disorders enshrined in official nosology can be detected in every culture where they have been sought, their prevalence varies widely. This may reflect methodological difficulties in applying diagnostic criteria as well as genuine variation in rates due to the influence in genetic, environmental, and social factors that influence incidence and course. As well, there is strong evidence for the cultural shaping of symptom experience and clinical presentations that can make it difficult to apply diagnostic criteria. There are many culture-related symptoms and syndromes not captured by official diagnostic nosology that may be a focus of concern for patients and contribute to distress and disability. Finally, and most importantly, the meaning of symptoms, illness, and suffering varies according to available cultural models and metaphors for affliction and this, in turn, is a major determinant of the individual and social impact of mental health problems.

Across cultures, people with severe mental illness are generally vulnerable to stigmatization and social exclusion (Fabrega 1991). Psychiatric diagnosis and treatment can both cause and mitigate the social processes of labeling and exclusion. However, the dynamics of labelling and stigma, and subsequent integration or exclusion, depend on cultural systems of meaning and social practices (Angermeyer et al. 2004). For example, in many parts of the world, some forms of psychotic experience may be viewed as divinely inspired, and the individual as having received spiritual gifts (Kirmayer et al. 2004). This may contribute to good outcome with potentially self-limited psychotic disorders. Replacing a religious explanation with an account in terms of disturbed brain chemistry may justify biomedical intervention but undermine the positive meanings and social support mobilized through religious or sociomoral explanations. At the same time, religious explanations may expose individuals to disturbing and disorienting interventions and, when these methods fail to achieve a cure, those afflicted may be blamed for their conditions and rejected. Mental health services can offer safe haven and advocate for individuals subjected to this moral blame, marginalization, or ostracism.

Psychiatry and human rights

The international institution of human rights built on earlier civil rights and liberties that emerged in Europe in the 18th and 19th centuries along with changing notions of the person and recognition of previously marginalized groups as sharing a common humanity (Hunt 2007). Nickel (2007) identifies six broad sets of human rights: security, due process, liberty, political participation, equality, and welfare. The last of these sets of rights speak directly to health—welfare is the basic goal of systems of health and healing, and equality is indirectly related to welfare in terms of equity. Social inequality itself is an important cause of illness (Marmot 2007). In the domain of psychiatry, human rights issues arise in several ways, each of which is shaped by local cultures.

Human rights aim to promote, preserve, and protect the well-being of the individual. By acting to restore individuals' functioning, mental health practices can therefore be an enabler of basic rights. Psychiatry aims to advocate on behalf of people with mental illness and invoking their human rights is one potentially effective strategy to promote social change. The problem of stigma, for example, can be framed as essentially a human rights issue of equality for people with disabilities or special needs. Classifying problems as 'psychiatric' may confer stigma and disqualify the moral autonomy and agency of the individual who is viewed as 'mad'. Insisting on a mental illness interpretation of a problem that was previously understood purely in religious or sociomoral terms can be liberating or debilitating depending on the cultural and social contexts and consequences.

Psychiatric research can document social and political situations that put people at risk for mental illness and identify the need for protection of human rights (e.g. detention of asylum seekers, oppression of women in patriarchal societies, vulnerability of children to sexual exploitation by adults, or the impact of child labor on development). This evidence can support efforts at advocacy for vulnerable individuals or groups. Psychiatric treatment, particularly psychotherapy, may offer possibilities for increasing individuals' agency and empowerment. This may allow individuals facing oppressive circumstances to assert their rights for autonomy either within the system or through some form of exit or escape.

Institutionally, psychiatry plays a social regulatory role acting on behalf of medical and state authority in *loco parentis* to involuntarily restrain, confine, and treat individuals deemed a risk to themselves or others. Although the aim of mental health professionals and psychiatrists is to act in the best interest of the vulnerable individual, at times professionals have colluded with forces of oppression. Human rights then are instruments for challenging abuses of psychiatric power.

Mental health problems are unequally distributed both within and across societies, with the poor and oppressed enduring higher rates (Desjarlais et al. 1995; Prince et al. 2007). To some extent, this reflects the fact that war, political conflict, and other forms of violence are more common in these regions. There is evidence that it is not poverty itself that is a cause of mental illness but the physical, psychological, and social impact of structural inequalities and injustices that are evident to all (Wilkinson and Pickett 2009). This impact of inequality is evident within developed countries as well, where those who face racism and discrimination and various forms of structural violence (often indigenous peoples and ethnoracial minorities) have higher rates of mental disorders (Kelly 2005). At the same time, those who are most afflicted have least access to services and may receive biased diagnosis and treatment (Smedley et al. 2003). This unequal distribution of illness and of access to services in itself constitutes a human rights challenge. Even if the unequal distribution of resources were addressed, however, a further challenge arises from the cultural embedding of mental health and illness. Equity in mental health care requires attention to these variations. Cultural psychiatry and psychology, as disciplines that systematically address the impact of culture on mental health, can be important vehicles to advance human rights.

Cultural relativism and human rights

The second question central to our concern is whether the concept of human rights is applicable across cultures. The assertion of human rights as universal rights would seem to answer this question prescriptively: human rights are meant to be applied across all cultures (Donnelly 2007). However, this universality has been challenged on both conceptual and political grounds. Conceptually, it has been claimed that the notion of human rights depends on specifically

Western notions of the person and cultural values that do not have the same meaning or importance in other cultural contexts. Politically, it has been claimed that human rights are used as a way
for Western societies to critique others, ignoring local values and priorities in favour of an agenda
that serves hegemonic political and economic interests.

Ironically, given its origins in concerns for justice, cultural relativism has been used to challenge
the universality of human rights. Relativism implies that moral values and judgments must always
be interpreted relative to a specific cultural system (Lukes 2008). Within anthropology, relativism
has its roots not in an attitude that 'anything goes' but in an attempt to counteract the racism and
oppression that devalued, discounted, and silenced others' cultural values and points of view (Engle
2002). In its strong or radical version, relativism argues that cultural worlds are 'incommensurable'—that is, they cannot be directly compared because they do not share any common measure
and can only be rightly understood, evaluated, and judged from within their own frameworks.

The cultural relativist critique of human rights makes certain specific claims: (1) that human
rights are rooted in Western traditions and therefore: (a) make sense only with that tradition;
(b) address issues that are peculiar to those traditions; (c) provide remedies that are workable or
effective only within that tradition; and (d) that the very notion of who or what is vulnerable
and of what constitutes human freedom and dignity is culturally determined; (2) that human
rights, because they have emerged from Western cultural traditions, carry and impose that culture
in ways that are corrosive to other traditions; and (3) that there are alternative ways to protect
vulnerable individuals in other traditions. While these arguments focus on the issue of the
cultural basis of human rights, a related set of arguments see human rights as handmaidens to
specific political systems or interests, with the corollary that human rights serve to protect
those interests (Ignatieff 2001).

Applied to the domain of human rights, cultural relativism argues that the concept of human
rights and its legitimation depend on specific notions of the person, cultural values, sociomoral
systems, and ways of life that vary across cultures. Rights, duties, and other ethical principles,
therefore, cannot be understood or enacted without attention to social and cultural context. More
fundamentally, certain rights, duties, and ethical principles cannot even be formulated or articulated without attention to these contexts and hence are irreducibly bound that way of life.

The claim that human rights are rooted in a Western tradition has been used to argue against
their universal applicability. Central to the argument is the observation that human rights are
founded on a distinctively European notion of the autonomy of the individual (Habermas 1998).
There is a close relationship between the political metaphor of self-government and the psychological metaphor of the mature person as an autonomous self-directed individual (Taylor 1989;
Hunt 2007). But other traditions argue for interdependence as the basic reality of human existence
and as a positive value throughout the lifespan (Critchley 2007). Emphasizing autonomy over the
values of connectedness and dependence then works to undermine the solidarity of community.
This critique questions the priority of rights over duties and emphasizes the value of community
over the atomizing effects of an individualistic social order. A community-based ethos subordinates individual autonomy to the group; in return, the group imbues life with meaningful
relationships and commitments through the medium of culture.

Although human rights as a social institution emerged in particular political and historical
contexts, and so would seem to be obviously linked to specific cultural values and forms of life,
there are many arguments as to why these rights can and should be asserted and applied across
diverse social and cultural contexts (Donnelly 2003; Nickel 2007).

The first argument rests on our shared humanity, which includes our common vulnerability as
well as similarities in processes of moral reasoning and intuition. While it is true that human

rights only can be articulated in relation to particular discursive formations that depend on cultural notions of the person, it does not follow that human rights are wholly contingent and relative, anymore than other basic human institutions. Although the content of moral reasoning varies substantially, we can recognize domains of the moral having to do with fairness, justice, and compassionate treatment of others across the range of human cultures. For example, Shweder and colleagues (1997) suggest that moral systems within societies may be divided into three types based on: (i) autonomy, individual rights and justice; (ii) community and hierarchy; and (iii) purity. These basic modes of moral experience are grounded in our evolutionary biology and in existential universals of human experience (Haidt 2007). Cultures differ in the relative emphasis given to these modes and to the social and psychological ramifications of each dimension, but compelling arguments for the protection of vulnerable persons can be made across cultures by appeal to basic moral intuitions. It is precisely because of our common vulnerability and interdependence that we need human rights, not only to preserve autonomy but to protect those bonds of dependence necessary for human flourishing.

The second argument involves a critique of the notion of culture and a clarification of its contemporary meanings. Historically, cultures have been viewed as homogeneous, self-justifying, closed worlds of moral meaning and practice. In reality, as we have noted, cultures are complex, open, hybrid, and contested from within and without. This makes it difficult to appeal to a cultural norm as part of a cohesive and consistent body of knowledge and practice adhered to by a community. Cultures are not finely tuned homeostatic systems that insure the well-being of all members of the community (Edgerton 1992). There may be conflict, inequities, and injustices within communities due to internal structures that advantage some members of a society while oppressing and exploiting others. This is particularly clear in the case of gender, age, or other forms of discrimination. Simply appealing to cultural tradition or collective values does not address the vulnerability of children, women, and minorities to systemic violence and injustice. Human rights offer a potentially useful strategy for the weak and vulnerable in any social system to gain support for challenges to the status quo. Rights language provides a way to speak back to power in social and political struggles that cut across diverse cultures.

The third argument has to do with the 'planetarization' of existence—that is, the fact that, in a globalizing and ecologically challenged world, the actions of one cultural community inevitably impact on all others. However much as we may live in separate cultural worlds, we all must coexist and this demands that we find ways to tolerate differences, maintain mutual respect, and adjudicate and resolve conflicts. Ultimately, this project of creating a safe home for humanity justifies the insistence of the universality of human rights as a prescriptive language for global development and peaceful coexistence.

The arguments against strong cultural relativism have been used by some to dismiss the relevance of culture to human rights but, in fact, they point the way toward addressing cultural difference as part of the political project of extending the reach of human rights to diverse societies and peoples. A weaker version of relativism as a method of understanding ethical problems in context is entirely compatible with human rights. This form of pragmatic relativism recognizes that cultural differences are important and seeks to trace their implications on a case-by-case basis without assuming that everything presented as culture or tradition is automatically sacrosanct and inviolable. This accords with the historical reality of cultures as constantly evolving in response to migration, growth, technological development, and the demands of changing social and political environments. Fixing a given moment of culture as an inflexible standard or tradition against which all future possibilities are to be measured (and rejected) precludes the creative dialogue with others that has always been part of the evolution of human societies.

Such rigidity usually serves the vested interests of those in power who are reluctant to change the status quo.

In its pragmatic and situated form, relativism makes the modest claim that understanding and evaluating a cultural or ethical system requires attention to its cultural frame or context. The meaning and values of specific actions depend on the perspectives of actors, who are all situated in specific social and cultural contexts. This situatedness of meaning and experience does not mean that moral worlds are incommensurable but simply that taking their proper measure requires close attention to the ways that contexts are defined by cultural values and practices, the position of actors within their specific social contexts, and the web of historical and ongoing relationships in which they are embedded (Freeman 2002).

Rights are not just a matter of rhetorical or discursive practices. There are no rights without corresponding social institutions. Rights exist not for naked human beings but for human beings embedded in a social world constructed of cultural meanings and institutions (that is to say, background assumptions and agreed-upon or enforced procedures for regulating others through social power). The debate over the universality of the application of human rights also is situated in these systems of power. Human rights are not invoked from a universal 'view from nowhere' but depend on appeals to principles of vulnerability, justice, dignity, and respect grounded in cultural and historical particulars (Nash 2009). Understanding cultural contexts, therefore, does not so much challenge the basis of human rights (which like every human construct, emerge from a specific cultural history) but gives us a way to work out the moral calculus when (as is the case in most situations) there is not a single right or value to protect but a complex and sometimes contradictory set of values with conflicting or competing costs, benefits, and tradeoffs.

Cultural notions of humanness, humanity, and the humane

The concept of human rights is a cultural and historical invention that was born of basic moral feelings, empathy, intuitions, and concerns toward specific groups of others, which has been generalized to successively broader circles of humanity following historical forces and political arguments (Hunt 2007). The key cultural concepts that underlie human rights are the notions of *humanness* (defining who or what is human); *humanity* (recognizing ourselves as all one species, kinship group, or community, and so supporting the extension of our compassion from those closest to us to all human beings); and the *humane* (identifying what is good, kind, virtuous treatment of each other, as exemplified by empathic concern and compassionate action in response to others' suffering).

Human rights are rights enjoyed simply by virtue of being human (Donnelly 2003). But being human is not as obvious a characteristic as it might first appear. Cultural definitions of the human are part of larger ontologies of personhood that may understand the individual primarily as an isolated autonomous being (individualism), or as fundamentally linked to others in community (collectivism), to the environment (ecocentrism), or to the world of spirits and ancestors (cosmocentrism; see Kirmayer 2007; Gone and Kirmayer 2010). Communal or collectivistic notions of the person emphasize the importance of relations with others as constitutive of the human being; hence maintaining these relationships is fundamental to individual well-being (Tu 1985). Cultures may also recognize certain types of non-human persons and extend rights to them. Thus, for some indigenous peoples, who were traditionally hunters, animals or animal spirits may be non-human persons deserving of respect and care to protect their dignity. The rights of animals and of the land itself for protection may figure in the moral calculus of such peoples. Similarly, in some cultures, ancestors who inhabit a spirit-world that intervenes in ordinary life are also important social presences who must be included in moral reasoning. The cultural concept of the person is used to frame ethical problems, identifying the relative balance of rights and duties, autonomy and dependence in the morality of everyday life. Cultural notions of the human include ideas about 'human nature' and these are often used to underwrite claims for the universality of human rights.

The massive violations of human rights in genocides and other forms of organized violence have been fueled by processes of dehumanizing the other as somehow not fully or really human (Baum 2008). We have psychological mechanisms for dehumanizing others as subhuman, primitive, and animalistic or non-human, machine-like, and devoid of the capacity for empathy (Haslam 2006). These processes of dehumanization pave the way to excluding others from the human community and allow acts of violence to proceed without the empathic recognition of the other as a vulnerable or suffering human being that might otherwise limit our aggression. In some communities, people may be ascribed inhuman qualities, for example, as witches or demons. These labels undermine the humanness of the accused and make it easier for others to attack them.

Global survival depends on the opposite process of extending our empathy, identification, and concern beyond local tribalisms to encompass humanity as a whole. Nationalism and ethnic loyalty may forge ties to a larger group but they define insiders and outsiders, 'us and them', in ways that can undermine our sense of connection to humanity as a whole (Kristeva 1993). The nation state affords new forms of belonging but also creates extraterritorial spaces, outside the system of legal and material protections. This extraterritoriality results in a new kind of vulnerability that requires special forms of protection, like those embodied in the UN conventions on refugees (Benhabib 2004; Gibney 2004). Refugees appeal to a transnational commitment to hospitality in the name of humanity, to a moral obligation to take in, protect, and engage the vulnerable and displaced other; this extends from providing safe haven, to recognizing and helping them to document human rights abuses, to respecting and supporting their individual and collective efforts to reconstruct identity and communal life after its violent disruption. To work, this commitment to humanity must be institutionalized as part of the culture of the institutions of the receiving society and members of the society must have knowledge of the cultural background of the refugees in order to make sense of their stories and respond appropriately (Kirmayer 2001).

The final cultural dimension to human rights concerns notions of the humane, of what constitutes dignified, respectful, and compassionate treatment of each other. Although this can be framed in abstract terms, any specification requires attention to specific cultural values and practices. What counts as inhumane treatment or indignity is clearly related to culture. For example, in the Indian Residential School system mandated by the Canadian federal government for over one hundred years to carry out a policy of forced assimilation, many Aboriginal children were taken from their homes, allowed only limited contact with their families, and forbidden to speak their language (Miller 1996). Accounts by survivors describe many forms of violence that are readily understood as inhumane treatment. Some men mention the fact that their hair was cut short to conform to Euro-Canadian styles and that this constituted a profound humiliation. Understanding the impact of this act requires an appreciation of the significance of hair as a cultural expression of manhood; as well, in some First Nations traditions, cutting the hair was a sign of mourning and boys who had their hair removed with little explanation worried that someone close to them had died. Though, as a general principle, dignified and humane treatment of another should include respecting culturally appropriate modes of dress and comportment, the seriousness of an assault on dignity can only be gauged with detailed cultural knowledge as well as an understanding of the individual's history.

The right to culture and community

Culture provides both the scaffolding of individual psychological development and much of its content. Cultural identity also provides the framework within and against which individuals articulate their identity. Respect for individual differences therefore necessarily entails respect for cultural differences. For all of these reasons, culture is essential to human flourishing, and international human rights declarations treat culture as a basic right (Holder 2006). Cultures, however, are not simply goods or commodities but ways of life that must be realized and enacted by social groups or communities.

Cultural identity also requires recognition by others within and outside the community. Hence, minority groups require a public space with opportunities for recognition by others in the larger society (Taylor 1992). Beyond mutual recognition, for cultures to be viable and have social power they must be engaged in dialogue with each other, founded on respect and open communication. This requires a dialogical situation where there is some common language, shared goal, or other basis to achieve a 'fused horizon' that expands each persons' vision of possibility (Gadamer 1969). This dialogical situation is also the place where human rights can be articulated and deployed to challenge oppressive forces within the community or the larger society.

The right to culture and community is equally important for individualistic and communalistic selves. The notion of the person as connected to community is not simply an alternative to the individualistic view but is complementary—identifying a basic truth about our nature as social beings for whom some degree of belonging is essential to well-being and the realization of personal strivings. 'Because even legal persons are individuated only on the path to socialization the integrity of individual persons can be protected only together with the free access to those interpersonal relationships and cultural traditions in which they can maintain their identities. Without this kind of "communitarianism", a properly understood individualism remains incomplete' (Habermas 1998:167). This makes the protection of communities a necessary concern of any system of human rights and, since culture is the medium through which communities are realized, with this right for community comes a right to culture. Indeed, the right to culture can be readily extended to many novel or emerging configurations of identity and community, including delocalized, transnational, hybrid, and virtual cultural communities.

Communal life is realized through culture but, in itself, this does not require any respect for or effort to preserve diversity—a single dominant culture would suffice. Diversity itself becomes a value when we recognize that each existing culture and community has a comparable claim to its own continuity and survival. There is also an argument on analogy to ecological diversity that sees in the diversity of cultures (and languages) the potential to adapt to new circumstances based on their unique knowledge, values, and practices (Harrison 2007).

There is continuing controversy over whether the protection of the right to participate in or belong to groups or communities (conferring specific identities, and realizing a way of life) necessarily requires group rights. The idea of group rights goes beyond the opportunity for individual freedom of association, to allow groups a measure of power and redress against oppressive forces. In so doing, group rights aim to preserve and protect groups as such, but this can readily come into conflict with individual rights. Nickel describes three kinds of group rights: 1) group security rights (the right to exist and be protected against genocide); 2) group representation rights (the right for political voice); and 3) group autonomy rights (the right for self-direction or governance) (Nickel 2007: 164).

The argument for group rights is based on the evidence that 'living within one's cultural group is a constituent part of some people's good (and not merely a means to that good). If so, for such people the survival of their group may have the same value as their own survival' (Nickel 2007: 165).

If the group is vulnerable to the power of the state or other larger forces applied to it as a group (rather than strictly through individuals), then it needs some mechanism to protect itself. Group rights have seen their strongest defense in response to the predicament of indigenous peoples. In the Declaration of the Rights of Indigenous Peoples, group rights are explicitly embraced, with rights attributed directly to 'indigenous peoples' rather than 'members of indigenous groups' (<http://www.un.org/esa/socdev/unpfii/en/drip.html>). These rights provide a basis for indigenous peoples to fight for the restoration of their traditional lands and for a degree of political autonomy. They also may create potential conflicts when groups exert cultural rights that challenge the autonomy of individuals within their own communities (Denis 1997).

Minority rights aim to address the vulnerability of ethnocultural, religious, or other groups living within a larger society with a dominant or majority group. The Universal Declaration of Human Rights explicitly includes minority persons among those who must enjoy rights without discrimination. Article 2 states 'Everyone is entitled to all the rights and freedoms set forth in this Declaration, without distinction of any kind, such as race, colour, sex, language, religion, political or other opinion, national or social origin, property, birth or other status' (<http://www.un.org/en/documents/udhr/>). The list is clearly not meant to be exhaustive but to recognize the major ways in which societies divide and discriminate between groups.

In general, approaches to minority rights have addressed group rights through the individual. This works because of the close link between cultural identity and individual well-being. However, in some instances, this may not be sufficient. The UN Convention on the Prevention and Punishment of the Crime of Genocide of 1948 speaks directly to the specific vulnerability of minority groups as such. Genocide is defined as the crime of killing, injuring, preventing births, or removing children 'with intent to destroy, in whole or in part, a national, ethnical, racial, or religious group, as such' (<http://www.hrweb.org/legal/genocide.html>). There are other human rights treaties that address minority rights either directly, or indirectly, under the rubric of more general principles (Nickel 2007:157ff). The UN International Civil and Political Covenant speaks of 'peoples', invoking the idea of distinctive if not wholly autonomous groups, and addresses minority rights explicitly: 'In those States in which ethnic, religious or linguistic minorities exist, persons belonging to such minorities shall not be denied the right, in community with the other members of their group, to enjoy their own culture, to profess and practise their own religion, or to use their own language' (<http://www.hrweb.org/legal/cpr.html>). Minorities here include ethnic, religious, and linguistic groups, that is, groups that have a distinct culture, religion, or language.

Beyond protection against direct threats to the survival of minorities, we have argued that basic issues of equity require efforts to make health services truly accessible and effective through systematic attention to issues to culture in mental health. Currently, this tends to be framed in terms of 'cultural competence' but models of service take different forms reflecting local demography, histories of migration, ideologies of citizenship, and the structure of the health care system (Kirmayer and Minas 2000). Equity in access and delivery of health services requires attention to the needs and values of cultural communities (Alegira et al. 2010).

Pluralism, multiculturalism, and interculturalism

The European conception of human rights implies a secularized political authority—or at least one committed to pluralism and to a democratic space for 'rational' debate where violators of human rights can be called to account (Lassman 2011). Hence, it stands against fundamentalism (which allows only its own truth) and dogmatism (which precludes rational debate). The space of pluralism allows for the coexistence of diverse cultures (multiculturalism) and their interaction and mutual transformation (interculturalism).

Multiculturalism aims to foster the coexistence of multiple cultures within one society and to make that diversity a defining feature of the collective (Kymlicka 1995, 2007). Benhabib (2002) grounds multicultural claims in three principles: egalitarian reciprocity, voluntary self-ascription, and freedom of association and exit. Beyond these basic political processes, multiculturalism involves a policy of public recognition and support for the institutions and practices (including those related to health care) of multiple ethnocultural communities within the same society (Kirmayer 2011).

Multiculturalism begins with an acceptance of the possibility of cultural difference in a common society. Maintaining islands of difference in a pluralistic system requires specific political efforts and provisions but these rest on particular cultural values or ideologies that embrace diversity (Kymlicka 2007). The persistence of minority communities may require a right of association or belonging and ways to elaborate their own intrinsic and relative values and protect their boundaries, for example, by teaching and using their own language or practicing their own religion, with all of its associated institutions.

At the same time, to protect individuals from the oppressive effects of groups, it is essential to insure the right of exit from a group or community. This is not a simply matter of preventing physical confinement and coercion, because there are psychological dynamics of attachment and belonging that may stand in the way of moving in or out of particular cultural communities. A pluralistic society provides options for continuing one's life outside the original cultural community. Pluralism itself therefore becomes the larger social context essential to insure the right of exit. Multiculturalism not only tolerates but actively supports alternative ways of life within a larger pluralistic society.

Some of the complexities of freedom of exit are illustrated by the Amish practice of *rumspringa* in which adolescents leave the community for a time to taste secular life and then are free to choose to rejoin the Amish community as a committed adult (Mazie 2005; Shachtman 2006). *Rumspringa* institutionalizes the right of exit; however, it also reveals some of the psychological and social complexities of 'freedom of choice.' To the extent that young people have been shielded from the secular world prior to adolescence, they may be ill-prepared to navigate their new-found freedom. As well, because their decision to leave the fold may involve severing ties with family and loved ones, the choice bears a substantial emotional cost. Thus, many individuals freely choose ways of life that are more constraining, whether because of the strength of affective bonds, the desire for meaningful structure in their lives, or other goals and convictions.

Multiculturalism has been criticized for viewing culture in terms of discrete community groups, conflating culture with ethnicity, and exaggerating the homogeneity of cultural identity and values (Modood 2007; Phillips 2007). Multiculturalism therefore runs the risk of trapping people within stereotypic and essentialized views of their cultural backgrounds. The argument for the virtues of communalism and connection is based on a romanticized view of community in small-scale societies, which becomes still more problematic in the context of nation states (Bauman 2001). A larger sense of belonging is needed to counter the divisive effects of identifying exclusively with an ethnically homogeneous cultural community (Kristeva 1993).

These same dilemmas apply to the uses of culture within the legal system. Thus, while Renteln (2004) has argued for the value of taking culture into consideration in legal processes, for Benhabib, 'the cultural defense strategy imprisons the individual in a cage of univocal cultural interpretations and psychological motivations; individuals' intentions are reduced to cultural stereotypes; moral agency us reduced to cultural puppetry' (Benhabib 2002:89). Treating culture as something that mitigates individuals' legal responsibility for their actions exaggerates the influence of culture on behaviour and undermines civil society. Nevertheless, systematic attention to culture can provide the contextual information essential to understand individual behaviour (which otherwise is judged against the implicit cultural norms of the dominant culture) and so can contribute to greater equity within the legal system (Kirmayer et al. 2007).

Much recent work has considered how to configure pluralistic societies in ways that respect and sustain cultural diversity while allowing for fluidity, hybridity, conflict, and contestation (Phillips 2007). In place of a multiculturalism that accepts strong incommensurability among communities with divergent values, Benhabib (2002) advocates intercultural dialogue, that allows for an 'inter-active universalism' (Bohman 2005). This recognizes that cultures and identities are formed through systems of dialogue that can be open at the boundaries to other ways of life. Democratic institutions make this dialogue possible (Habermas 1998). For Benhabib (2002, 2006), this dialogue reflects the reality that cultures are formed and reformed through interactions with other cultures. Dialogue requires not only tolerance of the other but active engagement.

There are a variety of political arrangements that can allow the tolerance and hospitality necessary for a dialogical process of encounter and exchange (Walzer 1997). Any regime of toleration, however, eventually meets its limits. For example, people willing to accept or even encourage others to maintain their distinctive style of dress (e.g. Sikh turbans, hijabs) may balk at tolerating genital cutting as a rite of passage for girls or young women (Shweder 2002). Yet even if it is clear that this is a medically harmful practice, it may have important cultural meanings that over-ride its health consequences for members of the cultural group. Thus, proscribing genital cutting without engaging the community in dialogue may erode communal authority and social institutions in ways that have unintended negative effects. Legal proscription sets limits on the tolerance of the other's cultural practices and so contributes to the (inevitable) process of culture change. Similar dilemmas occur in the more common cultural conflicts associated with migration, for example, intergenerational conflicts around adolescents dating, sexuality, or marital choices. A simple response of tolerance is not adequate because there are tensions within the community and adopting a 'tolerant' stance itself means taking one side in an argument within the community.

From an intercultural perspective, the aim then is to understand how particular practices are embedded in individual and collective identity and so, in enacting human rights legislation, to leave sufficient room for individuals and communities to work out transformations that preserve core values and maintain a necessary degree of cultural continuity. This speaks not to the basic principles or standards of human rights but to how they are enacted. Asserting and protecting human rights does not mean simply drawing a line in the sand and intervening forcefully in emergent situations, but depends on fostering a dialogue that includes the voices of the oppressed, those who desire change, and the conservative elements of a culture, community, or society that resist it. Human rights are instruments of change but must work with the cultural communities that give individual lives meaning and purpose.

In a pluralistic, democratic society, cultural exchange cannot be one-sided. Interculturalism means that the dominant or established groups allow themselves to be transformed by the other. The framework of pluralistic civil society, whether local, national, international, or global provides the arena for this interchange (Benhabib et al. 2006). The aim is not only basic respect for others in their cultural worlds as an end in itself, but the strengthening of the dialogical processes of encounter that can subserve the cultural transmission and institution building necessary to enact human rights. There is no doubt that human rights talk aims to transmit certain values and ideas and in so doing effects a transformation of culture (Nash 2009; Preis 1996). This need not be one-sided or imperialistic. Dialogue in an effort at moral persuasion can be founded on affirming our shared humanity and taking others seriously. Taking others seriously means recognizing not just their vulnerability but also their cultural allegiances and self-definitions. In so doing, we open ourselves to transformation through our encounters with others.

The two legs of human rights are a cosmopolitan understanding of the complexity and mobility of identities and a respect for and protection of local communities and their institutions as the holders and protectors of moral and cultural values (Sacks 2002). This demands what Appiah (2006) (borrowing from Ackerman 1994) has called a 'rooted cosmopolitanism' in which participants bring both their connections to specific traditions and their commitments to a pluralistic society that is realized through the process of dialogue and the institution of human rights. Within this pluralism, individuals and communities can allow themselves to encounter each other in ways that require their mutual transformation.

Conclusion: human rights in a globalizing world

Cultural communities are not isolated local worlds but increasingly embedded in global or planetary systems that offer new possibilities of identity and awareness and new scope for moral action. It is in this global context that we must understand the debates over the cultural relativity of human rights, and the problem of group versus individual rights. Human rights were devised to protect the individual from oppression and discrimination exercised by, or on behalf of, powerful groups or political entities. But human beings also are social beings who need to belong to groups—families, clans, communities, peoples—that preserve, protect, and confer meaning on a way of life. Thus, there is a tension between the needs for belonging and for autonomy. Efforts to advance human rights must consider how to negotiate tradeoffs when autonomy and belonging come into direct conflict.

In the domain of psychiatry, human rights have been used to address issues of unequal access to mental health care, bias and inequities in mental health treatment and outcomes, the exploitation of vulnerable groups and individuals in research, and the use of psychiatry as an agent of social control and political repression. These issues cut across cultural differences. However, attention to cultural context is needed to address the applicability of specific mental health policies and practices for particular populations or individuals.

Achieving equity in health care means not simply insuring access to services but also addressing their cultural appropriateness. If accessible and effective care demands attention to culture and engagement of the community, then the cultural safety and responsiveness of mental health services becomes a human rights issue akin to group or minority rights. The globalization of psychiatry itself also becomes a human rights issue as cultures are swallowed up by a form of cultural imperialism in which psychiatric knowledge and practices displace local frameworks of identity and systems of healing.

Although contemporary mental health professionals aim to ground their practice in scientific evidence, the 'psy' disciplines have their roots in Western cultural institutions (Rose 1996). There is a global hegemony of psychiatric knowledge largely derived from European and American traditions. Northern European and North American notions of individualism and autonomy underwrite much of psychiatric nosology, theory, and practice (Gaines 1992). The global economy that exports psychiatric knowledge and expertise also exports these values of individualism and corresponding ways of life. This may have a liberating effect by creating new options for people limited by illness or untenable social situations, but it also creates ethical conundrums. To act on behalf of the vulnerable, psychiatry must see beyond its complicity with the pharmaceutical industry and other economic and political interests that encourage mental health professionals and patients to frame problems in ways that exclude the social origins of suffering.

We need to explicitly address structural inequalities that are both the causes of psychiatric problems and the barriers to effective care. We need to work to ensure that the care people receive is effective. In intercultural clinical care, this includes addressing language differences with the use of interpreters, and differences in cultural explanations of illness with culture brokers. It also requires maintaining a pluralistic health care system with opportunities to make use of culturally consonant forms of assessment and treatment. This pluralism requires continued critical reflection on the cultural assumptions built into different systems of help and healing, including biomedicine and psychiatry.

Human rights are tools for building global civil society. Although they spring from particular cultural traditions, and cannot be justified on universally acceptable metaphysical grounds, they speak directly to major political dilemmas of the contemporary world. Because they rest on cultural assumptions about the worth and inviolability of individuals and the need to protect the most vulnerable among us, their spread and adoption depends on promoting culture change—not toward a single global culture but toward a pluralistic system that encourages diversity and makes mutual tolerance and respect paramount.

Globalization has led to new forms of citizenship characterized as transnational, postnational, and flexible. These demand rethinking the processes of protection of vulnerable individuals and groups. Among the notions that underwrite relationships between individuals and communities in this new era we can see a progression in political argument from concern with tolerance to notions of hospitality, pluralism, dialogue, and cosmopolitanism (Benhabib et al. 2006; van Hooft 2009).

Cosmopolitanism reflects the social changes wrought by globalization, including the erosion of national sovereignty, the growth of diasporic communities, and cultural hybridity. In addition to legal and political institutions to sustain global civil society, these changes call for a new set of 'cosmopolitan virtues' of irony and skepticism, self-reflectivity, recognition of and care for the other, and the willingness to be changed by the intercultural encounter (Turner 2006). The uses of human rights must be subjected to critical analysis as states accumulate new forms of power and surveillance and as transnational corporations assert their economic interests in ways that accentuate inequality and suffering (Cheah 2006; Tsing 2004). Mental health practitioners are part of the emerging global society and also must engage in critique of the cultural assumptions built into psychiatric theory and practice. Awareness of the cultural values inherent in mental health practices is essential to advance the aspirations for justice and equity that underlie the commitment to human rights.

References

Ackerman, B (1994) 'Rooted cosmopolitanism', *Ethics*, 104(3), 516–35.

Alegria, M, Atkins, M, Farmer, E, Slaton, E, and Stelk, W (2010) 'One size does not fit all: taking diversity, culture and context seriously', *Administration and Policy in Mental Health*, 37(1–2), 48–60.

Angermeyer, MC, Buyantugs, L, Kenzine, DV, and Matschinger, H (2004) 'Effects of labelling on public attitudes towards people with schizophrenia: are there cultural differences?', *Acta Psychiatrica Scandinavica*, 109(6), 420–25.

Appiah, A (2006) *Cosmopolitanism: ethics in a world of strangers*. New York: WW Norton.

Baum, S (2008) *The psychology of genocide*. Cambridge, UK: Cambridge University Press.

Bauman, Z (2001) *Community: Seeking safety in an insecure world*. Cambridge, UK: Polity Press.

Benhabib, S (2002) *The claims of culture: equality and diversity in the global era*. Princeton, NJ: Princeton University Press.

Benhabib, S (2004) *The rights of others: aliens, residents and citizens*. New York: Cambridge University Press.

Benhabib, S, Waldron, J, Honig, B, Kymlicka, W, and Post, R (2006) *Another cosmopolitanism*. New York: Oxford University Press.

Bohman, J (2005) 'Rights, cosmopolitanism and public reason: Interactive universalism in *The Claims of Culture*', *Philosophy & Social Criticism*, 31(7), 715–26.

Cheah, P (2006) *Inhuman conditions: On cosmopolitanism and human rights*. Berkeley, CA: University of California Press.

Critchley, S (2007) *Infinitely demanding: ethics of commitment, politics of resistance*. London: Verso.

Denis, C (1997) *We are not you: First Nations & Canadian modernity*. Orchard Park, NY: Broadview Press.

Desjarlais, R, Eisenberg, L, Good, B, and Kleinman, A (1995) *World mental health: Problems and priorities in low-income countries*. New York: Oxford University Press.

Donnelly, J (2003) *Universal human rights in theory and practice*. 2nd edn. Ithaca: Cornell University Press.

Donnelly, J (2007) 'The relative universality of human rights', *Human Rights Quarterly*, 29(2), 281–306.

Edgerton, RB (1992) *Sick societies: Challenging the myth of primitive harmony*. New York: The Free Press.

Engle, K (2002) 'From skepticism to embrace: Human rights and the American Anthropological Association from 1947 to 1999', in RA Shweder, M Minow, and H Markus (eds) *Engaging cultural differences: the multicultural challenge in liberal democracies*. New York: Russell Sage Foundation, 344–62.

Eriksen, TH (2001) 'Between universalism and relativism: A critique of the UNESCO concept of culture', in JK Cowan, M-B Dembour, and RA Wilson (eds) *Culture and rights: Anthropological perspectives*. Cambridge, UK: Cambridge University Press, 127–148.

Fabrega, H Jr. (1991) 'Psychiatric stigma in non-Western societies', *Comprehensive Psychiatry*, 32(6), 534–51.

Fredrickson, GM (2002) *Racism: a short history*. Princeton, NJ: Princeton University Press.

Freeman, M (2002) 'Anthropology and the democratisation of human rights', *The International Journal of Human Rights*, 6(3), 37–54.

Gadamer, H (1969) *Truth and method*. New York: Crossroad.

Gaines, AD (1992) 'From DSM-I to III-R: Voices of self, mastery and the other: A cultural constructivist reading of U.S. psychiatric classification', *Social Science and Medicine*, 35(1), 3–24.

Gibney, MJ (2004) *The ethics and politics of asylum: liberal democracy and the response to refugees*. New York: Cambridge University Press.

Gone, JP and Kirmayer, LJ (2010) 'On the wisdom of considering culture and context in psychopathology', in T Millon, RF Krueger, and E Simonsen (eds) *Contemporary directions in psychopathology: Toward the DSM-V and ICD-11*. New York: Guilford, 72–96.

Habermas, J (1998) 'Remarks on legitimation through human rights', *Philosophy and Social Criticism*, 24(2/3), 157–71.

Habermas, J (2006) *Time of transitions* (Cronin, C and Pensky, M, trans). Cambridge, UK: Polity.

Haidt, J (2007) 'The new synthesis in moral psychology', *Science*, 316(5827), 998–1002.

Harrison, KD (2007) *When languages die: the extinction of the world's languages and the erosion of human knowledge*. New York: Oxford University Press.

Haslam, N (2006) 'Dehumanization: an integrative review', *Personality and Social Psychology Review*, 10(3), 252–64.

Holder, C (2006) 'Culture as a basic human right', in AI Eisenberg (ed) *Diversity and equality: the changing framework of freedom in Canada*. Vancouver: UBC Press, 170–208.

Hollinger, DA (1995) *Postethnic America: Beyond multiculturalism*. New York: Basic Books.

Hunt, LA (2007) *Inventing human rights: a history*. New York: WW Norton & Co.

Ignatieff, M (2001) *Human rights as politics and idolatry*. Princeton, NJ: Princeton University Press.

Kelly, BD (2005) 'Structural violence and schizophrenia', *Social Science and Medicine*, 61(3), 721–30.

Kirmayer, LJ (1989) 'Cultural variations in the response to psychiatric disorders and emotional distress', *Social Science and Medicine*, 29(3), 327–39.

Kirmayer, LJ (2001) 'Failures of imagination: The refugee's narrative in psychiatry', *Anthropology & Medicine*, 10(2), 167–85.

Kirmayer, LJ (2006) 'Beyond the "new cross-cultural psychiatry": cultural biology, discursive psychology and the ironies of globalization', *Transcultural Psychiatry*, 43(1), 126–44.

Kirmayer, LJ (2007) 'Psychotherapy and the cultural concept of the person', *Transcultural Psychiatry*, 44(2), 232–57.

Kirmayer, LJ (2011) 'Multicultural medicine and the politics of recognition', *Journal of Medicine and Philosophy*, 36(4), 410–23.

Kirmayer, LJ, Corin, E, and Jarvis, GE (2004) 'Inside knowledge: Cultural constructions of insight in psychosis', in XF Amador AS David (eds) *Insight in Psychosis* (2 ed). New York: Oxford University Press, 197–229.

Kirmayer, LJ, and Minas, H (2000) 'The future of cultural psychiatry: an international perspective', *Canadian Journal of Psychiatry*, 45(5), 438–46.

Kirmayer, LJ, Rousseau, C, and Lashley, M (2007) 'The place of culture in forensic psychiatry', *Journal of the American Academy of Psychiatry and the Law*, 35(1), 98–102.

Kleinman, A (1988) *Rethinking psychiatry*. New York: Free Press.

Kraidy, M (2005) *Hybridity, or the cultural logic of globalization*. Philadelphia: Temple University Press.

Kristeva, J (1993) *Nations without nationalism*. New York: Columbia University Press.

Kuper, A (1999) *Culture: The anthropologists' account*. Cambridge, MA: Harvard University Press.

Kymlicka, W (1995) *Multicultural citizenship*. Oxford: Oxford University Press.

Kymlicka, W (2007) *Multicultural odysseys: navigating the new international politics of diversity*. New York: Oxford University Press.

Lassman, P (2011) *Pluralism*. Cambridge: Polity Press.

López, S and Guarnaccia, PJ (2000) 'Cultural psychopathology: Uncovering the social world of mental illness', *Annual Review of Psychology*, 51, 571–98.

Lukes, S (2008) *Moral relativism*. New York: Picador.

Marmot, M (2007) 'Achieving health equity: from root causes to fair outcomes', *The Lancet*, 370(9593), 1153–63.

Mazie, SV (2005) 'Consenting adults? Amish *Rumspringa* and the quandary of exit in liberalism', *Perspectives on Politics*, 3(4), 745–59.

Miller, JR (1996) *Shingwauk's vision: A history of native residential schools*. Toronto: University of Toronto Press.

Modood, T (2007) *Multiculturalism*. Cambridge; Malden, MA: Polity.

Nash, K (2009) *The cultural politics of human rights: Comparing the US and UK*. Cambridge, UK: Cambridge University Press.

Nickel, JW (2007) *Making sense of human rights*. 2nd edn. Oxford: Blackwell.

Phillips, A (2007) *Multiculturalism without culture*. Princeton, NJ: Princeton University Press.

Preis, AB (1996) 'Human rights as cultural practice: an anthropological critique', *Human Rights Quarterly*, 18, 286–315.

Prince, M, Patel, V, Saxena, S, Maj, M, Maselko, J, Phillips, MR, et al. (2007) 'No health without mental health', *The Lancet*, 370(9590), 859–77.

Renteln, AD (2004) *The cultural defense*. New York: Oxford University Press.

Rose, NS (1996) *Inventing our selves: psychology, power, and personhood*. New York: Cambridge University Press.

Sacks, J (2002) *The dignity of difference: how to avoid the clash of civilizations*. New York: Continuum.

Shachtman, T (2006) *Rumspringa: to be or not to be Amish*. New York: North Point Press.

Shweder, RA (2002) '"What about female genital mutilation?" And why understanding culture matters in the first place', in RA Shweder, M Minow, and H Markus (eds) *Engaging cultural differences: the multicultural challenge in liberal democracies*. New York: Russell Sage Foundation, 216–51.

Shweder, RA, Much, NC, Mahapatra, M, and Park L (1997) 'The "big three" of morality (autonomy, community, divinity) and the "big three" explanations of suffering', in A Brandt and P Rozin (eds) *Morality and Health*. New York: Routledge, 119–26.

Smedley, BD, Stith, AY, Nelson, AR, Institute of Medicine (US) Committee on Understanding and Eliminating Racial and Ethnic Disparities in Health Care (2003) *Unequal treatment: confronting racial and ethnic disparities in health care*. Washington, DC: National Academy Press.

Taylor, C (1989) *Sources of the self: The making of modern identity*. Cambridge, MA: Harvard University Press.

Taylor, C (1992) 'The politics of recognition', in A Gutmann (ed) *Multiculturalism and 'The politics of recognition': An essay by Charles Taylor*. Princeton, New Jersey: Princeton University Press, 25–73.

Tsing, AL (2004) *Friction: An ethnography of global connection*. Princeton: Princeton University Press.

Tu, Wei-Ming (1985) 'Selfhood and otherness in Confucian thought', in AJ Marsella, G Devos, and FLK Hsu (eds) *Culture and self: Asian and Western perspectives*. New York: Tavistock Publications, 231–51.

Turner, BS (2006) *Vulnerability and human rights*. University Park, PA: Pennsylvania State University Press.

van Hooft, S (2009) *Cosmopolitanism: A philosophy for global ethics*. Montreal & Kingston: McGill-Queen's Press.

Walzer, M (1997) *On toleration*. New Haven: Yale University Press.

Wexler, BE (2006) *Brain and culture: neurobiology, ideology, and social change*. Cambridge, MA: MIT Press.

Wilkinson, RG and Pickett, R (2009) *The spirit level: Why more equal societies almost always do better*. London: Penguin.

Wilson, RA (1997) 'Human rights, culture and context: An introduction', in R Wilson (ed) *Human rights, culture and context: anthropological perspectives*. London: Pluto Press, 1–27.

Chapter 5

Stigma and Discrimination
Critical Human Rights Issues for Mental Health

Jennifer Randall, Graham Thornicroft,
Elaine Brohan, Aliya Kassam, Elanor
Lewis-Holmes, and Nisha Mehta

Introduction

> Human rights violations are not accidents; they are not random in distribution or effect. Rights
> violations are, rather symptoms of deeper pathologies of power and are linked intimately to the social
> conditions that so often determine who will suffer abuse and who will be shielded from harm.
>
> *(Farmer 2005:7)*

'. . .we cannot avoid looking at power and connections if we hope to understand, and thus prevent, human rights abuses.' (Farmer 2005:16). In his book, *Pathologies of power*, Paul Farmer argues that when we expand our focus to the *ultimate* forces influencing people's lives, prescribing their choices, and limiting their opportunities, we can see that health outcomes are consequences of economic, political, historical, social, cultural, and geographic factors. His work with people with HIV and multi-drug resistant tuberculosis and other infectious diseases has demonstrated clear links between health and human rights and this perspective translates nicely into the field of mental health (Weiss 2008). For example, if we observe that a young woman from rural Haiti has become infected with HIV through a sexual encounter with a soldier, it is not only the single sexual episode which created this condition. The fact that she was forced to leave her hometown for the city to find work only to confront the reality that the only thing she could sell was her body, placed her at risk far before the single sexual episode. This same lens can also be used to understand the stigma and discrimination experienced by persons with mental disabilities. The fact that an increasing burden of mental disability now falls on those with less economic and social power indicates that certain populations are at differential risk for some health conditions.

The field of mental health learns a great deal about stigma and discrimination from the experiences of people working in the field of HIV and much of the work linking human rights and health has come from this area of research. Stigma and discrimination are part of the 'social conditions' which contribute and lead to poor outcomes for people infected with HIV just as it does for those with a diagnosis of a mental disability. Stigma and discrimination are part of this complex matrix and therefore can be considered within a human rights framework.

In a 2005 UNAIDS report, the authors present a simple schematic outlining the connections between stigma, discrimination, and human rights violations. Stigma causes discrimination which leads to violations of human rights which legitimates stigma. Left uninterrupted the cycle perpetuates and gains momentum. Interventions can target the cycle at three points: stigma reduction, anti-discrimination and human rights, and legal approaches. This schematic is also appropriate when considering mental health.

In just these ways, stigma contributes to the disability of many people with mental illness (Hinshaw and Cicchetti 2000; Thornicroft 2006) and many are subjected to systematic discrimination in most facets of their lives (Corrigan 2005; Corrigan et al. 2004). These forms of social exclusion occur at home, work, in their personal lives and social activities, in their consumption of health care, and in portrayals in the media (Wahl 1995). This chapter discusses: (i) definitions of stigma and their components; (ii) relevant international human rights conventions (iii) three Articles of a recent human rights convention to illustrate stigma as a critical human rights issue, and (iv) gives examples of the work of relevant international non-governmental organizations active in this field.

Defining stigma

Stigma can be broken into three related components:

- A problem of knowledge, namely *ignorance*
- A problem of negative attitudes, namely *prejudice*
- A problem of behaviour, namely *discrimination*

Ignorance: Even when societies have access to an unprecedented volume of information in the public domain, the level of accurate knowledge about mental illnesses (aka 'mental health literacy') is meagre (Crisp et al. 2005). In a 2003 population survey in England, 55 per cent of adults believed that the statement 'someone who cannot be held responsible for his or her own actions' describes a person who is mentally ill (Department of Health 2003). In the same study, 63 per cent thought that less than 10 per cent of the population would experience a mental illness at some time in their lives, while we know that one in four people will experience a mental health problem at some point in their lives.

Prejudice: People who do not have mental illness commonly feel fear, anxiety, and avoidance when reacting to people with mental illness. Likewise, people with mental illness, who anticipate rejection and discrimination, sometimes impose upon themselves a form of 'self-stigma' (Link et al. 2004). The majority act with prejudice in rejecting a minority group and this involves not just negative thoughts but also emotion such as anxiety, anger, resentment, hostility, distaste, or disgust. A recent study of terms used for mental illness among 14-year-old students in England found that they used 250 words or phrases to describe those with mental illness, none of which were positive (Rose et al. 2007).

Discrimination: Scientific evidence and strong messages from service users and advocates are clear: discrimination blights the lives of many people with mental illness, making marriage, childcare, work, and a normal social life much more difficult. Actions are needed to redress the social exclusion of people with mental illness, and to use the legal measures intended to support equality for all people with physical and mental disabilities (Peterson et al. 2007).

This chapter highlights discrimination because discrimination is a consequence of negative behaviour, and because human rights are largely associated with socially excluding behaviour.

Human rights framework: international conventions

So how do stigma and discrimination fit within a human rights framework? Why are stigma and discrimination critical human rights issues? Evidence clearly demonstrates that stigma is a significant factor in the suffering experienced by those who live with mental illness and some of this suffering constitutes human rights violations. While it is not the only factor propagating such atrocities, it is one which can be analysed within a human rights framework.

Since 1948 the world has witnessed the development of numerous international human rights conventions (see Table 5.1) and regional instruments (WHO 2012). These documents protect all people but are particularly important for vulnerable groups, e.g. people with mental illness and those involuntarily detained. They outline *protections* from abuse and *obligations* to states which ratify the convention. They establish a framework to support those who report breaches of human rights or who seek to end ill-treatment. They act as an integrating statement of the purpose for

Table 5.1 United Nations Conventions, Instruments, and Commentaries Relevant to Those With Mental Disabilities

---

Human Rights Conventions

- The Convention on the Prevention and Punishment of the Crime of Genocide (1948)
- The Convention relating to the Status of Refugees (1951)
- The Supplementary Convention on the Abolition of Slavery, the Slave Trade and Institutions and Practices Similar to Slavery (1956)
- The International Convention on the Elimination of All Forms of Racial Discrimination (1965)
- The International Covenant on Civil and Political Rights (1966)
- The International Covenant on Economic, Social and Cultural Rights (1966)
- The Convention on the Elimination of All forms of Discrimination against Women (1979)
- The Convention Against Torture (1984)
- The Convention on the Rights of the Child (1989)
- The International Convention on the Protection of the Rights of All Migrant Workers and Members of Their Families (1990)
- The Framework Convention on Climate Change (1992)
- The International Convention for the Protection of All Persons from Enforced Disappearance (1992)
- The Convention on the Rights of Persons with Disabilities (2006)

Other Related Instruments

- The World Programme of Action concerning Disabled Persons (1981)
- The Principles for the Protection of Persons with Mental Illness and the Improvement of Mental Health Care (1991)
- The Standard Rules on the Equalization of Opportunities for Persons with Disabilities (1993)
- The Declaration on the Rights of Disabled Persons (1995)

General Recommendations and Comments of convention monitoring bodies, including those pertaining to disability and health. Examples include:

- the Committee on the Elimination of Discrimination against Women, General Recommendation No. 18 (1994) on 'Disabled women'
- The Committee on Economic, Social and Cultural Rights, General Comment No. 5 (1994) on 'Persons with Disabilities'
- The Committee on Economic, Social and Cultural Rights, General Comment No. 14 (2000) on 'The Right to the Highest Attainable Standard of Health'
- The Committee on the Rights of the Child, General Comment No. 9 (2006) on 'The Rights of Children with Disabilities'

mental health services, and so assist in the development of local guidelines or laws and ensure that the ethical aspects of clinical practice are given sufficient emphasis to practitioners, and so reduce the likelihood of human rights abuses, including vilification (for example the latter is unlawful in Australia on grounds of race, religion, or sexual preferences but not on the grounds of mental health).

Those countries which have ratified these conventions are consequently obliged under international law to guarantee to every person in its territory, without discrimination, all the freedoms and entitlements enshrined within them. The impact of these documents depends largely on the local steps taken to implement the protections and obligations and the processes established to monitor their progress and compliance.

We highlight two important human rights documents: The European Convention on Human Rights (ECHR) and the Convention on the Rights of Persons with Disabilities (CRPD). The ECHR was drafted and signed in 1950 and is the main human rights document of the Council of Europe. The convention established the European Court of Human Rights (ECtHR) which monitors signatory states to the convention. The convention does reveal older and deeper prejudices against people with mental illness. Article 5 outlines conditions where persons of 'unsound mind', along with 'vagrants' and 'drug addicts', can be exempted from the right to liberty and security. Article 14 of the ECHR, its non-discrimination provision, states: 'The enjoyment of the rights and freedoms set forth in this Convention shall be secured without discrimination on any ground such as sex, race, colour, language, religion, political or other opinion, national or social origin, association with a national minority, property, birth or other status.' Breach of this is a violation of the convention. So, while mental illness related disabilities are not given as a specified ground, they are included in 'any ground', or 'other Status'. The ECHR has made decisions on over 100 cases involving persons with mental disabilities and is the highest legal recourse for people residing within the Council of Europe (Bartlett et al. 2007).

Turning now to conventions that refer to all countries, the most recent international human rights convention is the CRPD. This document marks a shift in the position of persons with disabilities within their societies. Persons with disabilities are not passive recipients of social welfare programs and support but are active participants with guaranteed rights and processes to protect those rights. While controversy still surrounds the exact interpretation of this document, the spirit of the convention is one of non-discrimination and equity. The convention was adopted by the UN in December 2006 and by February 2011 had been ratified by 98 countries.

The CRPD is composed of 50 Articles which outline provisions for those with disabilities and the responsibilities of nations in guaranteeing those rights. Nations have the responsibility to protect, respect, and fulfil the issues within these documents. We selected three Articles to illustrate how stigma and discrimination are critical human rights issues.

The right to health (Article 25 of CRPD)

According to the Universal Declaration of Human Rights as well as the CRPD, every person has the right to the highest attainable standard of health. Yet people with mental illness die prematurely and have significantly higher rates of medical co-morbidity, including higher rates of cardiovascular disease, diabetes, respiratory disease, and other illnesses (Felker et al. 1996; Harris and Barraclough 1998). This disparity is caused by a number of factors including structural barriers to care and explicit discrimination on the part of health care professionals through a process known as *diagnostic overshadowing* (Jones et al. 2008).

People with mental illness feel unwelcome because of certain settings or staff attitudes (Lauber et al. 2004; Lauber et al. 2006; Lawrie et al. 1998; Patel 2004). Although health care professionals are thought to hold attitudes that are positive, compassionate, and encouraging towards people with mental illness, this is often not the case as health care professionals may be ignorant about the possible outcomes of people with mental illness. This may be due to lack of knowledge in caring for people with mental illness which results from inadequate training (Hodges, Inch, and Silver 2001).

Health care practitioners also diagnose and treat people with mental illness differently. For example, people with mental illness are 'substantially less likely to undergo coronary re-vascular-isation procedures' compared to people without mental illness (Druss et al. 2000). Similarly, people with co-morbid mental illness and diabetes are less likely to be admitted to hospital for diabetic complications than those with no mental illness (Sullivan et al. 2006). People with schizophrenia are significantly less likely to receive important basic health checks such as blood pressure and cholesterol measurement (Roberts et al. 2007).

Diagnostic overshadowing is the process by which the physical needs of a patient are over-shadowed by their psychiatric diagnosis (Disability Rights Commission 2006). The person with mental illness has poorer physical health because health care professionals wrongly associate the physical symptoms to the mental illness. (Disability Rights Commission 2006). The concept of diagnostic overshadowing has been investigated in people with learning disabilities over the past 20 years; however, only recently has attention been given to this phenomenon occurring in people with mental illness (Disability Rights Commission 2006).

It is clear that people living with mental illness confront a number of barriers in asserting and achieving their right to the highest attainable standard of health. For example, they may lack sufficient organization or communication skills or social support systems to keep regular appoint-ments or to follow treatment plans. Pathways between health care professionals' lack of knowledge, stigmatizing attitudes, and discrimination towards people with mental illness contribute to their poor health.

In the United Kingdom, government organizations are addressing the physical health of people experiencing mental illness. For example, in Scotland a programme has been organized to pro-mote physical health equality for people with mental illness (Myers et al. 2005). This programme ensures that mental health services include or facilitate access to health promotion services as well as providing care and treatment for mental health problems. They are developing a register of people with severe mental illness to facilitate call and recall systems and regular communication between primary care professionals and the Community Mental Health Team (CMHT). Regular review/audit of care is required for every person with a severe mental illness and each should have an annual health check and be offered advice about reducing smoking (Cohen and Hove 2001). Indeed the Parliamentary Health Select Committee inquiry on the contribution of the NHS to reducing health inequalities is responsible for the physical health inequalities of people with men-tal illness.

Recently, the UK Disability Rights Commission (DRC) investigated the problem of diagnostic overshadowing and suggested necessary factors to overcome it (Disability Rights Commission 2006). They advocate for: (i) educating people with mental illness/learning disabilities on their rights and how to negotiate for services; (ii) training for clinicians to recognize and tackle diag-nostic overshadowing; (iii) equal recognition from the government for improved planning and commissioning to address these issues (Disability Rights Commission 2006).

The strategies outlined by the DRC for primary care practitioners and mental health service providers are in line with Article 25 CRPD which includes:

♦ The provision of quality, high-standard health care to people with disabilities.

♦ Early identification and intervention through health services in people with disabilities.

♦ The provision of such health care in people's communities so that it is 'in reach'.

- ◆ A requirement for health care practitioners to provide care that is of the same quality to all persons including people with disabilities whilst raising awareness of human rights, dignity, and autonomy of people with disabilities.
- ◆ Tackling discrimination against people with disabilities.

Raising awareness and evaluating the practice of the DRC recommendations and Article 25 to ensure they are in place and to a high standard should be the task of local, national, and international NGOs who are involved in this area. Providing an evidence base of what has worked in achieving such goals is important so that people with mental illness receive the physical health care they require and have a right to.

The right to work and employment (Article 27 of CRPD)

> The effects of disability-based discrimination have been particularly severe in fields such as education, employment, housing, transport, cultural life and access to public places and services. This may result from distinction, exclusion, restriction or preference, or denial of reasonable accommodation on the basis of disablement, which effectively nullifies or impairs the recognition, enjoyment or exercise of the rights of persons with disabilities.' (United Nations 2007)

Many countries have introduced legislation to address discrimination against people with disabilities. In the UK the Disability Discrimination Act (DDA) 2005 aims to address the problems of discrimination on the basis of disability in employment, access to education, goods and services, as well as buying or renting land or property. Within this Act, a person has a disability if '*he has a physical or mental impairment which has a substantial and long-term adverse effect on his ability to carry out normal day-to-day activities*'. The Act provides further information on the conditions that qualify as an impairment and with what is meant by 'long-term effects' and 'normal day-to-day activities' (Parliament 2005). Despite this legal protection, mental health service users' frequently report discrimination in the area of employment. The rest of this section will focus on this topic.

In a US survey, 61 per cent of participants (N=1,301) felt they had been turned down for a job for which they are qualified, when it was revealed that they are a mental health service user (Wahl 1999). In the UK, 56 per cent (N=411) believed that they had definitely or possibly been turned down for a job in the past because of their mental health problems (Mental Health Foundation 2002). In New Zealand, 34 per cent said that they had been discriminated against while looking for a job and 31 per cent felt that they had been discriminated against within the job (Peterson et al. 2007). Similarly, a recent international survey found that 64 per cent of participants (N=736) had stopped themselves from applying for work/training/education because of their mental illness diagnosis (Thornicroft et al. 2009). The four studies mentioned above all measure previously experienced discrimination, or reported events of being treated differently (Mental Health Foundation 2008), rather than expectations or feelings about oneself, which are more commonly assessed in the literature (Link et al. 2004). This is particularly interesting in the context of human rights as the participants felt that their status as a mental health service user had directly led to them failing to find or keep work.

This is supported by evidence that those with a diagnosis of severe mental illness are severely under-represented in the workforce. In the UK, approximately 75 per cent of adults are employed, 65 per cent of adults with physical health problems are employed, and 20 per cent of people with severe mental health problems are employed (Social Exclusion Unit 2004). It is not the case that people with mental ill health do not want to work, with estimates showing that 70–90 per cent of those with significant mental illness want to work (Rogers et al. 1991). Discrimination is present not only in finding employment but also in the wage differentials between employees with mental illness and those without a disability. A recent study linked participants' reports of stigma with econometric measures of discrimination in terms of wages received. Among workers with mental illness, those who did not report stigma had a wage of 85 per cent, and those who did report stigma had a wage of 72 per cent, of those with no mental illness. For those with psychotic disorders, the figures are 76 per cent and 46 per cent respectively. When wages were adjusted for functional limitations, the adjusted wage ratio comparing workers who had experienced stigma with those who have no mental illness was 69 per cent, indicating that other factors need to be considered. The adjusted wage ratio for workers with psychotic disorders was 17 per cent, indicating that in this illness group, a large proportion of variance in wage scores is unaccounted for by functional limitations (Baldwin and Marcus 2006). This provides evidence that self-reported stigma is linked to discrimination. It also emphasizes the point that legislation alone is not sufficient to end mental health service users' experience of discrimination.

Non-governmental organizations and human rights

In order to properly implement the idea and policies of these documents, effective monitoring and advocacy must occur in all countries. A number of non-governmental organizations (NGOs) are active in the field of mental health and human rights and continue to highlight the abuses and infractions as well as work to initiate change at local and international levels. The nature of their work varies within and between organizations.

The **Mental Disability Advocacy Centre** (MDAC) is an international NGO. This group works within the framework of the Council of Europe and has identified three key areas for change: guardianship, transparency, and prevention. People placed under guardianship are deprived of the right to make key life choices and are additionally subject to the discriminatory and stigmatizing views of the 'guardian'. Around the world human rights abuses occur behind the closed doors of institutions. MDAC fights for widespread *transparency* within psychiatric institutions and for closure of those failing to perform. MDAC is active is in the *prevention* of ill treatment and deaths within psychiatric care settings. The organization aims to ensure that deaths and ill-treatment are exposed and dealt with adequately by the legal and justice systems.

A second organization noted for its achievements in human rights and mental health is **Disability Rights International** (DRI) (formerly Mental Disability Rights International (MDRI)). The NGO is based in Washington DC and works internationally. Its stated aims are similar to those of MDAC. DRI investigates and publicizes human rights abuses, makes recommendations for reform, and works regionally to develop and promote concepts of lay advocacy within local populations and to spread its word through training and education.

Amnesty International (AI) is arguably the best-known human rights organization in the world, its remit encompassing all areas of human rights including issues concerning mental health. In 2001, AI partnered with DRI to highlight abuses in a state institution in Bulgaria where women with mental illnesses were imprisoned in cages. The NGO has also published a detailed report highlighting the need for better human rights for people with mental illness in Ireland and making practical and relevant recommendations for consideration by the Irish Government. In addition to these reports, AI regularly considers mental health a discrete issue within its other activities, reports, and campaigns.

Human Rights Watch (HRW) is another general human rights organization which incorporates mental health within its ambit. This organization has specifically considered issues of mental health and human rights abuses, for example highlighting the human rights issues surrounding US prisoners with mental illnesses. This approach is laudable for a relatively small NGO that aims to cover a greater breadth of human rights subjects. With this diverse group of organizations investigating these human rights situations, the world gains a more complete picture of the range conditions in which people with mental illness must survive. Their work highlights the gross negligence and abuse which can happen but human rights issues can also take on more nuanced consequences.

The significance of stigma and how it can be effectively reduced

How common is stigma and discrimination and how do they contribute to social exclusion? A recent global study used the Discrimination and Stigma Scale (DISC) in a cross-sectional survey in 27 countries, using language-equivalent versions of the instrument in face-to-face interviews between research staff and 732 participants with a clinical diagnosis of schizophrenia (Thornicroft et al. 2009). The most frequently occurring areas of negative experienced discrimination were: making or keeping friends (47 per cent); discrimination by family members (43 per cent); keeping a job (29 per cent); finding a job (29 per cent); and intimate or sexual relationships (29 per cent). Positive experienced discrimination was rare. Anticipated discrimination was common for: applying for work or training or education (64 per cent); looking for a close relationship (55 per cent); and 72 per cent felt the need to conceal the diagnosis. Anticipated discrimination occurred more often than experienced discrimination. This study suggests that rates of experienced discrimination are relatively high and consistent across countries. For two of the most important domains (work and personal relationships) anticipated discrimination occurs in the absence of experienced discrimination in over a third of participants. This has important implications: disability discrimination laws may not be effective without also developing interventions to reduce anticipated discrimination, for example by enhancing the self-esteem of people with mental illness, so that they will be more likely to apply for jobs.

Prejudice and discrimination by the public against people with mental illness are therefore common, deeply socially damaging, and are a part of more widespread stigmatization. Stigma against people with mental illness can contribute to negative outcomes as well as perpetuating self-stigmatization and contributing to low self-esteem. With a growing awareness about such stigma, a number of recent initiatives have been launched in the UK aiming to improve public attitudes. The Royal College of Psychiatrists 'Changing Minds' campaign in England ran between 1998 and 2003. It advertised websites, showed campaign videos in cinemas, distributed leaflets to the general public and health care professionals, and created reading material for young people for use in the curriculum (Crisp 2004; Crisp et al. 2004; Crisp et al. 2005). The Scottish government's 'See Me' campaign (2002–present) has a higher profile, is better funded, and more extensive. It aims to deliver specific messages to the Scottish population by using all forms of media as well as cinema advertising, outdoor posters, supporting leaflets in GP surgeries, libraries, prisons, schools, and youth groups It also has a detailed website containing interactive resources and its impact is regularly monitored and progress reported in the public domain (Dunion and Gordon 2005). The investment of public funds in government campaigns is an important step, and evidence suggesting that 'See Me' may have had a positive effect on attitudes in Scotland relative to England is encouraging (Mehta et al. 2009).

In terms of reducing public stigma, there are three main strategies: protest, education, and contact (Corrigan and Penn 1999). Protest is often applied against stigmatizing public statements, such as media reports and advertisements. Many of these protest interventions have successfully suppressed such public statements and for this purpose they are clearly very useful (Wahl 1995). However, protest is not effective to improve attitudes toward people with mental illness. Education aims to diminish stigma by replacing myths and negative stereotypes with facts and has reduced stigmatizing attitudes among a wide variety of participants. However, research on educational campaigns suggests that behaviour changes are often not assessed and effect sizes are limited and may fade quickly. The third strategy is personal contact with persons with mental illness. In a number of interventions with secondary school students education and contact have been combined (Pinfold et al. 2003b) and contact appears to be the more efficacious part of the intervention. There are a number of factors that create an advantageous environment for interpersonal contact and stigma reduction, including equal status among participants, a cooperative interaction, and institutional support for the contact initiative.

For both education and contact, the content of anti-stigma programmes matters. Biogenetic models of mental illness are often highlighted because viewing mental illness as a biochemical, mainly inherited problem may reduce shame and blame associated with it. Evidence supports this optimism in terms of reduced blame (Corrigan et al. 2003). On the other hand, a focus on biogenetic factors increases the perception of people with mental illness as fundamentally different and thus has been associated with increased social distance (Angermeyer and Matschinger 2005); with perceptions of mental illness as more persistent, serious (Phelan 2005); and dangerous (Jorm and Griffiths 2008); and with more pessimistic views about treatment outcomes (Phelan et al., 2006). Therefore, a message of mental illness as being 'genetic' or 'neurological' may be overly simplistic and unhelpful to reduce stigma.

Anti-stigma initiatives can take place nationally as well as locally. National campaigns often adopt a social marketing approach, whereas local initiatives usually focus on certain target groups such as employers, students, or police officers. An example of a big national campaign is 'Time to Change' in England (Henderson and Thornicroft 2009). It combines mass media advertising and local initiatives. The latter try to facilitate social contact between members of the general public and service users as well as target specific groups such as teachers. The programme is evaluated not only by public attitude and media surveys, but also by measuring the amount of experienced discrimination reported by people with mental illness. Similar initiatives in other countries, e.g. 'Like Minds Like Mine' in New Zealand (Vaughan and Hansen 2004), were successful.

Conclusion

In recent years, human rights violations against persons with mental disabilities have gained greater media and policy attention. The adoption of the CRPD and the debate about its implications evidences the importance of addressing these violations and inequities. NGOs across the world document and expose the abuses and failures in care provision currently happening behind the closed doors of mental health care settings. Lawyers and advocates have spent careers bringing those who commit them to justice. Those brought to courts and judged on their actions are perpetrators of human rights abuses; however, human rights are not only about atrocities and torture. Human rights law provides for protections and provisions to guarantee basic participation in society, i.e. the right to health and the right to work. Nested within the complex system which produces disparities in health and employment is stigma and discrimination. Its clear connections to differences in health and employment among those with mental disability makes this a critical human rights issue.

Within this context, measures which are known to be effective in reducing stigma and discrimination refer to interventions at the local level (where direct social contact with persons with mental illness is the most active ingredient) (Callard et al. 2008; Pinfold et al. 2003a; Pinfold et al. 2003b) and interventions at the national level (where the initial results of social marketing appear very promising) (Corrigan 2005; Hinshaw 2007; Pinfold et al. 2005; Sartorius and Schulze 2005;

Thornicroft 2006). A series of initiatives in Australia (including beyondblue, Mind Matters, Aussie Optimism, and the Resourceful Adolescent Program) (Jorm et al. 2005), New Zealand (Vaughan and Hansen 2004), and Scotland (Dunion and Gordon 2005) have demonstrated beneficial anti-stigma effects from such national programmes, and similar campaigns are now also underway in Canada and England.

Perceptions and ideas about persons with mental illness exact a measurable toll on those living with mental illness and their families, and the practitioners charged with caring for these people are sometimes themselves among the stigmatized of health care staff. Stigma is not the sole factor in this very multifaceted and complex system. This chapter therefore argues that there are clear benefits from bringing the issues of stigma and discrimination in mental health context into a human rights perspective, drawing on examples from two very important aspects of community participation: access to quality health care and opportunities for work and employment. Understanding the impact of stigma and armed with international conventions and treaties we can move forward in changing these injustices by improving the treatment, care, and opportunities available to people with mental health problems. In this sense, human rights is seen less as a set of abstract legal or moral entitlements, but more as a framework which directly and concretely contributes to the social inclusion of people with mental health problems.

References

Angermeyer, MC and Matschinger, H (2005) 'Causal beliefs and attitudes to people with schizophrenia. Trend analysis based on data from two population surveys in Germany', *British Journal of Psychiatry*, 186, 331–34.

Baldwin, ML and Marcus, SC (2006) 'Perceived and Measured Stigma Among Workers With Serious Mental Illness', *Psychiatric Services*, 57(3), 388–92.

Bartlett, P, Lewis, O, and Thorold, O (2007) *Mental Disability and the European Convention on Human Rights*. Leiden: Martinus Nijhoff.

Callard, F, Main, L, Myers, F, Pyonnonen, A-M, Thornicroft, G, Jenkins, R, Pinfold, V, and Sartorius, N (2008) *Stigma: a Guidebook for Action*. Edinburgh: Health Scotland.

Cohen, A and Hove, M (2001) *Physical Health of the Severe and Enduring Mentally Ill. A training pack for GP educators*. London: Sainsbury Centre for Mental Health.

Corrigan, P (2005) *On the Stigma of Mental Illness*. Washington, DC: American Psychological Association.

Corrigan, PW, Markowitz, FE, Watson, A, Rowan, D, and Kubiak, MA (2003) 'An attribution model of public discrimination towards persons with mental illness', *Journal of Health and Social Behavior*, 44(2), 162–79.

Corrigan, PW, Markowitz, FE, and Watson, AC (2004) 'Structural levels of mental illness stigma and discrimination', *Schizophrenia Bulletin*, 30(3), 481–91.

Corrigan, PW and Penn, DL (1999) 'Lessons from social psychology on discrediting psychiatric stigma', *American Psychologist*, 54(9), 765–76.

Crisp, A (2004) *Every Family in the Land: Understanding Prejudice and Discrimination Against People with Mental Illness*. London: Royal Society of Medicine Press.

Crisp, A, Gelder, MG, Goddard, E, and Meltzer, H (2005) 'Stigmatization of people with mental illnesses: a follow-up study within the Changing Minds campaign of the Royal College of Psychiatrists', *World Psychiatry*, 4, 106–113.

Crisp, AH, Cowan, L, and Hart, D (2004) 'The College's anti-stigma campaign 1998–2003', *Psychiatric Bulletin*, 28, 133–36.

Department of Health (2003) *Attitudes to Mental Illness 2003 Report*. London: Department of Health.

Disability Rights Commission (2006) *Equal treatment: Closing the gap*. Stratford upon Avon, UK: Disability Rights Commission, 1.

Druss, BG, Bradford, DW, Rosenheck, RA, Radford, MJ, and Krumholz, HM (2000) 'Mental disorders and use of cardiovascular procedures after myocardial infarction', *JAMA*, 283(4), 506–511.

Dunion, L and Gordon, L (2005) 'Tackling the attitude problem. The achievements to date of Scotland's "see me" anti-stigma campaign', *Mental Health Today*, (March) 22–25.

Farmer, P (2005) *Pathologies of power: health, human rights, and the new war on the poor.* London: University of California Press Ltd.

Felker, B, Yazel, JJ, and Short, D (1996) 'Mortality and medical comorbidity among psychiatric patients: a review', *Psychiatric Services*, 47(12), 1356–63.

Harris, EC and Barraclough, B (1998) 'Excess mortality of mental disorder', *British Journal of Psychiatry*, 173, 11–53.

Henderson, C and Thornicroft, G (2009) 'Stigma and discrimination in mental illness: Time to Change', *The Lancet*, 373(6), 1930–32.

Hinshaw, S (2007) *The Mark of Shame.* Oxford: Oxford University Press.

Hinshaw, SP and Cicchetti, D (2000) 'Stigma and mental disorder: conceptions of illness, public attitudes, personal disclosure, and social policy', *Development and Psychopathology*, 12(4), 555–98.

Hodges, B, Inch, C, and Silver, I (2001) 'Improving the psychiatric knowledge, skills, and attitudes of primary care physicians, 1950–2000: a review', *American Journal of Psychiatry*, 158(10), 1579–86.

Jones, S, Howard, L, and Thornicroft, G (2008) "Diagnostic overshadowing": worse physical health care for people with mental illness', *Acta Psychiatrica Scandinavica*, 118(3), 169–71.

Jorm, AF, Blewitt, KA, Griffiths, KM, Kitchener, BA, and Parslow, RA (2005) 'Mental health first aid responses of the public: results from an Australian national survey', *BMC Psychiatry*, 5(1), 9.

Jorm, AF and Griffiths, KM (2008) 'The public's stigmatizing attitudes towards people with mental disorders: How important are biomedical conceptualizations?', *Acta Psychiatrica Scandinavica*, 118(4), 315–21.

Lauber, C, Anthony, M, Ajdacic-Gross, V, and Rossler, W (2004) 'What about psychiatrists' attitude to mentally ill people?', *European Psychiatry: the Journal of the Association of European Psychiatrists*, 19(7), 423–27.

Lauber, C, Nordt, C, Braunschweig, C, and Rossler, W (2006) 'Do mental health professionals stigmatize their patients?', *Acta Psychiatrica Scandinavica, Supplementum*, 113(429), 51–59.

Lawrie, SM, Martin, K, McNeill, G, et al. (1998) 'General practitioners' attitudes to psychiatric and medical illness', *Psychological Medicine*, 28(6), 1463–67.

Link, BG, Yang, LH, Phelan, JC, and Collins, PY (2004) 'Measuring mental illness stigma', *Schizophrenia Bulletin*, 30(3), 511–41.

Mehta, N, Kassam, A, Leese, M, Butler, G, and Thornicroft G (2009) 'Public attitudes towards people with mental illness in England and Scotland, 1994–2003', *British Journal of Psychiatry*, Mar, 194(3), 278–84.

Mental Health Foundation (2002) *Out at Work. A Survey of the Experiences of People with Mental Health Problems within the Workplace.* London: Mental Health Foundation.

Mental Health Foundation of New Zealand (2008) *Fighting Shadows.* Wellington, NZ: Mental Health Foundation of New Zealand.

Myers, F, McCollam, A, and Woodhouse, A (2005), *National Programme for Improving Mental Health and Well-Being. Addressing mental health inequalities in Scotland: Equal Minds.* Edinburgh: Scottish Executive.

Parliament (2005) Disability Discrimination Act 2005. (UK legislation).

Patel, MX (2004) 'Attitudes to psychosis: health professionals', *Epidemiologia e Psichiatria Sociale*, 13(4), 213–218.

Peterson, D, Pere, L, Sheehan, N, and Surgenor, G (2007) 'Experiences of mental health discrimination in New Zealand', *Health & Social Care in the Community*, 15(1), 18–25.

Phelan, JC (2005) 'Geneticization of deviant behavior and consequences for stigma: The case of mental illness', *Journal of Health and Social Behavior*, 46(4), 307–22.

Phelan, JC, Yang, LH, and Cruz-Rojas, R (2006) 'Effects of attributing serious mental illnesses to genetic causes on orientations to treatment', *Psychiatric Services*, 57, (3), 382–87.

Pinfold, V, Huxley, P, Thornicroft, G, Farmer, P, Toulmin, H, and Graham, T (2003a) 'Reducing psychiatric stigma and discrimination—evaluating an educational intervention with the police force in England', *Social Psychiatry and Psychiatric Epidemiology*, 38(6), 337–44.

Pinfold, V, Thornicroft, G, Huxley, P, and Farmer, P (2005) 'Active ingredients in anti-stigma programmes in mental health', *International Review of Psychiatry*, 17(2), 123–31.

Pinfold, V, Toulmin, H, Thornicroft, G, Huxley, P, Farmer, P, and Graham, T (2003b) 'Reducing psychiatric stigma and discrimination: Evaluation of educational interventions in UK secondary schools', *British Journal of Psychiatry*, 182(4), 342–46.

Roberts, L, Roalfe, A, Wilson, S, and Lester, H (2007) 'Physical health care of patients with schizophrenia in primary care: A comparative study', *Family Practice*, 24(1), 34–40.

Rogers, ES, Walsh, D, Masotta, L, and Smith, K (1991) *Massachusetts survey of client preferences for community support services*. Final report. Submitted to the Department of Mental Health. Boston: Boston University, Center for Psychiatric Rehabilitation.

Rose, D, Thornicroft, G, Pinfold, V, and Kassam, A (2007) '250 labels used to stigmatise people with mental illness', *BMC Health Services Research*, 7, 97.

Sartorius, N and Schulze, H (2005) *Reducing the Stigma of Mental Illness. A Report from a Global Programme of the World Psychiatric Association*. Cambridge: Cambridge University Press.

Social Exclusion Unit (2004) *Mental Health and Social Exclusion*. London; Office of the Deputy Prime Minister.

Sullivan, G, Han, X, Moore, S, and Kotrla, K (2006) 'Disparities in hospitalization for diabetes among persons with and without co-occurring mental disorders', *Psychiatric Services*, 57, 1126–31.

Thornicroft, G (2006) *Shunned: Discrimination against People with Mental Illness*. Oxford: Oxford University Press.

Thornicroft, G, Brohan, E, Rose, D, Sartorius, N, and Leese, M (2009) 'Global pattern of experienced and anticipated discrimination against people with schizophrenia: a cross-sectional survey', *The Lancet*, 373(9661), 408–415.

United Nations (2007) Overview of International Legal Frameworks For Disability Legislation. Department of Economic and Social Affairs: Division for Social Policy and Development. Available at <http://www.un.org/esa/socdev/enable/disovlf.htm>.

Vaughan, G and Hansen, C (2004) '"Like Minds, Like Mine": a New Zealand project to counter the stigma and discrimination associated with mental illness', *Australasian Psychiatry*, 12(2), 113–117.

Wahl, OF (1995) *Media Madness: Public Images of Mental Illness*. New Brunswick, NJ: Rutgers University Press.

Wahl, OF (1999) 'Mental health consumers' experience of stigma', *Schizophrenia Bulletin*, 25(3), 467–78.

Weiss, MG (2008) 'Stigma and the social burden of neglected tropical diseases', *PLoS Neglected Tropical Diseases*, 2(5), e237.

World Health Organization, Mental Health Policy and Services: Mental Health Improvement for Nations Development: the WHO Mind Project. Mental health, human rights and legislation. <http://www.who.int/mental_health/policy/legislation/en/index.html>, accessed 9th April 2012.

Chapter 6

Genes, Biology, Mental Health, and Human Rights

The Effects of Traumatic Stress as a Case Example

Alexander C. McFarlane and Richard A. Bryant

Introduction

There have been enormous advances in recent years in our understanding of the biology of mental disorders. Exponential increases in the study of neuroimaging and genetics of psychiatric disorders have shed new light on the biological underpinnings of mental disorders and biological factors that render some people at risk for developing psychiatric problems (Hyman 2007). Although these advances have led to marked developments in terms of theoretical models of psychiatric disorders, enhanced assessment protocols, and more refined treatment options, they have also raised a raft of issues involving fundamental human rights. This chapter reviews some of the most recent biological developments in mental health that have direct human rights implications. We commence with a review of some of the major issues.

The issues

From an ethical perspective and human rights, the issue of free will and determinism are linked to the idea of individuals being in control of their mind and behaviour. This chapter will explore the impact of advances in genetics and neurobiology in terms of the potential risks and benefits such knowledge brings. In essence, the question arises as to whether the elucidation of the biological underpinning of psychiatric disorders may either create a greater obligation to benevolence or promote stigma and the misuse of information. In the absence of ethical consensus that determines how to balance competing courses of action, this domain requires careful elucidation (Beauchamp and Childress 2001). This chapter will not explore the controversial and challenging issues of physical treatments (such as ECT and psychosurgery), as such a discussion would be as much framed by the issue of past abuses as further potential for good. Rather, the chapter exemplifies the issues using the area of the effects of traumatic stress, a matter that has been subject to many ethical challenges in the legal, military, and migration arenas.

An optimistic view of the increasing knowledge about the role of genetics and biology and mental illness is that this body of knowledge may serve to reduce the stigma associated with psychiatric disorders (Spriggs et al. 2008). The ability to demonstrate neurophysiological abnormalities that underpin disorders in depression and anxiety highlights that these conditions do represent genuine alterations in one's biological profile (Etkin and Wager 2007) above and beyond the acceptance of the role of genetics and neurobiology in schizophrenia and bipolar disorder. In so doing, it is possible that the attitudes to people who are disabled by the symptoms will no longer simply be dismissed as people who lack strength of character (Shepherd 2001). Particularly in the domain of compensation (Roberts-Yates 2003), such evidence may strengthen the legitimacy of psychiatric disorders as matters that warrant equal concern and attention in the legislation as physical injuries (Austin and Honer 2005; Nuffield Council of Bioethics 1998). In so doing, the legal rights of individuals may be strengthened by demonstrating that self-reported psychiatric problems are associated with observable biological changes.

On the other hand, a more pessimistic perspective is that biological information which demonstrates an inherited predisposition to psychiatric disorder may increase the perception that individuals are judged to lack sufficient resilience relative to other people (Phelan 2002). Such a formulation can easily typecast some individuals into inferior or discounted positions when it comes to arguing for equal opportunities. Domains where individuals are likely to be particularly at risk are during the selection for particular employment roles and in settings where some liability arises if a person becomes unwell. Therefore, equal opportunities and human rights relating to the genetic and biological aspects of mental disorders in Western society are particularly likely to become issues in employment environments. The question will be asked, whether an employer has the right to demand that an individual has a genetic screening prior to be hired by that particular business.

Another domain where human rights may become an important issue is the role of genetic biology in disability and insurance matters (Korobkin and Rajkumar 2008). The aim of the insurance industry is to calculate actuarial risk and any tool that is available to improve the accuracy of prediction will be brought to bear. One of the challenges to individual human rights in this domain is that agencies with some responsibility to manage and prevent the adverse consequences of a risk factor are likely to seek and define those genetic characteristics that may mark elevated risk of developing particular mental disorders. Individuals may be disadvantaged because they are marked as possessing greater risk for liability because of genetic characteristics. For example, an individual who has a family history and a genetic predisposition to depression may be liable to have their life insurance premium weighted because of the risk of suicide and cardiac disease.

These are not new issues. Rather, the capability of biological and genetic sciences to better characterize the abnormalities associated with psychiatric disorders has become more sophisticated, which in turn makes these human rights issues more salient. The interaction of mental health and human rights has been debated for many years because the human rights of individuals labelled as mentally ill have frequently been violated in the past. We now turn to consider some of these issues from a historical perspective before turning to the current context.

Historical background

A brave new world of potential prejudice opened up when Charles Darwin published his theory of evolution. At the core of survival and emergence of a species was the notion of natural selection. The most successful species were those who could adapt to change and adversity and utilize this to their collective advantage. A less well-known aspect of Darwin's work was his fascination with the manifestation of emotion (Darwin 1872). He actively observed patients in mental institutions and was preoccupied by the similarities between some of the manifestations of their distress and the observed expressions of affect in the animal kingdom. One consequence of his theory was an increased interest in the role of heredity in mental illness (Kraepelin 1899). Even with those disorders where there was significant evidence about environmental determinants, such as traumatic neurosis, influential psychiatrists, such as Kraepelin, argued for the role of familial predisposition.

Some of the greatest abuses of human rights in the 19th and 20th centuries were argued on the basis of the biological theory. Colonial expansion in the 19th century was often justified on the basis of the inferiority of the coloured races of the African continent (Linqvist and Tate 1996). These beliefs allowed the imposition of social conditions and the deprivation of liberty that would never have been tolerated by a citizen of Europe. The justification of moral and ethical superiority allowed many practices which, in retrospect, are a cause of collective and cultural shame. The challenges and the potential to degrade moral and ethical standards were graphically captured by Conrad in 'the heart of darkness' (Conrad 2004). In European society, the same justifications were at times used to support the segregation and treatment of the mentally ill.

In the 20th century, intolerant and discriminatory attitudes to the mentally ill were often openly argued on the basis of the biological inferiority of those afflicted. Much of the interest in the Nazi regime has centred on the views about the racial superiority of the Aryans (Burleigh 1994). However, the first group who were systematically sterilized and killed by Hitler and his henchmen were the mentally ill. This persecution was based on a eugenics argument about the need to purify society and to protect it from the contamination with which these members allegedly threatened the 'superior race'. The outrage about this regime has arguably given inadequate consideration to the discrimination against the mentally ill. Similar attitudes existed within the German army, where the mentally unwell (defined as one who did not cope emotionally with battle) were at risk of being shot or allocated to 'stomach' battalions who were made to carry out extremely dangerous attacks with a very high risk of casualties (Shepherd 2001).

Similarly, the conclusions of the enquiries that were held after the First World War into the causes of shell shock largely blamed the individuals as having constitutional vulnerabilities, implying 'poor moral fibre' (Wessely 2006). The contribution of the extraordinary degree of danger and threat that individuals had to contend with in trench warfare was minimized. As a consequence, it was believed the problem of combat stress casualties could be resolved by adequate screening and excluding those who did not have the 'right stuff' (Shepherd 2001). An important aspect that would be considered in this approach was an individual's family history of a psychiatric disorder. In the early years of the Second World War, this meant that 25 per cent of the possible recruits in the US forces were excluded because they were seen to be unfit generally on psychological grounds (Ginzberg 1959). It did not take long for people to realize that the rates of combat stress disorders remained almost as high and that this programme had been ineffectual in resolving this problem. Increasingly, there was an acceptance of the importance of group morale and length of prolonged combat exposure, even in those who were deemed psychologically robust, as being primary determinants of psychological breakdown.

The field of social psychiatry emerged in the aftermath of the Second World War due to the emergence of a far greater belief in the importance and significance of the environmental determinants of psychiatric disorder relative to heredity. However, the discovery of the double helical structure of DNA by Watson and Crick was to open a new Pandora's box, eventually leading to the definition of the human genome (Inglis et al. 2003). The relentless search for specific genes that characterize the risk of particular illnesses has become a holy grail of science and also of the biotechnology sector. It has been hoped that advances in knowledge may better characterize the risk of particular psychiatric disorders for individuals who carry particular genes, and that these would foreshadow new treatments involving gene manipulation. To date, much of this promise is yet to eventuate: many illnesses arise from the effects of multiple genes rather than single large effects, thus reducing the practical likelihood of gene therapy. Nevertheless, the ethical issues are considerable.

Genetics and mental illness

The study of the familial risk of psychiatric disorders is not solely defined by molecular biology. Considerable effort has gone into conducting twin, family, and linkage studies to define the genetic basis for the full spectrum of mental disorders. Twin studies, which study the concordance between identical twins as compared with non-identical twins, would suggest that heritability of the common mental disorders, such as anxiety and depression, is approximately 40 per cent (Sullivan et al. 2000). In the case of schizophrenia, twin studies have yielded significantly higher estimates, in the range of 60–80 per cent, for the heritability of the disorder (Sullivan et al. 2003). In the field of gene identification, one of the most interesting findings has focused on the serotonin transporter gene which appears to mediate the risk of developing both anxiety and depression following exposure to environmental stress (Caspi et al. 2003). Equally, this body of research highlights the challenges in obtaining consistent findings.

The investigation of the chromosome's telomeres and the internal matrix of the chromosome has illuminated the problem of damage to the telomeres. This can be measured, and hints at the possibility of cumulative risk associated with constant stress exposure (Ulaner 2004). These mechanisms, which are a particular interest in ageing, may also improve the understanding of allostatic load, a construct important to a range of psychiatric disorders and phenotypic expression (McEwen 2000).

A series of ethical issues emerge in the course of conducting such studies and determining the optimal use of the information acquired. Firstly, the acquisition of the information from particular families creates unusual dilemmas in informed consent as the knowledge obtained may be to the disadvantage of the broader family. Equally, how should the information be fed back to the participants without stigmatizing those who have carried and transmitted the genes of importance? The predictive value of the information obtained has the potential to have a major impact on people's future and carries particular weight in how this should be provided (Morley et al. 2004).

Vulnerability to environmental stress

A major challenge posed by these domains to human rights includes the presumption that individuals with specific genetic predispositions are ineligible for certain opportunities. For example, an individual applying for a position in a high stress position, such as a police officer or a member of the armed forces, may be deemed inappropriate if they are found to carry the short allele of the serotonin transporter gene (Armbruster et al. 2009). It is conceivable that such an individual may be denied the right to apply for the position despite showing no signs of symptoms and being fully qualified otherwise to perform the role. Equally, if the person in such a position were monitored longitudinally and showed that they were accumulating a significant degree of genetic damage, such as telomere length, they could be discharged without compensation as they had no associated disability at that stage.

An example of risk factor modelling: PTSD

By way of example, we demonstrate the potential for misuse of recent empirical findings in relation to purported risk to the effects of environmental stress. Without doubt the major psychiatric condition associated with stress is post-traumatic stress disorder (PTSD) (Kilpatrick et al. 2007). The documented finding that only a minority of trauma survivors develop PTSD after exposure to a traumatic event raises the issue about variables that increase risk for PTSD development (Kessler et al. 1995). The capacity to identify people who are more prone to coping with extreme stress has been of extreme interest to military and emergency response organizations, for obvious reasons. Over recent decades, there has been much indirect evidence concerning risk for developing PTSD. Regarding pre-existing risk factors, prior psychological disturbance, family history of psychological disorders, abusive childhoods, and female gender are predictive of PTSD development (Breslau et al. 1998; Riggs et al. 1995). These findings have typically been achieved by measuring risk factors after trauma exposure and then calculating risk. An alternate approach adopted in recent years has been to assess people *prior to* trauma exposure and subsequently assess their adjustment after trauma exposure. This form of enquiry has focused on populations who are high-risk for trauma exposure (e.g. military or emergency service personnel) prior to their exposure to traumatic events.

Some datasets exist in which researchers have been able to identify documentation collected prior to trauma exposure and to link these data with subsequent reactions to trauma. Using this approach, there is evidence that pre-combat school problems, lower arithmetic aptitude, and lower heart rate predicts PTSD in military personnel (Pitman et al. 1991). Several researchers have found that personality variables measured before deployment to war zones, such as Hypochondriasis, Psychopathic Deviate, Paranoia, and Femininity predicted PTSD (Schnurr et al. 1993). There is also evidence that lower pre-deployment intelligence test scores predict PTSD in men who subsequently enter combat zones (Macklin et al. 1998).

Other studies have programmatically assessed high-risk populations using experimental paradigms. One of the most influential models of PTSD is based on fear conditioning mechanisms. Specifically, this model draws a comparison between the reactions of traumatized individuals and rats who experience fear conditioning paradigms. In a fear conditioning study, a rat may be exposed to an electric shock while also being presented with a light. In subsequent trials the rat will display a fear reaction to the light alone because it has developed a fear conditioned response in which it associates the light with an aversive consequence. When the rat is subsequently presented with trials when the light is presented without the electric shock, it learns that the light is harmless and it achieves new learning (extinction learning) that inhibits the initial fear conditioning response (Rauch et al. 2006).

A similar pattern has been observed in trauma survivors, such that exposure to a traumatic event (unconditioned stimulus) leads to a strong fear reaction (unconditioned response), which is experienced by most trauma survivors. In the following weeks and months, however, most people engage in extinction learning in which they learn that the many stimuli that were associated with trauma are no longer dangerous, and accordingly their fear reactions subside. In contrast, a minority of people develop strong conditioned responses such that when they are exposed to reminders of the trauma (conditioned stimuli), they experience strong fear reactions (conditioned response). (Charney et al. 1993). Consistent with this model, there is much evidence that people with PTSD display greater physiological reactivity to trauma reminders, consistent with marked fear conditioning to the traumatic event (Wessa and Flor 2007). In recent years, studies have assessed high-risk populations for their propensity to engage in conditioning and extinction learning as a risk factor for PTSD. Guthrie and Bryant (2006) found that fire-fighters' likelihood of developing acute stress reactions after trauma exposure was predicted by the magnitude of their startle reaction (a possible reflection of their unconditioned response) to an aversive tone prior to exposure (Bryant and Guthrie, 2005). A similar finding was observed in police officers, in which fear-potentiated startle prior to trauma was predictive of subsequent PTSD symptoms (Pole et al. 2009). Fire-fighters' impairment in extinction learning on a standard conditioning-extinction paradigm in a laboratory following conditioning to an electric shock accounted for 30 per cent of the variance of fire-fighters' post-traumatic stress six months after trauma exposure (Guthrie and Bryant, 2006).

These findings complement findings from twin studies. One study compared startle responses in pairs of Vietnam combat veterans and their non-combat-exposed monozygotic twins (Orr et al. 2003). This study found evidence of more slowly habituating skin conductance startle responses in veterans with PTSD and their non-combat-exposed co-twins, compared to veterans without PTSD and their non-combat exposed co-twins. This finding suggests that more slowly habituating skin conductance responses to startle stimuli may represent a pre trauma vulnerability factor for PTSD (Orr et al. 1993). Using magnetic resonance imaging to study monozygotic co-twins, Gilbertson et al. (2002) found that Vietnam veterans with PTSD were characterized by smaller hippocampi than were Vietnam veterans without PTSD, but that the co-twins of those with PTSD (but who had not served in Vietnam) had hippocampi that were just as small. These findings suggest that small hippocampal volume may constitute a vulnerability factor for PTSD among people exposed to trauma.

Another influential model for PTSD involves the cognitive mechanisms that drive the disorder. Cognitive models posit that PTSD is maintained by negative appraisals that catastrophizes about potential dangers in the world and how inadequate the survivor is in the aftermath of the experience (Ehlers and Clark, 2000; Foa et al. 1999). This perspective is supported by much evidence that PTSD is mediated, in part, by how one appraises one's reaction to the traumatic experience (Smith and Bryant 2000). Recent studies have also found that the tendency to engage in catastrophic thinking before trauma exposure predicts subsequent PTSD in fire-fighters (Bryant and Guthrie 2005; Bryant et al. 2007).

This increasing body of evidence raises intriguing issues concerning the appropriate use of evidence that certain biological, cognitive, and psychological markers can identify those who are at greater risk for developing PTSD. For example, should this evidence be used to exclude certain individuals from occupations that are high risk for trauma exposure? That is, should one be excluded from enlisting in the military on the basis of one's startle reaction or genetic predisposition? Many organizations around the world are keen to develop better screening measures to avoid inappropriate recruitment of people who may undergo very expensive training, and then be unsuitable for the tasks for which they were trained. Further, organizations have a responsibility to not place vulnerable individuals in positions in which they are at risk of developing psychiatric disorder if they are confronted with trauma.

Several caveats need to be considered with our current knowledge of risk factors for PTSD. First, the evidence base is currently very scant. Prospective studies have only commenced in recent years, and there is an urgent need for replication of the initial findings to determine the generalizability of these discoveries. At the current time it is premature to have strong conviction in any of the findings because they could be specific to particular cohorts, cultures, or experimental paradigms. Second, although each of these studies has demonstrated robust statistical effects in predicting PTSD symptoms after trauma, they have not achieved adequate sensitivity, specificity, or positive predictive power. Sensitivity refers to the proportion of trauma survivors who develop PTSD and satisfied a pre-existing marker, whereas specificity is the proportion of those who do not develop PTSD and do not satisfy the marker. Positive predictive power involves the proportion of people who satisfy the marker and subsequently develop PTSD. None of the studies reported to date have provided cut-offs that yield adequate sensitivity, specificity, or positive predictive power. Without these, any form of screening measures to identify people who are not appropriate for entry into an organization could be highly flawed. For example, excluding all potential recruits to an organization because of a specific risk factor would undoubtedly result in many people who could cope ably with traumatic experiences being rejected. The probable reason for the poor predictive capabilities of these markers is that the relationship between pre-existing vulnerability factors and subsequent functioning is not linear, and these vulnerability factors interact with many other variables to influence eventual adaptation to trauma. In this sense, it is possible that we may never achieve markers of risk that possess adequate accuracy.

Risk to parental rights

A further possibility exists, as the health-care cost increases and is less sustainable because of the ageing population, where health care is rationed. One form of rationing may be that people who carry a specific genetic risk of mental disorders, particularly if married to an individual who carries a similar risk, are prevented from having children. Whilst this could be seen to be providing people the opportunity to have informed reproductive decisions, equally, those who have significant genetic risks may be left with the costs of having to provide for the medical care of any child born with a significant disability.

As prenatal genetic testing becomes more sophisticated, the spectre of the more widespread use of abortion also emerges. Whilst this form of birth control is accepted in more liberal societies, the introduction of a genetic screen as a determinant will raise many complex ethical issues. A society could become obsessed by attempting to create the perfect child. Multiple pregnancies or the extrauterine cultivation of foetus may become standard practice until the optimal combination of genes emerges. In this way, the human rights of the unborn child may become the subject of considerable scrutiny and controversy.

A further challenge arises because of the need to differentiate a genetic vulnerability as against its phenotypic expression. There are many people who carry the genetic risk of particular conditions but these are never expressed. There are a few genes where there is 100 per cent expression of that characteristic. Many psychiatric disorders have multiple genes that contribute to their manifestation. Therefore, even though an individual had no symptoms, it is quite possible that the perception of others towards them could be significantly distorted. Particularly, if some form of early childhood screening had occurred it may distort a parent's perception of their child. This could lead to social subtle discrimination against those children who carry high genetic risk. Akin to this is the possible over-interpretation of positive test results such that the presence of some gene has a greater perceived risk that is actually the case. As has been the case with Huntington's disease, individuals who are found to be carrying a particular gene can adopt radically different views about their life that lead to inappropriate risk-taking or denial of future possibilities (Stout et al. 2001). In so doing, exposing individuals to genetic testing can take away their sense of a future, a basic human right in a free democratic society.

Conclusion

The dramatic developments in biological psychiatry, particularly in the domains of neuroimaging and genetics, pose many ethical challenges of the future. As we have demonstrated in the example of PTSD, it is now possible to model risk factors that predict how individuals may respond to extreme stress. Some of the greatest ethical challenges will emerge in populations who have a significant risk of being exposed to these types of events. It is in the situations of major environmental provocations that underlying biological risk factors have the greatest probability of being manifest. The way forward in dealing with the ethical issues arising from this emerging information is far from clear.

Precipitous and premature conclusions about risk have a significant potential to discriminate against individuals who are able to function at high levels of competency in difficult environments but may be excluded because of a theoretical risk profile. On the other hand, there is the possibility that individuals in positions of responsibility may see this ethical issue as being too challenging and hence avoid a consideration of the available information, which may reasonably allow some beneficial action. Ultimately, the resolution of these highly complex issues will involve a balancing of the costs and benefits to the individual as against the costs and benefits for the group and those in positions of responsibility. The ethical solution must consider the issues of prejudice and the ownership of some of the potential costs of this new knowledge by the broader society.

Once individuals can be categorized according to characteristics of desirability, it is easy to stigmatize and reject the supposedly inferior. It is important that any decisions about the use of biological risk factors in determining employability or access to other social roles are monitored by independent authorities that balance the rights of individuals as well as the social good. Those who have a particular vested interest in minimizing their responsibility for the health outcomes of individuals exposed to extreme environments may develop an entire new language to try and obfuscate the issues. Therefore, the values which are implicit in the communication of the biological constructs that underpin risk factors need to be carefully examined to ensure that new forms of prejudice do not come to pass unnoticed. This is a 'brave new world' and it is imperative that these exciting biological developments are matched by responsible advances in maintaining all people's fundamental human rights.

References

Armbruster, D, Moser, DA, Strobel, A et al. (2009) 'Serotonin transporter gene variation and stressful life events impact processing of fear and anxiety', *International Journal of Neuropsychopharmacology*, 12, 393–401.

Austin, JC and Honer, WG (2005) 'The potential impact of genetic counseling for mental illness', *Clinical Genetics*, 67(2), 134–42.

Beauchamp TL and Childress JF (2001) *Principles of Biomedical Ethics*. Oxford: Oxford University Press.

Breslau, N, Kessler, RC, Chilcoat, HD, Schultz, LR, Davis, GC, and Andreski, P (1998) 'Trauma and posttraumatic stress disorder in the community', *Archives of General Psychiatry*, 55(7), 626–32.

Bryant, RA and Guthrie, RM (2005) 'Maladaptive appraisals as a risk factor for posttraumatic stress: a study of trainee firefighters', *Psychological Science*, 16(10), 749–52.

Bryant, RA, Sutherland, K, and Guthrie, RM (2007) 'Impaired specific autobiographical memory as a risk factor for posttraumatic stress after trauma', *Journal of Abnormal Psychology*, 116(4), 837–41.

Burleigh, M (1994) 'Psychiatry, German society, and the Nazi "euthanasia" programme', *Social History of Medicine*, 7(2), 213–28.

Caspi, A et al. (2003) 'Influence of Life Stress on Depression: Moderation by a Polymorphism in the 5-HTT Gene', *Science*, 301(5631), 386–389.

Charney, DS, Deutch, AY, Krystal, JH, Southwick, SM, and Davis, M (1993) 'Psychobiologic mechanisms of posttraumatic stress disorder', *Archives of General Psychiatry*, 50, 294–305.

Clarke, H, Flint, J, Attwood, AS, and Munafo, MR (2010) 'Association of the 5-HTTLPR genotype and unipolar depression: a metal-analysis', *Psychological Medicine*, 40, 1767–78.

Conrad, J (2004) *Heart of Darkness*. Whitefish, MT: Kessinger Publishing.

Darwin, C (1872) *Expression of the Emotions in Man and Animals*. New York: Oxford University Press.

Ehlers, A and Clark, DM (2000) 'A cognitive model of posttraumatic stress disorder', *Behaviour Research & Therapy*, 38(4), 319–45.

Etkin, A and Wager, TD (2007) 'Functional neuroimaging of anxiety: a meta-analysis of emotional processing in PTSD, social anxiety disorder, and specific phobia', *American Journal of Psychiatry*, 164(10), 1476–88.

Foa, EB, Ehlers, A, Clark, DM, Tolin, DF, and Orsillo, SM (1999) 'The Posttraumatic Cognitions Inventory (PTCI): Development and validation', *Psychological Assessment*, 11(3), 303–314.

Gilbertson, MW, Shenton, ME, Ciszewski, A, et al. (2002) 'Smaller hippocampal volume predicts pathologic vulnerability to psychological trauma', *Nature Neuroscience*, 5(11), 1242–47.

Ginzberg, E (1959) *The Ineffective Soldier, Vol. 1: The Lost Divisions. Lessons for Management and the Nation*. New York: Columbia University Press.

Guthrie, RM and Bryant, RA (2006) 'Extinction learning before trauma and subsequent posttraumatic stress', *Psychosomatic Medicine*, 68(2), 307–11.

Hyman, SE (2007) 'Can neuroscience be integrated into the DSM-V?', *Nature Reviews Neuroscience*, 8(9), 725–32.

Inglis, J, Sambrook, J, and Witkowski, J (2003) *Inspiring Science: Jim Watson and the age of DNA*. Cold Spring Harbor, NY: Cold Spring Harbor Laboratory Press.

Kessler, RC, Sonnega, A, Hughes, M, and Nelson, CB (1995) 'Posttraumatic stress disorder in the national comorbidity survey', *Archives of General Psychiatry*, 52, 1048–60.

Kilpatrick, DG, Koenen, KC, Ruggiero, KJ, et al. (2007) 'The serotonin transporter genotype and social support and moderation of posttraumatic stress disorder and depression in hurricane-exposed adults', *American Journal of Psychiatry*, 164(11), 1693–99.

Korobkin, R and Rajkumar, R (2008) 'The Genetic Information Nondiscrimination Act—a half-step toward risk sharing', *New England Journal of Medicine*, 359(4), 335–37.

Kraepelin, E (1899) *Psychiatrie*. 6th edn. Leipzig, Germany: Verlag von Johann Ambrosius Barth.

Lindqvist, S and Tate, J (1996) *Exterminate all the brutes*. New York: New Press.

McEwen, BS (2000) 'The neurobiology of stress: from serendipity to clinical relevance', *Brain Research*, 886, 172–89.

Macklin, ML, Metzger, LJ, Litz, BT, et al. (1998) 'Lower precombat intelligence is a risk factor for posttraumatic stress disorder', *Journal of Consulting and Clinical Psychology*, 66(2), 323–26.

Morley, KI, Hall, WD, and Carter, L (2004) 'Genetic Screening for susceptibility to depression: can we and should we?', *Australian and New Zealand Journal of Psychiatry*, 38, 73–80.

Nuffield Council of Bioethics (1998) *Mental disorders and genetics: the ethical context*. London: Nuffield Council of Bioethics.

Orr, SP, Metzger, LJ, Lasko, NB, et al. (2003) 'Physiologic responses to sudden, loud tones in monozygotic twins discordant for combat exposure: association with posttraumatic stress disorder', Archives of General Psychiatry, Mar, 60(3), 283–88.

Orr, SP, Pitman, RK, Lasko, NB, and Herz, LR (1993) 'Psychophysiological assessment of posttraumatic stress disorder imagery in World War II and Korean combat veterans', *Journal of Abnormal Psychology*, 102(1), 152–59.

Phelan, JC (2002) 'Genetic bases of mental illness—a cure for stigma?', *Trends in Neurosciences*, 25(8), 430–31.

Pitman, RK, Orr, SP, Lowenhagen, MJ, et al. (1991) 'Pre-Vietnam contents of posttraumatic stress disorder veterans' service medical and personnel records', *Comprehensive Psychiatry*, 32(5), 416–22.

Pole, N, Neylan, TC, Otte, C, Henn-Hasse, C, Metzler, TJ, and Marmar, CR (2009) 'Prospective Prediction of PTSD Symptoms Using Fear Potentiated Auditory Startle Responses', *Biological Psychiatry*, 65(3), 235–240.

Rauch, SL, Shin, LM, and Phelps, EA (2006) 'Neurocircuitry models of posttraumatic stress disorder and extinction: human neuroimaging research-past, present, and future', *Biological Psychiatry*, 60(4), 376–82.

Riggs, DS, Rothbaum, BO, and Foa, EB (1995) 'A prospective examination of symptoms of posttraumatic stress disorder in victims of nonsexual assault', *Journal of Interpersonal Violence*, 10(2), 201–14.

Roberts-Yates, C (2003) 'The concerns and issues of injured workers in relation to claims/injury management and rehabilitation: the need for new operational frameworks', *Disability and Rehabilitation*, 25(16), 898–907.

Schnurr, PP, Friedman, MJ, and Rosenberg, SD (1993) 'Preliminary MMPI scores as predictors of combat-related PTSD symptoms', *American Journal of Psychiatry*, 150(3), 479–83.

Shepherd, B (2001) *A war of nerves: soldiers and psychiatrists in the twentieth century*. Cambridge, MA: Cambridge University Press.

Smith, K and Bryant, RA (2000) 'The generality of cognitive bias in acute stress disorder', *Behaviour Research and Therapy*, 38(7), 709–15.

Spriggs, M, Olsson, CA, and Hall, W (2008) 'How will information about the genetic risk of mental disorders impact on stigma?', *Australian and New Zealand Journal of Psychiatry*, 42(3), 214–20.

Stout, JC, Rodawalt, WC, and Siemers, ER (2001) 'Risky decision making in Huntington's disease', *Journal of the International Neuropsychological Society*, 7(1), 92–101.

Sullivan, PF, Kendler, KS, and Neale, MC (2003) 'Schizophrenia as a complex trait: evidence from a meta-analysis of twin studies', *Archives of General Psychiatry*, 60(12), 1187–92.

Sullivan, PF, Neale, MC, and Kendler, KS (2000) 'Genetic epidemiology of major depression: review and meta-analysis', *American Journal of Psychiatry*, 157(10), 1552–62.

Ulaner, GA (2004) 'Telomere maintenance in clinical medicine', *American Journal of Medicine*, 117(4), 262–69.

Wessa, M and Flor, H (2007) 'Failure of extinction of fear responses in posttraumatic stress disorder: evidence from second-order conditioning', *American Journal of Psychiatry*, 164(11), 1684–92.

Wessely, S (2006) 'Twentieth-century Theories on Combat Motivation and Breakdown', *Journal of Contemporary History*, 41(2), 268–86.

Chapter 7

Race Equality in Mental Health

Tristan McGeorge and Dinesh Bhugra

A 62 year old Chinese man was found wandering at Heathrow airport. He was perplexed and unable to communicate. Paramedics were called and he was taken to the hospital where emergency physical investigations were carried out which were normal. After the Chinese embassy opened and an interpreter was arranged it transpired that the patient was on his way to North America and got lost in transit. His perplexity and bewilderment was related to his having very limited English and becoming disorientated in the airport.

Introduction

With the advent of globalization, the major cities of the developed world have become increasingly multicultural and temporary movement of people across these cities has added another dimension. It has been reported widely that the rates of mental illness vary between different racial and ethnic minorities in the developed world. Although some of the research may be seen as of variable quality, with inconsistent findings, some minority groups have been found to have better mental health indices than the White majorities, whereas others have significantly worse. Considerable efforts have been made to understand the reasons for these differential rates of mental illness. An understanding of these differential rates will not only provide a means by which to ameliorate the situation of disadvantaged groups in society but it is hoped that this will also shed light on the causative mechanisms of mental illness itself.

Social and cultural factors in the pathogenesis of mental illness in minority groups are important. One of the key factors that has been seen as a possible contributor to the disparities in mental health and help-seeking is racial discrimination. This contribution could be mediated by a number of mechanisms. It could directly increase the amount of stress that individuals are exposed to, or alternatively, it could act indirectly through its associated effects such as socio-economic disadvantage.

An important means for reducing the impact of racial discrimination in society is the application of human rights principles. The mentally ill are stigmatized and discriminated against in all societies and are often a vulnerable group. Human rights principles have increasingly had a role in shaping how mental health services are delivered and provided a means of safeguarding the interests of people with mental illness. Individuals from racial and ethnic minorities who develop mental illness are exposed to discrimination on two fronts: their race and ethnicity, and the stigma of mental illness—sometimes called double jeopardy—further increasing the burden of psychological stress. Human rights law is well placed to provide a means of protecting the interests of individuals from minority groups who develop mental illness.

This chapter deals with race inequalities that exist in mental health and the extent to which discrimination may be contributing to them. The focus here is on the data from the United

Kingdom but it also includes relevant research conducted elsewhere. The first part of the chapter reviews the research on the rates of mental illness in black and ethnic minorities in the United Kingdom. In the second part, the impact of racism in the existing disparities in mental health is discussed. In the following section suggested strategies for improving race equality in mental health are described. Lastly, a review of existing human rights mechanisms that are relevant to reducing racial discrimination in mental health services is offered.

Disparities in mental health

In the UK, over the last two decades research has indicated that Black and ethnic minority groups have differential rates of mental illness.

a) Depression

A nationwide survey by Nazroo (1997) found that the prevalence rates for depression among Caribbean individuals were 60 per cent higher than the white group. Lower rates of depression and anxiety were reported in the South Asian group. However, the rates of these illnesses were higher for South Asians born in Britain or who had migrated at a relatively young age. The prevalence was higher amongst those who were fluent in English. Overall low rates of mental illness in the Chinese group and high rates amongst the minority white group were reported (Nazroo 1997).

A more recent study examining the rates of anxiety and depression in England found that the prevalence of these disorders was highest amongst Irish and Pakistani men aged 35–54 years, and Indian and Pakistani women aged 55–74 years. The differences were modest but statistically significant and were not altered by adjusting for measures of socio-economic status. Contrary to Nazroo's study, it did not find evidence of higher rates of depression and anxiety in African Caribbeans. However, these findings should be treated with caution. These differences in the rates of common mental disorders between ethnic groups are likely to be modest at best (Weich et al. 2004).

b) Psychosis

Early research indicated that the rates of psychosis in certain racial groups in the UK were significantly higher than in the white majority, particularly in African Caribbeans. However it was suggested that these higher rates were at least in part due to the methodological problems of the earlier treatment studies.[1] Nazroo (1997) found that there was no evidence that Caribbean men had higher rates of psychosis than white men. Caribbean women had rates twice that of white women but this finding did not reach statistical significance. The author suggested a number of reasons that could account for the discrepancy between these findings and those of earlier studies, but concluded that overall they were unlikely to have led to an underestimate of the rate of psychosis for the Caribbean group.[2]

---

[1] a) Use of western psychiatric measures to cross-cultural measurement of psychiatric disorder; b) Denominator problems where there was unreliable data on the size of the African Caribbean population from which hospital admissions were drawn; c) Number of African Caribbeans admitted to hospital with first episode psychosis was possibly overestimated; d) Differences in pathways to care resulted in more African Caribbeans being admitted; e) Differential treatment by healthcare workers resulted in an increased rate of diagnosis of African Caribbeans; f) Different symptom profile of African Caribbeans.

[2] The first was that African Caribbeans might experience a shorter duration of illness. The second was that his community survey might been less likely to include those with psychosis in the Caribbean group than the White group, given that young Caribbean men are more likely to be detained in institutions and to

The largest study to date on the incidence rates of psychoses in ethnic minority groups was carried out in 2006 (Fearon et al. 2006). The findings confirmed findings from earlier studies, which had reported a greatly increased risk of psychotic illness in African Caribbeans and black Africans in the UK.[3] Rates of psychotic illness in Asians were more modestly increased. It demonstrated, for the first time, that people of mixed race and non-British whites in the UK are also at an increased risk of psychosis, albeit this risk is lower. The risk of psychoses is not increased in the countries of origin (Hickling and Rodgers-Johnson 1995) and in those countries those that do develop the illness have lower rates of relapse and better outcome measures (Hickling et al. 2001). The risk of schizophrenia in migrants is inversely related to the size of the migrant community in the destination countries (Boydell et al. 2001).

On comparing the rates of psychoses for different generations of black and ethnic minority groups, a recent study noted that given the same age structure, the risk of psychoses in first and second generations of the same ethnicity is roughly similar. These authors suggested that socio-environmental factors operate differentially by ethnicity but not generation status while the exact specification of the stressors may differ across generations (Coid et al. 2008). When the risk of psychoses in black and ethnic minorities were compared, they remain elevated even when age, gender, and socioeconomic status are controlled for. Thus socioeconomic status by itself could not explain the elevated rates of psychoses in black and ethnic minority groups.

A number of hypotheses have been put forward to account for racial differences in psychiatric morbidity. One possibility is that schizophrenia may be misdiagnosed in this population. This might be the result of misdiagnosis by British psychiatrists unfamiliar with Caribbean beliefs or because African Caribbeans have a different symptom profile from the majority culture. There is no real evidence for this assertion as schizophrenia is a long term condition and, with same diagnostic tools used in the Caribbean based studies, rates were found to be lower there. Biological explanations include a genetic predisposition, a predisposition to migration, prenatal complications, childhood risk factors, and cannabis use. Psychological theories include differences in the interpretation of life events and attributional style. Social hypotheses include an urban effect, different views on psychiatric services, social disadvantage, and racism (Sharpley et al. 2001).

Pathways to care

It has been suggested that psychiatric services in the UK have failed in the increased rates of negative pathways to care of black patients relative to their white British counterparts (Nazroo 1998). Black patients are significantly more likely to come into contact with mental health services via negative and adversarial routes. These generally include police and courts and judicial system. Black and mixed race individuals were 3–4 times more likely to be admitted to hospital compulsorily (Commission for Healthcare Audit and Inspection 2005; Commission for Healthcare Audit and Inspection 2007).

Odds of compulsory admission are 3.5 times greater for African-Caribbean males than for white British males. Black African ethnicity was also found to be independently associated with increased likelihood of compulsory admission. Although diagnosis, perceived risk of violence, living alone, and being unemployed were all independently associated with compulsory admission, none of these factors could account for the excess of compulsory admissions among

---

refuse to participate in the sample. There was also the possibility that altering the PSQ for screening purposes may have affected the results.

[3] Incidence rate ratio schizophrenia 9.1, manic psychosis 8.0 in African Caribbeans; incidence rate ratio schizophrenia 5.8, manic psychosis 6.2 in black Africans.

African-Caribbean men or black African patients (Morgan et al. 2005). These authors also reported unequivocal differences in the pathways to care for different ethnic groups. Black patients were much less likely to have been referred by their GP and much more likely to have criminal justice agency involvement in bringing them to care. The duration of untreated psychosis did not affect either general practitioner or criminal justice agency referral. A diagnosis of manic psychosis decreased GP and increased criminal justice referral but did not account for ethnic differences in the source of referral. Although African-Caribbean families and friends were more likely than other ethnic groups to seek help initially from the police, adjusting for it weakened the association between ethnicity and the path of referral, but even this did not fully account for the differences (Chakraboty and McKenzie 2002).

The increased rate of adverse pathways to care has resulted in a more coercive relationship with mental health services (Morgan et al. 2004). A systematic review in 2007 suggested that that the relationship between black and minority ethnic patients and mental health services deteriorates over time as increasing detention rates are observed with subsequent admissions (Singh et al. 2007).

Racism and mental health

Racism is the process by which one race assumes power over another especially when related to status and advantages whether these are economic or practical. The concept of race emerged only in the 19th century with the British anthropologists and empire builders moving across the world. Racism occurs where negative attributions are made by people of one social group about another on the basis of putative biological characteristics (Bhugra and Ayorinde 2001). The underlying assumption is that people are to be treated differently because some groups are considered superior or inferior to others (Littlewood 2001). On the basis of biological superiority this notion of racism attributes a lesser moral and political worth to non-European groups. This allows a justification for allocating lesser resources, power, and responsibility (Littlewood 2001). Racism is associated with the overt and covert forceful establishment and maintenance of power by one social group over another. The creation of race is also linked with the creation of the Other who, by these characteristics, allows one's own identity to be established. Dominant cultural groups use race as a symbol disempowering people and to maintain their economic, political, and cultural domination (Moore 2000).

Racism exists in all aspects of life and has various forms depending on who is expressing it and who is experiencing it (Chakraboty and McKenzie 2002; Karlsen and Nazroo 2002). Discrimination, and therefore racial discrimination, has been divided into two main types: interpersonal and institutional (Karlsen and Nazroo 2002). Direct racial attacks are less common than perceived discrimination in interpersonal communications or inequity in the receipt of services or justice (Chakraboty and McKenzie 2002). Studies in the US have suggested that the darker a person's skin colour, the more racism they are likely to experience (McKenzie 2006).

Racism leads to poorer physical and mental health with physiological and cognitive changes identified in those subjected to it. However, its specific impact on mental health is complex and not easy to investigate due to its interaction with other risk factors (McKenzie 2006). Along with true instances of racial events, the appraisal of events as being caused due to racism have been associated with negative mental health outcomes (Klonoff et al. 1999). A UK survey found that a quarter of people from ethnic minority groups were worried about being racially harassed. These individuals were 61 per cent more likely to report their health as fair or poor compared to those who were not worried about racial harassment (Karlsen and Nazroo 2004). However, it has been recognized that the presence of mental disorder may result in an attributional style that places more emphasis on racism as a cause for negative events (Bhui et al. 2005).

A recent systematic review of the impact of self-reported racism and health in the US reported a strong and consistent association between self-reported racism and negative mental health. 72 per cent of negative mental health outcomes were significantly associated with self-reported racism. A strong sense of racial/ethnic identity and an active/expressive response to racism attenuated the association of self-reported racism and depression. Poor self-esteem, stressful events, and substance misuse intensified the detrimental effect of self-reported racism on mental health (Paradies 2006).

The relationship between racism and stress remains complex. An individual's perception of a society as racist results in chronic stress while overt acts of racism towards an individual constitute acute stressors (Chakraboty and McKenzie 2002; Bhugra and Cochrane 2001). Racism and racism-related stress are distinct concepts that may be independently related to health (Paradies 2006). Increasing levels of racial discrimination predict more psychiatric symptoms, including somatization, obsessive-compulsive, interpersonal sensitivity, depressive, and anxiety symptoms. In this study racism was a more powerful predictor of these symptoms than were general stressors and social status (Klonoff et al. 1999). Others have found increased rates of psychosis and delusional ideation in those who reported racial abuse (Karlsen and Nazroo 2002; Janssen et al. 2003).

Psychological consequences of racism have linked it with an increased rate in the onset of depression (Bhugra and Ayorinde 2001). Experiences related to racism include hopelessness, humiliation, and defeat as well as direct attacks on a person's self-esteem producing depression-like symptoms. Racial discrimination may also result in a sense of out-group status or exclusion that contributes to heightened levels of stress (Bhugra and Ayorinde 2001). An independent association between common mental disorders and the experience of racial insults and perception of unfair treatment at work has been reported indicating that perception itself may play a key role (Bhui et al. 2005). When investigating the role of racial discrimination in work stress it was noted that more African-Caribbean respondents reported high work stress than Bangladeshi or white respondents. Among African Caribbean females, the reported experience of discrimination at work was strongly associated with both perceived work stress and psychological distress (Wadsworth et al. 2007). Thus gender differences may play a role.

Both self-reported experience of interpersonal racism and perception of racism in wider British society have been shown to be independently associated with common mental disorders and psychosis. Experiencing racially motivated verbal or physical abuse has been shown to be associated with a two to three-fold increase in the risk of common mental disorders and psychosis. Reporting of an experience of employment-related discrimination was associated with an almost fifty percent additional risk (Karlsen et al. 2005).

It can be argued that the observation that racism causes an increased rate of psychotic illness through environmental stress would mean either that African Caribbeans have a special vulnerability to racism or that they experience greater levels of it because other racial minorities do not have the same elevated rates of the illness (Shashidharan 1993).

Institutional racism

Institutional racism was defined in the MacPherson Report (1999) as: 'The collective failure of an organization to provide an appropriate and professional service to people because of their colour, culture or ethnic origin. It can be seen or detected in processes, attitudes and behaviour which amount to discrimination through unwitting prejudice, ignorance, thoughtlessness and racist stereotyping which disadvantage minority ethnic people' (MacPherson 1999). It could also refer to discriminatory policies or practices embedded in organizational structures. Therefore, it tends to be more invisible than interpersonal discrimination (Karlsen and Nazroo 2002). Such an institutional racism is often indirect whereby the organization does not intend to be racist but it has this effect through its rules (Chakraboty and McKenzie 2002).

Statistics show significant racial disadvantage in many aspects of society. Cochrane has stated that mental health services are not immune from the values that pervade the rest of society (Cochrane 2001).[4] Other authors have referred to the evidence of ethnic differences in treatment approaches to mental illness (McKenzie and Bhui 2007a). Black and ethnic minority groups are less likely to be offered psychotherapy, more likely to be offered pharmacotherapy, and more likely to be treated by coercion, even after socioeconomic and diagnostic differences are taken account of (Bhui et al. 2003; McKenzie et al. 2001; Davies et al. 1996; Shashidharan 2003). It has been argued that the ideology of racism became incorporated into psychiatry resulting in an emphasis on individualized pathology with insufficient attention paid to social pressures such as race and culture (Chakraboty and McKenzie 2002; Fernando 1984). This view can be challenged in that social and cultural context of practice of psychiatry has always been very clear. Indeed social and cultural factors are included in understanding causation and management of psychiatric disorders.

Race of the patient and that of the clinician may affect diagnoses. A US study presented a group of psychiatrists with two patient vignettes: one of undifferentiated schizophrenia and the other with dependent personality disorder. They then altered the sex and race in the vignettes to determine the effect it would have on their diagnosis. They found that psychiatrists were more likely to diagnose paranoid schizophrenia and paranoid personality disorder in those they believed were African Americans. This was also true of the black psychiatrists in the study, though to a lesser extent. They also found that psychiatrists were more likely to perceive black patients as dangerous and violent (Loring and Powell 1988). A similar study in the UK altered the sex and race of patients in a vignette of psychotic illness. The respondents found the African-Caribbean case to be potentially more violent and thought criminal proceedings more appropriate. The British respondents also tended to diagnose cannabis psychosis and acute reactive psychosis more often and schizophrenia less often in African Caribbeans (Lewis et al. 1990). Doctors in the US had greater difficulty diagnosing black patients but did not observe their expected racial bias of a greater tendency to attribute schizophrenia or affective disorders to black patients (Sohler and Bromet 2003).

Higher rates of psychosis and detention in black patients in the UK have been attributed, at least in part, to institutional racism within services (McKenzie and Bhui 2007a; Patel and Heginbotham 2007; McKenzie and Bhui 2007b). The argument goes 'disparities reflect the way health services offer specific treatment and care pathways according to racial groups and therefore seem to satisfy the well-established and widely known definition of institutional racism' (McKenzie and Bhui 2007a). Others consider it a consequence of wider social factors (that might include racism) that black and ethnic minorities are disproportionately exposed to in the UK (Murray and Fearon 2007). Singh et al. (2007) found that, while racism and racial stereotyping of black and minority ethnic patients are the most common explanations offered for excess detentions, there is insufficient primary supportive evidence to justify the assertions. They acknowledged that racism may indeed play a part in the ethnic inequalities in mental health care, but they

---

[4] According to Cochrane, ethnic minorities are more likely to come into contact with mental health services through compulsory means; they are more likely to be misdiagnosed; they are more likely to receive less preferred treatments with high dose medication and fewer referrals for psychological treatment; more likely to be uncooperative and aggressive resulting in treatment in secure facilities; they are less likely to be compliant with treatment; and have lower levels of satisfaction with care.

argued that it needs to be scientifically explored rather than accepted as the only cause (Singh and Burns 2007; Singh et al. 2006).

Race and social class

Many psychiatric disorders have been shown to be more common in lower socioeconomic groups (Goldberg and Morrison 1963; Wiersma et al. 1983; Kelly 2003). The relationship is likely to be bidirectional with health affecting socioeconomic class and socioeconomic class affecting health (Kelly 2003; Lewis and Araya 2002). Higher social class is thought to buffer the exposure and effect of provoking agents thereby reducing difficulties (Bhugra and Ayorinde 2001). It is often argued that lower social class levels account for much of the variance in the health of ethnic minorities (Klonoff et al. 1999). It has been observed that longitudinally racism produces and perpetuates socioeconomic difference (Chakraboty and McKenzie 2002).

Nazroo (1997) showed a relatively uniform effect across ethnic groups. Class was inversely related to mental health for all outcomes (Nazroo 2007). Not only was social class an important predictors of mental health within ethnic groups it also contributed to the differences in rates of mental illness across groups. (Nazroo 1998). However these findings are not uniform as a recent study found that elevated rates of psychosis in black and ethnic minority groups could not be explained by socioeconomic status (Kirkbride et al. 2008).

Race equality in mental health

Significant disparities exist in the rates of mental illness and the patterns of service use of different racial and ethnic groups in the UK. However the causes for these discrepancies are still far from clear. Given the extent to which racism has affected humanity to date, it is safe to assume that it hasn't and will not necessarily just go away and it might be playing a role in the inequalities in mental health that exist.

There is a need to re-evaluate economic and social policy in response to the challenges facing mental health services from migration and the increased diversity of service users in the developed world (Kelly 2003). One of the key areas where policy changes can be effected is in education. It has been suggested that medical school training continues to produce homogeneity amongst doctors despite the fact that diversity in medical school students is increasing (Beagan 2000). There needs to be a greater emphasis on transcultural psychiatry in mental health curricula. There may be a particular role of psychiatrists and psychiatric institutions in education which may influence shaping policy (Kelly 2003).

The Royal College of Psychiatrists has been actively involved in promoting race equality since 1987 when it established a committee to review the issues. Subsequently in response to the duties introduced by the Race Relations (Amendment) Act 2000 it introduced a Race Equality Scheme. The College's Special Committee on ethnic issues contributed to the scheme's development and continues to oversee the College's efforts to meet its obligations under the Act until all these were mainstreamed and form part of all the activities in the College. The College has noted its awareness of institutional racism both within its own structures and in mental health services in general and continues to make press releases on related issues.[5]

Governmental organizations have also been active. The recognition of institutional racism in mental health led to the development of the Department of Health's policy on Delivering Race Equality (DRE) (McKenzie and Bhui 2007a; Department of Health 2005). This document

5 See Royal College of Psychiatrists website for details.

combined a five-year action plan for improving black and ethnic minorities' access to, experience of, and outcomes from mental health services with the government response to the inquiry into the death of David Bennett while in a psychiatric hospital as a result of restraint and control. Its aim was to achieve equality and tackle discrimination in mental health services for people of black and ethnic minority status. The programme is based on three 'building blocks': more appropriate and responsive services, community engagement, and better information. It was intended to assist the NHS with fulfilling its obligations under the Race Relations (Amendment) Act 2000. It set up a new black and minority ethnic (BME) Mental Health Programme Board to oversee the implementation of the action plan (Department of Health 2005).[6]

Improving access to services involves reducing stigma and removing fear of services in the community. There has been a call for informed commissioning of services to establish more appropriate services for black and ethnic minorities. This involves input from a range of providers to create a more integrated and coherent model, which would secure service user confidence. It has been suggested that if early intervention services engage effectively and consistently with local further education colleges this could reverse the trend of adverse care pathways for black and ethnic minority service users (Lau 2008), although there has also been a suggestion that on the line of women only services, segregated specialist services for ethnic minority groups could be helpful. However there is a danger that this may lead to a further isolation and alienation among the patients and their carers.

In the UK, another significant development has been the genesis of advocacy groups from within black and ethnic minority communities themselves. Black Mental Health UK (BMH UK) was established in 2006 to raise awareness and address the stigma associated with mental illness. It aims to reduce the inequalities in the treatment and care of people from African-Caribbean communities and inform these communities on how to influence the strategic development, policy design and implementation of services. The focus is on empowering African-Caribbean communities to improve the black service user experience and reduce the over representation of black people at the coercive end of psychiatric care.[7] BMH UK raised a number of human rights concerns over the amendment to the Mental Health Act 2007.

---

[6] The vision for DRE is that by 2010 there will be a service characterized by:

- less fear of mental health services among BME communities and service users;
- increased satisfaction with services;
- a reduction in the rate of admission of people from BME communities to psychiatric inpatient units;
- reduction in the disproportionate rates of compulsory detention of BME service users in inpatient units;
- fewer violent incidents that are secondary to inadequate treatment of mental illness; a reduction in the use of seclusion in BME groups;
- the prevention of deaths in mental health services following physical intervention;
- more BME service users reaching self-reported states of recovery;
- a reduction in the ethnic disparities found in prison populations;
- a more balanced range of effective therapies, such as peer support services and psychotherapeutic and counselling treatments, as well as pharmacological interventions that are culturally appropriate and effective;
- a more active role for BME communities and BME service users in the training of professionals, in the development of mental health policy, and in the planning and provision of services; and
- a workforce and organization capable of delivering appropriate and responsive mental health services to BME communities.

[7] Description taken from Black Mental Health UK website.

Human rights framework

Human rights law is important in the context of mental health because it is the only source of law that legitimizes international scrutiny of mental health policies and practices within a sovereign country (Gostin 2001). It expresses both fundamental prescriptions on behaviour and aspirational goals for society (Knowles 2001). Human rights principles have been increasingly employed to ensure and promote the rights of those with mental illness as a vulnerable group. Human rights law has the potential to address the inequalities that exist in mental health services especially towards black and ethnic minority groups, particularly where these are due to social inequalities and racism. Services could be challenged either through the generic protections against racial discrimination contained in international law or through the human rights principles contained in domestic law and mental health policy.

The MI Principles

In 1991 the General Assembly of the United Nations adopted Resolution 46/119: The UN Principles for the Protection of Persons with Mental Illness and for the Improvement for Mental Health Care, otherwise known as the MI Principles. These have been described as 'the first step in providing a global set of minimum standards for protecting persons with mental illness and improving mental health care' (Maingay et al. 2002). They include 25 principles for the treatment of people with mental disorder. Although they are not legally binding they are a useful system for monitoring the human rights status of persons with mental illness and provide a comprehensive guide for the development of appropriate mental services (Maingay et al. 2002). Of the 25 Principles, four in particular have potential relevance to institutional racism in mental health care. These are:

- Principle 1: Fundamental freedoms and human rights—All persons have the right to the best available mental health care, which should be part of the health and social care system.

- Principle 4: Determination of mental illness—'. . . determination of mental illness shall never be made on the basis of political, economic or social status, or membership of a cultural, racial or religious group, or any other reason not directly relevant to mental health status. . .' (Weich et al. 2004).

- Principle 7: Role of community and culture—Every patient shall have the right to treatment suited to his or her cultural background.

- Principle 9: Treatment—Every patient shall have the right to be treated in the least restrictive environment and with the least restrictive treatment.

These principles do not have the status of a formal international treaty so states are not required to use the principles to define minimum standards of care (Kelly 2001). However it has been argued that the best way to ensure that human rights in mental health are respected globally is to increase awareness and implementation of the MI Principles so as to inform legislative activity, psychiatric education, and service development (Kelly 2003).

International measures

The International Convention for the Elimination of all Forms of Racism and Racial Discrimination 1965 is the primary international instrument on race (Thornberry 2005). It states that parties to the convention condemn racial discrimination and undertake to pursue by all appropriate means and without delay a policy of eliminating racial discrimination in all its forms and promoting understanding among all races. Article 5 of the convention explicitly enjoins states parties to prohibit and eliminate racial discrimination in the enjoyment of the right to public health, medical care, social security and social services.[8]

Article 14 of the convention established the Committee on the Elimination of Racial Discrimination (CERD). States parties to the convention are required to provide reports to CERD, which it analyses and comments upon. It then engages in dialogue with the state party before making a number of concluding observations. Article 14 of the convention establishes a mechanism by which individuals or groups who claim to be a victim of a state violation of the convention can address their concerns directly to the committee. The committee has engaged in what is known as the 'effects' aspect of discrimination which includes disparities in the administration of justice, education, employment, life expectancy, and health (Thornberry 2005).

A submission to CERD is a potential option for those affected by racial discrimination in the provision of mental health services. In its response to an April 2007 report of the United States of America to CERD, the US Human Rights Network Prison Working Group (2008) referred to the 'over-representation of people of colour in the US prison system'. It made specific mention of mental illness and substance abuse in the disparities that affect the prison population. In a submission to CERD by the National Anti-Racism Council of Canada (2007), specific mention was made of the link between racism and mental illness. The Australian Non-Governmental Organisation's (2005) Submission to CERD recommended increased funding be allocated to indigenous health to redress serious health issues and increase access to services within that community.

Regional measures

A number of regional human rights instruments contain Articles, which protect against discrimination. The Council of Europe introduced the European Convention on Human Rights (ECHR) in 1950, which is overseen by the European Court of Human Rights. Article 14 of the ECHR requires that the exercise of the convention rights and freedoms be secured without discrimination on any one of 12 specific grounds which includes race (Moon 2003). This has been criticized because the protection against discrimination is dependent upon the other specific rights entailed in the convention. Protocol 12 extends the protection to any legal right recognized in the national law of state parties. However this has not been ratified by a number of countries including the UK.

In 2002 the Council of Europe's Commission against Racism and Intolerance (ECRI) adopted the General Policy Recommendation on National Legislation to Combat Racism and Racial Discrimination.[9] This allows for criticism of member states in ECRI reports for not taking sufficient action to combat racism.

The European Convention for the Prevention of Torture and Inhumane or Degrading Treatment or Punishment, which entered into force in 1989, signified a major step towards the enforcement of Article 3[10] of the ECHR established the European Committee for the prevention of torture and inhumane or degrading treatment of punishment (CPT) (Niveau 2004). The CPT visits closed psychiatric institutions in signatory countries to investigate their procedures, as mental health services are involved in the deprivation of liberty by a state authority (Harding 1989). It then provides reports with comments and recommendations to promote the reform of the establishments in order to promote human rights (Niveau 2004).

---

[8] UN GA Res. 2106A (XX) (1965).

[9] Recommendation CRI (2003) 8, ECRI, Council of Europe, 2003, Strasbourg.

[10] 'No one shall be subject to torture or inhumane or degrading treatment or punishment'.

Domestic measures

In the UK, the European Convention on Human Rights was enacted into domestic law with the Human Rights Act (HRA) 1998. The Act requires that all public bodies, and those private bodies which have public functions, ensure that their policies are compatible with the ECHR. Every new piece of legislation enacted in the UK must declare its compatibility with it. The HRA enables individuals to seek redress in local courts rather than having to go the European Court of Human Rights in Strasbourg. The other significant piece of legislation in the UK is the Race Relations Act 1976, which prohibits discrimination on grounds of race, colour, nationality, and ethnic origin. It was amended in 2000 to introduce a general statutory duty on public authorities to 'have due regard to the need (a) to eliminate unlawful discrimination; and (b) to promote equality of opportunity and good relations between persons of different racial groups'. Governmental bodies monitor issues pertaining to racial equality in the UK. These include the Race Equality Unit and UK Commission for Equality and Human Rights.

The third report of the Joint Committee on Human Rights in 2004 referred to the David Bennett Inquiry,[11] in acknowledging concerns expressed that restraint is used in a discriminatory way by police and in mental health custody. It stated that the possibility that racial stereotyping might be a contributory factor in at least some deaths in custody should be taken seriously as an alert to the risk of a breach of the ECHR and the obligations of police forces under the Race Relations Acts (1976 and 2000). The Joint Committee found that an obligation existed both under the Human Rights Act 1998 and the positive duty of the Race Relations (Amendment) Act 2000 to provide cultural awareness training to staff involved in the use of restraint.

References

Australian Non-governmental Organisations' Submission to the Committee on the Elimination of Racial Discrimination (2005) Australia: NACLC.

Beagan, BL (2000) 'Neutralising differences: producing neutral doctors for (almost) neutral patients', *Social Science and Medicine*, 51, 1253–65.

Bhugra, D and Ayonrinde, O (2001) 'Racial life events and psychiatric morbidity', in D Bhugra and R Cochrane (eds) *Psychiatry in Multicultural Britain*. London: Gaskell, 91–111.

Bhugra, D and Cochrane, R (eds) (2001) *Psychiatry in Multicultural Britain*. London: Gaskell.

Bhui, K, Stansfeld, S, Hull, S, Priebe, S, Mole, F, and Feder, G (2003) 'Ethnic variations in pathways to and use of specialist mental health services in the UK. Systematic review', *British Journal of Psychiatry*, 182, 105–16.

Bhui, K, Stansfeld, S, McKenzie, K, Karlsen, S, Nazroo, J, and Weich, S (2005) 'Racial/ethnic discrimination and common mental disorders among workers: findings from the EMPIRIC Study of Ethnic Minority Groups in the United Kingdom', *American Journal of Public Health*, 95(3), 496–501.

Boydell, J, van Os, J, McKenzie, K, et al. (2001) 'Incidence of schizophrenia in ethnic minorities in London: ecological study into interactions with environment'. *British Medical Journal*, 323(7325), 1336–8.

Chakraboty, A and McKenzie, K (2002) 'Does racial discrimination cause mental illness', *British Journal of Psychiatry*, 180, 475–7.

Cochrane, R (2001) 'Race, prejudice and ethnic identity', in D Bhugra and R Cochrane (eds) *Psychiatry in Multicultural Britain*. London: Gaskell, 75–90.

----

[11] David 'Rocky' Bennett was a 38-year-old African-Caribbean man who died on 30 October 1998 after being restrained in a medium secure psychiatric unit in the UK.

Coid, JW, Kirkbride, JB, Barker, D, et al. (2008) 'Raised incidence rates of all psychoses among migrant groups: findings from the East London first episode psychosis study', *Archives of General Psychiatry*, 65(11), 1250–8.

Davies, S, Thornicroft, G, Leese, M, Higgingbotham, A, and Phelan, M (1996) 'Ethnic differences in risk of compulsory psychiatric admission among representative cases of psychosis in London', *British Medical Journal*, 312(7030), 533–7.

Department of Health (2005) *Delivering Race Equality: an action plan for improving services inside and outside mental health care and the government's response to the independent enquiry of the death of David Bennett*. London: Department of Health.

Fearon, P, Kirkbride, JB, Morgan, C, et al. (2006) 'Incidence of schizophrenia and other psychoses in ethnic minority groups: results from the MRC AESOP Study', *Psychological Medicine*, 36(11), 1541–50.

Fernando, S (1984) 'Racism as a cause of depression', *International Journal of Social Psychiatry*, Spring, 30(1–2), 41–9.

Goldberg, EM, and Morrison, SL (1963) 'Schizophrenia and Social Class', *British Journal of Psychiatry*, 109, 785–802.

Gostin, LO (2001) 'Beyond moral claims: a human rights approach in mental health', *Cambridge Quarterly of Healthcare Ethics*, Summer, 10(3), 264–74.

Harding, TW (1989) 'Prevention of torture and inhuman or degrading treatment: medical implications of a new European convention', *The Lancet*, 1(8648), 1191–3.

Healthcare Commission (2005) *Count Me In. Results of a National Census of Inpatients in Mental Health Hospitals and Facilities in England and Wales*. London: Commission for Healthcare, Audit and Inspection.

Healthcare Commission (2007) *Count Me In. Results of the 2006 National Survey on Inpatients in Mental Health and Learning Disability Services in England and Wales*. London: Commission for Healthcare, Audit and Inspection.

Hickling, FW and Rodgers-Johnson, P (1995) 'The incidence of first contact schizophrenia in Jamaica', *British Journal of Psychiatry*, 167(2), 193–6.

Hickling, FW, McCallum, M, Nooks, L, and Rodgers-Johnson, P (2001) 'Outcome of first contact schizophrenia in Jamaica', *West Indian Medical Journal*, 50(3), 194–7.

Human Rights Network Prison Working Group (2008) *A Response to the Periodic Report of the United States of America April 2007*. USA: USHRNPWG.

Janssen, I, Hanssen, M, Bak, M, et al. (2003) 'Discrimination and delusional ideation', *British Journal of Psychiatry*, 182, 71–6.

Karlsen, S and Nazroo, JY (2002) 'Relation between racial discrimination, social class, and health among ethnic minority groups', *American Journal of Public Health*, 92(4), 624–31.

Karlsen, S and Nazroo, JY (2004) 'Fear of racism and health', *Journal of Epidemiology and Community Health*, 58(12). 1017–8.

Karlsen, S, Nazroo, JY, McKenzie, K, Bhui, K, and Weich, S (2005) 'Racism, psychosis and common mental disorder among ethnic minority groups in England', *Psychological Medicine*, 35(12), 1795–803.

Kelly, B (2001) 'Mental Health and Human Rights: Challenges for the New Millenium', *Irish Journal of Psychological Medicine*, 18(4), 114–5.

Kelly B (2003) 'Globalisation and Psychiatry', *Advances in Psychiatric Treatment*, 4, 464–74.

Kirkbride, JB, Barker, D, Cowden, F, Stamps, R, Yang, M, Jones, PB, et al. (2008) 'Psychoses, ethnicity and socio-economic status', *British Journal of Psychiatry*, 193(1), 18–24.

Klonoff, E, Landrine, H, and Ullman, J (1999) 'Racial Discrimination and Psychiatric Symptoms Among Blacks', *Cultural Diversity and Ethnic Minority Psychology*, 5(4), 329–39.

Knowles, LP (2001) 'The lingua franca of human rights and the rise of a global bioethic', *Cambridge Quarterly of Healthcare Ethics*, Summer, 10(3), 253–63.

Lau, A (2008) 'Delivering race equality in mental health services', *Advances in Psychiatric Treatment*, 14, 326–9.

Lewis, G, Croft-Jeffreys, C, and David, A (1990) 'Are British psychiatrists racist?' *British Journal of Psychiatry*, 157, 410–5.

Lewis, G, and Araya, R (2002) 'Globalisation and mental health', in N Sartorius, W Gaebel, JJ Lopez-Ibor, et al. (eds) *Psychiatry in Society*. Chichester: Wiley, 57–78.

Littlewood, R (2001) 'Psychiatry's Culture', in D Bhugra and R Cochrane (eds) *Psychiatry in Multicultural Britain*. London: Gaskell, 18–48.

Loring, M, and Powell, B (1988) 'Gender, race, and DSM-III: a study of the objectivity of psychiatric diagnostic behavior', *Journal of Health and Social Behaviour*, 29(1), 1–22.

MacPherson, SW (1999) *The Stephen Lawrence Inquiry*. London: Home Office.

Maingay, S, Thornicroft, G, Huxley, P, Jenkins, R, and Szmukler, G (2002) 'Mental health and human rights: the MI Principles—turning rhetoric into action', *International Review of Psychiatry*, 14, 19–25.

McKenzie, K (2006) 'Racial discrimination and mental health', *Psychiatry*, 5(11), 383–7.

McKenzie, K, Samele, C, Van Horn, E, Tattan, T, Van Os, J, and Murray, R (2001) 'Comparison of the outcome and treatment of psychosis in people of Caribbean origin living in the UK and British Whites. Report from the UK700 trial', *British Journal of Psychiatry*, 178, 160–5.

McKenzie, K and Bhui K (2007a) 'Institutional racism in mental health care', *British Medical Journal*, 334(7595), 649–50.

McKenzie, K and Bhui, K (2007b) 'Institutional racism in psychiatry', *Psychiatric Bulletin*, 31(10), 397.

Moon, G (2003) 'Complying with its international human rights obligations: the United Kingdom and Article 26 of the International Covenant on Civil and Political Rights', *European Human Rights Law Review*, 3, 283–307.

Moore, LJ (2000) 'Psychiatric Contributions to Understanding Racism', *Transcultural Psychiatry*, 37(2), 147–83.

Morgan, C, Mallett, R, Hutchinson, G, and Leff, J (2004) 'Negative pathways to psychiatric care and ethnicity: the bridge between social science and psychiatry', *Social Sciences Medicine*, 58(4), 739–52.

Morgan, C, Mallett, R, Hutchinson, G, et al. (2005) 'Pathways to care and ethnicity. 1: Sample characteristics and compulsory admission. Report from the AESOP study', *British Journal of Psychiatry*, 186, 281–9.

Murray, R, and Fearon, P (2007) 'Institutional racism in psychiatry', *Psychiatric Bulletin*, 31(10), 398.

National Anti-Racism Council of Canada (2007) *Racial Discrimination in Canada*. Canada: NARCC.

Nazroo, J (1997) *Ethnicity and Mental Health; Findings from a National Community Survey*. London: Policy Studies Institute.

Nazroo, J (1998) 'Rethinking the relationship between ethnicity and mental health: the British Fourth National Survey of Ethnic Minorities', *Social Psychiatry and Psychiatric Epdemiology*, 33, 145–8.

Niveau G (2004) 'Preventing human rights abuses in psychiatric establishments: the work of the CPT', *European Psychiatry*, 19(3), 146–54.

Paradies Y (2006) 'A systematic review of empirical research on self-reported racism and health', *International Journal of Epidemiology*, 35(4), 888–901.

Patel, K, and Heginbotham, C (2007) 'Institutional racism in psychiatry', *Psychiatric Bulletin*, 31(10), 397–8.

Sharpley, M, Hutchinson, G, McKenzie, K, Murray, RM (2001) 'Understanding the excess of psychosis among the African-Caribbean population in England. Review of current hypotheses', *British Journal of Psychiatry. Suppl.*, 40, s60–8.

Shashidharan, SP (1993) 'Afro-Caribbeans and schizophrenia: the ethnic vulnerability hypothesis reexamined', *International Review of Psychiatry*, 5, 129–44.

Shashidharan, SP (2003) *Inside Outside: Improving Mental Health Services for Black and Ethnic Communities in England*. London: Department of Health.

Singh SP, and Burns, T (2006) 'Race and mental illness: there is more to race than racism', *British Medical Journal*, 333, 648–51.

Singh, SP, Greenwood, N, White, S, and Churchill, R (2007) 'Ethnicity and the Mental Health Act 1983', *British Journal of Psychiatry*, 191, 99–105.

Sohler, NL, and Bromet EJ (2003) 'Does racial bias influence psychiatric diagnoses assigned at first hospitalization?' *Social Psychiatry and Psychiatric Epidemiology*, 38(8), 463–72.

Thornberry, P (2005) 'Confronting Racial Discrimination: A CERD Perspective', *Human Rights Law Review*, 5(2), 239–69.

Wadsworth, E, Dhillon, K, Shaw, C, Bhui, K, Stansfeld, S, and Smith, A (2007) 'Racial discrimination, ethnicity and work stress', *Occupational Medicine (London)*, 57(1), 18–24.

Weich, S, Nazroo, J, Sproston, K, et al. (2004) 'Common mental disorders and ethnicity in England: the EMPIRIC study', *Psychological Medicine*, 34(8), 1543–51.

Wiersma, D, Giel, R, De Jong, A, and Slooff, CJ (1983) 'Social class and schizophrenia in a Dutch cohort', *Psychological Medicine*, 13(1), 141–50.

Chapter 8

Mental Health Economics, Mental Health Policies, and Human Rights

Roshni Mangalore, Martin Knapp, and
David McDaid

Introduction

Mental disorders often have devastating effects because of their impact on the quality of life of individuals with these disorders and their families, and because of the societal reactions to them, including human rights abuses. They can also have enormous *economic* consequences, since there are close and enduring links between mental illness and economic hardship, and because of the costs of providing treatment and support.

Consider, for example, the most commonly expressed policy concerns regarding mental health. Across much of the world, these concerns would include:

- the continued reliance in many countries on the old and discredited asylums;
- the complex task of developing good community-based care to replace them;
- the need to build better detection and treatment of mental health problems into primary care systems;
- the controversial question of compulsory treatment;
- the challenge of coordinating activity across health, social care, housing, criminal justice, employment, and other service systems;
- the search for effective treatments and support services, and then ensuring that people in need can get access to them;
- the elusive desirability of good preventive arrangements that can stop mental health problems arising in the first place; and
- the huge and pervasive challenges of stigma and discrimination.

As is clear from other chapters, many of these concerns stem from the realization that the opportunity to maintain good mental health is a basic human right. But while none of them is specifically 'economic', any actions taken to address them will inevitably have economic implications. When mental health problems lead to contacts with health care systems they can result in quite substantial demands for support, and can also exact a heavy toll on other service systems. Poor mental health generally adversely affects productivity and participation in the labour force, which can strain an individual or family's financial resources, while also generating losses for businesses and the national economy.

In seeking to address the broad policy concerns listed above, a country therefore needs to commit (probably considerable) resources, but because there will never be enough resources to meet all needs, it will also need to find some way to ration those resources between competing demands. And in seeking to allocate scarce resources, it will need to employ some (hopefully widely agreed) principles of efficiency and equity. We discuss these topics in this chapter.

Economics and human rights

The conceptualization of mental health as a human right implies that states have an obligation to go beyond the provision of psychiatric treatments to the provision of a broad array of services, including the promotion of mental well-being, as well as the prevention and early identification of mental health problems, for the entire population. This could include providing decent economic conditions and social welfare services necessary for maintaining good mental health. A key issue is how to ensure this right in the face of limited resources.

While traditional economic approaches did not have a basis in human rights or individual civil liberties, recent advances have changed the way economists think. Nobel Laureate Amartya Sen has been especially influential. Basic rights and liberties are now at the forefront of theoretical and empirical economics of development, for example. Two concepts important for mental health economics in the modern context are *basic capabilities* and *needs*. The paths to equity and efficiency of resource use can be defined by reference to them.

Basic capabilities

The central idea of the capability approach as set out by Sen (1999) is that fairness of social states depends not only on how human beings actually function, but on their having the *capability*, which is a practical choice, to function in important ways if they so wish. Functional capabilities (or 'substantial freedoms') such as the ability to live to old age, engage in economic transactions, or live a healthy life are emphasized. Poverty is considered by Sen to be capability-deprivation. Similarly, mental health problems can result in capability-deprivation as they can restrict the freedom one has to achieve and enjoy positive mental health, which can result in further deprivation such as the ability to engage in productive economic activities or to have an active political or social life. These restrictions are due both to the symptoms of poor mental health, as well as the environments in which people with mental health problems live and the way in which they are often viewed negatively by society. For instance in some countries, including the UK, individuals with enduring mental health problems still face the prospect of being barred from political office or be denied the right to vote (All Party Parliamentary Group on Mental Health 2008).

A good example of the operationalization of the basic capabilities concept which has great relevance for people with mental health problems is the set of proposals put forward by the Equalities Review in the UK (2007). Examples from their core list of capabilities are included in Box 8.1.

Clearly, mental illness can deprive an individual of some, or all, of these capabilities. Ensuring the right to good mental health would mean that when it is possible to remedy such capability-deprivations through appropriate and reasonable interventions, society has the responsibility to provide such interventions. The aim of public policy should be recognition of the factors that might cause capability-deprivation and making concerted efforts to equalize capabilities or, given that not all mental health problems are avoidable or fully ameliorable to treatment (e.g. dementia), make necessary compensations when it is not possible to do so (e.g. by giving free and easy access to good long-term care facilities).

One could assert that every individual has a right to 'positive mental health', and that the state and society have a duty to honour this 'right' as best they can, helping to facilitate opportunities to

Box 8.1: Core capabilities

- ◆ To have the right to life
- ◆ To live in physical security
- ◆ To be healthy and knowledgeable
- ◆ To understand and reason and have the skills to participate in society
- ◆ To enjoy a comfortable standard of living with independence and security
- ◆ To engage in productive and valued activities
- ◆ To enjoy individual, family, and social life
- ◆ To participate in decision-making, have a voice and influence, of being and expressing oneself
- ◆ Having the self-respect of knowing that one will be protected and treated fairly by the law

improve the quality of life of people with mental health problems, for instance through access to better treatments and/or social or vocational support. This can help society move towards the goal, albeit aspirational, of as much equalization as possible in the capability to achieve 'positive mental health'. For those with severe debilitating mental health conditions which cannot be altered significantly by medical or alternative interventions, their health deficiency becomes a parameter in their health-production function and therefore also in their basic capabilities. The policy aim should be to find ways of avoiding or reducing such misfortunes for future generations. It may also be necessary to spend more on social and economic elements for those with intrinsically disabling disorders in order to compensate for the endogenous effects of the illness.

The basic capabilities approach has expanded the frontiers of empirical economics by incorporating new concerns that reflect the instrumental value of fundamental freedoms and human rights in the analysis of economic processes and arrangements. A useful summary of Sen's proposals in this regard can be found in Vizard (2005). We suggest a few examples for expanding such empirical analyses in the mental health context:

a. *Examining individual entitlements*: Sen's approach would require developing an analytical framework for assessing the sensitivity of the rights-structure prevailing in a particular society to poverty, hunger and starvation. Analysis of how mental health interacts and affects these variables would be a useful extension.

b. *Capabilities and functioning*: Conceptualization could be attempted of basic rights and freedoms as the primary objectives of social and economic arrangements, leading to the development of approaches to poverty and inequality that focus both on preventive actions to help reduce the risk of developing mental health problems (e.g. access to fair credit), as well as on reduction of capability deprivation because of mental illness through an equitable system of provision of clinical treatment. Analysis of inequalities in capability achievement by different population groups (e.g. defined by gender, ethnicity, or nationality) would especially be very useful in this context.

c. *Freedom of choice and opportunity freedom*: Proposals for capturing and formalizing the idea of the right to choose and the nature and scope of individual choices and constraints in mental health care provision and finance would also be insightful.

Need

The correct interpretation of 'need' for care is important, for many and various definitions have been developed in the health economics literature. Bradshaw (1972) provided the following very useful and widely cited classification of needs:

- Normative need (defined by an expert or professional)
- Felt need (what people want)
- Expressed need (equivalent to demand made upon health services)
- Comparative need (identified by comparing populations)

Distinguishing between these four types of needs should aid economic analysis of equity and efficiency in the health domain. Equity or social justice demands satisfaction of the 'normative need' for services, providing good health and equal opportunity for healthy living. At the same time, resource efficiency calls for analysis of the costs and benefits of interventions, meeting only those needs where net benefits are positive. We may term these 'economic needs', as they will not necessarily match the perceptions of care providers, users of mental health services or the general public. A widely discussed concept in this regard is *capacity to benefit*, which is a measure of how far the quality and length of life of an individual can be increased by intervention (Culyer and Wagstaff 1991). This concept has actually created more confusion than clarity in the debate about what is to be considered as 'need' for care. Conflict between equity and efficiency goals and the reluctance to move beyond the neoclassical economic interpretations of efficiency is a major problem here. According to this (improperly conceived) concept, need is assumed to exist only when there is an effective treatment or measurable health gain. The assumption underlying this concept that the only valid benefits are those that can be measured, or fitting the dominant paradigm, poses serious concern in the context of mental health where benefits can be intangible. Moreover, the ability to benefit from health care will be influenced by several factors that influence service uptake, including inequalities in access to care, perhaps due to the costs of care or perhaps due in part to the stigma associated with mental illness. Society might therefore decide that it is willing to sacrifice some potential efficiency gains (i.e. meeting only 'economic needs') in order to focus more resources on 'normative needs' of those with severe mental health problems even if the gains are intangible.

In surveys relating to psychiatric morbidity, we often find that individuals report many symptoms but that they do not make use of services or are not considered by the system to be in need of services. It may be useful to recognize that when problems are reported by individuals or their families, there is likely to be a 'felt need' for services or some alternatives that can reduce the capability-deprivation. The levels and standard of such felt needs may also depend on comparative need. But often these felt needs are not translated into 'expressed needs' or demand for services due to various reasons. The international human rights framework provides the basis for making comparative needs legitimate in relation to mental health. The lack of resources, mental health policies, and the political will to address the felt as well as comparative needs (besides the normative needs) of people with mental health problems in high-, middle- and low-income countries might be regarded as a contravention of the principles of human rights and therefore appropriate government actions may be necessary to create the environments for meeting these needs.

We now turn to three key areas where economic arguments intersect with mental health and human rights: promoting equity, ensuring that there is an appropriate level of resourcing, and using economic evaluation to ensure that these resources are targeted to where they may best help promote and maintain mental health.

Equity

In health economics policies and decisions, efficiency in the use of scarce resources is often viewed as a primary objective. However, equity remains an important goal. It may not be possible to both maximize efficiency and attain equity, for instance if investment in the most efficient way of maximizing overall population health also leads to a widening of inequalities in health status between different groups in society. In ensuring opportunities for positive mental health and access to mental health services as a human right and in acknowledging mental health as a basic capability, the equity objective is clearly of critical importance.

Equity in the health context has been conceptualized and defined in several ways. A brief review of various theories and principles of distributive justice and their suitability for defining equity in a mental health context is provided by Mangalore and Knapp (2006). The central view is that 'need', suitably defined, can form an acceptable basis for distributive justice in the mental health field. A theory which has great appeal in this context is John Rawls' (1973) Maximin Theory. He proposes the following general conception of justice: 'All social primary goods—liberty and opportunity, income and wealth, and the bases of self-respect—are to be distributed equally unless an unequal distribution of any or all of these goods is to the advantage of the least favoured.' The 'least favoured' or the 'worst off' are recognized as having greater need. Application of this principle of justice to the distribution of mental health care would mean that an equitable distribution is one that maximizes the welfare of those with the lowest level of health. This principle is more appealing than some others such as the Utilitarian principle of the 'greatest good of the greatest number' or the Entitlement Theory, which sees health care as a market commodity. Sen's capability approach reiterates the importance of 'needs' in deciding distributive justice. Need, thus, is something that links human rights, basic capabilities, resource allocation, and equity in mental health:

> . . . to have an unfulfilled need is to have a kind of claim against the world, even if against no one in particular . . . Such claims, based on need alone, are 'permanent' possibilities of rights, the natural seed from which rights grow (Feinberg 1970:249).

For achieving equity in resource allocation in the mental health field, the emphasis should be on establishing the role of needs and capabilities in attaining the functioning of positive mental health.

While the principle of Maximin (maximizing the level of health of the one with the minimum level) can be seen as a useful decision rule in mental health contexts, the concept of a 'decent minimum' put forward by Fried (1976) can also be seen as deserving more attention in this domain. Equality of access to health care is also a major equity goal in many countries. However, it is important to recognize that, while equality of access to needed care is vital, it is only a part of the resource equality that is essential for equity in mental health. This will be clear if we understand that there is difference in the need for positive mental health and the need for mental health care. For example, for the purposes of empirical analysis, *equity in [mental] health* is 'the absence of potentially remediable, systematic differences in one or more aspects of health across socially, economically, demographically or geographically defined population groups' (Starfield 2001:546). *Equity in mental health services* implies that 'there are no differences in use of, or access to health services where health needs are equal (what is usually called horizontal equity) or that enhanced health services are provided where greater health needs are present (vertical equity)'. Equity in the latter may not result in equity in the former as there are many factors other than health care that contribute to mental health.

We argue that an equitable mental health policy should ensure that everyone will have an 'equal probability' of reaching a certain desirable level of positive mental health, irrespective of (say) age, gender, ethnicity, wealth, religion, sexual orientation, educational qualifications, employment status, or other differential factors affecting individual circumstances and life-time opportunities for health and welfare. Empirical analyses of equity in mental health contexts could then helpfully examine the distributions of psychiatric morbidity and access to treatment/support by income, socio-economic group, ethnicity, gender, or place of residence, but conditional, of course, on other demographic factors which are likely to be correlated with mental health.

Another very significant problem that warrants attention is that of self-exclusion from the utilization of services because of stigma. Individuals do not want to be labelled as having mental health needs. As the World Mental Health Surveys indicate in settings across the world, regardless of whether or not there are financial barriers to access, no more than one-third of people with mental health problems make use of services, a rate much lower than that for most other health problems (Wang et al. 2007).

It is also important to look at who exactly does make use of mental health services. Standardized methods for measurement of equity and inequalities have been developed for such analysis. One such tool, the concentration index, has wide acceptance in contemporary research (Van Doorslaer et al. 2004). It can be used to quantify the degree of income-related or living standards-related inequality, as well in the use of a specific health service. It can capture the effect of both the distribution of living standards or income, as well as the distribution of health, and gives an indication of the level of capability-deprivation of the population studied. This tool was employed in recent research on the examination of income-related inequality in the distribution of psychiatric disorders in Great Britain (Mangalore et al. 2007). Using data from the Psychiatric Morbidity Survey 2000 for Britain, it was found that there is marked inequality in the distribution of mental illnesses across income groups. Those in lower income groups had a greater share of mental disorders than the rest and the extent of such inequality increased with the more severe disorders such as psychosis. Since much of the observed inequality was due to factors associated with income and not to the demographic composition of the income quintiles, it could be stated that these inequalities are potentially 'avoidable'. In the words of human rights and basic capabilities, there are deficiencies that need to be addressed through appropriate policies aimed at lower income groups.

In a linked study using the same approach, wide variations were found in income-related inequalities in common mental disorders among the different ethnic groups in Britain (Mangalore 2009). Inequality unfavourable to the poor was found to be quite marked among the Irish, White, and Black Caribbean communities. Inequality within the three Asian communities studied—Indian, Bangladeshi, and Pakistani—was less clearly defined. However, when inequalities were compared *across* ethnic groups the result was striking in that the adverse effect of lower income on mental health and in the use of services was more pronounced if the person was a member of the Bangladeshi, Pakistani, or Black Caribbean group. Although in general the lower income groups are more intensive users of services, the important finding was that when use of services were compared to the needs, those in lower income groups among these ethnic minorities had utilization rates that were lower than what would be appropriate for their level of needs. Differences between ethnic communities can be the result of differences in perceptions of needs, as well as from disparity in responses to needs from the services. It must be pointed out, however, that since the data were cross-sectional, it is not possible to explain causality which can only be revealed from a study of longitudinal data.

For an insightful equity analysis in the domain of mental health, it would be necessary to examine both normative and felt needs, and also to see how these needs compare between different population groups, defined by economic and other distinguishing characteristics. Legislation could become one potent tool for advancing equity for people with mental health problems as it could set out legally enforceable anti-discriminatory legislation which might help ensure that individuals with mental health needs have the same entitlements to make use of health care services if they so choose as those with physical health needs, regardless of socio-economic status. Minimum quality standards for care might also be set out in legislation, while provisions might also be made to ensure the right to advocacy when considering what services, if any, to use.

Resources

As mentioned earlier, mental health problems can often have very damaging consequences for individuals, families, local communities, and nations. Moreover, these difficulties are often enduring (e.g. many children with mental health problems grow up to have mental health problems in adulthood) and 'transmitted' (e.g. poor maternal mental health may have long-term adverse consequences for offspring, limiting their own lifetime opportunities) (Prince et al. 2007). Each of those negative consequences may be more marked and more challenging in lower- than in higher-income countries, because of the lower levels of personal resources and the absence or under-development of social protection safety nets, compounded by high levels of stigma and superstition.

Much literature suggests that there is an association between poverty and poor mental health worldwide (e.g. Patel et al. 1999). This view however is not uncontested: one recent analysis across five low income countries contends that factors such as poor physical health and widowhood may be more important triggers for poor mental health (Das et al. 2007). Nonetheless practical steps to tackle poverty such as maintaining employment in individuals following the onset of illness have been shown to help facilitate improvements in mental health (Boyce et al. 2009)

Needs and inadequate responses

Under-funding of mental health care and associated systems is a major factor, but simply throwing resources at these systems is unlikely adequately to address the challenges of poor mental health and attendant human rights abuses. In fact, a number of resource challenges (or barriers) have been suggested (Knapp et al. 2006).

We should start with the most fundamental challenge: mental health services are universally under-funded relative to the potential to alleviate and prevent mental health problems. This *resource insufficiency* is a greater problem in countries where the proportion of national income devoted to health care is low, as in most low-income countries. In high-income countries, while between 7 per cent and 14 per cent of national budgets are typically allocated to health, it should not be assumed that a reasonable proportion of this budget will be allocated to mental health. While some countries such as England allocate around 13 per cent of their total health budget to mental health services, elsewhere in the European Union funding proportions are much lower, e.g. in Portugal mental health receives only 3 per cent of the health care budget (Knapp et al. 2007). Countries accounting for more than 2 billion of the world's population spend less than 1 per cent of their total public sector health care budgets on mental health (Saxena et al. 2006). Moreover, the state of the economy in these countries means that the actual cash amounts going to mental health services are tiny.

According to the WHO Atlas (Saxena et al. 2006), only 51 per cent of the world population in low-income countries have access to any community care services. Evidence on utilization of mental health services is limited; indeed, there is now plenty of evidence from low- and middle-income countries of desperately low commitment of resources to mental health (Saxena et al. 2007), alongside the longstanding problem of self-exclusion.

Another aspect of resource insufficiency is limited access to drug therapy: the WHO Atlas describes the low utilization of even quite basic psychopharmacological treatments. Enforcement of the World Trade Organization's Trade Related Intellectual Property Rights (TRIPs) agreement that bans cheap generic bioequivalent versions of patented drugs (WTO and WHO 2002) will only exacerbate the situation. There are some exemptions to these WTO rules to cover national emergencies and diseases which are life-threatening, but there are no exemptions for mental disorders.

Resource barriers

Increasing the resources available for mental health care would help overcome the challenges that many countries face, but even when resources are committed, available services might be poorly distributed or available only to certain population groups. These barriers—like TRIPs—could be seen as contributing to the curtailment of the right to good mental health.

Resource inappropriateness is a related challenge: available services do not match what is needed. Treatment or care may be rigidly or inflexibly organized, leaving little scope for a care system to respond to individual circumstances. Conservative, narrowly constructed practices and a general reluctance to embrace new service and treatment models, even when they are strongly evidence-based, are strong impediments. One of the most powerful such constraints is the long-term investment in hospital-based services which has held back the development of more appropriate, more flexible, and more effective community-based models of support (Desjarlais et al. 1995). For example, most East European countries relied heavily for many years on large, often remote, and usually under-resourced hospitals to deliver mental health services, but there was considerable resistance to change (Tomov 1999).

Attitudes can erect other barriers. The low priority accorded mental health in allocating health expenditure might be partly because decision-makers do not appreciate the true prevalence and disabling burden of mental health problems, or are unaware that effective (and affordable) treatments exist. Of course, decision-makers understandably want to give priority to treating life-threatening conditions, and most mental health problems are not of that kind, but deep-rooted stigma and discrimination are highly influential in shaping attitudes.

Financing mechanisms can also place major barriers in the way of access. In most low-income countries, prepayment financing arrangements such as social insurance (where an individual pays into a fund, perhaps on the basis of expected future risk of ill-health, rather than paying for health services as they are used)—which are widely held to be more equitable and efficient than other forms of financing—are either completely absent (often because the necessary employment and infrastructures are not in place) or affordable only by wealthier people. In the absence of insurance or any state-funded health system (paid for out of tax revenues), out-of-pocket payments will be the primary source of finance. Around 40 per cent of low-income countries reported out-of-pocket payments to be the primary method for financing mental health care in the WHO Atlas, compared with only 3 per cent of high-income countries (Saxena et al. 2007). Even this figure of 40 per cent is undoubtedly conservative, as it does not take account of costs incurred through consultation with traditional healers. Reliance on out-of-pocket payments is inefficient and inequitable, as it discourages service utilization by people with a low income—a double jeopardy given the close links between poverty and morbidity.

Available resources in low- and middle-income countries are often heavily concentrated in urban areas. Enormous distances may have to be travelled to reach a community-based mental health facility. Resources may also be distributed inefficiently across disorders: for example, depression has been a lower priority than schizophrenia within the health systems of most low-income countries.

Low policy priority

The focus of health policy (and international donor assistance) in most low- and middle-income countries has been overwhelmingly on communicable diseases that lead to premature mortality, notably HIV/AIDS, malaria, and tuberculosis. The Millennium Development Goals explicitly recognize the contribution of good health towards economic growth, and include several health-related targets. However, mental health is notable by its absence from these goals.

This low perceived priority is exacerbated by stigma and negative attitudes among decision-makers and the public, in turn leading to lack of resources, poor staff morale, decaying institutions, lack of leadership, inadequate information systems, and inadequate legislation (McDaid 2008). There are a few encouraging signs of a reversal of these tendencies. Chile, Belize, and parts of Argentina, for example, have developed impressive mental health plans and are investing in structures and interventions. At supra-national level, the recent Mental Health Pact from the European Commission demonstrates a strong commitment to meeting needs and urges national governments to pay proper attention to human rights (European Commission 2008).

Optimizing use of available resources

Information is a further resource in limited supply: better evidence is needed on the basic epidemiology of mental health problems, and on the effectiveness and cost-effectiveness of preventive strategies and interventions to treat and support people who are ill. Evidence on successful ways to tackle discrimination is urgently needed. Plugging these information deficits would go some way to strengthening the arguments for better mental health.

It is important also to expand the role of economic analysis to evaluate initiatives to tackle economic risk factors for poor mental health, such as poor living conditions, financial insecurity, poorly managed debt, rapid economic transition, and poor educational attainment. For instance, what benefits to mental health might be achieved through the operation of fair credit schemes in low-income countries?

We now turn to the linked question of how economic analyses can be used to help make the best use of scarce resources to help facilitate the development and implementation of good mental health policies and practices.

Rationing and the use of economic evaluation

While there is a strong moral argument for investing in mental health systems, pursuing these aims is always constrained by available resources. For example, limitations on money, trained staff, inpatient beds, therapy sessions, and medications mean that no mental health system, even if it is perfectly designed and efficiently managed, can meet all mental health needs. Rationing of resources is a permanent feature of all mental health systems. Difficult choices have to be made between alternative uses of the same resource, whether it is a hospital bed day, attendance at a day service, or an hour of clinician time.

Economic evaluation can help decision-makers to make those choices. It can be thought of as 'the comparative analysis of alternative course of action in terms of both their costs and consequences' (Drummond et al. 2005). A number of different techniques are available: all measure costs in monetary terms but differ in outcome measurement.

The most widely used approach, cost-effectiveness analysis, measures outcomes using a natural (e.g. disease-specific) measure, such as a reduction in the symptoms of depression. While intuitively easy to understand, it is difficult to compare potential investments in mental health with other areas of health care.

Cost-utility analysis theoretically overcomes this limitation by measuring all health-related outcomes using a common metric, such as the Quality Adjusted Life Year (QALY) or Disability Adjusted Life Year (DALY). Both adjust the value of years of life lived to take account either of the quality of life of those years or the level of disability experienced during that time period. Another alternative is cost-benefit analysis, which measures both costs and benefits in monetary terms, allowing comparisons to be made between investments in health and other sectors such as education. A positive net benefit (i.e. where the value of the benefits is greater than the costs incurred to achieve them) would merit investment. However, this cost-benefit approach is rarely used for mental health interventions because of the difficulty of converting outcomes into monetary measures.

One of the limitations of all but the cost-benefit approach is that unless a new intervention is both less costly and more effective than the existing situation policymakers must make a value judgement as to whether the new intervention is worthwhile. All of this will be influenced by the resources and infrastructure available, as well as by cultural norms; what may be deemed cost-effective in France may not be viewed as cost-effective in Tajikistan or Uganda. This, some people contend, allows economic evaluation to be used to discriminate against segments of society, as in the case of drugs to treat dementia. Moreover, they argue that it is morally inappropriate to ration access to treatments on the basis of the length and quality of future life (Harris 2005, 2006). The focus of much economic evaluation in mental health on narrow measures of clinical symptoms may also discriminate against treatments whose principal benefits (e.g. to help improve an individual's circumstances) may be more difficult to measure (Berghmans et al. 2004).

In fact, far from being a way of discriminating against people with mental health needs, economic evaluation as one input into the health policy decision-making process can be used to overcome some of the prejudice against mental health and justify a much greater level of investment in the growing range of interventions that are cost-effective in low-, middle- and high-income countries (Chisholm 2005). Indeed it might be argued that the failure to use economic evaluation in the decision-making process can itself be unethical, as it may mean that resources are consumed in ways that are ineffective, thus denying others the opportunity to benefit from help and support (Maynard and McDaid 2003).

It is important to recognize that the use of economic evaluation is not a value-free process. Inevitably, normative judgements have to be made, such as on the appropriateness of treatments for different groups of individuals, the importance of what service users feel about the appropriateness of treatments, the extent to which side-effects are acceptable, and the value of non-clinical outcomes such as social inclusion. In addition, every decision to invest in a specific mental health-related intervention potentially means that resources are not available to invest elsewhere in the health system. In turn, this might impinge on the rights of others to maintain their health status. Thus it is critical that decisions on investments within and external to the health system are not made on the grounds of cost-effectiveness alone. Other considerations need to feature in these deliberations; perhaps most prominently human rights (given the unique nature of mental health care whereby individuals can sometimes be involuntarily detained and treated), as well as issues of distributive justice, ethics, fairness and the local political context. What is needed is more attention to the use of cost-effectiveness and similar evidence to support arguments to develop mental health systems from their current low base to a situation where human rights are protected and promoted.

Conclusion

Policy makers are keen to identify and address economic issues raised by mental health problems. In this chapter we have focused on three areas where economics plays a key role—equity, resources, rationing—to illustrate and emphasize the interactions between human rights and economics in the formulation of fair mental health policies and practices. These interactions can usefully be built on contemporary economic thinking that allows us to view mental health as a substantive right. Procedural rights in relation to the treatment of mental health patients (which is dealt with in some other chapters) was not the subject matter here.

Investment in mental health, which can be described as a *basic capability,* can generate economic as well as quality of life benefits to individuals and families, and these benefits are likely to have a positive impact on the mental health of future generations as well. The experience of many countries, however, suggests that even when substantial additional funding for mental health services is made available, overcoming the challenges in this field is not easy. Wide-ranging policy developments and a multi-dimensional strategy are required to ensure the basic human right of good mental health to all individuals and to ensure a better quality of life for those with mental illness. Cost-effectiveness analysis of interventions can play a role in this process: in particular in justifying investment in low-income countries faced by stark problems such as resource insufficiency, resource inappropriateness, the low policy priority accorded to mental health, and physical as well as psychological barriers to use of services.

The links that were explored in this chapter from human rights to equity and efficiency of resourcing for mental health provide further food for thought. The main points to carry forward in policy, practice, and further research can be summarized briefly.

Positive mental health is essential for the achievement of basic vital goals of decent living (survival). In economic terms, this is a basic capability, i.e. the practical freedom of choice to function in important ways if one so wishes. Since mental health problems can impact on an individual's ability to reach these basic vital goals, it is a capability-deprivation in much the same way as is poverty. Many of the arguments for poverty reduction as an essential goal for human development globally will, therefore, apply in the context of mental health as well.

Although deprivation of basic capability in relation to mental health may be exacerbated by many factors such as stigma, government oppression, human rights abuse, or ignorance, the fundamental lack of resources remains a major concern globally. Innovative ways are needed to overcome some of the barriers to fair funding and the better allocation of health and societal resources to address mental health needs. When it is possible to remedy capability-deprivation through appropriate policy and practice, there should be no hesitation to make the necessary changes based on careful assessment of needs and the appropriateness of interventions in different settings and contexts.

Equity in mental health and health care is as important as efficiency in resource use. In distributing mental health care (or relevant alternatives), need in the sense of curtailment of basic capabilities should be properly defined and appropriately measured using standardized methods. In this respect it is important to recognize the differences between equity and efficiency as objectives. Efficiency objectives often lead to decisions that conflict with equity considerations. For example, cost-effectiveness analysis of interventions which has become the main 'mantra' of health economists looks to maximize health gains for a given level of resource. Importantly, as we have indicated, the determination of what is considered cost-effective is a normative value judgement. Considerations of equity may point toward the importance of other factors such as equality of access to care, long-term support arrangements for people with severe disabilities, as well as the fundamental need to protect dignity and human rights. It is therefore essential to understand that economic evaluation is just one input into the decision-making process, albeit an increasingly important one. Equity considerations and other factors such as service users' views should be additional inputs to that process.

A basic question that policy makers should ask in this context is this: With current socio-economic conditions, current levels of expenditure in the mental health sector, and current technology and availability of services, does everyone have an 'equal probability' of having and maintaining positive mental health? An equitable policy should aim to neutralize the differential effects of non-biological factors within cohorts, thus ensuring the opportunity to enjoy good mental health for all. And it should ensure that treatment and support services are equally accessible to all individuals, subject of course to the overall supply constraint and the need for some targeting on individuals with higher needs. Actions taken in policy and practice settings, driven by the kinds of economic consideration discussed in this chapter and of course by non-economic considerations too, should reflect these concerns and objectives.

References

All Party Parliamentary Group on Mental Health (2008) *Mental health in Parliament. Report by the All Party Parliamentary Group on Mental Health.* London: APPGMH.

Berghmans, R, Berg, M, van den Burg, M, and ter Meulen, R (2004) 'Ethical issues of cost effectiveness analysis and guideline setting in mental health care', *Journal of Medical Ethics*, 30, 146–50.

Boyce, W, Raja, S, Patranabish, R, Bekoe, T, Deme-der, D, and Gallupe, O (2009) 'Occupation, poverty and mental health improvement in Ghana', *European Journal of Disability Research*, 3, 233–44.

Bradshaw, J (1972) 'A taxonomy of social need', in: G McLachlan (ed) *Problems and Progress in Medical Care: Essays on Current Research*. 7th Series. London: Oxford University Press, 69–82.

Chisholm, D, on behalf of WHO-CHOICE (2005) 'Choosing cost effective interventions in psychiatry: results from the CHOICE programme of the World Health Organization', *World Psychiatry*, 4, 36–44.

Culyer, AJ and Wagstaff, A (1991) *Need, equality and social justice, Discussion paper 90*. York: Centre for Health Economics, University of York.

Das, J, Do, Q-T, Friedman, J, McKenzie, D, and Scott, K (2007) 'Mental health and poverty in developing countries: revisiting the relationship', *Social Science and Medicine*, 65, 467–80.

Desjarlais, R, Eisenberg, L, Good, B, and Kleinman, A (1995) *World Mental Health: Problems and Priorities in Low Income Countries*. Oxford: Oxford University Press.

Drummond, MF, Schulpher, MJ, Torrance, GW, O'Brien, BJ, and Stoddart, GL (2005). *Methods for the economic evaluation of health care programmes*. 3rd edn. Oxford: Oxford University Press.

Equalities Review (2007) *Fairness and Freedom: the final report of the Equalities Review*. London: HMSO.

European Commission (2008) *European Pact for Mental Health and Well-Being*. Brussels: European Commission.

Feinberg, J (1970) 'The nature and value of rights', *Journal of Value Enquiry*, 4, 243–57.

Fried, C (1976) 'Equality and Rights in Medical Care', *Hastings Center Report*, 6, 303–19.

Harris, J (2005) 'It's not NICE to discriminate', *Journal of Medical Ethics*, 31, 373–75.

Harris, J (2006) 'NICE is not cost effective', *Journal of Medical Ethics*, 32, 378–80.

Knapp, M, Funk, M, Curran, C, Prince, M, Gibbs, M, and McDaid, D (2006) 'Mental health in low- and middle-income countries: economic barriers to better practice and policy', *Health Policy and Planning*, 21, 157–70.

Knapp, M, McDaid, D, Mossialos, E, and Thornicroft, G (eds) (2007) *Mental Health Policy and Practice across Europe*. Maidenhead: McGraw-Hill.

Mangalore, R and Knapp, M (2006) 'Equity in Mental Health', *Epidemiologia E Psichiatria Sociale*, 15(4), 260–66.

Mangalore, R, Knapp, M, and Jenkins, R (2007) 'Income-related inequality in mental health in Britain: the concentration index approach', *Psychological Medicine*, 37(7), 1037–46.

Mangalore, R (2009) *Equity in mental health and mental health care in Britain; concept, definition and empirical evidence*. Saarbrücken: VDM Verlag.

Maynard, A and McDaid, D (2003) 'Evaluating health interventions: exploiting the potential', *Health Policy*, 63(2), 215–26.

McDaid, D (2008) *Countering the Stigmatisation and Discrimination of People with Mental Health Problems in Europe*. Brussels: Directorate General Employment, Social Affairs and Equal Opportunities.

Patel, V, Araya, R, de Lima, M, et al. (1999) 'Women, poverty and common mental disorders in four restructuring countries', *Social Science and Medicine*, 49, 1461–71.

Prince, M, Patel, V, Saxena, S, et al. (2007) 'No health without mental health', *The Lancet*, 370, 859–77.

Rawls, J (1973). *A Theory of Justice*. Oxford: Oxford University Press.

Saxena, S, Sharan, S, Garrido, M, et al. (2006) 'WHO's Mental Health Atlas 2005: implications for policy development', *World Psychiatry*, 5, 179–84.

Saxena, S, Thornicroft, G, Knapp, M, and Whiteford, H (2007) 'Scarcity, inequity and inefficiency of resources: three major obstacles to better mental health', *The Lancet*, 370, 878–89.

Sen, A (1999) *Development as Freedom*. New Delhi: Oxford University Press.

Starfield, B (2001) 'Improving equity in health: a research agenda', *International Journal of Health Services*, 31(3), 54–56.

Tomov, T (1999) 'Central and Eastern European countries', in G Thornicroft, and M Tansella (eds) *The Mental Health Matrix: a Manual to Improve Services*. Cambridge: Cambridge University Press, 216–27.

Van Doorslaer, E, Koolman, X, and Jones, AM (2004) 'Explaining income-related inequalities in doctor utilisation in Europe', *Health Economics*, 13, 629–47.

Vizard P (2005) *The contributions of Professor Amartya Sen in the field of human rights, Paper No. CASE091*. London: The Centre for Economic Performance, LSE.

Wang, PS, Aguilar-Gaxiola, S, Alonso, J, et al. (2007) 'Use of mental health services for anxiety, mood, and substance disorders in 17 countries in the WHO world mental health surveys', *The Lancet*, 370(9590), 841–50.

World Trade Organization & World Health Organization (2002) *WTO Agreements and Public Health*. Geneva: World Trade Organization.

Chapter 9

HIV, Mental Health, and Human Rights

Catherine Esposito and Daniel Tarantola

Introduction

HIV and mental disability are recognized as issues of global importance. The relationship between HIV and mental disability is circuitous and confounding; mental disability can generate vulnerability to HIV and reduce capacity to mitigate its deleterious impact, whilst having HIV infection can create somatic or functional disorders among those infected compromising their quality of life. Despite growing recognition of the interaction and the behavioural and societal factors that mediate this reciprocal relationship, HIV and mental health care for those affected is sorely lacking.

This chapter will propose the application of a human rights framework as a valuable tool for explaining and attending to individual, programmatic, and societal level issues that create vulnerability to HIV and mental illness and the disability they create. It will describe the history and nature of the bidirectional relationships between HIV and mental health, HIV and human rights, and then mental health and human rights. It will then, through a rights-based approach, suggest how HIV, mental health, and human rights are inextricably linked and propose a pathway of action to minimize risk, vulnerability, and impacts of HIV and mental illness to ensure individuals can achieve the highest possible standard of physical, mental, and social well-being.

The reciprocal interplay of HIV and mental health: a disease-focused perspective

HIV and mental health

In 2008, 33.4 million people were living with the HIV virus and 2 million had died from AIDS (UNAIDS 2009). HIV challenges the economies, security, and social stability of nations (Piot et al. 2009). As an individual experience, it has the capacity to engulf identities, disrupt and destroy relationships, radically alter life patterns, and submerge the human spirit. While much has been documented on the aetiology, manifestations, and impact of HIV, it is only in the past decade that there has been growing recognition of the interplay between mental illness and HIV (Collins et al. 2006). As previously noted, the relationship between HIV and mental illness is multifaceted.

HIV impacts on mental health

The psychological burden created or exacerbated by the virus is significant. The virus can directly affect the central nervous systems causing neuropsychiatric complications (Dube et al. 2005), mania or cognitive disorders or impairment (Maj et al. 1994). The prevalence of HIV-1-associated dementia among asymptomatic subjects is estimated to be 15–30 per cent in the United States (Heaton et al. 1995; White et al. 1995).

In high-income countries, where the majority of research has been undertaken, there has been an increased focus on the mental health needs of HIV populations and evidence that the prevalence of mental illnesses among people living with HIV is higher than in the general population (Ciesla and Roberts 2001). This has been echoed in a growing number of studies in low-and middle-income countries. In the largest of these studies employing a control group, depression averaged 6 per cent among asymptomatic subjects and 17.8 per cent among symptomatic HIV populations in four sites within developing countries (Maj et al. 1994).

Some of the correlates of mental illness such as depression among HIV populations include other serious medical illnesses (Evans 2005), substance abuse (Goodkin et al. 1996), younger age (Emlet 2006), female gender (Moore et al. 1999), perceptions of HIV related stigma (Emlet 2006) and social isolation (Catz et al. 2002), and exposure to stress and traumatic events (Esposito et al. 2009). The rate of suicide attempts remains higher in people living with HIV than in other comparable populations (Carrico 2010). Most of these data are generated from high-income countries yet these risks may be heightened in low- and middle-income countries due to higher levels of poverty, political instability, exposure to trauma, and lower access to services and treatment.

HIV treatment impacts on mental health

Studies researching the psychological impact of HIV treatment document both treatment specific and global mental health improvements resulting from anti-retroviral therapy (Rabkin et al. 2000). The rate of suicidal intent has been documented to be lowered by the introduction of Highly Active Anti Retroviral Therapy (HAART), and this was partly attributed to improved health status although this rate remains higher than in comparable populations of non-HIV infected individuals. (Rabkin et al. 2000; Carrico 2010). Studies have shown a connection between HAART regimes that include protease inhibitors on sexual dysfunction in men (Wynn et al. 2004). Some of the drugs used in HAART, particularly efavirenz, have been associated with a range of psychiatric side effects including cognitive disorders, anxiety, mood disorders, and suicidal ideation (Lochet 2003).

Mental illness impacts on the spread and effects of HIV

The presence of mental illness has the potential to impact on behaviours related to HIV transmission and treatment adherence. A multi site study within the United States reported HIV prevalence rates of between 2 per cent among people with serious mental illness residing in rural areas and 5 per cent among those within the large metropolitan sites (Rosenberg et al. 2001). Rates were highest among those who were also homeless and or had a substance abuse disorder. Fuelled by factors such as hyper-sexuality, self-destructive behaviour, or impaired appreciation of risk, people with serious mental illness have also been found to engage in behaviours enhancing risk and vulnerability to HIV infection, including multiplicity of sexual contact, infrequent condom use, and unsafe injecting practices (Meade et al. 2005; Wright and Gayman 2005). Serious mental illness has the power to mediate adherence to HIV treatment regimes (Horberg et al. 2008) and/or influence HIV disease progression and AIDS related mortality (Ironson 2005).

HIV and mental health services are neglected

In spite of increasing understanding of the impact of the interactions between HIV and mental illness, there has been little evidence of public health interventions to reduce co-morbidity and the disability it creates (Prince et al. 2007). As a result, the bulk of mental illness among people living with HIV goes undiagnosed and untreated (Asch et al. 2003).

Studies analyzing structural barriers to improved and utilized mental health services commonly note that lack of political will at a national and international level is a major impediment to the individual, societal, and global changes needed to promote mental health and reduce mental morbidity (Saraceno et al. 2007). Reasons for this lack of interest include limited knowledge of the cost-effectiveness of mental health care, perceptions of insufficient gains from investment in mental health, challenges associated with the decentralization and institutionalization of mental health care, and the fragmentation of mental health advocacy efforts (Saraceno 2007). Given these structural barriers, re-examining HIV and mental health through a human rights lens is particularly suited and adds value to a disease-focused approach to HIV and mental health.

Examining HIV and mental health through a human rights lens

A human rights perspective on HIV and mental health builds on the evidence borne out of the study of the drivers of health, and examines these systematically against international human rights principles, norms, and standards. This perspective adds to traditional public health approaches the value of linking health policies, programmes, and outcome to an extensively documented set of obligations states have committed to deliver under international human rights treaties they have ratified. The 'value-add' of human rights to traditional public health approaches finds at least three justifications.

Firstly, human rights, as a framework for analysis and action, provides a conceptual framework and vocabulary for describing and connecting the individual, societal, and programmatic sources of vulnerability to, and impacts of, HIV and mental illness, and outlines the essential conditions required for good physical and mental health and well-being.

Secondly, when states ratify and sign up to standards detailed in human rights treaties such as the International Covenant on Civil and Political Rights (ICCPR) (UN-ICCPR 1966) and the International Covenant on Economic, Social and Cultural Rights (ICESCR) (UN-ICCPR 1966), they are required to adhere to and periodically report on progress made in meeting the standards outlined in the treaties (Gruskin and Tarantola 2005; OHCHR 2011). The requirements on states to report publicly on progress towards the realization of human rights means that duty bearers can be held accountable for their action or inactions. Accordingly, human rights transform traditional passive 'beneficiaries' into legitimate claim holders who can hold governments and non-state actors accountable through formal mechanisms at state or international level.

Thirdly, a human rights perspective on HIV and mental health includes but extends far beyond the right to health. Human rights bring into play structural factors driving or impeding progress in health. In contrast, traditional state-driven public health approaches tend to examine health issues independently from one another and fail to reveal and address the roots of ill health as the lack of fulfillment or the deliberate neglect of human rights.

Both HIV and mental health are historical examples of how a human rights perspective can deepen the understanding of the roots of ill health and how they can help shape the responses brought against them. It is therefore appropriate to recognize how the reciprocal links between HIV and human rights, on the one hand, and mental health and human rights, on the other, emerged in the academic and public discourse; how human rights approaches to HIV and mental health and human rights can be conflated; and how such approaches can help shape more effective public policy and programmes towards better health outcomes.

HIV and the rise of human rights as a public health strategy

Traditional public health approaches acknowledged the notions of risk, vulnerability, and impact (Mann and Tarantola 1996; Tarantola 1998) and the power of social milieu over an individual's control of health. Yet, it was unable to provide a common vocabulary for describing the commonalities and interconnectedness that underlie the specific situations of vulnerable people around the world, or a course of action and clarity about the necessary direction of health-promoting societal change (Mann 1999).

The confrontation with HIV, in the mid-1980s, was pivotal in elucidating these links between HIV and human rights. The development of the Global Strategy for the Prevention and Control of AIDS, led by Jonathan Mann and produced by the World Health Organization in 1987, was the first strategy to be founded on and include specific reference to human rights principles and practices (WHO 1987). The importance of this strategy was that it was adopted by the member states of WHO—one of the inter-governmental organizations concerned with the protection and promotion of human rights articulated in the UN Charter, the UDHR, and various covenants and declarations, thus placing HIV 'within the realm of international human rights law' (Gruskin et al. 2007a).

This was responding to concerns over the abuses people with HIV suffered and the role stigma and discrimination played in driving infected individuals underground and away from prevention care and support programmes (Mann and Tarantola 1998). This prompted an earlier pragmatic questioning of traditional public health approaches such as the Theory of Reasoned Action (Fishbein and Middlestadt 1989) which inferred that once people knew about modes of HIV transmission and protection methods they would change their individual risk behaviour. The AIDS experience highlighted the inadequacies of such approaches as the availability of information, education, and an ensured condom supply did not enable women to control the sexual behaviour of their husbands or allow them to refuse unprotected or forced sex (Mann and Tarantola 1998). Qualitative inquiries attributed women's vulnerability to HIV infection to the key issue of the poor status of women (Kapiga 1994) linked, in turn, to the denial of women's human rights (Rahman and Pine 1995).

Based on these inherent difficulties in responding to the HIV epidemic, Jonathan Mann and colleagues suggested that the human rights framework allowed for an analysis of the complex issues of power, culture, history, economics, or society underlying health. It identified duty bearers responsible under international human rights law for ensuring that these structural drivers and processes work to protect and promote the health and well-being of all people (Mann et al. 1994). However, perhaps more importantly, human rights principles, norms, and standards provided a convenient framework applicable to the development of HIV-related policies, the design of programmes and the monitoring of progress (Mann and Tarantola 1998).

Mental health approaches grounded in human rights

A large body of evidence has shown that human rights violations such as torture or involuntary institutionalization can generate mental disabilities whilst prejudices associated with mental illness may marginalize people with mental disability and deny them the opportunity to participate equally in society and exercise their rights (CPT 2003) As mentioned in previous chapters, the human rights movement within mental health emerged in the late 1960s in response to rights violations within institutional settings and to mental health legislation that increased discretionary powers of professional psychologists over the wishes of the patients (Brown 1992). In the 1970s the movement established that people with intellectual disabilities had the same rights as others, claiming that these rights could not be restricted without due process (Gostin 2000). The development and ratification of the United Nations Convention on the Rights of Persons with Disability in 2007 is seen by many as the culmination of the human rights struggle of people with disabilities (Jones 2005) as it locates mental disability within society and does not regard those affected as merely objects of welfare or medical treatment (UN 2007).

Understanding the human rights dimensions of HIV and mental health

The introduction of human rights to the separate fields of HIV and mental health suggest they are equally relevant to people vulnerable to or living with HIV and mental illness and, more generally, to all stigmatizing conditions including cancer, tuberculosis, or disability. Building on these historical experiences and the early works describing the relationships between health and human rights,[1] three fundamental relationships between human rights, mental illness, and HIV emerge.

The first relationship is that inappropriate HIV and mental health laws, programmes, and practices can jeopardize the enjoyment of human rights. For example, people with serious mental illness are often unnecessarily confined to mental health hospitals (Saxena et al. 2007). Under such circumstances, patient's rights to autonomy, bodily integrity, privacy, and liberty are deliberately restricted. Decisions to institutionalize an individual may have been made by family or care practitioners for the intended benefit of patients, but in too many instances without establishing grounds and applying due processes for determining capacity and competence and seeking less restrictive alternatives.

Similarly, in many parts of Asia, drug users, at high risk of HIV infection, are placed within mandatory drug treatment facilities (WHO 2009), or in 'Rehabilitation Centers', often without access to a due legal process. Despite the likelihood of mental illness and HIV prevalence among people within these closed settings, research has shown that mental health, HIV, or drug treatment programmes are lacking (Gruskin 2004) and that detainees are unable to assent or dissent to such imposed measures as HIV testing on admission, drug substitution, or abstinence-based treatment (WHO 2009). This policy and programme of non-voluntary treatment may be considered a breach of the detainee's right to liberty and security of persons (ICCPR Article 9) or the right to be treated with humanity and respect for their dignity (ICCPR Article 10) (UN-ICCPR 1966). Moreover, incarceration in the absence of HIV or mental health programmes denies the men their right to health and specifically to participate in the development and execution of programmes directly affecting their physical and mental health (UN-CESCR 2000 General Comment 14 Para 54).

The second relationship is that human rights violations, such as discrimination directed towards people with HIV and mental illness, can impact on people's risk and vulnerability to HIV and mental illness. For example, stigmatizing attitudes of or discrimination perpetrated by health care providers may exacerbate or generate mental distress among people living with HIV and deter them from seeking support for mental health problems. Similarly, assumptions that people with mental illness and or substance abusers are unable to digest and comprehend information on HIV prevention or adhere to treatment regimes (Stoff et al. 2004) effectively denies them equal access to information and resources needed to reduce vulnerability to and mitigate the impact of living with HIV.

Women living with HIV are more likely to report exposure to stressors, such as sexual or physical assault, from an early age and repeatedly over time (Kimerling et al. 1999). Exposure to such trauma combined with the lack of access to appropriate information and counselling services concerning issues such as safe termination of pregnancies or about HIV protection may result in emotional distress and development of mental disorders such as major depression or post-traumatic stress disorder (Varma et al. 2007). Stressors for drug users associated with incarceration and the absence of mental health programmes has been associated with elevated levels of

---

[1] The relationships between human rights and health were laid out by Jonathan Mann and co-authors in the first volume of *Health and Human Rights* (1994, vol 1, 6–23).

depression and post-traumatic stress disorder (Esposito et al. 2009). Likewise, given that mental health hospitals can facilitate HIV transmission via the shaping of individuals' sexual networks, the commonly observed lack of reproductive and sexual health programmes within mental hospitals creates vulnerability to HIV infection among an already marginalized population (Wright and Gayman 2005).

A third relationship between human rights, HIV, and mental health emerges from the recognition that human rights are indivisible, interrelated, and interdependent, as was underscored by the Vienna Declaration borne out of the World Conference of Human Rights (UN 1993). Put simply, the three areas interconnect in a mutually reinforcing manner that has a positive and additive effect on mental and physical health and the realization of human rights. The Universal Declaration of Human Rights and international human rights treaties and declarations are explicit about the obligations of states to create the conditions favourable for people to, *inter alia*, respect, protect, and fulfill the rights to information, education, employment, free movement, food, housing, safe environment, and property, and to marry and found a family. These are some of the rights that merely illustrate the array of civil, political, economic, social, and cultural rights, which drive the attainment of the highest standard of physical and mental health (UN-CESCR 2000 General Comment 14 Para 3; Yamin 2008). Although still insufficiently explicated in the context of human rights, the 'Social and Economic Determinants of Health' documents the reciprocal relationship between any of these factors and the state of individual and public health, and calls for the adoption of rights based approaches to address issues of gender inequities, childhood development, and the inclusion of disenfranchised individuals and groups (WHO 2008).

This third relationship between HIV, mental health, and human rights suggests that, just as vulnerability to mental health and HIV is rooted in rights denial, the power to reduce vulnerability is rooted in government's ability to deliver on its human rights obligations. The lack of state response to these issues owes partly to the lack of structures and services, and the lack of human rights awareness among health practitioners (Hunt 2007; Friedman 2009) and their reluctance to engage in multi-disciplinary work. The tripartite relationships described above is yet to be considered in a systematic and comprehensive manner within HIV and mental health responses, applied to the development of policies and programmes, and implemented in practice.

Moving forward: creating synergy between HIV, mental health, and human rights

One way in which to create synergy between HIV, mental health, and human rights is through the application of a rights-based approach. Gruskin et al. (2007b) suggest that there is no one application or definition of a rights-based approach, rather elements that are common core components of a variety of approaches: 'the core components of rights-based approaches include: examining the laws and policies under which programmes take place; systematically integrating core human rights principles such as participation, non-discrimination, transparency, and accountability into policy and responses; and focusing on key elements of the right to health—availability, accessibility, acceptability, and quality when defining standards for provision of services.' (Gruskin et al. 2007b).

The next section will briefly highlight each of these components and provide illustrative examples of interventions to create a synergistic interaction across the domains of HIV, mental health, and human rights.

Policy and legal context

A supportive policy and legal environment that acknowledges rather than ignores the relationship between HIV, mental health, and human rights is crucial to reducing the psychosocial burdens of

HIV and ensuring that those with co-morbidity are able to enjoy the same human rights and freedoms afforded others.

Policy and law should ensure people living with or at risk of HIV and mental disorders can access mental health and HIV prevention and treatment care (including access to essential drugs) on an equal basis as physical care. Such services could include a comprehensive package of community-based HIV and mental health care.

Law and policy should guarantee people with HIV or mental illness freedom from exploitation, violence and abuse and that they have access to recovery, rehabilitation, and reintegration services. Abuses should also be denounced, investigated, and the means of redress made available. There should be safeguards for people who commit prohibited acts related to HIV due to the presence of a mental disorder and provisions for referring mentally ill perpetrators of HIV-related crimes to mental health services. The enhanced risk of mental health and HIV co-morbidity associated with institutionalization in closed settings should be unveiled and the need for public health programmes within and on release from these institutions addressed.

To facilitate the inclusion and participation of individuals with HIV or mental illness, law and policy should provide for the freedom of association for those affected and their informal social-support networks. HIV, mental health, and human rights literacy programmes are needed for affected individuals and the state agencies responsible for their care and support.

To help achieve the above approaches, policy and law should be informed by evidence of the nature and prevalence of the main interactions between HIV and mental health. From an HIV perspective, this dictates more rigorous longitudinal studies to explore the impact of mental health treatment interventions on the effectiveness of HIV prevention efforts, the efficacy of antiretroviral therapy programmes on both HIV and mental health, and barriers to service utilization by those with mental disorders. From a mental health perspective, researchers should consider the effectiveness of cognitive or skill based interventions on reducing HIV risk generating behaviours (e.g. unprotected sex) or risk situations (e.g. sexual abuse) among people living with mental illness, and the effect of HIV treatment or lack thereof has on mental health status. Human rights research should seek to identify factors creating vulnerability to mental health and HIV and assess their combined impacts, using government's human rights obligations as an analytical framework.

The right to health

The right to the highest attainable physical and mental health, commonly referred to as 'The Right to Health', is laid out in Article 25 of the Universal Declaration of Human Rights and Article 12.1 of the ICESCR. The core content of the right to health, as described within General Comment 14 (UN-CESCR 2000) requires that HIV and mental health services must be available, affordable, accessible, and of good quality. These standards apply to both physical and mental health care as well as to related support services (Hunt 2005).

To help ensure that mental health and HIV goods, facilities, and services are available, there is a need to increase the number of HIV professionals and lay people able to detect mental disorders and provide care or refer patients to skilled care providers when necessary. There is an equal need for mental health providers to acquire and apply the skills needed for the prevention of HIV infection, the management of anti retroviral therapy (ART), or the referral to skilled colleagues. Primary care providers within district and community health centers and within HIV facilities need to be trained in the assessment and treatment of common mental disorders such as depression, and substance use disorders including the overlap between somatic and HIV consistent symptoms (Patel 2001; Freeman et al. 2005). Stress management interventions should be available given their ability to significantly improve mental health and quality of life of HIV populations

(Scott-Sheldon et al. 2008). Mental health staff should be able to identify HIV-related risks and feel comfortable and equipped to discuss HIV prevention issues including reproductive health, sexuality, and substance abuse. In the longer term however, initiating and scaling up mental health care within the HIV response and vice versa will require more than just increasing the number and capacity of people available. Across health systems, it will require mechanisms and incentives for two-ways referral between services dedicated to HIV, mental health, sexual and reproductive health, and substance use services.

Mental health and HIV services need to be located within the geographic reach of those in need, in particular most-at-risk populations as determined by needs mapping. Not only do services have to be physically accessible, they have to be culturally acceptable too. There are two reasons why a primary health carecare approach would respond to these needs. Firstly, the establishment or extension of community-based services would bring services closer to where people live and work. Secondly, the role of specialists such as psychiatrists, psychologists, or mental health nurses working within the public system needs to be redefined to include training and supervision of primary care and non-formal providers within the community. HIV and mental health training for families and peers of people living with HIV and mental illness will help establish a supportive environment and make certain that caregivers are able to recognize symptoms of co-morbidity and help alleviate its impacts.

Mental health and HIV care also needs to be economically affordable for people affected. Given the capacity of mental disorders and HIV to impact negatively on employment and income, any user charges for mental health or HIV services will be highly inequitable and counterproductive. People living with HIV and mental disorders are unlikely to benefit from public financing due to generally low levels of mental health financing and the lack of coverage afforded to people with common mental disorders under health insurance policies (Saxena et al. 2007). Overcoming the economic barriers to accessing mental health and HIV services is a complex issue that requires reform of financing mechanisms within the context of general health systems and within the system of prevention and control of HIV. However, given that people living with or vulnerable to HIV and mental illness have a reduced capacity to pay for the often chronic and high costs of treatment, services that include both pharmacological treatment and psychotherapy should be available free of charge, be subsidized by the government, or covered by social health insurance.

Mental health and HIV care also needs to be of good quality. This will require HIV and mental health professionals skilled in differential diagnosis and the subsequent provision of appropriate and evidence-based psychosocial and pharmacological interventions.

To ensure people living with HIV and mental illness have equal opportunity to access and use health facilities, goods and services, policies, and programmes need to address the persistent discrimination encountered by people with HIV and or mental illness from health care providers. To achieve this, general and specialized health practitioners may benefit from human rights training to increase their awareness of the rights of people living with HIV and/or mental illness and alert them about human rights obligations required of them as state actors, including policy and service requirements to maximize mental and physical health, and protect against unhealthy and unjust conditions.

Mental health and HIV care also needs to address the requirements for mental health located outside of the health care system. This claim is supported by the state's core obligation under the right to health to ensure access to basic shelter, housing sanitation and an adequate supply of potable water (UN-CESCR 2000 General Comment 14 Para 43(c)). Social service programmes addressing housing, employment, or financial assistance may be key to eliminating exposure to stressful or potentially traumatic events associated with HIV infection and mental disorders

(Brief et al. 2004). Those involved in delivering programmes outside the health sector should similarly be aware of their human rights obligations.

Participation

International human rights law confirms the right of people to take part in cultural life (ICCPR Article 15(a)) and to take part in the conduct of public affairs (Article 25(a) UN-ICCPR 1966). General Comment 14 states that an important aspect of the right to health 'is the participation of the population in all-health related decision-making at the community, national and international levels' (General Comment 14 Para 11 UN-CESCR 2000). Participation is also recognized as a component of or a means to achieve other rights impacting on health.

Mental health literacy campaigns for people living with HIV who are vulnerable to or affected by mental disorders will help ensure access to the information they need to participate in decisions related to their physical and mental health. Such programmes are also one of the first steps required to initiate a mental health and HIV advocacy movement aimed at changing the major structural and attitudinal barriers to achieving positive mental and physical health outcomes (Hickie 2004). Similar programmes for family members would enable them to provide the vital physical and emotional supports that people with co-morbidity need to participate. In cases where mental disability or HIV negatively affects individual's ability to communicate their preferences, family members or friends can become their advocates. They can raise awareness of the importance of mental health to the lives of people living with HIV and vice versa, denounce poor access to services, provide mutual support for other mental health caregivers, and become involved in the planning and implementation of services.

Non-discrimination

Social inequities, fuelled by stigma and discrimination related to HIV and mental illness, shape the distribution of co-morbidity. The adoption of anti-discrimination legislation and policy proposed within the preceding section on law and policy is a sound measure to combat discrimination and can be achieved with a minimum of resources (ICESCR) (General Comment 14 Para 10 UN-CESCR 2000). In addition to legislation, the provision of judicial remedies and other means of recourse need to be available for people who experience discrimination. To assist this process, redress mechanisms available for people living with HIV need to ensure information is appropriate and accessible to people with mental illness while similar services for people with mental illness should be cognizant of possible forms of and remedies for HIV related discrimination. This would involve sensitizing lawyers to the human rights relevant to issues of HIV and mental illness and assisting people with co-morbidity to communicate their experiences of discrimination and compensation required.

To combat discrimination to which people with HIV and mental illness are exposed requires states to meet their tripartite obligations: to respect rights (i.e. to refrain violating human rights in their own policies, laws, and actions as would be the case if illegitimate restrictive measures were imposed on people living with HIV or mental health); protect rights (i.e. ensure that non-state actors such as the industry, employers, private care providers, or non-governmental voluntary organizations do not violate human rights); and fulfill (i.e. putting in place the laws, policies, programmes, services, and resources adequate to promote human rights, receive complaints, and provide redress).

Accountability

Human rights obligations give shape to the nature of services and outcomes expected of governments and their need to develop plans to achieve obligations for which they are accountable.

As national monitoring systems supporting accountability in health and human rights terms are often shaped by international standards of 'best practice' and international human rights law, this section will begin by highlighting some international monitoring requirements and practices. It will subsequently examine the implications of these to country-based systems of accountability.

Global treaties and declarations related to HIV, mental health, or human rights are complemented by monitoring mechanisms and instruments (often containing indicators of achievement) and reporting processes. Not all international monitoring mechanisms impose similar demands on reporting states. UN charter-based bodies, including the Human Rights Council, and bodies created under the international human rights treaties and made up of independent experts are mandated to monitor state parties' compliance with their treaty obligations. Among these Treaty Monitoring Bodies (TMBs) are: the Committee on Economic, Social and Cultural Rights monitoring the implementation of rights embodied in the ICESC (UN-ICESCR 1966), including the right to health encompassing activities related to mental health and HIV; the Human Rights Committee monitoring the implementation of the ICPPR (UN-ICCPR 1966), including discriminatory policies and laws and the denial of access to fair judicial processes. Likewise, the implementation of the Convention on the Rights of Persons with Disabilities (UN-CRPD 2009) and the Convention on the Elimination of Discrimination against Women (UN-CEDAW 1979) is monitored by dedicated Committees of the same name. These TMBs monitor progress towards state obligations spelled out under international human rights treaties and associated optional protocols on the basis of reports received periodically by states along with reports submitted by non-state actors (so-called shadow reports). In addition to these mandated reporting processes, there are non-mandated reporting mechanisms to which state (and non-state actors) contribute as a sign of their commitment to non-binding UN General Assembly resolutions and declarations. Particularly relevant to the topic of this chapter are the Declaration on the Millennium Development Goals (MDGs)—one of which is related to halting and reversing the spread of HIV—(UNGA 2001), monitored by the United Nations Development Programme (UNDP); and the Declaration of Commitment on HIV/AIDS passed at the United Nations General Assembly Special Session on HIV/AIDS (UNGA 2001), monitored by the United Nations Joint Programme on HIV/AIDS (UNAIDS). In both instances, the declarations were followed by the development of monitoring instruments and periodic reporting to the UN General Assembly.

An examination of these accountability processes and reports shows a general lack of attention to the issue and impact of HIV/mental health co-morbidity. For example, the Declaration of Commitment to HIV and monitoring framework does not call for mental health information, and consequently no information exists about rates of mental morbidity or suicide among people living with HIV. In a similar vein, the monitoring reports and indicators used to track progress towards achievement of the MDGs focus on narrowly defined health outcomes (e.g. HIV, maternal and child health) but do not refer to mental health. Neither of these reporting mechanisms generates information on people with mental illness, for example concerning the rates of access to HIV prevention and care services, condom use, or safe injecting practices. Finally, the mandated reporting on the CRPD only requires information pertaining to the provision of HIV information in Braille but not to a format accessible to people with mental disability (UN-CRPD 2009).

Because these accountability mechanisms ignore the interaction between HIV, mental health, and human rights, government performance in relation to the tripartite relationship goes unreported and unnoticed (Miranda and Patel 2005). Given the diversity of global health priorities and the effort involved in developing and obtaining consensus on declarations, treaties, and accompanying monitoring documents, it is unrealistic to expect that one single mechanism can simultaneously address the interactions and impacts of HIV, mental health, and human rights. Moreover, in countries where HIV prevalence is low, this may not be viewed as a priority.

However, in countries with high rates of HIV or mental illness, there is a need and opportunity to harmonize current monitoring mechanisms in order to allow for a combined accountability in HIV, mental health, and human rights terms. This could be achieved in two ways. Firstly, at a global level, existing monitoring documents and indicators could be modified to include one of the missing domains. For example, reports on the Declaration of Commitment to HIV could include the number of people screened for mental disorders during voluntary counselling and testing processes. The CESCR could expand its monitoring requirement on the 'Right to the Highest Attainable Standard of Physical and Mental Health' to include not only separate information on HIV and mental health, but also information on co-morbidity and the extent to which states are responding to this dual need.

Secondly, country level monitoring mechanisms such as HIV strategies and national plans of action should examine and respond to the prevalence of mental disorders among populations recognized as most-at-risk of HIV infection while mental health plans should address the need for public health initiatives that include HIV prevention, care, and treatment for people with serious mental illness, especially those within closed settings.

The embryonic nature of the HIV, mental health, and human rights dialogue suggests that it will take time and effort to modify existing information generation and management mechanisms; develop a common understanding, stimulate to commitment, and enhance capacity among professional and advocacy groups currently dedicated to either of these fields; and increase combined accountability. Until such time, the movement must rely on occasional research projects that produce the evidence of compounded vulnerabilities induced by the interplay between HIV, mental ill-health, and the lack of realization of human rights.

Conclusion

Mental health and HIV are important public health issues each taking a substantial independent share of the global burden of disease. Their contribution to despair and disability among those affected is equally significant. Mental illness has the potential to alter the course of the HIV epidemic and undermines the responses brought against it. The spread of HIV among people with mental illness further compromises their health, social insertion, and quality of life.

This chapter explained the reciprocal relationship between HIV and mental health but also highlighted how, especially within resources-constrained settings, the neglect or overt violations of human rights create vulnerabilities to HIV and mental illness and deny those affected the knowledge, skills, and services needed to mitigate their impact. The current paucity of data on the nature and impacts of the relationship between HIV, mental health, and human rights support the need for enhanced efforts to build the evidence required to induce changes in policies, laws, and practice. However, the empirical evidence already accumulated and the application of internationally agreed principles, norms, and standards relevant to public health and human rights should be applied by default to people living with co-morbidity as they should to all human beings. They are sufficient to dictate priorities and generate the needed impetus for action. This means seeking and creating a synergy between the three domains of mental health, HIV, and human rights inspired by and building on the historical evidence of human rights as an effective public health strategy. Such an approach implies overcoming disciplinary barriers and bridging the existing structural, systemic, and financial obstacles which currently preempt comprehensive and effective responses to compounding vulnerabilities to co-morbidity where human rights neglect and abuses are the norm. A rights-based approach to HIV and mental ill-health creates the common vision, vocabulary, and methodology needed to move forward. It provides a systematic and pragmatic way to actively involve clinicians, lawyers, civil society, and people living with HIV and mental illness in initiatives aimed at bridging these two challenges to health and well-being.

References

Asch, SM, Kilbourne, AM, Gifford, A, et al. (2003) 'Underdiagnosis of depression in HIV: Who are we missing?', *Journal of General Internal Medicine*, 18, 450–60.

Brief, D, Bollinger, AR, Vielhauer, M, et al. (2004) 'Understanding the interface of HIV, trauma, post-traumatic stress disorder, and substance use and its implications for health outcomes', *AIDS care*, 16 (Supplement 1), S97–S102.

Brown, GR, Rundell, JR, McManis, S, Kendal, S, Zachary, R, and Temoshok, L (1992) 'Prevalence of Psychiatric Disorders in Early Stages of HIV Infection', *Psychosomatic Medicine*, 54, 588–601.

Carrico, AW (2010) 'Elevated suicide rates among HIV-Positive persons despite benefits of Antiretroviral therapy: Implications for a stress and coping model of suicide', *American Journal of Psychology*, 167, 117–119.

Catz, SL, Gore-Felton, C, and McClure, J (2002) 'Psychological distress among minority and low income women living with HIV', *Behavioral Medicine*, 28, 53–60.

Ciesla, JA, and Roberts, JE (2001) 'Meta-analysis of the relationship between HIV infection and risk for depressive disorders', *American Journal of Psychiatry*, 158, 725–50.

Collins, PH, Freeman, M, and Patel, V (2006) 'What is the relevance of mental health to HIV/AIDS care and treatment programs in developing countries? A systematic review', *AIDS*, 20(12), 1571–82.

Dube, B, Benton, T, Creuss, D, and Evans, D (2005). 'Neuropsychiatric manifestations of HIV infections and AIDS', *Journal of Psychiatry Neuroscience*, 30(4), 237–246.

Emlet, CA (2006) 'An examination of social networks and social isolation in older and younger adults living with HIV/AIDS', *Health & Social Work*, 31, 299–308.

Esposito, C, Steel, Z, Tran, G, Tran, H and Tarantola, D (2009) 'The Prevalence of Depression Among Men Living with HIV Infection in Vietnam', *American Journal of Public Health*, 99(Supplement 2), S439–S444.

European Committee for the Prevention of Torture and Inhuman or Degrading Treatment (CPT) (2003) *CPT Standards: 'substantive' section, CPT General reports, CPT/IN/E 2002 1-Rev.2003*. Brussels: Council of Europe.

Evans, P, Charney, D, Lewis, L et al. (2005) 'Mood Disorders in the medically ill: Scientific reviews and recommendations', *Biological Psychiatry*, 58, 175–89.

Fishbein, M and Middlestadt, S (1989) 'Using the Theory of Reasoned Action as a Framework for Understanding and Changing AIDS-Related Behaviors', in VM Mays, GW Albee, and SF Schneider (eds) *Primary Prevention of AIDS: Psychological Approaches*. Thousand Oaks, CA: SAGE, 93–110.

Flowers, P, Davis, M, Hart, G et al. (2006) 'Diagnosis and stigma amongst HIV and black Africans living in the UK', *Psychology and Health*, 21, 109–22.

Freeman, M, Patel,V, Collins, PY, and Bertolote, J (2005) 'Integrating mental health in global initiatives for HIV/AIDS', *British Journal of Psychiatry*, 187, 1–3.

Friedman, E (2009) 'Building Rights-Based Health Systems: A Focus on the Health Workforce', in A Clapham and M Robinson (eds) *Realizing the Right to Health*. Geneva: Swiss Human Rights Books, 421–435.

Goodkin, K, Forstein, M, Beckett, A et al. (1996) 'HIV-related neuropsychiatric complications and treatments', in American Psychiatric Association, *AIDS and HIV Disease: A mental health perspective*. Washington, DC: AIDS Program Office, American Psychiatric Association.

Gostin, L and Gable, L (2000) 'Human Rights of Persons with Mental Disabilities', *International Journal of Law and Psychiatry*, 23(2), 125–59.

Gruskin, S (2004) 'Current Issues and concerns in HIV testing: a health and human rights perspective', *HIV/AIDS Policy Law Review*, 9, 99–103.

Gruskin, S and Tarantola D (2005) 'Health and Human Rights', in S Gruskin, M Grodin, G Annas, and S Marks (eds) *Perspectives on health and human rights*. New York: Routledge, 3–57.

Gruskin, S, Ferguson, L and Bogecho, O (2007a) 'Beyond the numbers: using rights based perspectives to enhance antiretroviral treatment scale up', *AIDS*, 21(Supplement 5), S13–S19.

Gruskin, S, Mills, E, and Tarantola, D (2007b) 'Health, Human Rights 1: History, principle and practices of health and human rights', *The Lancet*, 370, 449–54.

Heaton, RK, Grant, I, Butters, N, et al. (1995) 'The HNRC 500–neuropsychology of HIV infection at different disease stages. HIV Neurobehavioral Research Center', *Journal of the International Neuropsychological Society*, 1, 231–51.

Hickie, I (2004) 'Can we reduce the burden of depression? The Australian experience of beyond blue: the national depression initiative', *Australasian Psychiatry*, 12(Supplement), S38–40.

Horberg, HS, Bartemeier, M, Hurley, L, et al. (2008) 'Effects of Depression and Selective Serotonin Reuptake Inhibitor Use on Adherence to Highly Active Antiretroviral Therapy and on Clinical Outcomes in HIV-Infected Patients', *Journal of Acquired Immune Deficiency Syndrome*, 47, 384–90.

Hunt, P (2005) *Report of the Special Rapporteur on the right of everyone to the enjoyment of the highest attainable standard of physical and mental health, 11 February 2005, UN Doc E/CN.4/2005/51.* New York: United Nations.

Hunt, P (2007) *Report of the Special Rapporteur on the right of everyone to the enjoyment of the highest attainable standard of physical and mental health, 17 January 2007, UN Doc.A/HRC/4/28.* New York: United Nations.

Ironson, G, O'Cleirigh, C, Fletcher, MA, et al. (2005). 'Psychosocial factors predict CD4 and viral load change in men and women with human immunodeficiency virus in the era of highly active antiretroviral treatment', *Psychosomatic Medicine*, 67(6), 1013–21.

Jones, M (2005) 'Can international law improve mental health? Some thoughts on the proposed convention on the rights of people with disabilities', *International Journal of Law and Psychiatry*, 28(2), March-April 2005, 183–205.

Kapiga, S (1994). 'Risk Factors for HIV Infection among women in Dar-es-Salaam Tanzania', *JAMA*, 7(3), 301–9.

Kimerling, R, Calhoun, KS, Forehand, R, et al. (1999) 'Traumatic stress in HIV-infected women', *AIDS Education and Prevention*, 11, 321–30.

Lochet, P, Peyriere, H, Lotthe, A, Mauboussin, J, Delmas, B, Reynes, J (2003) 'Long-term assessment of neuropsychiatric adverse reactions associated with efavirenz', *HIV Medicine*, 4, 62–66.

Maj, M, Satz, P, Janssen, R, et al. (1994) 'WHO neuropsychiatric AIDS Study, cross sectional Phase II: neuropsychological and neurological findings', *Archives of General Psychiatry*, 51, 51–61.

Mann, J (1999) 'Human Rights and AIDS: The Future of the Pandemic', in J Mann, S Gruskin, G Grodin, and G Annas (eds) *Health and Human Rights: A Reader*. New York: Routledge, 216–226.

Mann, J and Tarantola, D (1996) 'Societal vulnerability: contextual analysis', in J Mann and D Tarantola (eds) *AIDS in the World II*. New York: Oxford University Press, 444–62.

Mann, J and Tarantola, D (1998) 'Responding to HIV/AIDS: a historical perspective', *Health and Human Rights*, 2, 5–8.

Mann, J, Gostin, J, Gruskin, S, Brennan, T, Lazzarini, Z, Finberg, H (1994) 'Health and Human Rights', *Health and Human Rights*, 1(3), 6–23.

Meade, C and Sikkema, K (2005) 'HIV risk behaviour among adults with severe mental illness: A systematic review', *Clinical Psychology Review*, 25, 433–57.

Miranda, JJ and Patel, V (2005) 'Achieving the Millennium Development Goals: Does Mental Health Play a Role?', *PLoS Medicine*, 2(10), e291.

Moore, J, Schuman, P, Schoenbaum, E, Boland, B, Solomon, L, and Smith, D (1999) 'Severe adverse life events and depressive symptoms among women with, or at risk for, HIV infection in four cities in the United States of America', *AIDS*, 13, 2459–2468.

OHCHR, Human Rights Bodies, <http://www.ohchr.org/EN/HRBodies/Pages/HumanRightsBodies.aspx>, accessed 24 October 2011.

Patel, V (2001) 'Poverty, inequality and mental health in developing countries', in D Leon and G Walt (eds) *Poverty, inequality and health*. Oxford: Oxford University Press, 247–62.

Piot, P, Timberlake, S, and Sigurdson, J (2009) 'Governance and Response to AIDS: Lessons learned for Development and Human Rights', in A Clapham and M Robinson (eds) *Realizing the Right to Health*. Geneva: Swiss Human Rights Books, 331–345.

Prince, M, Patel, V, Saxena, S, et al. (2007) 'No Health without Mental Health', *The Lancet*, 370, 859–77.

Rabkin, JG, Ferrando, S, Lin, SH, et al. (2000) 'Psychological effects of HAART: a 2-year study', *Psychosomatic Med*, 62, 413–22.

Rahman, A and Pine, RN (1995). 'An International Human Right to Reproductive Health Care: Toward definition and accountability', *Health and Human Rights*, 1(4), 400–427.

Rosenberg, S, Goodman, L, Osher, F, et al. (2001) 'Prevalence of HIV, hepatitis B, and hepatitis C in people with severe mental illness', *American Journal of Public Health*, 91, 31–37.

Saraceno, B, Van Ommeren, M, Batniji, R, et al. (2007) 'Barriers to improvement of mental health services in low-income and middle-income countries', *The Lancet*, 370, 1164–74.

Saxena, A, Paraje, G, Pratap, S, Karan, G, and Sadana, R (2006) 'The 10/90 Divide in Mental Health Research trends over a ten year period', *British Journal of Psychiatry*, 188, 81–81.

Saxena, S, Lora, A, Van Ommeren, M, Barret, T, Morris, J, and Saraceno, B (2007) 'WHO's Assessment Instrument for Mental Health Systems: Collecting Essential Information for Policy and Service delivery', *Psychiatric Services*, 58(6), 816–21.

Scott-Sheldon, L, Kalichman, S, Carey, M, Fielder, L (2008) 'Stress Management Interventions for HIV+ Adults: A Meta-analysis of randomized Control Trials 1989–2006', *Health Psychology*, 27, 129–39.

Stoff, D, Mitnick, L, and Kalichman, S (2004) 'Research issues in the multiple diagnoses of HIV/AIDS, mental illness and substance abuse', *AIDS Care*, 16(Supplement 1), S1–S5.

Tarantola, D (1998) *Expanding the Global Reponse to HIV/AIDS through focused action. UNAIDS Best Practice Collection*. Geneva: UNAIDS.

UNAIDS and World Health Organization (2009) *Global Facts and Figures 09*. Geneva: UNAIDS.

UN-ICCPR (1966) *United Nations: International Covenant on Civil and Political Rights. GA Resolution 2200 (XXI) UN GAOR 21st session, Supplement No 16 at 49, UN Document A/6316*. New York: United Nations.

UN-CEDAW (1979) *United Nations: Convention on the Elimination of All Forms of Discrimination Against Women. GA Resolution 34/180 adopted on 18 December 1979*. New York: United Nations.

UNCESCR (2000) *United Nations Committee on Economic, Social and Cultural Rights General Comment No 14 (twenty-second session) The right to the highest attainable standard of health E/C.12/2000/4*. Geneva: United Nations.

UN-CRPD (2009) *Guidelines on treaty-specific document to be submitted by states parties under article 35, paragraph 1, of the Convention on the Rights of Persons with Disabilities. 2nd session 19–23 October 2009. UN Doc CRPD/C/2/3*. Geneva: United Nations.

UN-ICESCR (1966) *United Nations: International Covenant on Economic, Social and Cultural Rights GA Resolution 2200 (XXI), UN GAOR, 21st session, Supplement No 16, at 49 UN Document A/6316*. Geneva: United Nations.

United Nations (1993) *United Nations General Assembly: Vienna Declaration and programme of action. World Conference on Human Rights, Vienna 14–25 June 1993. UN Document A/CONF.157/23*. New York: United Nations.

United Nations Enable (2007) *Convention on the rights of persons with disabilities and optional protocol*. http://www.un.org/disabilities/default.asp?navid=14&pid=150, accessed 3 November 2011.

United Nations General Assembly (2001) *Special session on HIV/AIDS. Declaration of Commitment on HIV/AIDS—'Global Crisis-Global Action'*. Geneva: United Nations.

Varma, D, Chandra, S, Thomas, T, and Carey, M (2007) 'Intimate Partner Violence and Sexual Coercion among Pregnant Women in India: Relationships with Depression and Post Traumatic Stress Disorder', *Journal of Affective Disorders*, 102, 227–50.

White, DA, Heaton, RK, and Monsch, AU (1995) 'Neuropsychological studies of asymptomatic human immunodeficiency virus-type 1 infected individuals. The HNRC Group. HIV Neurobehavioral Research Center', *Journal of the International Neuropsychological Society*, 1, 304–15.

World Health Organization (1987) *Global strategy for the prevention and control of AIDS. Res WHJA 40.26 World Health Organization World Health Assembly 40th session*. Geneva: World Health Organization.

World Health Organization (2008) *Commission on the Social Determinants of Health: Closing the gap in a generation: health equity through action on the social determinants of health. Final report of the Commission on Social Determinants of Health*. Geneva: World Health Organization.

World Health Organization (2009) *Assessment of compulsory treatment of people who use drugs in Cambodia, China, Malaysia and Vietnam: An application of selected human rights principles*. Geneva: World Health Organization Western Pacific Region.

Wright, E and Gayman M (2005) 'Sexual networks and risk of people with serious mental illness in Institutional and community-based care', *AIDS and Behaviour*, 9, 341–57.

Wynn, G, Zapor, MJ, Smith, BH, et al. (2004) 'Antiretrovirals, Part 1: Overview, History and Focus on Protease Inhibitors', *Psychosomatics*, 45, 262–70.

Yamin, A (2008) 'Will we take suffering seriously? Reflections on what applying a rights framework to health means and why we should care?', *Health and Human Rights*, 10, 45–59.

Chapter 10

Universal Legal Capacity as a Universal Human Right

Amita Dhanda

Introduction

Universality, indivisibility, interdependence, and interrelatedness are key values which contribute to the rhetoric of human rights. The value of universality contributes to the rhetoric in two ways. One, it underscores the commonness of all humans irrespective of differences be they of region, religion, ethnicity, or culture. And two, it emphasizes that human rights are those rights which must be available to all humans by reason of their being human (Donnelly 2003). The significance of the value of universality in this rhetoric is that it causes all of humanity to rally behind the rights of every human person. In this manner the value of universality significantly contributes to the moral force of human rights.

The above said claims on the necessity of universal human rights have not been without contest. Whilst postmodernism negates the possibility of universal values, subaltern studies and feminist theories expose the occidental and patriarchal bias of the values claimed as universal. It is beyond the scope of this chapter to examine the promise and limitations of postmodernism; I refer to that body of thought only to refer to the technique of deconstruction employed by postmodern theorists in order to expose the submerged biases of universal formulations. The technique of deconstruction has been used by feminists to show how often so called universal norms are male values in disguise. Insofar as rights are a means of protecting people in vulnerable positions from people in power, it is important to ensure that rights are not used as shields by people in authority to perpetuate their powerful positions. Every challenge mounted against claims of universality, whether by women, children, or indigenous people has only demonstrated that, unless human rights are inclusive in purport, any claims of universality made with regard to them are false and hollow (Brens 2001).

The claim of universality made in human rights instruments once again came into dispute when persons with disabilities demonstrated the exclusionary impact of the instruments on them. Persons with disabilities were not expressly excluded in the text of the human rights instruments; they were, however, factually excluded. This is because the human rights regime was made keeping the non-disabled person in view. Since the 'universal' in the Universal Declaration of Human Rights was constructed without taking into account the difference of disability, and it did not in addition conceptualize human rights for disabled persons and extend rights to them, it necessarily discriminated against persons with disabilities.[1] In order to remedy this exclusion and to advance

---

[1] This manner of inclusion was in evidence in Article 23 of the Convention on the Rights of the Child which made express provision for the child with disability.

the cause of inclusive universality, the United Nations has adopted the Convention on the Rights of Persons with Disabilities (hereinafter CRPD).[2]

The CRPD is the first hard international instrument which spells out the rights of persons with disabilities. This articulation, by enhancing the inclusive content of human rights and clarifying the obligations under prior instruments, deepens the universal content of human rights. This deepened content has however not ceased the tension between the universal and the particular. Before the adoption of the CRPD this tension subsisted between disabled and non-disabled persons. During the negotiation, adoption, and enforcement of the CRPD this tension has surfaced, especially in the submissions of some state parties, towards persons with certain kind of impairments and thereby introduced distinction between persons with disabilities. This difference between persons with disabilities has been articulated in two kinds of ways: one of which is empowering, and the other which is excluding. The empowering initiative acknowledged that there were certain persons with disabilities who experienced multiple discriminations, and to obtain equality of outcome for them the CRPD would need to grant more to get the same. In order to achieve this objective in the CRPD, it was suggested that a twin track approach may be adopted, whereby the concerns of women and children with disabilities could be mainstreamed in relevant core articles of the convention, along with dedicated Articles which recognized the rights of women and children with disabilities (Dhanda 2008). This emphasis was in no way exclusionary as it is accompanied with a right to equality and non-discrimination which guarantees all rights for all persons with disabilities.

The exclusionary mode came into play when questions around the universal application of some rights were raised. Should all the rights guaranteed in the CRPD be available in the same manner, to all persons with disabilities? Or should persons with certain kinds of disabilities, not be a part of this universal regime? This question surfaced in an implicit and inarticulate manner during the negotiations on the right to liberty, integrity, independent living, and right to home and family. It was more explicitly raised when legal capacity was negotiated, wherein it was asked whether the right to legal capacity in Article 12(2) extended the capacity to bear rights and the capacity to act to all persons with disabilities. Or were there some categories of persons with disabilities who could be bearers of rights but could not have the capacity to act (Dhanda 2007)? Since some persons with disabilities could exercise their legal capacity with minimal support, and others would be even unable to seek support, would it be appropriate to accord similar kind of treatment to both kinds of persons? Was it appropriate to recognize the legal capacity of persons with disabilities with such high support needs? Persons with disabilities were generically constructed in the CRPD[3] and the negotiations of each Article were largely informed by this generic person with disabilities. In the negotiations on legal capacity, however, this generic identity receded and discussion started to make explicit references to the constraints experienced by persons with intellectual disability, psychosocial disability, persons with high communication constraints, and persons in coma. The last category was often mentioned during the CRPD deliberations as a conclusive example of the need for exclusion from the standard of universal legal capacity.

---

[2] The convention was adopted by the General Assembly in December 2006. It was opened for signature on 30 March 2007 and came into force after obtaining the requisite 20 ratifications on 3 May 2008.

[3] Article 1 of the CRPD, which outlined the purpose of the convention, defined persons with disabilities to 'include those who have long term physical, mental, intellectual, or sensory impairments which in interaction with various barriers may hinder their full and effective participation in society on an equal basis with others'.

My contention in this chapter is that the CRPD has adopted the paradigm of universal legal capacity, whilst providing for the differences between persons with disabilities, through strategies such as reasonable accommodation and support. I further argue that a universal adoption of legal capacity is necessary, if the rights guaranteed by the CRPD are to be available to all persons with disabilities, and if all persons with disabilities are to have an equal opportunity for capability development, and if a human society informed by the principles of empathy and solidarity is to be constituted. It is in this context that this chapter examines the various arguments set up against the paradigm of universal legal capacity; and the various strategies adopted by state parties to subvert this paradigm. By setting up the argument for universal legal capacity in this chapter, I do not deny either the difference in disability or the variations in socio-cultural contexts. Consequently, the chapter also elaborates on how the reality of difference can be accommodated within the paradigm of universal legal capacity. The chapter concludes by showing how the value of universalism in legal capacity advances the human rights of all, and why, whilst room should be given to difference, space should not be conceded to prejudice and stereotypes in the name of difference. This insight is of special relevance to this book which is examining the realm of mental health and the rights of persons living with mental illness. The central argument of this chapter of the book is that the recognition of universal legal capacity should aid in the enactment of human rights consonant with mental health laws. To establish this contention I firstly elaborate on the mandate of Article 12 of the CRPD.

The mandate of Article 12

Article 16 of the International Covenant on Civil and Political Rights (hereinafter ICCPR) laid down that everyone shall have the right to recognition everywhere as a person before the law. This Article found inclusion in the ICCPR primarily to deal with the aftermath of colonization whereby colonizing countries had often denied colonized people recognition before the law. The text of this provision ostensibly also applied to persons with disabilities due to the all inclusive ambit of the pronoun 'everyone'. Nevertheless, no questions were raised by treaty bodies on the impact of Article 16 on the legal recognition of persons with disabilities. This was because persons with disabilities were not within the contemplation of the treaty body monitoring the implementation of ICCPR. This deduction is further strengthened by the fact that, even as the ICCPR (as also the International Convention of Social Economic and Cultural Rights) has an elaborate outlining of grounds of discrimination such as race, colour, sex, language, religion, political or other opinion, national or social origin, property, and birth, it makes no mention of disability. Thus the only category under which discrimination on the basis of disability can find inclusion is the residuary ground of other status.

Yet Article 12(1) of the CRPD relies on the textual capaciousness of ICCPR and proceeds on the basis that 'everyone' in Article 16 included persons with disabilities; consequently in this clause state parties reaffirm that persons with disabilities have the right to recognition everywhere as persons before the law. This clause of Article 12 accords identity to persons with disabilities, which is a significant precondition for recognizing the legal capacity of persons with disabilities.

Article 12(2) of the CRPD lays down that 'state parties shall recognize that persons with disabilities enjoy legal capacity on an equal basis with others in all aspects of life'. It is significant to note that the ICCPR makes no mention of legal capacity. The convention proceeds on the presumption that once the identity of a person is recognized before the law then such person necessarily possesses the requisite legal capacity to act in furtherance of his or her rights. The only human rights instrument which refers to legal capacity is the Convention on the Elimination of Discrimination against Women (hereinafter CEDAW) which recognized women as having legal capacity on an equal basis with men.[4]

State parties needed to make explicit provision on the legal capacity of women in CEDAW because CEDAW was negotiated in the background of umpteen national laws and customs which expressly denied legal capacity to women. Persons with disabilities are in a comparable position, insofar as there are laws denying legal capacity to blind persons in some regions of the world, and persons with intellectual disability, as also persons living with mental illness, across jurisdictions. The nature of the deprivation varies from country to country depending upon how the laws providing for denial of legal capacity have been formulated. Whilst some laws attributed lack of legal capacity to the fact of impairment itself, others attributed legal incapacity if impairment was coupled with an inability to perform a specified function, and still others reached a finding of incapacity if persons with disabilities reached socially unacceptable decisions. It is necessary to know that these inadequacies in the definition of legal capacity resulted in a number of reform efforts to be launched, to guard against the wrongful attribution of lack of capacity to persons with disabilities (Grisso 2003). Even as there were studies that conceded to the harmful side effects of a legal attribution of incapacity, the next logical move of exorcising the concept of incapacity from the law was not made. It was in such like legal circumstances that Article 12(2) of the CRPD recognized the legal capacity of all persons with disabilities.

Article 12(2) not only recognized legal capacity of all persons with disabilities, it reconstituted the person in the person with disabilities. Whilst the ICCPR conceptualized person as free, independent, and autonomous, a more interdependent conception of the human was made in CRPD. It was by reason of this interdependent conception that Article 12(3) obligated state parties to take appropriate measures to provide access by persons with disabilities to the support they may require in exercising their legal capacity. The idea of support was aimed to underscore that, whilst all persons with disabilities have the right to self-determination, all of them may not be able to exercise this right without support. The extent of the support provided may vary from person to person; however, the fact of seeking support would not negate the presence of legal capacity.

Whilst the first three clauses of Article 12 constructed the paradigm of legal capacity with support, the safeguards to prevent the abuse of support were provided in clause 4 of Article 12. Since the safeguards were to be proportional to the extent of the support, the regime of safeguards were so constructed that the higher the degree of support, the greater the extent of oversight. Thus, all support needed to be provided respecting the rights, will, and preference of persons with disabilities, without conflict of interest and undue influence. However, the provision of high support was made subject to regular review by a competent independent and impartial authority or judicial body.

As already mentioned, the deprivation of legal capacity happened on an uneven scale across jurisdictions. The freedom to own, inherit, or manage property, control their own financial affairs, and have access to bank loans, mortgages, and other forms of financial credit were, more often than not, denied to persons with disabilities across jurisdictions. Consequently clause 5 of Article 12 explicitly requires state parties to take all appropriate and effective measures to ensure these rights to all persons with disabilities.

The above narration on the mandate of Article 12 has, however, not been without controversy. Whilst the recognition of legal capacity for persons with disabilities is generally accepted, it is not universally conceded. The argument on the other side is that there are persons with severe

---

[4] Article 15(2) of CEDAW states that 'states parties shall accord to women in civil matters, a legal capacity identical to that of men and the same opportunities to exercise that capacity'.

intellectual disability or psychosocial disability or communication difficulties who cannot exercise capacity even with support; hence substitution arrangements must be made for them. It is important here to recall the postmodern critique of universalism, which demonstrated how dominant perceptions are presented as exclusive outlooks and thereby accorded universal status. As a consequence of this critique any version of the universal which is exclusionary in impact is per se problematic. The power dynamic at play in the creation of the universal is further problematized by feminist thought, which seeks credence for personal narrative and lived experience as valid bodies of knowledge. Truth is thus not something which is objectively discovered by the unbiased external observer; it can also be something which is found by the lived experience of the subject. Epistemological understanding of truth is further deepened by theorists who point to the situation bound genealogy of truth.

I refer to these philosophical positions only to underscore that arguments of incapacity are primarily posited when certain persons with disabilities do not meet the non-disabled standard of capacity. Evaluation of the competence of persons with disabilities is again being undertaken by externalized objective standards; the subjective experience which would significantly determine the well-being of the person with disabilities stands rejected. Legal capacity has a close relationship with self determination rights and, if it is my self that I have the right to determine, then how can this right of determination be decided on the standard of another's self? The only argument that can be put forth for the adoption of this externalized standard is the argument of social expectations and third party interests. Since legal capacity is about the freedom to act in a social milieu, a totally subjective, valid for me alone standard, would be socially unworkable. If the reason for not recognizing legal capacity in some persons with disabilities arises from the practical necessities of social functioning, then it is only correct that such practical necessities have balancing relevance and not trumping status (Pound 1940; Dworkin 1977). To elaborate, the practical needs of social functioning can be accommodated by creating legal entities that could co-facilitate or be joint decision-makers with the person with disability; such an arrangement can work without denying the right of self-determination to persons with disabilities (Bach M, Personal Communication, 2009).

Why is universal legal capacity required?

The above analysis demonstrates that the principle of universal legal capacity can be put into practice even for persons with high support needs. For state parties to seek and work such a solution, it is necessary for them to accept the inherent merit in the paradigm of universal legal capacity with support. In this segment, therefore, I outline the reasons for organizing law and policy upon the premise of universal legal capacity. The merit of this course of action can be justified on the basis of three kinds of reasons. One kind focuses on how universal legal capacity is required for capability development of society generally and persons with disabilities particularly. The second kind shows how a model of selective legal capacity would necessarily be over inclusive and hence cannot challenge the stereotypical association between disability and incompetence. Further the incompetence attributed to persons with disabilities is not peculiar to them; hence any singling out of persons with disabilities would infringe the CRPD mandate of equality and non-discrimination. Consequently if factual incompetence has to be a ground of exclusion then it cannot be restricted to persons with disabilities and would necessarily have to include all incompetent persons. The third kind will demonstrate that legal capacity is a *sine qua non* for all persons with disabilities to claim all their rights under the CRPD.

The primary distinction between the presence and absence of legal capacity is that, whilst the former entitles a person to retain agency of his or her life, the latter robs this authority from the individual and gives it to another. Insofar as doing is an integral part of learning, those persons with disabilities who are denied the freedom to do are also deprived of the freedom to learn. Such a conclusion can be drawn if Deci's work on the value of self-determination to human well-being (Deci 1980; Ryan and Deci 2000), growth, and development is read in conjunction with Seligman's study on learned helplessness (Seligman 1975; Garber and Seligman 1980). Bruce Winck draws such a connection in his study on the side effects of incompetence labeling and its implication for mental health (Winck 1995).

The value of self determination to human happiness has been demonstrated in relation to other vulnerable constituencies. Thus people working on poverty alleviation have found that the poor accord greater value to those programmes which are participatory, and respectful of the choices and dignity of the poor (Streeten 1995:28–53). Similar kinds of findings arise from studies evaluating the value of support networks. Those networks which operated in consultation with the person supported were accorded greater value than un-consulted unilateral support (Brown et al. 1997).

A primary reason for the enactment of the CRPD was to facilitate persons with disabilities to take their place as integral members of humanity. This inclusion has to happen in such manner that it promotes the growth and development of the person with disabilities. Insofar as universal legal capacity compels interaction with the person with disabilities, it accords opportunity to the person with disabilities to grow and develop in accordance with his or her genius. Selective legal capacity, on the other hand, by designating some persons with disabilities as lacking in legal capacity denies them the opportunity to grow and develop and such deprivation would be in contradiction with the universal ambit of human rights.

An integral feature of universal legal capacity is that it promotes social interaction between all members of society, disabled and non-disabled. This inclusive mode of social relationship creates opportunity for the capabilities of empathy and social solidarity to be developed. The development of these capabilities is required for peaceful co-existence in society.[5]

Persons arguing for the retention of the model of selective legal capacity with substitution, constantly assert that this model would only apply in the rarest of rare cases, after all alternatives of recognizing capacity with support have been exhausted. This remedy of compromise is suggested without realizing how the exception could swallow the rule. Once the law permits the argument of incompetence to be raised against persons with disabilities then it cannot prevent the leveling of the allegation of incompetence against all persons with disabilities. Consequently, whilst only some persons with disabilities may in fact lose the opportunity of organizing their own lives, all persons with disabilities are put at risk of such loss. The rarest of rare argument does not take on board the deprivation of process, which a provision of incapacity inflicts upon all persons with disabilities. This processual deprivation reinforces the stereotype of incompetence associated with persons with psychosocial and intellectual disabilities.

It could be argued that the above reasoning is sacrificing at the altar of the rights of persons with disabilities, generally, the concerns of those persons with disabilities who have high support needs. Such a course of action would be in conflict with the inclusive universalism advocated in this chapter, insofar as the needs of the few are being sacrificed for the needs of the many. Earlier in this segment, I have referred to Deci's work on self-determination where he has found the fulfillment of the innate psychological needs of competence, autonomy, and relatedness result in

---

[5] I am thankful to Gabor Gombos for pointing me to this dimension of capability development. This reasoning has been employed by the Disabled Peoples Organization in Hungary in their open letter to the President advocating requisite state initiatives on creation of support in furtherance of the mandate of universal legal capacity.

enhanced self motivation and mental health. These consequences do not only ensue for those persons with disabilities who have little or no need for support, they hold good for all. Thus the adoption of the paradigm of universal legal capacity with support mandates engagement with all human beings to determine their choice and will irrespective of the extent of impairment. Insofar as the person in coma is often put forth as the reason for retaining a regime of substitution, it may be worthwhile to refer to this category of persons with disabilities to sharpen the above point.

A recent news item in the *Guardian* newspaper reports the case of a person who suffered an all limbs paralysis which was misdiagnosed as coma (Connolly 2009). Since he was diagnosed as a person in coma, the doctors and carers stopped any kind of interaction and communication with the person. A whole series of interventions which the person found grossly unsuitable were practiced on him and what he needed he could not obtain as no one was talking with him since he was in coma. After a long period of time, it was discovered that there was a misdiagnosis and the person was not in coma. Upon this finding being made, the friends and relatives impelled upon the doctors to devise a mechanism by which communication could be established between the alleged person in coma and the rest of the world. What the case shows is that if there had not been a label of incompetence appended on people in coma, the doctors would have stayed in communication with the so-called comatose person and discovered their misdiagnosis way earlier—surely a consequence which is to the benefit of all and not just persons in coma.

The above examples, it could be said, only address the case of misdiagnosed coma or labelled incompetence; they do not address the situation of persons who are in fact in coma or incompetent. To ask this question is to miss the point of this chapter. I am not contending that all persons have either a similar standard of competence or that all people can do all things with equal competence. Evidently the opportunity to develop capabilities and to evolve capacity is required. It is this opportunity which is taken away when the label of incompetence is affixed on an individual, be it a person in coma, a person with cerebral palsy and communication difficulties, or a person with a very low intelligence quotient. The law, I hold, should operate on the presumption of competence of all as that presumption advances the interest of all. And if there is desire to provide protection to those who require it by reason of any vulnerability, then such protection should also be constructed in universal terms. Any other mechanism of addressing alleged incompetence would necessarily be in breach of the right of equality and non-discrimination.

The paradigm of universal legal capacity also merits adoption because it would challenge the present privileging of cognitive faculties and allow for the recognition of multiple intelligences (Gardner 1999, 1993). Current standards of legal capacity primarily revolve around the cognitive faculties of knowledge and understanding, even as these are not the only faculties which are relied upon for decision-making. And yet persons who are possessed of deficient cognitive faculties could be termed legally incapable, because the faculties or intelligences possessed by them are not taken note of by the law to construct legal capacity.

This miscued construction of the law is further aggravated by labels of competence and incompetence as was demonstrated by the MacArthur and Appelbaum study on treatment competence. The MacArthur treatment competence study evaluated the decision-making capacities of people who are hospitalized with mental illness. The study found that 'most patients hospitalized with serious mental illness have abilities similar to persons without mental illness for making treatment decisions. Taken by itself mental illness does not invariably impair decision making capacities' (MacArthur Treatment Competence Study 1995). At the same time, they found 'a substantial percentage of hospitalized patients—up to half in the group with schizophrenia when all four types of abilities considered—show high levels of impairment'. Since a substantial number of persons living with mental illness were found to be incompetent in the MacArthur study, it can be credibly argued on the strength of these findings that the legal attribution of incompetence was not prejudicial and unscientific. Such a conclusion cannot be offered primarily due to the findings of the Grisso–Appelbaum study (Grisso–Appelbaum 1995). The Grisso–Appelbaum study relied upon the same parameters of decision-making competence as employed in the MacArthur study to evaluate patients seeking treatment in a general hospital setting. Grisso–Appelbaum found a large number of general hospital patients lacking in competence. And yet, since the law does not attribute a lack of competence to persons living with other illnesses, their legal capacity is not questioned and they continue to take their own decisions. On the other hand, even those people living with mental illness who possess decision-making capacities are denied legal capacity.

The advocacy for universal legal capacity is often challenged on the fact that it only stresses the deprivations imposed on persons with disabilities; whilst the accommodations made in the shape of the defense of insanity are generally ignored. This contention seems to be advanced on the premise that criminal responsibility is an all or nothing affair for non-disabled persons. Even a preliminary study of criminal justice systems would establish the falsehood of this assumption. The affixation of criminal responsibility requires that the prosecution prove that the wrongful act was committed with the wrongful intention and none of the general defenses such as mistake or necessity or self defense is applicable. Once universal legal capacity is recognized, persons with disabilities would also function in this regime and hence will be able to seek benefit of these general defences along with non-disabled persons. These defences, once accepted, result in clear acquittal and discharge of the person with disabilities. The defence of insanity, in contrast, even when accepted results in a technical acquittal alone; actual discharge is often indefinitely postponed. Studies (Szasz 1989:138–48; Dhanda 2000) show how the uncertain benefits of the defence are outweighed by the heightened social protection costs extracted from persons acquitted on grounds of insanity who are often kept in detention for periods longer than for which they could be punished.

Irrespective of these practical inadequacies, it is next contended, the sub-competent status of persons with intellectual and psychosocial disabilities is life saving in countries which retain the death sentence. It is only as recent as 2002 (*Atkins v Virginia* 536 US 304) that the United States Supreme Court reversed its ruling in *Penry v Lynaugh* (492 US 302) and found by majority of 6:3 the execution of persons with intellectual disabilities to be unconstitutional. Yet whether this protection will be available to an individual person with intellectual disability will depend upon whether the accused person is or is not considered to be of intellectual disability. The recent execution of Teresa Lewis on 23 September 2010 in Virginia is a case in point. Both the defence of insanity and commutation of death sentence for persons with intellectual and psychosocial disability create a systemic impression of fairness which curtains off the unfairness experienced by the individual person with disability. The paradigm of universal legal capacity with support will hopefully cause the question of criminal responsibility to be examined afresh and replace standard form guidelines with individuated procedures.

The CRPD recognizes a range of rights from education to rehabilitation; from freedom of speech and expression to political participation; from right to home and family to independent living and life in the community for persons with disabilities. The paradigm of universal legal capacity and support would require that each of these rights be appropriately customized for persons with disabilities who have high support needs. On the other hand, the paradigm of selective legal capacity and substitution would appoint a surrogate to take the place of the persons with disabilities and act for him or her. Several of the above named rights in the CRPD would be rendered redundant in this kind of arrangement, a consequence which is not in harmony with the universal discourse of human rights.

Arguments and strategies to undermine universal legal capacity

The previous segments detailed the mandate of Article 12 and why universal human rights required the adoption of universal legal capacity. The coherence of reasoning and the cogency of an argument does not ensure its acceptance. The paradigm of universal legal capacity is primarily up against the barriers of the mind. It is only the existence of these attitudinal barriers which can explain why certain states kept coming back to the paradigm of selective legal capacity and substitution. The following narration of state resistance to the paradigm of universal legal capacity is being undertaken, in order to show the lengths to which states travelled to avoid recognizing the legal capacity of all persons with disabilities.

The elaboration on legal capacity began with the working group text, which admitted to loss of capacity in exceptional cases, and allowed for the appointment of a personal representative after observance of fair process safeguards. In the ensuing negotiations, there was constant conflict between this paradigm of selective capacity with provision for substitution and the paradigm of universal capacity with support. Ultimately, the persistent tussle between the two paradigms was resolved, and consensus was reached in the shape of the Article 12 text which was analyzed above.

However this consensus did not come without its hiccups. State parties continued to make direct and indirect efforts to deny universal legal capacity. Thus to the text of Article 12 agreed upon in the front rooms of the ad-hoc committee, a long forgotten footnote was added in the negotiating backrooms. Consequently, in order to retain the consensus arrived at for all the other Articles of the convention, the ad-hoc committee agreed to the addition of a footnote to Article 12 which stated that 'in Arabic, Chinese and Russian, the term legal capacity refers to legal capacity for rights instead of legal capacity to act'. This undermining of the universal content of the CRPD evoked protests from both states and civil society. It was the persistent lobbying by states and disabled people's organizations which caused the footnote to be dropped from the text which was adopted by the General Assembly in December, 2006 (Dhanda 2007).

The deletion of the footnote, however, did not wipe out the resistance to universal legal capacity. States continued to use explicit and oblique strategies to get around the mandate of Article 12. Thus, states need to take special care to ensure that the text of Article 12 was not inaccurately translated to use terminology which signified capacity for rights instead of capacity to act.[6] In order to promote universal content whilst allowing local variations, Article 46 of the CRPD allows states to enter reservations provided they were compatible with the object and purpose of the convention. The above analysis demonstrates that a reservation on Article 12 is equivalent to a reservation on the convention. Hence, it is a moot point whether such reservation would be permissible. It is, however, necessary to appreciate that a state that enters reservations on Article 12 recognizes that the Article has adopted the paradigm of universal legal capacity and finds itself unable to subscribe to it generally because the Article was not in conformity with the national laws of the reserving state. Such reasoning seems specious and opposed to Article 4 of CRPD which requires ratifying states to amend, repeal or modify their national laws and customs to bring them in conformity with the CRPD.

---

6 Thus, for example, it is important that 'cselekvőképesség' (capacity to act) and not 'jog-illetőleg cselekvőképesség' (capacity to have rights and/or capacity to act) is used in Hungarian and that in Croatian and Slovenian 'psolovna sposobnost' (capacity to act) is used instead of 'pravna sposobnost' (capacity to have rights). And appropriate that 'Handlungsfähigkeit', (capacity to act) 'handelingsbekwaamheid' (capacity to act) is used in German and Dutch respectively.

Since Article 46(2) allows a state to withdraw a reservation at any time, a reservation retains room for dialogue and change of mind. A number of states, however, have also entered interpretative declarations, whereby they have through a process of interpretation attempted to superimpose the compulsions of substitution on the universal legal capacity model of Article 12.

The above noted strategies of inaccurate translations, reservations, and interpretative declarations on Article 12 show the extent of resistance expressed by state parties even after the prejudicial denial of legal capacity was rectified by the CRPD.

Accommodating difference in the paradigm of universal legal capacity

The paradigm of universal legal capacity invited two kinds of resistance: one, which dismissed the recognition of legal capacity for all as an impossible proposition and hence not worthy of serious consideration; and the other, which conceded to the basic justness of the proposition but pointed to the difficulties of realization.

The first kind of resistance is primarily born from prejudicial understanding and needs to be addressed like all other prejudicial perspectives through awareness building, sensitization, and education. Since these attitude change exercises are being required in order to ensure that all persons with disabilities obtain their basic human right of full legal capacity, it is imperative that such mind change operations should be mandated by the law. Such a law would be in furtherance of the obligations placed in Article 8 of the CRPD on state parties. In order to demonstrate the non-negotiability of universal legal capacity, it is imperative that it be first incorporated in the law through necessary legal amendments. And then in order to create conducive environment for the operation of the new paradigm programs of attitude change and awareness building should be conducted.

The second kind of resistance is more a verbalization of people's apprehension on the feasibility of a cataclysmic change. A number of these apprehensions also bring to the fore the varied support needs of persons with different disabilities in varied social context and for different situations.

These apprehensions could be addressed by allowing for a range of support to be developed which varies from person to person, and takes into account the socio-political context within which a person with disability would need to undertake different kinds of tasks. In the context of the central argument of this chapter, the point that is being made is that, whilst the legal capacity of all persons with disabilities requires universal recognition, the support that may be needed to exercise this capacity could be locally devised. Thus, whilst people's entitlement to support would be a universal proposition, the nature of the support could vary, depending upon the social, cultural, and economic resources available (Gombos and Dhanda 2009). Similarly, the need to devise safeguards to prevent abuse of support should be a universal proposition but there could be differences in the construction of the safeguards.

Conclusion

This chapter has operated on the premise that the value of universalism enriches the discourse of human rights provided it is inclusive in import and does not privilege the choices and preferences of dominant groups. This tenet of universality needs to be respected when humans are being addressed, whether generally or denominationally. Thus a convention addressing the rights of persons with disabilities cannot introduce a hierarchy between persons with disabilities.

This chapter has made a case for universal legal capacity as a universal human right. Even as the chapter has only made interstitial references to persons living with mental illness and mental health law, these references have been made with the clear understanding that the question of legal capacity and its absence are of central significance to mental health law. In order to seek appreciation of the larger human rights costs which ensue on the deprivation of legal capacity, this chapter has addressed the issue of universal legal capacity generically without limiting itself to the particular arguments that get to be raised in mental health treatment settings. This disassociation has been practiced to underscore the commonality between the mental health sector and the other sectors in the reasons put forth to deny persons living with mental illness legal capacity. Severity of the illness, lack of insight, and dangerousness of the condition are the reasons that are routinely offered to deny choice to persons with psychosocial disability. The above analysis makes it imperative on the mental health sector to reflect on the prejudicial underpinnings of these justifications. Also, it is important to ask as to whether the denial of capacity and the presence of force and compulsion have impeded the capability development of the mental health profession who, due to the easy presence of force, have not felt the need to develop skills of dialogue, persuasion, and understanding. The necessity of these skills is brought home by the testimonies of psychiatric users and survivors who have narrated the diminishing and traumatizing effects of no choice and force (WNUSP and Bapu Trust 2006).

The chapter has advocated for universal legal capacity with support on the strength of the CRPD. Even as capacity has to be universal, support can be customized to meet up the needs of different sectors, functions, and situations. One such arena is the realm of mental health treatment. For this support to be non-oppressive, it is essential that it be developed in close consultation with the persons seeking support. For example, persons with psychosocial disabilities would be the key stakeholders in the mental health sector. Even as the paradigm of universal legal capacity with support would assist in the building of social and individual capabilities, it will encounter direct and indirect resistance. In order to overcome this attitudinal resistance, it is necessary that awareness-raising programs accompany law reform efforts. The law is required to ascribe a non-negotiable status to universal legal capacity and to ensure that prejudice does not pass off as difference.

References

Brens, E (2001) *Human Rights: Universality and Diversity.* Netherlands: Kluwer International.

Brown, I, Raphael, D, and Renwick, R (1997) *Quality of Life—Dream or Reality? Life for People with Developmental Disabilities in Ontario.* Toronto: Quality of Life Research Unit, Centre for Health Promotion, University of Toronto.

Connolly, K (2009) 'Trapped in his own body for 23 years—the coma victim who screamed unheard', *The Guardian,* 23 November 2009, available at <http://www.guardian.co.uk/world/2009/nov/23/man-trapped-coma-23-years>.

Deci, E (1980) *Psychology of Self Determination.* Lexington, MA: Lexington Books.

Dhanda, A (2000) *Legal Order and Mental Disorder.* New Delhi: Sage Publications.

Dhanda, A (2007) 'Legal Capacity in the Disability Rights Convention: Stranglehold of the Past or Lodestar for the Future', *Syracuse Journal of International Law and Commerce,* 34(2) 429–62.

Dhanda, A (2008) 'Sameness and Difference : Twin Track Empowerment for Women with Disabilities', *Indian Journal of Gender Studies,* 15(2), 209–32.

Donnelly, J (2003) *Universal Human Rights in Theory and Practice.* Ithaca, NY: Cornell University Press.

Dworkin, R (1977) *Taking Rights Seriously.* Cambridge, MA: Harvard University Press.

Garber, J and Seligman, MEP (eds) (1980) *Human Helplessness: Theory and Applications.* New York, NY: Academic Press.

Gardner, H (1993) *Frames of Mind. The Theory of Multiple Intelligences.* New York, NY: Basic Books.

Gardner, H (1999) *Intelligences Reframed Multiple Intelligences for the 21st Century.* New York, NY: Basic Books.

Gombos, G and Dhanda, A (2009) *Catalyzing Self Advocacy: An Experiment in India.* Pune: Bapu Trust.

Grisso, T (2003) *Evaluating Competencies: Forensic Assessments and Instruments.* New York, NY: Kluwer Academic/Plenum Publishers.

Grisso, T and Appelbaum, PS (1995) 'The MacArthur Treatment Competence Study III : Abilities of Patients to Consent to Psychiatric and Medical Treatment', *Law and Human Behaviour,* 19, 149–74.

MacArthur Treatment Competence Study (1995) Available online at <http://www.macarthur.virginia.edu/treatment.html>, accessed 20 December 2009.

Pound, R (1940) *Contemporary Juristic Theory.* Claremont, CA: Claremont Colleges.

Ryan, RM and Deci, EL (2000) 'Self Determination Theory and the Facilitation of Intrinsic Motivation, Social Development and Well Being', *American Psychologist,* 55, 68–78.

Seligman, MEP (1975) *Helplessness: On depression development and Death.* New York, NY: WH Freeman.

Streeten, P (1995) *Thinking About Development.* Cambridge, UK: Cambridge University Press.

Szasz, T (1989) *Law, Liberty, and Psychiatry.* Syracuse, NY: Syracuse University Press.

Winck, BJ (1995) 'The Side Effects of Incompetency Labeling and the Implications for Mental Health', *Psychology, Public Policy, and Law,* 1, 6–42.

WNUSP and Bapu Trust (2006) *First Person Stories on Forced Interventions and Being Deprived of Legal Capacity.* Pune: Bapu Trust.

Commentary 1

Thinking about Human Rights

Eugene B. Brody

This book's size, multiplicity of authors, and diversity of content affirm the concept of human rights as a social construct. The idea of human rights is not a new product of human thought. Declarations about the 'rights of man' or some equivalent thereof have emerged on many occasions throughout recorded history. Typically, they represent the consensus of an elite group, or the thinking of an enlightened leader or philosopher about privileges and protections which express the respect accorded the dignity of human status. Following Kant we might say that the capacity for self-legislation through the exercise of reason gives a rational being a particular kind of dignity which requires respect.

Assertions about this inherent dignity derive from a view of the meaning and nature of being human. Humans everywhere share assumptions about their own nature and that of others who resemble them. Central, in addition to approximations of the ideas of inherent worth and dignity, is awareness of one's status as a person, a self-reflective sentient being with unique talents and history. In pre-literate societies the quality of uniqueness was often invoked by the self-designation of group members, in contrast to all others, as 'the' people. The essence of humanity not shared by other creatures is often considered a divine spark.

At the personal level, introspection suggests the idea of human rights as a creation of individuals searching for a sense of purpose and meaning through a focus on the mysteries of identity and personhood. What is the essence of being human, in contrast to non-human? To what freedoms does my identity as a human person entitle me? To what material resources should I be entitled simply by virtue of being human? Do other creatures, such as the anthropoid apes, with evidence of self-awareness or reflective thinking merit such respect as well?

Answers to such existential questions do not come easily. It is no surprise that some historically significant rights proclamations reflect the dominant religious beliefs of their authors or the populations they represented. The founding documents of the United States attribute universal and 'inalienable' rights to a Creator. Their authors, however, were not consistent in their application. They did not extend such rights protection to their slaves or to those owned by their constituents. Since then the relegation of human beings to the status of slaves has become a source of official discomfort if not universal action. The Slavery, Servitude, Forced Labour and Similar Institutions and Practices Convention of 1926, sponsored by the League of Nations, tried to outlaw slavery. Despite its support by a significant number of governments it was not officially adopted by the United Nations until April 1957 (Supplementary Convention on the Abolition of Slavery, the Slave Trade and Institutions and Practices Similar to Slavery of 1956). In the 21st century, slavery although not always acknowledged as such, continues as an aspect of human interaction.

The concept of universal human rights implies loyalty to the well-being of all persons, regardless of nationality, minority, or stigmatized status. American psychiatrist Harry Stack Sullivan introduced the idea of 'world loyalty' to the first UNESCO conference in 1947 on *Tensions That*

Cause Wars (Sullivan 1950). Brock Chisholm, later to become the first Director General of WHO, introduced it to the International Committee on Mental Hygiene, predecessor of the World Federation for Mental Health (WFMH) (Brody 1998). At the Third World Congress on Mental Health at which WFMH was founded, he declared that if the concept of world loyalty were adopted it would 'be one of the great historical occasions of the world' (Chisholm 1948). In keeping with this theme the WFMH founding proclamation on 20 August 1948 was entitled *Mental Health and World Citizenship.* 'The ultimate goal of mental health' it concluded is 'to help [people] live with their fellows in one world.' It defined 'world citizenship' as 'an informed, reflective, responsible allegiance to mankind as a whole. . . a world community built on free consent and. . . respect for individual and cultural differences' (Brody 1987).

Despite these brave attempts it has been difficult for humans to move from the idea of universal and inalienable rights to its practical application. Even in the window of hope and optimism following the Second World War, whole-hearted agreement about what constituted such a right was not achieved. The signatories to the 10 December 1948 United Nations *Universal Declaration of Human Rights* formally approved its reference to the rights of 'all members of the human family' in a manner reminiscent of the WFMH proclamation. However, its Article 18, asserting rights to freedom of thought, conscience, and religion, including the right to change one's religious beliefs, remained controversial. Some UN member states regarded it as an inappropriate imposition of Western and Judeo-Christian values upon non-Western cultures, indeed a form of cultural imperialism. Islamic countries, while assenting reluctantly to the declaration, objected to its including freedom of religious choice. The 'Western' nations, moving spirits in forming the declaration, under the guidance of Eleanor Roosevelt (Glendon 2001), were mainly the industrial democracies which placed highest value on individual self-determination and independence of thought and action. But in 1948 the bulk of the world's inhabitants, living in still-agrarian economies, embraced collective values granting highest value to family, lineage, tradition, and community. At particular issue was the matter of individual freedom of expression versus collective well-being requiring communal order. Less affluent and more authoritarian nations, such as the Soviet Union, objected to granting political freedom the status of a right in circumstances of insufficient resources. Instead, they attached highest value to such entitlements as food, shelter, and employment, ranking them as pre-eminent among the rights.

Interpretations of the rights concept become complicated to the degree that it is understood in moral terms as a statement of what a community regards as correct or good, in contrast to what is wrong or bad. In this sense it represents a code of behavior indicating what is approved or condemned in the treatment of one human being by another. Behavioral codes, voluntarily adopted or invested with the force of law, may be regarded as attempts to ensure social harmony, and to encourage order and cohesion instead of chaos and disorder. Yet, their progress has been uneven. Their interpretation depends upon who invokes them and in what socio-economic and political context. In some instances circumstances may lead to apparent conflict between rights.

Historically, societies have met the demands of universal human rights by limiting the categories of individuals classified as human. Individuals otherwise committed to the rights concept may accept the limitation of human status. A minister who often professed his belief in the worth and dignity of every human being once asked me if I would attribute such worth to a rapist and murderer of children. US advocates of the death penalty do not consider execution of a criminal to be a human rights violation. Populations excluded from human status by governments or pervasive custom have included psychotic or mentally impaired individuals, slaves, cultural minorities, and infants prior to the age of nine days. In societies under stress, strangers have been particularly vulnerable to being dehumanized. Wartime dehumanization of the enemy has been commonplace, making it easier for socialized civilians to become killers. In the 20th century, exclusion from full human status was epitomized by the Nazi designation of Jews, Gypsies and others as 'life unworthy of life.' 'Ethnic cleansing' of dehumanized persons from communities other than one's own continues into the 21st century. Also in this century, the Geneva Conventions' prohibitions of such massive identity violations as the torture of suspected enemies have become open to interpretation by democratic authorities because of the possibility that they might yield information necessary to save the lives of potential victims.

The appearance of a book of this kind is in part an effort by the scholarly community to clarify the understanding and use of the international and national documents enshrining the human rights concept. Human rights are invoked with increasing frequency to condemn violations of personal freedom or integrity, or the lack of resources necessary for personal development. In this last instance, where resources are simply unavailable, an unfulfilled right to material support may be regarded as a claim, valid despite the absence of resources necessary to fulfill it.

Contemporary usages of the human rights concept reflect the vicissitudes of social life influenced by a potentially infinite host of factors. Recent are the consequences of globalization. Most prominent, perhaps, especially in the long run, are scientific and technological advances with special reference to the practice of biomedicine (Brody 1993). Systematic international attention to this latter area began with a 1985 symposium sponsored by UNESCO and organized by the International Social Science Council on 'The Effects on Human Rights of Recent Advances in Science and Technology.' This and subsequent discussions recognized the individual right embodied in the UN declaration to access to the fruits of scientific research and to 'a standard of living adequate for the well-being of himself and of his family including. . . medical care and necessary social services.' The 1985 symposium specifically noted the lack of access of underprivileged and marginalized groups to the benefits of science and technology as well as their vulnerability to medical screening with eugenic aims, loss of privacy, impaired right to work in certain jobs, and impaired capacity to obtain insurance. At the same time there was concern that the protection of human rights should not impose unjustified restrictions on research.

In the late 20th century advancing biological technologies, especially of artificial reproduction including cloning, complicated perceptions of what is uniquely human. They have generated conflict about the developmental point at which a fertilized egg or a fetus should be granted full human status with its associated civil and legal rights. This is only the most recent instance of technologies of family planning leading to conflict about reproductive rights and whether or not women have a right to manage their own fertility (Brody 1976).

The new technologies of life-support and extension including organ transplantation have given rise to rights regarding decisions previously resolved by nature. Among them are rights to refuse treatment, to die, to doctor-assisted suicide, and to utilize human embryos as a source of cells, tissues, or organs for therapeutic use. The right to informed consent has been raised in regard to needy subjects of experimental treatments or drug trials who depend for a living upon 'volunteering' as a paid subject. Similarly, questions about freedom of choice were raised when the government of India offered transistor radios to impoverished young men willing to be sterilized. In both instances the right to informed consent and a free choice were in conflict with societal needs for illness management in the former and for population control in the latter.

Public health specialists now propose that the realization of global health goals requires attention to population based research on the interaction of rights and disease (Beyrer and Pizer 2007). The AIDS epidemic in particular illustrates the way in which limited rights, restricted information, press censorship, and deliberate governmental malfeasance can impair needed medical care.

Non-biological scientific advances have also influenced the perception of human rights. Rapidly evolving communications technologies have created new dimensions to rights of privacy.

As media monopolies control the transmission of information, the possibilities of 'brain washing' with loss of the freedom to arrive at independent political decisions become greater. The ultimate impact of the internet upon human freedoms is still unfathomed.

The consequences of globalization for human rights are only beginning to be recognized. The immense population mobility attendant upon new forms of mass transportation has raised questions about whether or not to respect customs, such as genital mutilation (female circumcision), traditional in the homeland, but conflicting with the ethical (human rights) codes of the new country. Concern is increasing about the working conditions of persons, including children, in less developed countries who are producing goods for the international corporations based in the more developed world. The rights of these workers are violated when they labour under unhygienic conditions with minimal rest and inadequate pay by US standards. Yet, the workers themselves often feel that the higher wages gained by such work are an ample reward for the discomfort and hazards involved.

Many psychiatrists and mental health specialists are introduced to the rights question in their treatment of people perceived as non-conforming, especially those diagnosed as mentally ill. The widespread bias against and stigmatization of such persons has been exploited for political reasons. An extreme exploitation of such public fear and distrust has been the forceful incarceration of political dissidents in mental hospitals and their definition as mentally ill in order to deprive them of status as rational beings with views deserving attention. In 1970 I visited the Soviet Union as one of a group of American psychiatrists invited to discuss the treatment of schizophrenia. There I discovered that our Soviet colleagues had invented a new diagnosis which allowed them to deflect accusations of human rights violations against them. It was 'sluggish schizophrenia', the pathognomonic feature of which was anti-state behavior. Initially, I assumed that the physicians who were active in such diagnostic abuse were agents of an oppressive government. However, I learned that they, like everyone else, were creatures of their culture. When a Soviet psychiatrist in a relaxed mood over late night drinks said, 'Don't you think that someone who leads a demonstration in Red Square must be a psychopath?' I realized that I might feel the same way.

The main focus of American concern about patients' rights has been involuntary hospitalization or commitment. However, every psychiatric encounter, as it aims to constrain the behavior of these individuals, and thus their autonomous decision-making, threatens a personhood already impaired by emotional distress or illness. The encounter is made more difficult by the disparity in social power of clinician and patient. People of unequal means cannot relate to each other on an egalitarian basis. This difference is magnified with patients who are socio-economically less advantaged, ethnically different from, or culturally alien to, the power-holders of society.

Psychiatrists have been made aware of these issues by the rise of a consumer movement among psychiatric patients and their families. Through this movement, citizens have accused psychiatry of depriving nonconforming individuals of their rights and demanded therapies not perceived as violating individual personhood, autonomy, or psycho-social integrity. Survivors of psychiatric hospitalization have asserted that mental health is more a human rights rather than a medical issue, most effectively maintained by protecting personal dignity and the capacity for self-determination. The fundamental challenge persists: how to foster individual dignity and freedom and the patient's right to autonomy while at the same time respecting his need for the protection which requires some limitations on his freedom (Brody 1985).

Years before I entered medical school, prolonged contact with a chronically delusional neighbour of my own age taught me an important fact: he needed to be recognized as having qualities and an identity other than those of a powerless, traumatized, disturbed person. In other words, he needed to be recognized as human. The complexity of the idea that being recognized as human is a fundamental right, essential to personal integrity, came to me most forcefully in late 1946.

At that time I was a medical officer, a psychiatrist with the United States army in Germany, transferred from the old Herman Goering Luftwaffe Hospital near European Command head-quarters in Frankfurt to the 385th Station Hospital in Furth, a suburb of bombed-out Nuremberg. There I learned that in addition to American soldiers I would be seeing Nazi prisoners of the International Military Tribunal. I was a 26-year-old American invested with military power at the trials of cultural strangers, 'foreigners', accused of committing crimes against humanity. Older than I, they had occupied powerful positions in the Nazi hierarchy.

I soon discovered how difficult it is to preserve one's own humanity while dealing with the per-ceived inhuman, yet someone to whom the dignity of human status must be accorded. My intro-duction came in the person of a *gauleiter*, a military governor, accused of ordering the deaths of several thousand innocent civilians. He was admitted to my ward with pneumonia following a suicide attempt with barbiturates smuggled into the prison. He was in his late forties, a former university professor, fluent in English. But when he reached out to me, wanted to hold my hand and talk, I recoiled. It was not only that he was, in my view, a mass murderer. He also reminded me of what we had come to regard as the Nazi stereotype, obsequious to authority with power over him, and brutal to those beneath him in the hierarchy. Even as I recognized his depression and the likelihood of another suicidal attempt, I denied him the compassionate care which he craved. This was not deliberate on my part; it stemmed from the revulsion I felt for what he had done. Then, one night, while I was away from the unit, the Latvian refugee soldiers assigned to guard him took him to the latrine, handed him the cord from his robe which had been confiscated, and allowed him to hang himself.

The thought that I had failed to recognize the prisoner, also my patient, as human came only later. In 1948, once more a civilian, I was talking with a professor at the Yale Divinity School about the discrepancies in power between doctor and help-seeking patient. He reminded me of Hegel's sense of the interaction between master and slave fueled by the mutual requirement of each for recognition by the other as human. Looking back over the span of approximately sixty years I have been unable to come up with another resolution of the dilemma posed by the enemy, prisoner, or free. The only way to preserve one's own humanity, and to embrace the idea of human rights, is to recognize and somehow address the humanity of the other, even when the other is perceived as the embodiment of evil.

References

Beyrer, C and Pizer, HF (eds) (2007) *Public Health and Human Rights. Evidence-Based Approaches.* Baltimore: Johns Hopkins University Press.

Brody, EB (1976) 'Reproductive freedom, coercion and justice: Some ethical aspects of population policy and practice', *Social Science & Medicine*, 10, 553–57.

Brody, EB (1985) 'Patients' rights. A cultural challenge to Western psychiatry', *American Journal of Psychiatry*, 142, 58–62.

Brody, EB (1987) *Mental health and world citizenship.* Austin, TX: Hogg Foundation for Mental Health.

Brody, EB (1993) *Biomedical Technology and Human Rights.* Hants, England: Dartmouth Press. (with the sponsorship of the International Social Science Council, UNESCO, and WFMH).

Brody, EB (1998) *The Search for Mental Health. A history and memoir of WFMH. 1948–1997.* Baltimore: Williams and Wilkins.

Chisholm, G Brock (1948) Minutes, International Committee on Mental Hygiene, April 26.

Glendon, Mary Ann (2001) *A World Made New: Eleanor Roosevelt and the Universal Declaration of Human Rights.* New York: Random House.

'Slavery, Servitude, Forced Labour and Similar Institutions and Practices Convention of 1926. League of Nations Treaty Series, Vol. 6, p. 253; entered into force on 9 March 1927', in David Weissbrodt and

Anti-Slavery International, *Abolishing Slavery and its Contemporary Forms*, HR/PUB/02/4. New York and Geneva: Office of the United Nations High Commissioner for Human Rights, 4–5. Available at <http://www.ohchr.org/Documents/Publications/slaveryen.pdf>, accessed 9 November 2011.

Sullivan, Harry Stack (1950) 'Tensions interpersonal and international. A psychiatrist's view', in H Cantril (ed) *Tensions That Cause Wars: Common Statement and Individual Papers by a Group of Social Scientists Brought Together by Unesco (1947)*. Urbana, Il: University of Illinois Press, 79–138.

'Supplementary Convention on the Abolition of Slavery, the Slave Trade and Institutions and Practices Similar to Slavery of 1956. United Nations Treaty Series, vol. 226, p. 3; entered into force on 20 April 1957', in David Weissbrodt and Anti-Slavery International, *Abolishing Slavery and its Contemporary Forms*, HR/PUB/02/4. New York and Geneva: Office of the United Nations High Commissioner for Human Rights, 4–5. Available at <http://www.ohchr.org/Documents/Publications/slaveryen.pdf>, accessed 9 November 2011.

Gene Brody: a personal memoir

Senior academics who devote their time to mentoring the young and to advocating for social causes are in short supply in the modern world. Sadly, Gene Brody may have been one of the last in the line of this great tradition.

After his illustrious career as Professor of Psychiatry at the University of Maryland, Gene devoted his time to championing good causes and progressive organizations, particularly the World Federation of Mental Health (WFMH). He also promoted, nurtured, and supported the next generation of professionals and academics working at the intersection of human rights and mental health. He bravely resisted the modern trend that favours biological psychiatry over other fields by continuing to encourage submissions on cultural, social, and human rights aspects of psychiatry to the Journal of Nervous and Mental Disease which he edited.

I first met Gene when he visited Sydney, Australia in the early period of my career in Refugee and Post-conflict Mental Health. He soon added me to his informal list of "adoptees", lending a helping hand whenever called on to support our work in Sydney and around the world. His wry humour, his deep humanistic convictions, his towering intellect, and his encyclopaedic knowledge blended to produce a harmonious mix of wisdom and worldliness that is rarely observed in leaders nowadays.

There are many anecdotes I could tell about Gene Brody but the one that stands out in my mind was the festschrift that the Harvard Program in Refugee Trauma and my unit at the University of New South Wales organized for him when he retired as Secretary General of the WFMH. Gene was at his very best, graciously accepting the "roasting" that is traditional at Harvard on these occasions. In his right to reply, he pointed out in his inimitable fashion that great men without an Achilles heel belong in heaven where, ironically, there is no demand for their talents!

Gene was a truly great man; leaving us with some of his most personal experiences and thoughts in his posthumous contribution to this volume; a fitting tribute to a man who was unsparing in his willingness to share his time and wisdom with others.

Derrick Silove

Global Mental Health and Social Justice[1]

Ezra Susser and Michaeline Bresnahan

The neglect of people with mental disorders has deep social roots, and pertains across many spheres of social life including health care and public health. People with severe mental illnesses such as schizophrenia suffer intense discrimination and stigma. In recent history, probably the most flagrant example was in Nazi Germany when more than 200,000 people with schizophrenia and other severe mental illnesses were systematically selected for the gas chambers, a fate that later befell Jewish people and other victims (Alexander 1949; Lifton 1986; Kater 1989; Strous 2007; Fuller Torrey 2010). In contemporary societies, people with severe mental illness have basic human rights enshrined in international agreements (UN 2008), but these are widely ignored (see Global Initiative on Psychiatry <http://www.gip-global.org> and Disability Rights International (formerly Mental Disability Rights International) <http://www.disabilityrightsintl.org/>). In some spheres, and in particular in health care, this injustice extends to people with common mental disorders such as depression and anxiety. A landmark series of papers in *The Lancet* documented the extent of the neglect of common mental disorders in health care and public health across the globe (Andrews and Titov 2007; Chisholm et al. 2007; Horton 2007; Prince et al. 2007; Sartorius 2007; Saxena et al. 2007; Thornicroft 2007; Wang et al. 2007).

The neglect of mental health is not immutable and in the present time it is being challenged as never before (NIMH 1999; WHO 2001). In this commentary, we aim to contribute to this change by stimulating the proponents of global health and social justice to revisit and revise their own understandings of the history of public health and its connections to social justice. The contributions and the experiences of groups that suffer discrimination are often minimized in the written histories of health and other professions. Certainly, in public health, the contributions of people with mental illness, and of studies of mental illness, have received little recognition. In addition, the historically significant role of mental health in population health has often been overlooked. To illustrate the potential for remedying this situation, we select historical examples from four eras (adapted from Susser and Susser 1996a and Susser and Stein 2009): Embryonic (approx 1760–1820): Sanitarian (approx 1820–1880); Infectious disease (approx 1880–1940); and Chronic disease (approx 1940–2000).

Embryonic era

Why should we think that people (not just our 'own kind') have basic rights (Hochschild 2005); and that this includes a right to mental health, or to any other kind of health, for that matter? In the Western world, this idea emerged in the Enlightenment, and was institutionalized for the first

---

[1] Adapted from E Susser, *WG Armstrong Oration*, University of Sydney, 2007.

time in the French Revolution (Ackerknecht 1948; La Berge 1992; Rosen 1993; Weiner 1993; Barnes 2006; Quinlan 2007). In 1790–91, the Revolutionary government established the Poverty Committee which was charged with ensuring the citizen's right to health (Weiner 1993). Mental health was included.

Probably the most influential person involved in the care of people with mental illness during the French Revolution and the Napoleonic era was Philippe Pinel, who gave his lecture on 'Memoir on madness: A contribution to the natural history of man,' to a revolutionary audience in 1794 (see translation by Weiner 1992), and then expanded it and published it as a book in 1801 (Pinel 1983). Striking in his work is the human dignity that he accorded to people with mental illness. He talked to patients and listened to their stories; and he wrote about patients with tenderness, sometimes admiration, conveying their humanity. This was in itself a radical departure from the past. Pinel deplored the conditions in the institutions where insane people were kept, and embarked on a campaign to reform these conditions. Thus the French Revolution crystallized the idea of health and mental health as a right, and in its aftermath, Pinel and his colleagues put forward the idea that people with mental illnesses should be treated with respect and dignity (something we still haven't achieved in most of the world).

A famous painting by Robert-Fleury in the Charcot Library of the Salpêtrière Hospital Medical School in Paris (and a similar picture by another artist depicting the same act at Bicêtre Hospital) purports to show Pinel freeing mental patients from their chains. These paintings are not, however, historically accurate (Weiner 1979). The man who did free the patients from their chains was Jean-Baptiste Pussin. Citizen Pussin was a former patient at Bicêtre who later sought employment at the hospital and subsequently rose through the ranks to become supervisor on the ward of the incurably mentally ill. Having been a patient himself, Pussin had access to the lived experience of the patients, and their humanity was readily apparent to him. When Pinel was appointed Physician of the Infirmaries at Bicêtre in 1793 and then Physician-in-Chief at Salpêtrière, he had the chance to tap Pussin's depth of knowledge about the patients' lives, and was stimulated to start listening to the patients directly. According to Pinel, his distinctly humanitarian perspective on psychiatric care was fashioned by these experiences (Weiner 1979). Pinel is a legendary figure in psychiatric history, deservedly so, and he did have a pivotal role in removing mental patients from bondage in many of the asylums of France. Nonetheless, it is worth noting the contrast with Pussin. Although the former patient Citizen Pussin actually carried out the act depicted in these paintings, and stimulated Pinel's insights about psychiatric patients, his contribution is virtually unknown.

Sanitarian era

During the Industrial Revolution in the 19th century, it was evident that the social world was changing rapidly, and that the health and diseases of the population were changing along with it (Villermé 1826). The reforms advocated by most public health leaders in this period involved societal change. In England, for instance, Edwin Chadwick and others succeeded in passing legislation mandating the development of sanitation systems in urban areas (Chadwick 1843; La Berge 1988). Most of these public health leaders mistook the mechanisms by which poor sanitation led to disease. Yet, the public health measures that they introduced—and which were later emulated elsewhere—have led to substantial improvements in the health of populations thereafter (Szreter 1988; Morabia 2007; Oppenheimer and Susser 2007).

In this era, we can turn to the contributions of William Farr, one of the forefathers of the profession of epidemiology (Farr 1975; Eyler 1979). He is best known for his work in the Registrar General's office, where he began and maintained the systematic collection of vital statistics for the British population. Farr thought deeply about social justice and health. He looked beyond the individual citizen—whose right to health was proclaimed in the French Revolution—to consider the health of the population. He and others in the sanitarian era explicitly placed value on the health of the population and on improving the health of populations through societal intervention. That was a novel perspective at the time and is still central to public health today.

Less known, William Farr placed great value on mental health, and especially, on humane care of people with mental illness. He documented and drew attention to the appalling mortality rates among mental patients in asylums. '. . . the annual mortality . . . [is] as high as the mortality experienced by the British troops upon the western coast of Africa, and by the population of London when the plague rendered its habitations desolate!' (Farr 1975:430). Even in the good asylums the annual mortality was 10 to 20 per cent (Farr 1975). Some of his most innovative work pertained to people with mental illness. A good example is his study of the Hanwell asylum. John Connolly, resident physician at Hanwell, instituted a policy of non-restraint beginning in 1839. To examine the benefits of humane care and treatment, Farr compared the annual mortality of patients discharged from Hanwell with that of patients discharged from other asylums (Farr 1975:428). The study was innovative in many ways. It included the use of a comparison group in a quasi-experimental design; an embryonic version of survival analysis; and an attempt to control for social class. The main result was that Hanwell had some beneficial effect, though not as large as the effect of social class; paupers had a higher death rate than non-paupers in all settings.

We also offer an example of how population statistics on mental illness were (mis)used to reinforce social *in*justice. Although this episode is known to few people in public health, it was significant and influential in social history. The 1840 census in the United States involved the first attempt by any nation to enumerate the number of insane individuals in the population (Deutsch 1944). Census takers were asked to record, along with other information, the individuals suffering from insanity in every household. The data revealed an association between race and insanity that was stunning (though wrong, see below). Among whites in both the north and the slave-holding south, about one in a thousand were 'insane'. Among free blacks in the north, however, about one in 150 were insane, a six-fold higher prevalence compared to Whites. Among black slaves in the south only about one in 1550 were insane. The common interpretation of these results is reflected in this quotation from *The Southern Literary Messenger*: 'Slaves are not only far happier in the states of slavery than freedom but we believe the happiest class on this continent. . .the free Negroes of the northern states are the most vicious persons on the continent perhaps on the earth. . .they furnish little else but materials for jails, penitentiaries and madhouses' (1843). A quotation from the *American Journal of Insanity* (forerunner of the *American Journal of Psychiatry*) shows that the interpretation by the psychiatric profession was similar: 'There is an awful prevalence of idiocy and insanity among the free blacks over the whites and especially over the slaves' (1851). The 1840 census provided the slave-holding states with one of their most compelling arguments that slavery was a better state for blacks than freedom (Deutsch 1944).

Initially Edward Jarvis, the forefather of psychiatric epidemiology in the United States, made a similar interpretation of the census results: 'Slavery has a wonderful influence upon the developments of moral faculties of the intellectual powers. . .it saves them from some of the liabilities and dangers of acts of self-direction' (Jarvis 1842a) Fortunately for the field of psychiatric epidemiology, Jarvis subsequently inspected the census data in detail. He found that they were riddled with blatant errors. In Limerick, Maine, for example, there was no coloured population, yet there were four coloured insane people; similarly, in Scarborough, Maine, there was no coloured population, yet there were six coloured insane people; and so forth. To his great credit, Jarvis had the courage and integrity to proclaim to the public that he had been wrong.: 'As it now stands we are disappointed and mortified we had looked at this with eager hope as the most extensive statistical report on insanity presented by any nation' (Jarvis 1842b). Jarvis and others made a concerted effort to persuade the US government to correct the 1840 census. But a lot of damage had already been done and much of it was not remediable. Their efforts were blocked by the legislators from the Southern states, and the census results stood uncorrected. Thus, according to the official results of the United States 1840 census, slavery was a happier state than freedom for blacks.[2]

Infectious disease era

Following the discovery of microbes in the late 19th century, the sanitarian era gave way to the 'infectious disease era.' For a long period, the main focus of epidemiology was on identifying the microbial agent that caused a disease, and finding ways to control it. In its heyday in the early 20th century, virtually every disease was thought to be infectious, and epidemiology was often defined as the study of infectious diseases. As they trained their eyes ever more sharply—and success-fully—on identifying germs and understanding their transmission, epidemiologists and public health practitioners diminished their emphasis on societal reform. Yet one of the best epidemiological investigations during that era pertained to pellagra, a disease that wasn't infectious, and evolved into a campaign for social justice.

Around the turn of the 20th century, there was an apparent epidemic of pellagra in the south of the United States. (We use the qualifier 'apparent' because it is not clear to what degree the epidemic was due to increasing recognition of the disease). There were also alarming reports of outbreaks of pellagra, especially in institutions such as orphanages and psychiatric hospitals. Pellagra is now known to be caused by a nutritional deficiency, but at the time, almost every expert in the United States thought it was an infectious disease.

The work of Joseph Goldberger on pellagra in the early decades of the 20th century has become legendary in the history of public health (Goldberger 1964; Kraut 2003). With courage and exceptional insight, he postulated and systematically demonstrated that the proximate cause was a nutritional deficiency.[3] Goldberger initially studied people in orphanages and insane asylums and prisons, and later together with Edgar Sydenstricker he studied entire communities. At each stage, he conducted innovative observational studies and experiments which advanced the methods of epidemiology.

What is often overlooked is that Goldberger's work on pellagra was intertwined in many ways with the care and prevention of mental illness (Goldberger 1964; Etheridge 1972; Kraut 2003). First, pellagra was a cause of significant mental illness. The classic sign was a 'butterfly rash,' but pellagra also commonly had effects on cognition and behaviours. Like syphilis, pellagra was one of the leading causes of insanity in this era (Etheridge 1972; Kraut 2003; also see the Museum of the Insane Asylum of San Servolo, at <http://www.fondazionesanservolo.it/html/home.asp>). Within an insane asylum in the south of the United States there would typically be large numbers of patients who were there because of the consequences of pellagra. Second, confinement for mental illness exposed patients to the risk of pellagra. Some of the major outbreaks which drew the public's attention to pellagra occurred in psychiatric hospitals. Third, owing to these interconnections with mental illness, psychiatrists played a large role in the investigations of pellagra, and

---

[2] It is easy to jump to the conclusion that the 1840 census data were falsified to produce the desired result for slaveholders. According to researchers who have studied them, this was probably not the case (Cohen 1982). Rather it appears that the errors were due to the poor methods of the census—for example, minimal training of census takers, unreliable ratings of insanity, and multiple errors in data entry and transcription—and that the resulting bias was systematic.

[3] Ultimately it turned out that a B vitamin could prevent pellagra. Goldberger didn't discover the vitamin before his death, though he postulated its presence and tried to discover it in laboratory studies.

were key collaborators in Goldberger's studies. Finally, Goldberger's key insight was partly the result of observing the lives of patients with mental illness. It was believed that pellagra couldn't have a nutritional cause because in psychiatric hospitals, unlike some other institutions, the staff were served the same food as the patients, yet the outbreaks tended to affect patients and not staff. Goldberger solved this puzzle by actually visiting the asylums and observing how people lived. He saw that the diets of patients and staff were not the same; staff tended to take the best foods for themselves and give the remainder to the patients.

Goldberger, like Farr, perceived a connection between social justice and public health. After showing that insufficient diet caused pellagra, he went on to study milltowns in the south where pellagra was endemic, and tried to understand what social conditions produced the insufficient diet. At this stage he joined up with Edgar Sydenstricker,[4] an economist and social scientist, who applied his skills to develop a sophisticated study of the milltowns, which included not only a survey of household diets, but also an analysis of their economies and social networks and how food was distributed. At the end of these classic studies, Sydenstricker concluded: '. . .It may appear at first glance that any attempt to remove the conditions that are fundamentally responsible for the prevalence of pellagra would involve a revolution of the dietary habits and of the entire economic and financial system as it now exists' (Sydenstricker 1974). Later, after Goldberger's death, Sydenstricker advanced the concept of disability, established the famous Hagerstown study, and elaborated a broad vision of public health: 'Society has a basic responsibility for assuring all its members, healthful conditions of housing and living, a reasonable degree of economic security, proper facilities for curative and preventive medicine and adequate medical care—in fact the control, so far as means are known to science, of all the environmental factors that affect physical and mental wellbeing' (Sydenstricker 1935). This elegant statement about public health and mental health was made in 1935 and we believe it holds true today.

Risk factor era

'Chronic disease' or risk factor epidemiology became dominant in the middle of the 20th century. The approach crystallized in response to emerging epidemics of lung cancer, cardiovascular disease, peptic ulcer, and other 'chronic diseases' that defied explanation in terms of an infectious agent.[5] The essence of the approach is to design studies to identify within a population the factors that make one person more at risk of disease than another. The underlying premise is that a cause may be neither necessary nor sufficient, but nonetheless result in an increased risk of disease (Susser 1973). The demonstration that smoking cigarettes was a cause of lung cancer was the most definitive early success and helped establish the dominance of this approach. The application of these methods has led to countless advances in public health. Nowadays, the designs most often employed to identify risk factors—case control and cohort studies—are familiar to everyone in the health sciences.

Many of the people who initiated chronic disease epidemiology were centrally concerned with social justice (Davey Smith 2001; March and Susser 2006). A notable pioneer was Jerry Morris, who wrote the first epidemiology textbook of this era (Morris 1957). He proposed that

---

4 Edgar Sydenstricker was the brother of Pearl S. Buck, a Nobel prize winning author. He was probably the first social scientist to fully integrate his work with that of epidemiologists.

5 It was named chronic disease epidemiology, but it was later discovered that some of these chronic diseases, notably peptic ulcer, indeed were related to an infectious agent. In addition, the leading infectious diseases of our time (HIV and TB and malaria) are chronic conditions. Hence we prefer the term risk factor epidemiology.

epidemiologists should advocate for improving the health and mental health of the population, and for improving the standard of living of the population as required to sustain health for all. Mervyn Susser (father of ES) was of this ilk, and he put it thus: 'Equity will elude any society that does not weigh the questions before it in terms of their higher professional values—that is, the right to health of the people at large' (Susser 1993). Many of them were also concerned with mental health, and the application of epidemiology to psychiatric disorders took root early on (Morris 1957; Susser 1968; Cooper and Morgan 1973).

Building upon this early work, the methods of risk factor epidemiology were systematically elaborated into a full fledged discipline. Its maturation is represented in an elegant and influential textbook by Kenneth Rothman published in 1986 with the title *Modern Epidemiology*. In terms of the ties that bind epidemiology to social justice and mental health, however, this period of maturation was a period of retrenchment. Rothman, for example, took the view that social justice is not part of the field of study in epidemiology (Rothman 1986; Rothman et al. 1998). Mental health is hardly to be seen among the examples in his textbook. Psychiatric epidemiology continued to develop, but along somewhat different lines from the mainstream of epidemiology, and was increasingly marginal to the discipline as a whole (Susser et al. 2006). The retrenchment was, however, soon undermined by historical events (March and Susser 2006). One of these was the advent of the HIV/AIDS epidemic in the 1980s. Another was the accumulating evidence that while health was improving overall in majority world countries, social inequalities in health were stubbornly persistent and sometimes increasing.

In the risk factor era, the reduction of cigarette smoking was a capstone achievement of epidemiology and public health. Cigarette smoking was arguably the dominant preventable cause of non-communicable diseases in the 20th century in high-income countries (Peto et al. 1992, 1996; Brandt 2007). The proliferation of findings from epidemiologic studies on the manifold harmful effects of cigarette smoking (and of environmental tobacco exposure or 'passive' smoking) played a central role in public health campaigns to reduce cigarette smoking.

Cigarette smoking is inextricably intertwined with mental health. It is an addictive behavior, which most often starts in youth, after which it is difficult to quit smoking. Cigarette smoking has effects on the brain and on mood and is very strongly associated with common (as well as other) mental disorders (Glassman et al. 1990; Glassman 1993; Wilhelm et al. 2006, Wilhelm et al. 2004). Yet the dimension of mental health received scant attention in the classic debates and political struggles which ultimately led to (partially) successful interventions to reduce cigarette smoking. Consequently, public mental health was peripheral to this landmark achievement of epidemiology and public health, when it could have been central, and had much to contribute. In retrospect, this is difficult to comprehend. The failure to recognize that cigarette smoking is in the sphere of public mental health can only be partly explained by the low priority given to mental health by mainstream epidemiology and public health, and by the efforts of tobacco companies to deny and/or downplay the addictive potential of cigarettes. There was another important factor; leaders in public mental health were unable to either realize or assert that they had a central role to play.

One reason to draw attention to the neglect of public mental health in this central arena of public health is that it remains relevant today. Cigarette smoking is still a major determinant of health in high-income countries, and it looks destined to become one of the leading determinants of health in low- and middle-income countries in this century (Peto et al. 1999). Therefore within the global health movement today, we still have the opportunity to draw the connections of cigarette smoking to mental health, and thereby enhance the effectiveness of research and public health policy in this domain.

Conclusion

In the 21st century we have entered a new era, which is clearly different than the risk factor era, but is not yet well defined. We have referred to it as 'eco epidemiology' and have elaborated our perspective in previous publications (Susser and Susser 1996b; Susser 2004; Susser et al. 2006; March and Susser 2006). Most relevant here, epidemiologists and public health practitioners are increasingly concerned with the relationship between social life and disease; with the connections between public health and social justice (McCord and Freeman 1990); and with global health.

Non-communicable diseases are the largest cause of mortality in the world today, and that trend is likely to continue over the coming decades (Leeder 2002; Yach et al. 2004; Yach et al. 2005). This does not imply that the resources to combat HIV/AIDS (and other infectious diseases such as tuberculosis and malaria) should be reduced; the challenge of HIV/AIDS remains a benchmark of our times, because it is devastating entire nations in the poorest region of the globe. It does mean, however, that we cannot afford to be complacent about the non-communicable disease epidemics which are now emerging in middle-income and low-income countries, and the changing profiles of non-communicable disease in high-income countries. To adequately confront the future of public health in the 21st century, we need to think globally, and we need to recognize the dominance of non-communicable disease across the globe.

As longevity increases, it is also apparent that we need to think beyond mortality to disability: the quality as well as the duration of our lives. This perspective can be traced back at least as far as Sydenstricker, but it has only recently been quantified and given the imprimatur of the WHO. One of the best known approaches is to compute Disability Adjusted Life Years or DALYs in order to answer the question: what diseases take away more years of our life due to either death or disability? (Murray and Lopez 1996; Murray and World Health Organization 2002). When one sets the goal as reducing disability as well as mortality, something very surprising happens; one sees a dramatic change in the ranking of health domains. Notably, mental disorders are leading causes of DALYs (Murray and Lopez 1997).[6] A large share of this is accounted for by common mental disorders such as depression, but long term disorders such as schizophrenia and autism also make a substantial contribution.

The significant impact of mental disorders is apparent in all societies. It is often said that the neglect of people with mental illness and of mental health care is due to the fact that they cannot be a priority—especially in developing countries—until the major causes of mortality are brought under control. As long as one focuses narrowly on mortality, this argument carries weight. But as soon as one takes a broader perspective, and considers what causes morbidity and disability, impacts family caregivers, causes loss of productivity, and interferes with socioeconomic development, the argument is no longer tenable. The neglect of mental disorders constrains the advance of health and wealth in all countries.

The WHO, the CDC in the United States, and other national and international public health agencies have documented the discrimination and neglect of people with mental illness and offered guidelines in calls to redress it (WHO and Department of Mental Health and Substance Abuse 2005; Ustun 1999; WHO 2001; NIMH 1999). Yet the public health community has been

---

[6] The exact ranking depends partly on the assumptions made in the computation. A legitimate critique can be made of the methods of computing DALYs, as well as of the estimates of the frequency and disabling consequences of mental disorders. Thus one should not place too much weight on the specific ranking of health domains. What is indisputable, however, under any reasonable method of computation, is that mental disorders are among the most important causes of disability.

slow to take up the call. For example, in the United States, the major schools of public health have not put mental health at the centre of their agenda. One might argue, then, that change begins at home. Until the public health community itself acknowledges and redresses its own historical and ongoing neglect of mental health, the public is unlikely to do so.

There are many ways for public health practitioners to raise the profile of mental health within public health. One is to encourage and support advocacy groups, a method that made a pivotal contribution to placing the treatment of HIV/AIDS at the forefront of the global health agenda (Siplon 2002; Stockdill 2003; Gruskin et al. 2007). Another is to train public health professionals to be concerned with mental health, in low-, middle-, and high-income countries. A practical programme must be devised to ensure that in the course of their education epidemiologists and other public health professionals are socialized to recognize that 'there is no health without mental health' (Thornicroft 2007). As a corollary, we need to teach students that the pursuit of social justice cannot be not limited to reducing inequalities in health and wealth across the general population. It must also include attention to social groups who are excluded from civic life, neglected and discriminated against, and considered to be less than full human beings, as is the case for people with severe mental illness today.

References

Ackerknecht, EH (1948) 'Hygiene in France, 1815–1848', *Bulletin of the History of Medicine*, **22**, 117–55.

Alexander, L (1949) 'Medical Science Under Dictatorship', *New England Journal of Medicine*, 241, 39–47.

Andrews, G and Titov, N (2007) 'Depression Is Very Disabling', *The Lancet*, 370, 808–809.

Anonymous (1843) 'Reflections on the Census of 1840', *Southern Literary Messenger* IX (June 1843). APS online, 340–352.

Anonymous (1851) 'Startling Facts About the Census', *American Journal of Insanity as reprinted from the New York Observer*, 8, 53–55.

Barnes, DS (2006) *The Great Stink of Paris and the Nineteenth-Century Struggle Against Filth and Germs*. Baltimore: Johns Hopkins University Press.

Brandt, A. (2007) *The Cigarette Century: The Rise Fall and Deadly Persistence of the Product That Defined America*. New York: Basic Books.

Chadwick, E (1843) *Report on the Sanitary Condition of the Labouring Population of Great Britain: A Supplementary Report on the Results of a Special Inquiry into the Practice of Interment in Towns*. London: W. Clowes and Sons for HM Stationery Office.

Chisholm, D, Flisher, AJ, Lund, C et al. (2007) 'Scale Up Services for Mental Disorders: A Call for Action', *The Lancet*, **370**, 1241–52.

Cohen, PC (1982) *A Calculating People: The Spread of Numeracy in Early America*. Chicago: University of Chicago Press.

Cooper, B and Morgan, HG (1973) *Epidemiological Psychiatry*. Springfield: Charles C. Thomas.

Davey Smith, G (2001) 'The Uses of "Uses of Epidemiology"', *International Journal of Epidemiology*, 30, 1146–55.

Deutsch, A (1944) 'The First U.S. Census of the Insane (1840) and its Use as a Pro-Slavery Propaganda', *Bulletin of the History of Medicine*, 15, 469–82.

Disability Rights International : <http://www.disabilityrightsintl.org/>.

Epstein, H (2007) *The Invisible Cure: Africa, the West, and the Fight Against AIDS*. New York: Farrar, Straus and Giroux.

Etheridge, EW (1972) *The Butterfly Caste: A Social History of Pellagra in the South*. Westport, CT: Greenwood Pub. Co.

Eyler, JM (1979) *Victorian Social Medicine: The Ideas and Methods of William Farr*. Baltimore: Johns Hopkins University Press.

Farr, W (1975) *Vital Statistics: A Memorial Volume of Selections From the Reports and Writings of William Farr*. MW Susser and A Adelstein, (eds). Metuchen: The Scarecrow Press, Inc.

Fuller Torrey, E and Yolken, RH (2010) 'Psychiatric genocide: Nazi attempts to eradicate'. *Schizophrenia Bulletin*, 36, 26–32.

Glassman, A (1993) 'Cigarette smoking: Implications for psychiatric illness', *American Journal of Psychiatry*, 150, 546–553.

Glassman, A, Helzer, JE, Covey, LS et al. (1990) 'Smoking, smoking cessation, and major depression', *JAMA*, 264, 545–49.

Global Initiative on Psychiatry : <http://www.gip-global.org>.

Goldberger, J (1964) *Goldberger on Pellagra*. Baton Rouge: Louisiana State University Press.

Gordon, D (1975) 'The Inaugural W.G. Armstrong Lecture: Social and Preventative Medicine—The Nature of the Beasts', *Bulletin of the Post-Graduate Committee in Medicine, University of Sydney*.

Gruskin, S, Mills, EJ, Tarantola, D (2007) 'History, Principles, and Practice of Health and Human Rights', *The Lancet*, 370, 449–55.

Hochschild, A (2005) *Bury the Chains: Prophets and Rebels in the Fight to Free an Empire's Slaves*. Boston: Houghton Mifflin.

Horton, R (2007) 'Launching a New Movement for Mental Health', *The Lancet*, 370, 806.

Jarvis, E (1842a) *Boston Medical and Surgical Journal. APS online*, 281, 27, 281.

Jarvis, E (1842b) *Boston Medical and Surgical Journal. APS online*, 116, 27, 116.

Kater, MH (1989) *Doctors Under Hitler*. Chapel Hill: University of North Carolina Press.

Kraut, AM (2003) *Goldberger's War: The Life and Work of a Public Health Crusader*. New York: Hill and Wang.

Kuller, LH (2004) 'Commentary: Hazards of Studying Women: the Oestrogen Oestrogen/Progesterone Dilemma', *International Journal of Epidemiology*, 33, 459–60.

La Berge, AF (1988) 'Edwin Chadwick and the French Connection', *Bulletin of the History of Medicine*, 62, 23–41.

La Berge, AF (1992) *Mission and Method: The Early Nineteenth-Century French Public Health Movement*. Cambridge: Cambridge University Press.

Lawlor, DA, Davey Smith G, and Ebrahim, S (2004) 'Commentary: the Hormone Replacement-Coronary Heart Disease Conundrum: Is This the Death of Observational Epidemiology?', *International Journal of Epidemiology*, 33, 464–67.

Leeder, SR (2002) 'Public Health Change and Challenge: an Academic (and Personal) Response', *WG Armstrong Lecture*.

Lifton, RJ (1986) *The Nazi Doctors: Medical Killing and the Psychology of Genocide*. New York: Basic Books.

March, D and Susser, E (2006) 'The Eco- in Eco-Epidemiology', *International Journal of Epidemiology*, 35(6), 1379–83.

Marmot, M and Wilkinson, R (eds) (1999) *Social Determinants of Health*. Oxford: Oxford University Press.

McCord, C and Freeman, HP (1990) Excess Mortality in Harlem. *New England Journal of Medicine*, 322, 173–77.

Morabia, A (2007) 'Epidemiologic Interactions, Complexity, and the Lonesome Death of Max Von Pettenkofer', *American Journal of Epidemiology*, 166, 1233–38.

Morris, JN (1957) *Uses of Epidemiology*. Edinburgh: Livingstone.

Murray, CJ and Lopez, AD (1997) 'Global Mortality, Disability, and the Contribution of Risk Factors: Global Burden of Disease Study', *The Lancet*, 349, 1436–42.

Murray, CJL and Lopez, AD (1996) *The Global Burden of Disease: a Comprehensive Assessment of Mortality and Disability From Diseases, Injuries, and Risk Factors in 1990 and Project to 2020*. Cambridge: Harvard University Press.

Murray, CJL and World Health Organization (2002) *Summary Measures of Population Health: Concepts, Ethics, Measurement, and Applications.* Geneva: World Health Organization.

Museum of the Insane Asylum of San Servolo : <http://www.fondazionesanservolo.it/html/home.asp>.

National Institute of Mental Health (1999) *Mental Health: A Report of the Surgeon General.* Rockville, MD: National Institute of Mental Health.

Oppenheimer, GM and Susser, E (2007) 'Invited Commentary: The Context and Challenge of Von Pettenkofer's Contributions to Epidemiology', *American Journal of Epidemiology,* 166, 1239–41.

Peto, R, Lopez, AD, Boreham, J, Thun, M, and Heath, C (1992) 'Mortality from tobacco in developed countries: indirect estimation from national vital statistics', *The Lancet,* 339, 1269–78.

Peto, R, Lopez, AD, Boreham, J, Thun, M, Heath, C and Doll, R (1996) 'Mortality from smoking worldwide', *British Medical Bulletin,* 52, 12–21.

Peto, R, Chen, ZM, and Boreham, J (1999) Tobacco—the growing epidemic. *Nature Medicine,* 5, 15–21.

Pinel, P (1983) *A Treatise on Insanity.* Birmingham, AL: The Classics of Medicine Library.

Prince, M, Patel, V, Saxena, S, et al. (2007) 'No Health Without Mental Health', *The Lancet,* 370, 859–77.

Quinlan, SM (2007) *The Great Nation in Decline: Sex, Modernity, and Health Crises in Revolutionary France C.1750–1850.* Aldershot, England: Ashgate.

Rosen, G (1993) *A History of Public Health.* Expanded edn. Baltimore: Johns Hopkins University Press.

Rothman, KJ, Adami, HO, and Trichopoulos, D (1998) 'Should the Mission of Epidemiology Include the Eradication of Poverty?', *The Lancet,* 352, 810–813.

Rothman, KJ (1986) *Modern Epidemiology.* 1st edn. Boston: Little, Brown.

Sartorius, N (2007) 'Stigma and Mental Health', *The Lancet,* 370, 810–811.

Saxena, S, Thornicroft, G, Knapp, M, and Whiteford, H (2007) 'Resources for Mental Health: Scarcity, Inequity, and Inefficiency', *The Lancet,* 370, 878–89.

Siplon, PD (2002) 'Us and Them: AIDS As a Foreign Policy Issue' in *AIDS and the Policy Struggle in the United States.* Washington, DC: Georgetown University Press, 111–34.

Stockdill, BC (2003) *Activism Against AIDS at the Intersection of Sexuality, Race, Gender, and Class.* Boulder, Col: Lynne Rienner Pub.

Strous, RD (2007) 'Psychiatry During the Nazi Era: Ethical Lessons for the Modern Professional', *Annals of General Psychiatry,* 6, 8.

Susser, E (2004) 'Eco-Epidemiology: Thinking Outside the Black Box', *Epidemiology,* 15, 519–20.

Susser, E, Schwartz, S, Morabia, A, and Bromet, E (2006) *Psychiatric Epidemiology: Searching for the Causes of Mental Disorders.* New York: Oxford University Press.

Susser, M (1968) *Community Psychiatry: Epidemiology and Social Themes.* New York: Random House.

Susser, M (1973) *Causal Thinking in the Health Sciences: Concepts and Strategies of Epidemiology.* New York: Oxford University Press.

Susser, M (1993) 'Health As a Human Right: an Epidemiologist's Perspective on the Public Health', *American Journal of Public Health,* 83, 418–26.

Susser, M and Stein, Z (2009) *Eras in Epidemiology: The Evolution of Ideas.* New York: Oxford University Press.

Susser, M and Susser, E (1996a) 'Choosing a Future for Epidemiology: I. Eras and Paradigms', *American Journal of Public Health,* 86, 668–73.

Susser, M and Susser, E (1996b) 'Choosing a Future for Epidemiology: II. From Black Box to Chinese Boxes and Eco-Epidemiology', *American Journal of Public Health,* 86, 674–77.

Sydenstricker, E (1935) 'The Changing Concept of Public Health', *The Milbank Memorial Fund Quarterly,* 13, 301–310.

Sydenstricker, E and Kasius, RV (ed) (1974) *The challenge of facts: selected public health papers of Edgar Sydenstricker.* New York: PRODIST.

Szreter, S (1988) 'The Importance of Social Intervention in Britain's Mortality Decline C. 1850–1914: a Reinterpretation of the Role of Public Health', *Social History of Medicine,* 1, 1–38.

Thornicroft, G (2006) *Shunned: Discrimination Against People With Mental Illness.* Oxford: Oxford University Press.

Thornicroft, G (2007) 'Most People With Mental Illness Are Not Treated', *The Lancet*, 370, 807–808.

Unknown artist (1837) Depiction of Slave in Shackles, appearing next to John Greenleaf Whittier's poem, 'My Countrymen in Chains!' *Rare Book, Broadside Collection, portfolio 118, no. 32A. Library of Congress.*

United Nations (2008) UN Convention on the Rights of Persons with Disabilities (UN CRPD). <http://www2.ohchr.org/english/law/disabilities-convention.htm>.

Ustun, TB (1999) 'The Global Burden of Mental Disorders', *American Journal of Public Health*, 89, 1315–1318.

Villermé, l (1826) *Rapport fait par M. Villermé, et lu à l'Academie Royale de Médicine, au Nom de la Commission de Statistique, sur une Serie de Tableaux Relatifs au Mouvement de la Population dans les Douze Arrondissements Municipaux de la Ville de Paris pendant les Cinq Années 1817, 1818, 1819, 1820, et 1821. Archives Genérales de Médicine*, 10, 216–45.

Wang, PS, Aguilar-Gaxiola, S, Alonso, J et al. (2007) 'Use of Mental Health Services for Anxiety, Mood, and Substance Disorders in 17 Countries in the WHO World Mental Health Surveys', *The Lancet*, 370, 841–50.

Weiner, DB (1979) 'The Apprenticeship of Philippe Pinel: a New Document, "Observations of Citizen Pussin on the Insane"', *American Journal of Psychiatry*, 136, 1128–34.

Weiner, DB (1992) 'Philippe Pinel's 'Memoir on Madness' of December 11, 1794: a Fundamental Text of Modern Psychiatry', *American Journal of Psychiatry*, 149, 725–32.

Weiner, DB (1993) *The Citizen-Patient in Revolutionary and Imperial Paris.* Baltimore: Johns Hopkins University Press.

Wilhelm, K, Arnold, K, Niven, H, and Richmond, R (2004) 'Grey lungs and blue moods: smoking cessation in the context of lifetime depression history', *Australian and New Zealand Journal of Psychiatry*, 38, 896–905.

Wilhelm, K, Wedgewood, L, Niven, H and Kay-Lambkin, F (2006) 'Smoking cessation and depression: current knowledge and future directions', *Drug and Alcohol Review*, 25, 97–107.

World Health Organization (2001) *The World Health Report 2001: Mental Health: New Understanding, New Hope.* Geneva: WHO.

World Health Organization Department of Mental Health and Substance Abuse (2005) *Mental Health Atlas.* Geneva: WHO.

Yach, D, Hawkes, C, Gould, CL, and Hofman, KJ (2004) 'The global burden of chronic diseases', *JAMA*, 291, 2616–2622.

Yach, D, Leeder, SR, Bell, J, and Kistnasamy, B (2005) 'Editorial: Global Chronic Diseases', *Science*, 307, 317.

Part 2

Human Rights Abuses, Psychiatry, Nation States, and Markets

These chapters principally focus on the role of nation states, though the final chapter in this section, on psychiatrists and the pharmaceutical industry, illustrates the relevance of our topic in the context of multinational corporations and markets.

Michael Dudley and Fran Gale use the background of contemporary human rights abuses by mental health professionals, and the enduring legacies of the Holocaust, to examine the actions of Nazi doctors and psychiatrists, and the lasting outcomes of the Nuremberg medical and other trials for human rights and mental health. The main focus of the chapter, however, concerns motives for harming, bystanding, and helping that these events highlighted, the understanding of which underpins human rights abuses and also their remediation.

Robert van Voren describes and analyses totalitarian political abuses of psychiatry. In the former Soviet Union, he notes how dissent and 'grandiose reformism' were repressed through expanding psychiatric diagnosis and incarcerations in Special Hospitals, and how science and clinical practice bowed to state power as key psychiatrists knowingly developed and implemented this system on Party and KGB orders. For many Soviet psychiatrists this system seemed logical (to give up everything for such fundamentally different convictions seemed 'madness') and avoided difficult questions with authorities. The World Psychiatric Association suspended Soviet membership in the 1980s until abuses were halted; the subsequent discussions on medical and psychiatric ethics resulted in WPA declarations. In China, dissidents reported psychiatric abuses in the Falun Gong crackdown from 1999. However, China's officially published psychiatric and legal literature indicates large-scale political abuse of psychiatry from the 1950s and 1960s, increasing enormously during the Cultural Revolution, thereafter emulating that in the Soviet Union. A network of high security forensic psychiatric institutions managed a sizeable percentage of political cases, which recently may have decreased. Information restrictions would prevent most Chinese psychiatrists knowing this. Paradoxically and separately, a lack of state control over psychiatry has resulted general psychiatric hospitals increasingly incarcerating 'petitioners' or whistleblowers in cases that may not have political connotation. Chinese media increasingly report these abuses, which are aggravated by deficient uniform psychiatric training and national mental health legislation protecting patients' rights. The Ministry of Public Security has recently

(May 2010) emphasized that monitoring mechanisms must be established for mental hospitals, which must avoid giving of private favors during legal validation procedures, and not admit anyone who is not a mental patient.

Derrick Silove, Susan Rees, and Zachary Steel review the modern international movement that sought to abolish torture and support refugee survivors, culminating in the 1984 Convention Against Torture whose prohibition is absolute. They discuss arguments against torture, including risks of torturing the wrong person, for wrong reasons, and/or eliciting wrong information; and the empirical finding that torture is a potent cause of PTSD, to a lesser degree of depression, and in final analyses remains the strongest factor predicting PTSD risk. Whether the staple of post-torture treatment is psychotherapy for trauma or a broad-based, multidisciplinary psychosocial approach, focusing on resettlement, acculturation, language acquisition, and building resiliency, is debatable. The unraveling consensus against torture in the 'war on terror' after '9/11' is described, the qualified support of leading academics, and the US Bush Administration's subversion of the Geneva Conventions, pursuing enhanced interrogations while denying these caused physical or psychological harm. Steps leading societies towards torture include the role of political leaders, propaganda and dehumanizing language, overriding normal judicial processes for 'national security', attacking critics, and offering plausible excuses afterwards, including deniability. The authors particularly review the lack of evidence that supports mental health professionals assessing and monitoring torture.

James Welsh explores the death penalty in human rights law and ethics, its implementation and the role of health and mental health professionals. Executing people with serious mental illness or intellectual disability contravenes norms of justice and rational penal policy. The death penalty is a cruel and inhuman punishment that provokes and worsens mental disorder and suffering of the condemned and his or her family, and has a brutalizing effect on those carrying out the penalty and society in general. While international standards exempt children and people with mental and intellectual disabilities, in practice these groups are not always spared this punishment. The American Medical Association holds the only ethical involvement is in supporting the patient, not facilitating the execution. Welsh documents the challenge posed to mental health professionals, since mental competence is relevant to standing trial, to terminating appeals, for 'qualifying' for execution. Treating to restore competence for execution is unethical, while intervening in attempted suicide on death row to allow the state to do the job soon after raises ethical challenges. Not identifying mental impairments in those accused and subsequent disregard for their rights is evident at each step. The issue raises questions about wider social issues: the quality and availability of mental health services, and the need for mental health professionals to speak out for abolition.

Danny Sullivan and Paul Mullen consider the rights of those doubly stigmatized as mentally disordered and criminal. Citizens committing serious criminal offences and mentally ill people unable to protect themselves or others both forfeit some civil rights. Offending and mental illness curtail rights in the name of justice and therapy. Deinstitutionalization, intended to end coercion and exclusion, preceded a trend towards compulsory hospital admissions and community treatment orders, thus perpetuating coercion in less forbidding places. Forensic psychiatry services and secure hospitals have grown substantially. Minimal standards for these services and for mentally ill offenders are sometimes deflected by populist media outrage. The authors consider the relationship between prisons and asylums (or hospitals), and for secure mental health institutions, and the tensions between therapeutic and custodial goals and cultures. Civil commitment necessitates diagnostic or dysfunction criteria, and/or incapacity to consent, treatment refusal, treatability, and other thresholds, such as harm to self or others, least restrictive environment, and *parens patriae*. The authors discuss capacity-based commitment, arguments against commitment, coercive cultures, and the situation of the mentally abnormal offender: the problems of (especially compulsory) treatment in prisons, transfer to hospitals, sexuality, and political dissent. The challenges for mental health professionals of providing care are scrutinized.

Alan Rosen, Tully Rosen, and Patrick McGorry, in reviewing the rights of people with serious and persistent mental illness, examine the significance and origins of the mental health and human rights advocacy movement, its political setting, and 'reforms' with different, even opposing agendas. Concerning the debate over involuntary treatment, tensions between rights are discerned: the right to autonomy (or to refuse treatment) encounters the right to treatment and/ or access to health care, and also encounters the right of others to health and safety. Selfdetermination, undergirded by the UN Principles (1991), includes participation in decisionmaking, civic life, and citizen roles, and should not be confused with 'dying with one's rights on' — civic abandonment that opposes paternalism on the pendulum of injustice. The authors distinguish dominant from alternative paradigms: prevailing individualistic international approaches in mental health and rights are contrasted with collectivist, multifaceted models. Alternative formulations attempt to bridge medical and social domains, and include indigenous healing systems. To effect change, the authors engage with and affirm complex, layered understandings. Stakeholder miscommunications are reviewed. Systemic abuses and neglects of psychiatry occur in authoritarian regimes, but also with coercive treatments, including for forensic patients and those in police custody. Improvements include increasing media scrutiny and public information access, advances in early intervention, minimizing and regulating involuntary treatment, adopting user-focused definitions of recovery including quality of life, advance directives, shared decision-making, and collectivist as well as individualistic solutions. To enhance social inclusion, the authors advocate including all stakeholder groups in service participation, overturning laws that breach rights, and addressing power imbalances. Significantly, they outline and strongly advocate for the application of a comprehensive repertoire of many of these strategies, including interactive consultative methods, which if systematically applied within mental health services, could substantially reduce and obviate the need for much involuntary treatment and care.

Jonathan Marks draws on cognitive and behavioural psychology to provide an account of how health professionals became complicit in the abuse of detainees in the 'war on terror'. It recognizes that health professionals did not act in isolation, and highlights the role of both macro (social, political, and cultural) and meso (organizational and community) factors that may have contributed to their behaviours. Drawing on the same body of social science research, the chapter also offers some potential measures to address and prevent the complicity of health professionals. These measures include constructing counternarratives, debiasing, acculturating human rights in social and institutional frameworks, developing ethics and policy guidelines, education and mentorship in ethics and human rights, and structural reforms. The role of accountability mechanisms is also discussed, and recommendations made for further qualitative and quantitative research to test and enrich the explanatory account, and to help refine and tailor more effective efforts at prevention and remediation.

Reviewing coercive psychiatry, Thomas Kallert notes inconsistencies in mental health legislation in European countries, the greater effectiveness of the European Convention of Human Rights regarding unwanted treatment than access to treatment, and inequities in individual access to the European Court of Human Rights depending on the degree of democracy in the applicant's country and access to legal assistance. Some psychiatrists and psychiatric bodies have advanced proposals to address legal discrimination against those with severe and persistent mental illness. Clinically, patients report various coercions (restrictions on movement, forced medication, patronizing communication, property confiscated, not knowing one's legal status), and sometimes involuntary commitment and treatment are not distinguished. Reducing coercion requires leadership and policy to reduce and regulate seclusion and restraint, incident management systems and data reporting, staff training, independent patient advocates, emergency response teams, reducing unit sizes, improving patient-staff ratios, using second generation antipsychosis medications, and increasing non-pharmacological treatments. Re-institutionalization may promote complacency about standards. Stakeholders differ about the CRPD's implications, but the ability of mental health systems and laws to reduce coercion requires re-examination, as also coercion in non-psychiatric residential settings, non-Western countries, and totalitarian regimes. There is a need for further discussions between all parties whatever their positions.

Philip Mitchell examines the challenge to the reputation of psychiatry arising from its aberrant relationship with pharmaceutical companies. There has been public, media, and institutional concern about this relationship. Proceeding from the assumption that it is not the relationship per se but how it operates, the chapter considers how it is dysfunctional and may be reformed. The chapter reviews general literature on the relationship of doctors to industry, specific points of contact, why psychiatrists are in the dubious lead, and how various bodies are responding, through professional organizations, medical schools, medical journals, and pharmaceutical industry organizations. The challenge of integrity and transparency is one that affects credibility and confidence in the profession.

In their commentary, Vikram Patel, Arthur Kleinman, and Benedetto Saraceno observe that while the rights of people with mental disorders are violated in all regions of the world, and while headway has been made towards addressing these in many Western settings, this is not so for the majority of people with mental disorders residing in developing countries. The authors underscore their horrifying abuse using de-identified images as well as text. The authors closely examine the ethics of using such images. These portray forgotten people, denied basic care, often robbed of the ability to protest their grievances, stripped of rights and dignity. There is reason to believe that the practices portrayed — privations, restraints, seclusion, abuses, neglect — are common or certainly not unrepresentative, rather than aberrations. These circumstances prevail, not only in mental institutions but in homes and communities. The authors highlight the origins in several factors, notably stigma, institutional cultures, lack of community mental health initiatives, and the silence of the global health and mental health communities. They contend that combatting this shameful situation is the single most important priority for global mental health. They have declared a call to action on this issue, in the form of a global mental health movement.

Meg Smith provides a historical perspective with sharp contemporary relevance, as she details what it was like to be treated for a major mental illness in New South Wales in the 1980s. She describes the vagaries of legislation regarding compulsory detention and treatment, including lack of requirement for corroborating evidence of mental illness, lack of legal representation or medical attendance at hearings, and failure to consult with relatives and carers. She notes in hospitals the lack of protection against assault, lack of recognition and response regarding iatrogenic effects of medication, automatic takeover of one's financial affairs with assets used to pay fees, and the contemporaneous tragic scandal of Chelmsford Hospital's deep sleep programme. She recalls how, following the method of Rosenhan's classic study, her postgraduate psychology class admitted themselves to mental hospitals with fictitious symptoms of mental illness, and how she did not have to do the class exercise because she got academic credit for being a real patient. She details the advent of consumer movements and community care, legislative reforms and official enquiries that began to change these trends, noting that while the law has improved in several ways, there is much to do strengthening social resources.

Chapter 11

Through a Glass, Darkly

Nazi Era Illuminations of Psychiatry, Human Rights, and Rights Violations

Michael Dudley and Fran Gale

Introduction

This chapter and its companion (Chapter 38) evaluate the lessons and legacies of the Nazi era for human rights and mental health: specifically, understandings, practices, and remedial and preventive responses related to genocide, mass human rights violations, and state-based abuses of psychiatry and mental health.

Nazism is not a closed episode. Like nuclear war and environmental destruction, it warrants universal concern. Mental health and helping professionals have played key roles in waging the 'war on terror'. A British doctor recently (2007) attempted to bomb Glasgow airport. Che Guevara, Radovan Karadjic, and doctors supporting Hamas provide other examples of doctors or psychiatrists allied to state violence. Though it is imperative that helping professionals ponder professional abuses and their origins, contemporary bioethics generally neglects this record (Caplan 2007:70–71). Individual professionals may exploit patients in a manner universally regarded as criminal or in breach of codes, but also may follow political–institutional or state-based rules without necessarily knowing (or perhaps 'knowing'—that is, they are denying at some level) that their behaviours are abusive. Such systemic abuses frequently involve loyalties divided between patients and third parties—in this case, the state. (Corporations are considered elsewhere (Philip Mitchell, Chapter 18)).

This first chapter initially notes how mental health professionals abused human rights in the 'war on terror'. Against this contemporary setting, we examine the actions of Nazi doctors and psychiatrists, the lasting outcomes of the Nuremberg medical and other trials for both human rights and mental health, and most significantly, the motives and reasons for harming, bystanding, and rescuing.

We chose the Holocaust because of its historical significance for human rights, and because it is a pure case of genocide that has been researched in great detail and therefore is instructive about the causes and remediation of human rights abuses. Motivating questions include: 'What prevents today's doctors, psychiatrists, and helping professionals falling from grace in comparable ways?' and 'Given the Holocaust's interplay of individual, situational, and social factors, where should the emphasis in prevention lie?' The answers matter greatly for states, institutions, and professional and other communities that must safeguard against recurrence. Chapter 38 further explores the inheritance of the Nazi era for psychiatrists and other helping professionals. It considers the helping professional as a positive socially engaged agent; justice, reconciliation, and mental health concerns in response to rights violations; and the prospect of genuine change based in professional reforms and social movements. Psychiatrists and doctors are most in focus, because of the wealth of evidence, but also other mental health and helping professionals.

The contemporary setting: human rights abuses specific to mental health

The 'war on terror' has damaged the human rights achievements that followed the Second World War. The US G.W. Bush Administration produced this result through 'renditions' of suspects to places of torture, through undermining the International Criminal Court, and by using notorious centres such as Guantanamo Bay and Abu Ghraib prison (the former site of Saddam Hussein's tortures, murders, and experiments) (Ehrenfreund 2007:209–213).

Multiple investigations into Abu Ghraib expose that it was overcrowded and un-sewered, its staff and prisoners frequently killed or traumatized by constant shelling. Sweeps and checkpoints collected blameless civilians and families, and fear of their joining the insurgency and absence of administrative authority foiled their release. Missing was leadership by its new inexperienced commander and other principals; staff training, supervision, accountability and co-ordination; and any capacity to care for prisoner children and inmates with contagious diseases or mental illness (Zimbardo 2007).

Frustrated higher commanders determined to extract 'actionable intelligence' from suspected insurgents. Major General Geoffrey Miller, visiting from Guantanamo Bay, stated he wanted Abu Ghraib's prisoners 'treated like dogs' (Karpinski 2004, 2005). Post-Korean war programmes, developed to enable military personnel to survive interrogations, were modified. They included long-term isolation, threats, exploitation of phobias, inducement of fear (including through use of dogs), severe (including sexual) humiliation and sometimes sexual assault, degrading 'trophy photography', and sleep deprivation (Sontag 2003; Bloche and Marks 2005; Zimbardo 2007: 362–365). Both military and civilian suspects were held indefinitely, and their Geneva Convention rights to fair trial and freedom from 'cruel, inhuman and degrading' treatment were brushed aside. Abu Ghraib's civilian interrogators were anonymous and lawless, sometimes killing with impunity.

Philip Zimbardo rejects the emphasis on individual character which blamed a minority of low-ranking individuals ('bad apples'). Instead he highlights situational and wider social contexts (the 'bad barrel' and 'bad barrel makers' respectively) (Zimbardo 2007). His interviews with Sergeant Chip Frederick, a key operations manager whom he was asked to help defend, reveal that untrained army reservists despised by fellow-soldiers committed the abuses. Lack of actionable intelligence led to further pressure to break prisoners. Frederick, who previously acted as a guard in a low security prison, had no record of violence or antisocial behaviour, and his personality testing was unremarkable. Yet he was responsible for attaching electrodes to a hooded prisoner who was forced to stand on a box and told that if he moved he would be electrocuted. While Frederick received a severe sentence, heads of state and senior 'architects' (politicians, lawyers, security chiefs), military leaders, and medical personnel, escaped prosecution (Zimbardo 2007:324–443).

US Department of Defense documents show that health professionals worked in behavioural science consultation teams to facilitate coercive interrogations. They formulated general and individual interrogation approaches, allowed interrogators to exploit detainees' medical records, certified detainees' fitness, monitored interrogations, falsified medical records and death certificates, and failed to report abuses and to provide basic medical care (Miles 2004; Zimbardo 2007).

Not only did higher command not authorize and check tactics, but directives for health professionals diverged from human rights standards. Some argued that as they were not operating as clinicians, patient ethical codes did not apply. Ethical guidelines from the US Presidential Task Force on Psychological Ethics and National Security did not prohibit psychologists' participation, nor require their adherence to international human rights law regardless of interpretation by military authorities (Bloche and Marks 2005). The American Psychological Association initially endorsed interrogation up to a 'sub-torture threshold', and was accused of dispensing with traditional ethical standards outside the strictly therapeutic context, by separating clinical from non-clinical duties. However, such coercive, deceptive procedures depart from the doctor–patient relationship with its precondition of voluntary, informed consent. Even if physicians did not participate directly, their presence legitimated and sanitized it. The American Psychiatric Association stated that not only should psychiatrists not participate in torture, but should not be part of interrogations; and that they have a responsibility to report situations of torture. However, Abu Ghraib's psychiatrist was employed not to meet the needs of mentally ill detainees or staff, but to help make interrogations more effective (Zimbardo 2007: 362). Moreover, there is no indication that doctors have the kind of skills that are useful in interrogation per se. Silove and colleagues, and Marks consider this issue in their chapters.

Enduring legacies of the Holocaust

The Nazi era arguably represents the nadir of modern Western history. At its heart are six million Jewish victims, not counting other murdered groups, and actions so enormous, cruel, and intricate as to be unbelievable. Surviving and remembering such horrors forever changes feeling, thinking, imagination, and memory (e.g. Levi 1987; Higgins 2003, 2006). The death camps are another universe, defying speech (Adorno 1955 (1967)). SS militiamen taunted their prisoners with this prospect of denial and disbelief as they worked to destroy all traces of evidence. Fortunately their quest failed (Levi 1987:1–2). The Holocaust is a thoroughly documented historical event, as well as a universal symbol for radical evil, and a yardstick for crimes against humanity (Alexander et al. 2009). US Prosecutor Robert Jackson stated in his opening address at the first Nuremberg trial, 'The wrongs which we seek to condemn and punish have been so calculated, so malignant and so devastating that civilisation cannot tolerate their being ignored because it cannot survive their being repeated'.

Mirroring and harnessing Western modernity, Nazism used technology and bureaucracy to pursue its ideologically driven, murderous racism (Bauman 1989; Bauer 2001). Its economic, environmental, and public health emphases are familiar, captivating, and confronting (Dudley and Gale 2002). Holocaust analysts divide populations by their responses: perpetrators (numbering around two million), bystanders (numbering 100s of millions), and rescuers, maybe a few tens of thousands (Bauer 2001). These categories, while heuristically useful, are not watertight. Bavarian peasants, for example, dealt with Jewish cattle dealers despite Nazi attempts to prevent this, yet often approved anti-Semitic laws (Kershaw 2000:193). In the camps' 'grey zone', victims sometimes were accomplices (*kapos*, etc) to perpetrators, though perpetrators were not victims (Levi 1987). Despite the Nazi state's genocide and criminality, the actors were neither angels nor demons, but ordinary people (Bauer 2001; Browning 1998). Holocaust remembrance continues for victims and survivors, and for nations, communities, and professions to prevent amnesia and protect against recurrence.

Nazi doctors and psychiatrists: activities

A particular breach of trust occurs when physicians abandon their special responsibilities (Lifton 1986; Grodin and Annas 2007; Annas and Grodin 1992). That doctors as helping professionals should act as architects, leaders, and auxiliaries of mass murder, conducting lethal experiments on behalf of a transgressive state, may beggar belief: yet after the Second World War, prosecution investigators at the Nuremberg and other medical trials exposed and thoroughly documented such activities on a large scale (Alexander 1948, 1949). These transgressions of doctors, psychiatrists, and other professionals under Nazism have been extensively examined (see Grodin and Annas (2007); Schmidt (2006); Weindling (2006); Baum (2008); Dudley and Gale (2002); and Markusen (1997) for examples of recent bibliographies). Such a debacle was unprecedented. Education and professional status rather than conferring immunity, generally facilitated the Nazi agenda. Medicine in particular was united to the Nazi state, with psychiatry the chief medical specialty represented in the killing programmes (Dudley and Gale 2002): without them the Holocaust would have failed (Weindling 2006:94–95; Markusen 1997).

As the Nazis removed moral restraints, they quickly ceased to ratify advanced Weimar Republic legislation on human experimentation (Hanauski-Abel 1996). However, clinicians and scientists then decisively abandoned medical and psychiatric ethics when they promoted and participated in compulsory sterilization. Doctors, psychiatrists, welfare, church, and community groups supported the 1933 law, which required mandatory reporting and was widely enforced. Lawyers, doctors, and psychiatrists manned courts which heard cases in secret and allowed few successful appeals. The law encompassed those suffering from schizophrenia, manic depressive insanity, hereditary epilepsy, alcoholism, and Huntingdon's chorea, as well as hereditary blindness, hereditary deafness, severe deformity, and congenital feeble-mindedness. The last, a vague, flexible category, captured social deviance (such as prostitution under 'moral feeble-mindedness'), and accounted for three-quarters of cases, including many in poverty. Sterilization also allowed asylum directors to discharge patients and cut costs. Many patients died of surgical complications (Lifton 1986:25; Bock 1997:161–2; Evans 2006:507–511).

From 1939 in occupied Poland, adults with mental disabilities were killed, including with poisoned gas, the first trial of this method. In Germany, doctors, psychiatrists, nurses, and other helping professionals and staff joined with administrators in the Tiergartenstrasse (T4) so-called 'euthanasia' programme for children. Gassing was extended to adults with mental disabilities. Hitler authorized the T4 programme outside law in a few lines on his private letterhead (Kershaw 2008:40). The criteria for killing were both 'eugenic' (including 'non-Aryan') and economic, related to potential productivity, but in practice were sacrificed for quotas and administrative efficiency. As an open secret, which claimed 200,000 victims, 'euthanasia' had many accomplices: the myth of a small group of fanatical perpetrators hoodwinking a public who knew nothing is untenable (Friedlander 1995; Bauer 2001; Evans 2006:507–511; Evans 2009:72–101).

This dress rehearsal provided senior expertise to killing centres in the occupied territories, for the so-called '14f13' programme that claimed approximately 50,000 concentration camp victims (Lifton 1986; Schmidt 2006:271). Then from mid-1941, doctors and psychiatrists oversaw the 'Final Solution', manning camps, performing executions and selections and providing ideological justifications (Lifton 1986; Proctor 1992:27). In all phases, they exploited the murdered and the living for medical research. Coerced inmates underwent at least 26 types of experiments including ice water immersion, high altitude decompression, high dose radiation, and making seawater drinkable, and often died in the search for better killing methods or through callous disregard (Caplan 2007:67; Schmidt 2006:160ff). While most experiments were scientifically useless (Weindling 2006:4), the possible exceptions (e.g. hypothermia and decompression) raised sharp ethical questions about using knowledge obtained by such means (Moreno 2007; Muller-Hill 1988).

The motives of perpetrators—among which peer pressure, duress, authoritarianism, careerism, and ideology featured prominently—are explored below. Specifically, Nazi pseudo-science ('race hygiene', 'scientific racism', and eugenics) and its biomedical engineering project for a *judenrein* utopia dovetailed perfectly with the experimental ambitions of scientists, doctors, and psychiatrists, whose careers prospered. Few psychiatrists resisted and no letters survive from psychiatrists on behalf of their patients to the authorities (Dudley and Gale 2002). As noted, nurses (McFarland-Icke 1999) participated in killings, while psychologists (Mandler 2002) were also implicated in the Nazi debacle.

When the war ended, the ensuing trials and plethora of psychiatrist and physician suicides confirmed the debasement of German medicine. A US de-nazification report estimated that about half of German physicians were 'proven Nazis' (about 24,000, against the profession's later view of only 350 criminal doctors) (Weindling 2006:38–39). What had gone wrong, and how, was too complex for a trial which piloted new international law (Schmidt 2006:3, 168).

Doctors and medical scientists denied complicity by representing themselves as victims of Nazism. Unrepentant Nazis, conservatives, and leading physicians disparaged the trials as 'victors' justice', and suppressed publications by the trial's medical observers (Weindling 2006:5, 39, 43, 211–217). German medical associations avoided examining their Nazi past (Pross 1992; Kater 1997) and exonerated individuals by blaming socialized medicine and excessive state powers, while insisting on professional autonomy (Weindling 2006:6; Schmidt 2006:266). Cold War priorities (strategic research and intelligence) also protected those who were implicated. (Contemporaneously, US authorities gave Japanese Unit 731, which also conducted biological warfare experiments accounting for 270,000 victims, immunity from prosecution (Weindling 2006:309, 342)). In the 1980s, a research-granting agency which funded Robert Ritter's project (see under 'Nazi doctors and psychiatrists: motivations and reasons'), refused to acknowledge that its precursor financed the genocide (Müller-Hill 2007:59). Medical institutes and researchers used materials from murdered victims before this was outlawed and the remains reburied in 1989 (Müller-Hill 2007:61; Hanauski-Abel 1996). Nazi influence also affected the World Medical Association, which virtually ignored the Nuremberg Code (see under 'Positive outcomes from the doctors' trials: the Nuremberg Code and its successors') (Kater, 1997; Schmidt 2006:266).

Human rights outcomes of the Nuremberg trials

The post-war Nuremberg trials of the Nazi leadership (1945–49) were landmark events, defining new standards of international justice with far-reaching significance for human rights. An International Military Tribunal defined crimes such as conspiring against peace, waging aggressive war, and a new category, crimes against humanity, and tried the former Nazi military leaders for these and for war crimes. The trials of Nazi doctors, the *Einsatzgruppen* (killing squads), jurists and industrialists, the war crimes trials in the separate zones of occupation, and national prosecutions in various German-occupied countries followed (Ehrenfreund 2007). All four occupying powers exercised sovereignty and tried the German accused for crimes against pre-Nazi German law.

The trials overthrew, at least partially, the principle of national sovereignty (established in the Treaty of Westphalia in 1648) which bestowed immunity on state functionaries within state borders. States and other authorities could not wilfully disregard individuals' rights. The trials also demolished the defence of superior orders, and the 'tu quoque' ('you did it too') defence, thus re-asserting the principle of individual moral responsibility, eroded by authoritarian leadership (Schmidt 2006:250). They affected the rules of war and treatment of prisoners. International trials, bridging gulfs of language, nationality, custom, and procedure, proved feasible. For grave crimes, the principle of universal jurisdiction held that any country where they are committed could judge and punish an individual for the international community. The trials of Nazi industrialists foreshadowed lawsuits against businesses accused of human rights abuses (Ehrenfreund 2007:107–110, 215–219).

Furthermore, the extensive, authoritative documentation of Nazi atrocities '[established] these perceived "incredible" events by clear and public proof, so that no one can ever doubt that they were fact not fable' (US Prosecutor Telford Taylor, quoted by Schmidt 2006:174). This inaugurated Holocaust history, belied future Holocaust denial, and shaped German democracy.

Raphael Lemkin coined the word 'genocide' to describe the German authorities' systematic murder of ethnic and religious groups defined as degenerate. Arguing that genocide should denote the motivation to commit such crimes, he criticized the new category 'crimes against humanity' for neglecting this motivation. How much the medical trials applied this reasoning is a moot point (Weindling 2006:3, 102); Telford Taylor regarded the experiments as pilot studies for genocide (Weindling 2006:5; Schmidt 2006:161).

The Nuremberg trials (and for medicine the Nuremberg Code) were three great contemporaneous reforms, together with the formation of the United Nations (1945) and the Universal Declaration of Human Rights (1948). Collectively, they helped launch the international human rights movement and frameworks, including the Convention on the Prevention and Punishment of the Crime of Genocide, the Geneva Conventions on laws and customs of war, the European Court of Human Rights, the Bill of Rights, and subsequent rights treaties and institutions. They are relevant not just for medicine and mental health, but civil society and planetary survival (Robertson 2006; Ehrenfreund 2007).

However, enforcement has been piecemeal. During and after the Cold War, no international machinery underwrote human rights protections. Genocide continued: today, perpetrators in places like East Timor and Darfur remain free. The United States circumvented international standards in its 'war on terror'. The charge of 'victors' justice' (made by Hermann Goering at Nuremberg) endures: the Allies were not tried for dropping the atom bomb, for example. Nevertheless, the Nuremberg legacy endures in the Pinochet, Milosevic, and Tadic trials, the advent of the International Criminal Court, and recent international actions to address genocide—the Kosovo bombings and the tribunals or special courts for the former Yugoslavia, Rwanda, Sierra Leone, and Cambodia (Ehrenfreund 2007:153–196; Robertson 2006).

Positive outcomes from the doctors' trials: the Nuremberg Code and its successors

While the patient's health and protection from harm date from Hippocrates, informed consent and non-therapeutic experimentation only emerged in 19th century codes of ethics and pre-Nazi (1900 and 1931) German documents that thoroughly discussed these issues (Grodin 1992; Winau 2007).

The Nuremberg doctors' trial ended with a declaration about permissible medical experiments. In Europe and the US however, frequent dangerous medical experiments continued. Re-discovery of the 'Nuremberg Code' in the 1960s as the first global, comprehensive reflection on the nature, purpose, and limits of human experimentation was vital to identifying and addressing this area (Weindling 2006:340–343; Perley et al, 1992; Grodin 1992).

Pre-eminently the Code (<http://www.ushmm.org/research/doctors/Nuremberg_Code.htm>) requires voluntary informed consent. It mandates qualified researchers, socially beneficial intent, scientific design, and results unobtainable by other methods. Benefits must outweigh risks, harm must be minimized, and risk to life prevented (except when researchers experiment on themselves). Subjects must be allowed to withdraw at any time. Researcher responsibility for participants' well-being is paramount.

The Code's successors, not comprehensively discussed here, assert the rights of health research participants. They include the World Medical Association's Declaration of Helsinki (DoH) (1964, revised 1975, 1983, 1989, 1996, 2000, 2008, with clarifications 2002, 2004), which has formed the cornerstone of human research ethics. For vulnerable populations such as children, prisoners, and military personnel, the DoH emphasized physician responsibility (Schmidt 2006:283) and softened the Code's absolute requirement of voluntary informed consent, instead requiring consent by legal guardians ('responsible relatives' for children; minors should consent where possible). Nevertheless the first DoH revision (1975) confirmed that the interests of science and society should never take precedence over the well-being of the subject (paragraph III. 4), and decreed that research ethics committees (or equivalent) must oversee research, initiating what is now widespread practice (Williams 2008).

The Council for the International Organizations of Medical Sciences (CIOMS), formed by the World Health Organization (WHO) and UNESCO, also developed the International Ethical Guidelines for Biomedical Research Involving Human Subjects (1982; CIOMS-WHO 1993), which despite some inconsistencies with DoH (Macklin 1999), were also informed by the Code. In communal and non-Western research settings, they noted difficulties with informed consent, research knowledge, funding, and governance (Perley et al. 1992). Successive DoH revisions have fired controversies about principled versus pragmatic approaches to research ethics in the developing world (Lurie and Wolfe 1997; Lie et al. 2004; Social Medicine Portal 2008; Rennie 2008; Sharma 2004).

Motives and reasons for harming by individuals and groups: the Nazi example

The Holocaust like other great evils was inhuman, yet humans were responsible. Social science lexicons rarely discuss evil, and behavioural scientists and clinicians reluctantly examine it, thus magnifying its apparent incomprehensibility. Some consign evil to the province of philosophers and theologians, or alternatively (and positivistically) reduce it to behaviour, biology, or mental illness. This dishonours those with a genuine mental illness and relieves culprits of responsibility (Rosen 2011). Actually the political and military elite of the Third Reich rarely suffered overt mental illness, though the fact that these were 'ordinary men' (Browning 1998) does not mean they were mentally healthy. Clinical science however cannot exclude (im)moral acts from its purview, nor reduce them to judgements about (ab)normality. Like morality, it assays not just events and causes, but who we are, should be, and take ourselves to be (Glas 2006). Patients may interpret professional neutrality on such matters as indifference.

Evil encompasses moral wrongness as an end (the intent to harm) or a means to an end (Oxford English Dictionary), and extreme harm, through acts disproportionate to any instigation or provocation. Bandura (1975) refers to 'moral disengagement', which involves suspending proactive humane behaviour and abandoning restraints on harmful behaviour. Some note the persistence of such acts, victims' helplessness, levels of perpetrator responsibility, and sometimes the 'magnitude gap' between damage to victims and benefits accruing to perpetrators (Berkowitz 1999; Hamilton and Sanders 1999; Staub 2003:47–51). Omission may also be evil. Card's (2002:3) definition of evils as 'foreseeable intolerable harms produced by culpable wrongdoing' leaves open the question of intent, which may be complex, even impenetrable (Staub 2003:49). Noting humanity's potential for good and evil, this perspective bypasses essentialist dichotomies.

As well as Holocaust history, other genocides (not considered in detail here), and experimental psychology reveal that recurring individual, socio-cultural, and situational factors contribute to mass human rights violations. Theories about the origins of Nazi doctors and psychiatrists' actions must not only consider these levels of action, but the wider German national situation. In the following sections, the Nazi example and experimental evidence are reviewed to shed light on motives and reasons for harming, bystanding, and helping. To direct prevention, it is also important to decide where the 'engine-room' is located.

Personality

Early researchers considered innate characteristics: Adorno and colleagues (1955) described the 'authoritarian personality' (characterized by conventionalism, authority submission, aggression, projection, and anti-introspection) self-selecting for the Party and SS. Rather than one (authoritarian) Nazi personality, unsurprisingly a range exists. For example, Robert Lifton (1986) describes SS doctor Josef Mengele's scientific detachment, flamboyance, and fanatical cruelty, chief Auschwitz doctor Eduard Wirths' meticulousness and obedience, gynaecologist and mass sterilizer Carl Clauberg's arrogant ambition. A frequent theme, noted with Lifton's doctor Ernst B, and Gitta Sereny's studies of Franz Stangl, the commandant of Treblinka (1974) and Albert Speer, Hitler's architect and from 1942 munitions/armaments minister (1995), is of people emotionally starved or abused as children, struggling to make human connections and seeking liveliness in movements of national regeneration. Stangl feared resistance and was intimidated. Despite Speer's burden of guilt, his wish for transformation and to make amends, his narcissism prevented him empathizing with the humanity of his slave labourers or the Jews whom he saw deported from Berlin, and even reciprocating the love of those close to him (Sereny 1996; Kubarych 2005). Speer's problem with denial is treated under 'Language, and the problem with and function of denial'.

Interplay between personality, group, situational, and social determinants

However, Adorno and colleagues postulated a relationship between authoritarian personality and the group and/or social environment (Baum 2008:2). Studies of mass human rights violations highlight how cultures of obedience, whether populist, authoritarian, collectivist, or fundamentalist, reject social diversity and dissent. Frequently male-dominated, they avoid critical thinking, prize loyalty, honour, and death for the group, and identify and punish their enemies. Institutional and informational control, indoctrination, creating fear and agonizing uncertainty, destruction of family and social bonds, and brainwashing children (e.g. as soldiers) all enable radical, utopian actions: violence against family, intimates, moral codes (Glover 1999; Cohen 2001; Pina e Cunha et al. 2010). Women are often particularly vulnerable (Baum 2008:48–49). In Nazism, personality and situational determinants both contributed to the outcome of racist ideology. While individual doctors and scientists were centrally responsible, sponsored by the Nazi state, the failure of German society and institutions and the force of situations and social roles must also be understood.

Hitler is the most striking example in point. In the 1980s 'historians' debate' (Mason, 1989; Baum 2008:26), intentionalists (e.g. Dawidowicz 1975) emphasized the importance of Hitler's master plan as expressed in 'Mein Kampf', while functionalists minimized Hitler's role. They stressed anarchic forces, such as opportunism from Nazism's lower ranks, and bureaucratic chaos and infighting which drove improvisation and increasingly radical agendas (e.g. Browning 1998, 2004). A more nuanced synthesis of intentionalism and functionalism now prevails (Bauer 2001). Thus, Hitler's charismatic authority (Kershaw 2008) backed actions, however radical or inhumane, which furthered his ideological obsessions. His non-interventive style permitted party bosses, bureaucrats, and professionals full scope for initiative in implementation. Since opportunities abounded for expansion, power, status, and enrichment, there was never any shortage of chaotic rival schemes or willing participants. One might denounce neighbours to the Gestapo, slur a business competitor's 'Aryan' credentials, or nominate patients for the euthanasia programme: this was all 'working towards the Fuhrer' (Kershaw 2008; Bankier 1988; Michman 2010).

Adolf Eichmann's rise from obscurity to managing the 'Final Solution' follows this trajectory (Kershaw 2008). Hannah Arendt (1963) diagnosed Eichmann's 'banality of evil'; his incapacity to introspect and lack of inner language inclined him to unquestioning obedience to his assigned task, like a cog in a machine. Eichmann however was not devoid of ideological drivers. Though not radically anti-Semitic as a young man, he joined the party late as a bourgeois careerist and swiftly took on its programme (Berkowitz 1999; Cesarani 2006).

Yet the influence of individuals like Hitler on groups and wider society was also inevitably mutual. As we shall see, for example, in order to further pursue their programme the Nazis depended on public adulation or inertia and lack of resistance.

Socio-cultural and national–historical factors

Socio-cultural and national–historical factors contribute significantly to mass human rights violations (Zimbardo 2007:273–5; Staub 1989, 2003:352–353, 358). At a personal or cultural level, tribalism and ethnic nationalism can nurse old narratives that maintain enmity. Past victimization, enduring wounds, even early child-rearing may trigger reactive withdrawal or compensatory anger. Severe, persistent life conditions and struggle for resources may frustrate basic needs such as security, attachment, positive identity and role, effective control, justice, and meaning (Maslow 1987; Silove 2000). When an individual or group's self-concept is vulnerable, setbacks overwhelm collective and personal self-worth. Defensive superiority then forms a compensatory identity that diminishes and scapegoats others. Leaders who share the group's culture, life situations and often unhealed wounds (Staub 2003:302), may then propagate destructive ideologies to gain followers or consolidate a following (Allport 1954).

From its foundation in 1871, Germany was a weak (and ultimately a failed) state (Moore 1966; Steinmetz 1997; Kershaw 2008; Higgins 2006), and a non-existent state in the Third Reich period, as Franz Neumann (1967) pointed out contemporaneously. Its ideologies of 'race hygiene' and scientific racism, and the Great War's bitter legacies, were primers for eventual genocide. Defeat, revolution, and the Versailles Treaty's war guilt clauses fed the myth that Jews, socialists, communists, and war profiteers stabbed Germany in the back. Colossal reparations, foreign occupation of the Ruhr, and hyperinflation fuelled economic depression and social chaos. Hitler promised to redeem Germany by modernization, racial purification, and imperial conquest (Kershaw 2008:20). In the earlier Nazi years, many Germans experienced mystical, exalted states associated with nationalism (Soelle 2001), expressed in the resurgent economy, the spectacle of the Nuremberg rallies, the victories of German athletes at the Berlin Olympics, and Hitler's achievements in foreign affairs (Friedlander 2007). Psychiatrist Carl Jung, who loved pagan symbolism and myth, valorized the German peoples' revitalization under National Socialism (Noll 1997:264). With the coming of the Third Reich, however, state deliberative decision-making also completely disappeared, civilized standards collapsed, and barriers to state-sanctioned inhumanity were rapidly removed (Mommsen 1997; Kershaw 2008). Race hygiene replaced social and sexual health clinics. Waves of repression and violence descended on Jews and other minorities. Political opponents held in the new Dachau concentration camp were murdered (Evans 2004; Lifton 1986:25). Most Germans, however, were insulated from the experience of these groups.

The role of anti-Semitism is disputed. Earlier historians traced a lineage from Luther through Christian anti-Semitism to the Third Reich (e.g. McGovern 1973). However, several authorities suggest that anti-Semitism was weaker in Germany than in other Western countries (such as France), and certainly weaker than in Eastern Europe. For instance, from emancipation in 1848 till the Weimar Republic, German Jews did not die of anti-Semitic violence. During the Weimar period, polarization occurred between Jewish integration and intensifying anti-Semitism among various organizations and political parties, especially just after the First World War and also the years immediately preceding the Third Reich, but not the period in between.

From 30 January 1933, a cascade of disastrous policy, legal, and social developments overtook Jews (Abrahams-Sprod 2006). Hitler's anti-Semitism, 'calculation and fanaticism' (Bullock 1992) inspired these, and institutions, bureaucracies, and professions willingly implemented them.

However, Daniel Goldhagen's famous (1996) thesis that anti-Semitism among ordinary Germans enabled Holocaust killing has been strongly contested. Some thought it massively simplified and demonized German popular motivations, others noted the lack of comparison with Nazi-occupied countries (Baum 2008:27), and as the sole cause of popular participation in genocide it was widely discounted. While anti-Semitism permeated German national culture, Nazi propaganda (at least to 1941) apparently failed to bolster public support for anti-Jewish policy and provoked concerns about the illegality of these measures and possible repercussions. Ultimately it produced distancing, alienation, and (from 1941) a buffer between the regime and a war-weary populace, who wanted to know little and who because of their pre-existent anti-Semitic attitudes, did not protest. Thus popular anti-Semitism may have directly motivated murder but also indirectly and probably more frequently contributed to the radical Nazi programme's success by promoting non-intervention, that is bystanding, towards Jews (Bankier 1988; Michman 2010; Kershaw 2008).

Zygmunt Bauman (1989) also highlights the Holocaust's origins in modernity, and particularly its trademark: instrumental rationality, which is characterized by segmentation of labour, categorization, and procedures. Although modernity does not explain all genocides, for example Rwanda (Kershaw 2008:22), instrumental rationality plays a vital role.

Instrumental rationality, group dynamics, and 'othering'

Bauman (1989) notes that administrative or organizational evil depends on deficient ethical frameworks, with efficiency paramount, conscience captive to authority, information diffused, and responsibility fragmented. Attention to task, technique, rules, and limited morality separates actions from emotion (Cohen 2001:95). Harms are even easier to commit when one is an intermediary, neither giving orders nor carrying them out (Kilham and Mann 1974), when one is anonymous or disguised (Zimbardo 2007:297–323; Staub 2003), and when one is removed from the consequences of one's actions, as modern technological warfare (Glover 1999) and the Milgram experiments (see under 'Motives and reasons for harming') demonstrate. Eichmann and other 'desk murderers', using the railway tourist fare schedule, could therefore organize 'removal transports' to effect a 'change of residence' of Jews to Auschwitz (Glas 2006:178–179). Bureaucratization and progressively sophisticated means of killing, such as Zyklon-B gas chambers rather than shooting, maximized efficiency and psychological insulation: perpetrators did not face their victims, who became non-human legitimate targets (Browning 1998; Glover 1999:64–68; Russell and Gregory 2005; Bauman 1989). Each agent's task is plausibly deniable. As a good manager or employee, effective, efficient and legal, one can still (un)wittingly commit evil acts (Adams and Balfour 2004; Pina e Cunha et al. 2010). Contemporary examples include international corporations that deal in destruction and death: international small arms traders, the tobacco lobby (Bandura 1999), multinational polluters, and the Hardie asbestos scandal (Peacock 2009).

Likewise in overt war, terrorism, and genocide, group allegiance and absolution facilitate killing; and situational and group roles, and cultural and organizational arrangements, channel the emotions and proclivities of perpetrators. Fundamental needs to survive and belong mean accepting group norms and cooperation (Staub 2003; Zimbardo 2007). Promoting soldiers' connections with comrades also enhances their willingness to act for them and their operational effectiveness against enemies (Grossman 1996).

Interviewing Nazi killers, Lifton and psychiatrist Henry Dicks (1972) underscored their normality rather than pathology (Berkowitz 1999:249). Collective, diffused, or displaced responsibility allows people to behave more cruelly than if acting alone, to relinquish responsibility for victims' life and welfare, and makes bystander helping less probable (Bandura 1999:198, Staub 2003:330). Christopher Browning, studying the trial documents of Reserve Police Battalion 101, comprising 'ordinary' middle-aged working class men from the social democratic city of Hamburg, emphasized such variables: group and tribal loyalty, peer pressure, assigned roles, and obedience to authority. Ordered to murder Jews in a Polish village, the men could choose to opt out, but less than 15 of 500 did so. Not initially heartless, they became progressively desensitized, eventually murdering 70,000–80,000 people (Browning 1998).

De-humanization involves stripping people of human qualities, thus denying likeness, empathy, and obligation. Social group research demonstrates that in-groups rate themselves as more human than out-groups and strangers (Haslam et al. 2005). Thus moral principles apply to 'us', but not 'them' (Staub 1989, 2003:305). 'Just-world' thinking assumes the world is just, therefore suffering people invited their fate by their actions or character: hence perpetrators devalue people they have harmed (Lerner 1980; Staub 2003). In wars and actions against 'undesirable' minorities, state propaganda portrays enemies as greedy, cruel, godless, raping, murdering, criminal, mindless savages or barbarians or 'gooks', demonic, or dangerous animals (Keen 2004, Zimbardo 2007:313; Glover 1999).

As Primo Levi's Nazi camp commandant explained, rather than being pointlessly cruel to those who would die, dehumanizing victims enabled perpetrators to kill (Levi 1987). Nazism sought to influence public perception through propaganda films that portrayed Jews, Roma, homosexuals, and people with mental disabilities as vermin or as vicious, lascivious, sinister, grotesque, or otherwise subhuman. Such films popularized 'natural selection', and promoted voluntary and involuntary 'euthanasia' (Burleigh 1994; Gallagher 1990:92; Friedlander 1995:88–93). Blaming victims by staging incidents where they stand accused as provocateurs (as the Nazis did to Jews on *Kristallnacht* or Hitler did to Poland at the outbreak of the Second World War) absolves the perpetrator and justifies further aggression and marginalization. Zimbardo (2007) shows how institutional power without safeguards leads to abuse. Contagion of emotions may spread with mobs. For some, psychological mechanisms such as sadism, sensational thrill-seeking, and threatened egotism may play into this (Baumeister and Campbell 1999). In short, dehumanizing people enables torture and murder.

Language, and the problem with and function of denial

Denial (specifically knowing yet not-knowing), which operates at personal, cultural, and official levels (Cohen 2001), is the sine qua non of mass human rights violations. Denial is literal ('nothing is happening'), interpretive ('what is happening is not what it seems'), or volitional ('it's got nothing to do with me') (Cohen 2001:7–9).

Exculpatory or neutralized language is intrinsic to rights violations. Harms are often justified by invoking higher moral principles (just war theories and rhetoric rationalize making war to resist oppression, save humanity, or secure peace), or by using euphemistic or non-agentic phrases (e.g. 'collateral damage', 'surgical strikes', 'friendly fire') (Bandura 1999). Nazi deceptive or distancing language (e.g. 'selection', 'special operation', 'resettlement', 'Final Solution') facilitated denial for observers and victims, enabling perpetrators to split off and disown personal acts (Arendt 1963; Cohen 2001:79). The term 'Final Solution' stood for mass murder without sounding like it, keeping the focus on problem-solving (Zimbardo 2007:215; Lifton 1986:420–455).

For Hitler, compartmentalization was vital. Personally, he avoided physical and visual contact with the consequences of his murderous orders, and actively prevented others telling him the truth. Collectively, Hitler strictly separated his life with Himmler, Goebbels, his Generals, and staff from his intimate personal circle. He also required compartmentalization by others. A notice on every wall read: 'Every man need only know what is going on in his own domain'. Compartmentalization involved not only activities but also thinking. Speer observed that linked with his secrecy order, this meant much more than Hitler's wanting people to concentrate their minds—it meant it was dangerous not to (Sereny 1996:184; Kubarych 2005).

Albert Speer exemplifies individual denial. While denying lifelong that he knew the Jews were being exterminated, Speer affirmed that he was blind by choice, not ignorant. Noticing the obvious destruction of *Kristallnacht* and Jewish evictions, he avoided knowing the reasons. He eluded recognizing the barbarous conditions of his slave labourers. A friend advised him never to visit Auschwitz: what he saw there he was not permitted to describe and could not describe. Speer avoided querying him or anyone, evading evidence that would confirm his suspicions that crimes had been committed. He admitted he was 'inescapably contaminated morally; from discovering something which might have made me turn from my course, I had closed my eyes' (Sereny 1996:463; Kubarych 2005). On tough questions, he generalized about specifics and admitted a little to deny a lot. It was not that Speer did not want to know, but (more strongly) that he wanted not to know (Kubarych 2005; Sereny 1996:148).

German collective denial was expressed and examined after April 1945, when the widely publicized liberation of the Bergen-Belsen concentration camp shocked the world. As events unfolded, many Germans claimed 'We knew nothing about this' (*Davon haben wir nichts gewusst*). Though Germans knew of Nazi murderousness towards Jews through propaganda (Johnson 2005), awareness of genocide (which began after the invasion of Russia) had come gradually for the Allies and Germans. Except for civilians and soldiers in close proximity to the *Einsatzgruppen*, the concentration camps in German-occupied lands or extermination camps in Poland, there were rumours and guesses (Sereny 2000). German historian Peter Longerich comments that '"*Davon*", meaning "about this", implies knowledge and unwillingness to openly address the subject further. The verb "gewusst", implying knowledge, is carefully chosen, not excluding rumours and partial information that was uncertain. People accordingly employed this strategy to distance themselves from responsibility' (Richards, 2006). The Holocaust therefore was an open secret in real time (Cohen 2001). The question of knowledge and accountability has been central to recent German history (see Chapter 38). After the war many asserted that Germans had been misled (Schmidt 2006:268) or were uninformed. Defendants concealed, distorted, or justified their roles, for example citing obedience and community loyalty during war (Schmidt 2006:157), or were self-righteously indignant (Weindling 2006:161). Neurologist Julius Hallervorden who removed brains from murdered children with cerebral palsy, told Leo Alexander that 'there was wonderful material among those brains, beautiful mental defectives. . . [but] how they came to me was none of my business' (Weindling 2006:70; Alexander 1949:4).

Gradualism

People and societies change for worse (or better) through stepwise actions (Zimbardo 2007; Staub 2003:29, 303). Prefacing big requests with related smaller requests (the 'foot-in-the-door' tactic) is effective (Staub 2003:326; Milgram 1963; Zimbardo 2007). Learning through participation is critical—for harming, gradually inducting, and capturing people in practices they normally find morally abhorrent. Thus exposure and step-wise change overcomes resistance, altering values, self-concept, and behaviours. 'Teachers' who shock errant 'learners' increase shock intensity as learner performance declines (Bandura et al. 1975). Some observe the role of learned perversity or unleashed sadism, based on an emerging culture of freedom from constraints that is associated with absolute power, or the removal or suppression of negative consequences for undertaking increasingly cruel acts upon others (Rosen 2011).

Under the Nazis, Jewish assimilation and the German-Jewish symbiosis was destroyed through progressive exclusion (dismissal from jobs, expropriation, disenfranchisement, prohibition of marriage and sexual relations), terrorization (the *Kristallnacht* pogrom), stigmatization (wearing yellow stars), and finally removal and extermination (Staub 2003:291–324; Abrahams-Sprod 2006). The 'euthanasia' programmes pioneered Holocaust technologies, and effected psychological and institutional changes that facilitated it (Dudley and Gale 2002; Staub 2003:304). Eichmann acclimatized to genocide through ethnic cleansing of Poles in 1939. When first exposed to bodies of massacred Jews, he reacted with revulsion: however, Nazi ideology, Fuhrer loyalty, his need to belong and careerism, made him continue and ignore his distress, which gradually extinguished (Arendt 1963). Stangl was also drawn into genocide in a stepwise fashion (Sereny 1974). For members of Police Battalion 101, police force career choice and training, increasing Jewish persecution, and prior participation in Nazi violence, may have aided their desensitization (Staub 2003:18–19). Greek torturers were not selected for sadism but non-deviancy, identification with the political regime, and obedience. Training bound them together through initiation rites, isolation, new values, and elitist language; de-individuation and prevention of thinking; and exposure to frequent, group, controlled violence (Gibson and Haritos-Fatouros 1986). Forms of contractual obligation are created, meaningful roles are played, and apparently reasonable rules become binding. Preventing exit, and offering an (ideological) end to justify the means (Staub 2003) are also important. The induction of executioners (Haney et al. 1997; Robertson 2006; Welsh, this volume), the 'normalization' of executions in various countries, and the evolution of terrorists (Bandura 1999) exemplify the same gradualism. In war, indoctrination, humiliation, and distancing and the killing or wounding of comrades may provoke explosive retaliation and excitement, a wish to go on killing (Glover, 1999:47–57). Glover (1999) convincingly documents a stepwise progression in the shift to killing at distance, from the British naval blockade in World War One to the use of the atomic bomb, and details the institutional momentum, moral inertia, diffused responsibility, and moral sliding that made it possible. The role of miscommunication, Hobbesian fear, and military drift should also not be underestimated.

Nazi doctors and psychiatrists: motivations and reasons

All the above factors are evident when considering the motivation of Nazi doctors and psychiatrists. Illich and Foucault chart the dangers inherent in medical power and biological knowledge (Weindling 2006:5). Technical knowledge can facilitate both healing and killing (Lafleur et al. 2007). Unsurprisingly, similar motives and reasons emerge in medical and helping contexts: as noted above, the criteria for 'euthanasia' for example were ideological ('eugenic', anti-Semitic, and economic), practical (related to administrative efficiency), and achieved through bureaucratic routine, peer pressure, evasive or metaphorical language and propaganda, and inducements (Evans 2009:101).

At Nuremberg, Nazi doctors and psychiatrists multiplied excuses. These included: following orders, 'tu quoque' (as noted above), acting for public health or national security, total war demands extreme measures (Proctor 1992), the captives would be killed anyway, prisoners who volunteered for experiments were offered freedom (there was no evidence of this) or might expiate their 'crimes' (i.e. minority group status or political beliefs), scientists lacked moral or 'values' expertise, or that the few could be sacrificed for the many (Caplan 2007:66–70; Schmidt 2006, Weindling 2006). The post-war medical trials admitted none of these justifications. Moreover, the claim that the Nazis enforced psychiatric cooperation is a half-truth at best. Despite pressure from peers and superiors, higher ranking and direct perpetrators were seldom simply coerced into transgression. Doctors were not coerced, insane, psychopathic, demonic, or incompetent, but frequently pillars of the establishment (Caplan 2007:65). German medicine affiliated to the Nazi party early (Weindling 2006:5), enthusiastically—it actively welcomed the Nazis—(Dudley and Gale 2002), and in greater numbers than any other professional group (Proctor 1988). The SS was the chief perpetrator organization, which recruited a high number of professional culprits, especially doctors. Anti-semitic ideology, obedience, and more authoritarian personality orientation distinguished SS members (Dicks 1972; Merkl 1980; Elms and Milgram 1966; Staub 2003:300–301). Scientists were not bystanders or pawns: many helped construct Nazi racial policies (Proctor 1992:29), which progressively subverted discussions of human experimentation in ethics journals (Frewer 2007:30–45).

German psychiatry, which was somatically focused, state-dominated, and objectified patients (Pross 1992:38; Weindling 2006:7), had aided the pursuit of compulsory sterilization and 'euthanasia'. Eugenics and 'race hygiene' resulted in compulsory sterilizations in several countries. German authorities argued the War sacrificed the best genes, while medicine supported the weak, leaving the worst to proliferate. Purging such 'epidemics' would redeem and regenerate Germany. Many Nazis therefore endorsed medical 'counterselection' of 'degenerate' individuals and 'useless eaters' (those with various physical, mental, and intellectual disabilities, or belonging to certain cultural groups) for euthanasia (Lifton 1986; Zimbardo 2007:313; Gallagher 1990; Friedlander 1995; Weindling 2006:99, 158; Dudley and Gale 2002). Hitler conceived the German nation as a body to which every true German was indissolubly joined but from which the Jewish 'bacillus' in particular was to be extirpated. Thus genocide was an immune response to illness in the body politic (Koenigsburg 2009). Robert Ritter, psychiatrist with the German National Institute of Health, also viewed 90 per cent of gypsies as descendants of the lowest European criminal sub-proletariat, dispatching many for killing (Müller-Hill 2007:59; Weindling 2006:188–189; Pross 1992:37). The supposed subhuman status of live subjects also facilitated coerced experiments. Commitment to public health and alternative medicine contrasted with denial of the social causes of poverty (Pross 1992:38).

Interviewing Nuremberg medical defendants and others, Alexander (1948, 1949) concluded that indoctrination, group seduction, and sanctioning led to denial of individual responsibility and reality. He speculated that the Nazi regime's enforcement of *Blutkitt* ('blood putty'), the collective commission of crimes contrary to one's personal values, confirmed extraordinary service in the 'greater cause' or 'sacred mission', proving and reinforcing party allegiance and loyalty. Thus Himmler, famously addressing the SS perpetrators, pardoned them in discharging their 'heroic duty'. Doctors and psychiatrists were often committed Nazis, who 'selected' for national health. For doctors and psychiatrists, the language of eugenics, and the metaphor of surgical extirpation of the ulcer of Jewry and other 'degenerates' from the body of German humanity, represented murder as a public service (Friedlander 1995:11; Graham 1977:1138–1139; Evans 1997:73). Ferocity and hardness replaced Judeo-Christian compassion (Gallagher 1990:198; Glover 1999). Among camp doctors, Lifton noted 'doubling', whereby a portion of the self becomes the whole (or 'Auschwitz self'), enabling self-deception and adaptation to evil environments. Irrespective of this construct's validity (Burleigh 1994; Cohen 2001; Gaita 1999:225–226), the separation of roles characterized T4 psychiatrists.

In contrast to the notion of a 'duty to kill', embodied in medical writings of the time (Dudley and Gale 2002) is the motive of venality. As noted above, opportunism and careerism were rampant as the Nazis offered non-Jewish doctors, who did not demur, improved earnings, assets, research opportunities, and status as Jewish colleagues were ousted (Proctor 1992). Self-interest such as financial incentive, career advancement, or expropriation are common motives in genocide and mass murder (Staub 2003:291–324; Baum 2008:31). Zealots also participated eagerly in exterminations, others performed required duties more or less methodically, others again participated reluctantly (Lifton 1986:194).

Holocaust bystanders

Bystanding rarely receives sufficient attention including research, compared with perpetrators, victims, and rescuers. Bystanding encompasses a number of heterogeneous responses. Some bystanders may be guilt-ridden. Others may fear consequences, be in denial, suppressing uncomfortable knowledge (Speer fits this description), be morally indifferent, or tacitly approve or be complicit in what is occurring (Kershaw 2008:11).

In the Third Reich, many were passive bystanders or even active participants, boycotting Jewish businesses, benefiting from expropriations of Jewish property or firing Jewish employees, breaking off friendships (Abrahams-Sprod 2006). Deception and obfuscation determined the 'language rules' (Goldhagen 1996; Arendt 1963; Cohen 2001). As noted, Jewish and non-Jewish doctors were pitted against each other. The Berlin Psychoanalytic Institute, re-named after Goering, accommodated psychoanalytic concepts to Nazi ideology (Staub 2003:306–307). Psychiatrists enhanced their lowly status by accepting the task of identifying and excluding inferior Germans (Muller-Hill 1988:22; Friedlander 1995:123–124). German psychiatrist Oswald Bumke asserted in 1945 that though killing people with mental illness was meant to be top secret, 'the sparrows were whistling it from the rooftops' (Schmidt 2006:92).

Underpinning bystanding are situational risks that are judged insuperable, and the wish for normality, predictability, and social acceptance. Numbing and avoidance of critical thinking are common. Depending on social conditions, bystanders may become temporary perpetrators or rescuers (Baum 2008:153–180).

Bystanders however have power to influence events. To act against Jews, the Nazi leadership needed a reliable substrate of anti-Semitism. They were apprehensive about popular reactions, but surprised and emboldened by the lack of response, and also popular action against Jews (Hilberg 1961; Dawidowicz 1975; Staub 1989, 2003:309). Arendt (1994:10–11) spoke of 'the empty space' forming around friends and loved ones when the Nazis came to power, in the wave of coordination, not yet the pressure of terror. Thus bystanders—nice enough men and women whose moral sense was blunted—made the Holocaust possible (Gryn 2000).

As bystanders, many nations facilitated the Holocaust. Anti-semitism existed in Western nations. They supported the 1936 Berlin Olympics. American corporations traded with Germany throughout the 1930s (Wyman 1984). In May 1939, the SS St Louis carried 937 Jewish refugees from Hamburg to Cuba, which denied them entry. So, despite appeals, did the United States. Britain, France, Belgium, and Holland finally admitted them but subsequently many died in Nazi gas chambers, a consequence of collective international indecision and policy failure regarding Jewish refugees (Thomas and Morgan-Witts 1974). The Rwandan (Staub 2003:341–350) and Darfur genocides (among others) also exemplify the effects of bystanding.

Motives and reasons for harming: experimental models

A number of experimental paradigms have modelled elements of perpetrator behaviour, shedding light on Holocaust events as well as later genocides. Stanley Milgram's famous experiments (1963, 1974) examined how obedience to authority and conformity might violate people's basic moral beliefs. Milgram was inspired by Asch's conformity experiments. These demonstrated that individual participants' visual comparisons of different line lengths with a reference line could be influenced by peers' false responses. Dissenting peer responses reduced the likelihood of conformity (Asch 1956), but collectivist cultures increased it (Bond and Smith 1996). The Holocaust and contemporaneous Eichmann trial primed Milgram's work.

In New Haven, Connecticut, 1000 adults aged 20–50 years from numerous occupations and educational backgrounds became unwitting subjects for Milgram's purported study of memory and learning. A white-coated, impassive experimenter ordered them to teach a pleasant volunteer stranger a series of word pairs, using a generator that supposedly administered increasingly painful and hazardous shocks when errors were made. The learner, out of sight in another room, was the experimenter's confederate, and though increasingly distressed sounds were pre-recorded and played for each shock level, no shocks were actually given. The experimenter met participants' distress, questioning, and wish to discontinue with reassurances that he would assume all responsibility and there was no permanent damage, but increasingly assertive demands that they continue.

Beforehand, Milgram polled professionals' predicted outcomes. All 14 Yale University senior psychology majors believed that very few (average 1.2 per cent) would inflict maximum voltage. Thirty-nine psychiatrists predicted that most would not exceed 150 volts (where the victim first pleads to be released), only 4 per cent would permit 300 volts (an intense shock), and only 0.1 per cent would administer maximum voltage. The actual results starkly discredited these predictions. Despite personal distress, when pressed almost two-thirds of participants obeyed to the end (three administrations of 450 volts). Women and men were equally obedient. The experiment delivered similar results in Princeton, Rome, South Africa, Australia, and Munich (where 85 per cent of subjects obeyed until the end) (Milgram 1974). High compliance (69 per cent) occurred when peers complied, the experimenter was adjacent, the learner was in another room, distress sounds were absent, and the warning was only written on the shock generator. Thus avoiding personal sensory awareness of the impact of harmful acts was crucial. Conversely, the experimenter's reduced physical proximity (e.g. instructing via phone), the learner's distress sounds or increased proximity (e.g. having to hold the learner's arm on a shock plate), conflicting authority (e.g. incompatible orders of equal status experimenters), and peer rebellion (e.g. observed disobedience of other teachers (actually actors)) reduced obedience. Perhaps non-strangers (family, friends) as learners reducing emotional distance would have decreased obedience, while the procedural impersonality of the shock generator facilitated it (Russell and Gregory 2005). Choosing to please rather than confront the experimenter, most participants relinquished personal responsibility and delegated: administering word-pair tests while another participant administered shocks ensured high (93 per cent) compliance. Milgram (1974:121–122) associated this with modern bureaucracy, which absolves most from directly destructive actions, employing small numbers of 'the most callous and obtuse' for 'dirty work'. For those who resisted, personalities, feelings of competence, values, and (sometimes) group cultures were important (Milgram 1974; Staub 2003:9).

Albert Bandura et al. (1975), purporting to study the effects of punishment on decision-making, derived similar findings. 'Supervisors' who were told to administer electric shocks to unseen subjects who made faulty decisions, increased the intensity of 'shocking' behaviour if responsibility was collective rather than individual, and if recipients were negatively labelled. (No electric shocks were actually given). As performance declined, shock intensities increased, creating further failures that were taken as further evidence of culpability. Self-exonerating justifications prevailed.

The also famous Stanford Prison Experiment (SPE) (Zimbardo 2007; Haney et al. 1973) explored the effects of situational variables (including duress and peer pressure) on individual behaviour. Role-playing life in a simulated prison, 24 white middle class young males selected for apparently normal psychological adjustment were randomly assigned to the parts of warders or prisoners. The experiment intentionally reproduced the worst features of prisons, including de-individuation (warders) and dehumanization (prisoners). Warders received military uniforms, wooden batons, and reflective glasses (minimizing eye contact), and worked in shifts, returning home off hours. Prisoners donned smocks without underpants, thongs, and ankle chains, were assigned identifying numbers, and booked in by actual police cooperating with the experiment at its inception. Loss of personal identity facilitated learned helplessness, with prisoners suffering and accepting sadistic and humiliating treatment from guards—physical punishments, arbitrary controls including deprivation of privacy, food, and sleep, and degrading practices, e.g. enforced nudity, cleaning toilets with bare hands. Some resisted, others became zealous models, many developed uncontrollable crying or disorganized thinking. As with the Nazi doctors (Lifton 1986), guards were zealous, methodical, or reluctant, though even the latter failed to challenge the situation (Zimbardo 2007:208). Inadequate supervision abetted prisoner abuse. The experiment had to be abandoned after six days of the projected fortnight.

Contrary to expectation that individuals facing moral dilemmas would follow their conscience, Milgram's experiment showed that directives from authorities overwhelmed the morality of most individuals who are in no way evil (Milgram 1974; Blass 2002). Zimbardo et al's experiment (and also that by Bandura et al.) similarly revealed the importance of individual, situational, and systemic factors, including de-individuation and dehumanization, in understanding institutional abuses (Zimbardo 2007:297–323, 330; Staub 2003). Taken together, these experiments illustrate the influence of experimentally induced authority, peers, institutional ideology ('the slogan that legitimises the means to attain the goal'—Zimbardo 2007:226) and onlookers, on individual behaviours. Ordinary people, performing tasks without particular hostility, can act destructively even without physical coercion. Obedience to authority can lead to verbal abuse, sexual assault (strip-search scams provoked by anonymous 'police officers' in US fast-food restaurant chains), or death (e.g. doctors' power over nurses in drug ordering, airline pilots' authority over first officers) (Zimbardo 2007:278ff). Schoolteachers favouring students with blue eyes or brown eyes can transform classrooms into totalitarian, abusive, and exclusive environments (Peters 1985). This 'situational' paradigm, rather than formal mental illness, repeatedly supports torture and mass murder, as exemplified by the Third Reich's camp guards, Rwandan and former-Yugoslavian genocides, terrorists, and suicide bombers (Zimbardo 2007:293; Baum 2008:76–78) and destructive cults (Jim Jones People's Temple, Aum Shinrikyo). Role identification and compartmentalization can produce dire results, as the camp guards who played Bach while they murdered Jews illustrates (Gaita 1999:225–226).

Milgram (1974:6) believed his results confirmed Arendt's conception of 'the banality of evil'. However, direct authority does not fully explain the sanctioning of harms in everyday situations, where authority is often deliberately diffused, and where ideology is vital (Bandura 1999).

This is not to excuse individuals' reprehensible actions, or to minimize their accountability. But investigators differ in interpreting individual vulnerability to antisocial behaviours and 'moral disengagement'. Bandura (1999) cites parenting failures, abuse and neglect, early aggression, failure to recognize and cultivate prosocial behaviour, lack of guilt, rumination over personal injustices and retaliation, and lack of perceived efficacy to withstand peer pressure. Zimbardo (2007) argues that these experiments show the potential corruptibility of anyone (including our kin and ourselves) given the right situational and/or systemic (socio-cultural) forces, and difficulty predicting behaviours under stress even with prior knowledge of people's innate, apparently 'normal', dispositions. Baum (2008:4–5, 44–45, 88) however responds that this does not account for individual rescuing, and emphasizes the predictive importance of personal emotional development.

Motives and reasons for helping

Social psychology emphasizes the power of social situations: under conducive conditions, ordinary decent people can do appalling things. However, the situational paradigm begs the question about why some people behave well, heroically, and sometimes repeatedly, in dire situations (Bernstein 2002; Baum 2008). Milgram found a sizeable minority resisted pressure, displaying moral courage and imagination (Bandura 1999). Against self-interest, without expectation of gain, and often in prolonged peril, rescuers of Jews in the Holocaust frequently acted for acquaintances or strangers. Such active behaviour (those honoured by Yad Vashem under-represent those who rescued) was often crucial to outcome in Nazi-occupied Europe. Typically, they minimized their contribution, rather than seeing it as heroic. Their actions and motives have been frequently described (e.g. Tec 1986; Oliner and Oliner 1988; Paldiel 1988; Fogelman 1994; Gilbert 2002).

Helping can be situationally influenced. For example, the more people who witness an emergency, the less likely they will help (Darley and Latane 1968). Diffusion of responsibility may explain this (Zimbardo 2007:315), because helping is more likely when needs are clear, great, impactful and focused, costs are affordable, and the behaviour required is socially acceptable (Staub 2003:125, 131). Time pressure (Darley and Batson 1973) and the prior relationship are also relevant. In Milgram's experiments, as noted, situational determinants, like being personally responsible for and witnessing harms one causes (Milgram 1974; Bandura et al. 1975), affected obedience.

However, this is notwithstanding the importance of character, competencies in crises, and the capacity of situations to shape character. Crime interveners have a sense of capability founded on training and subjective personal strength (Hudson et al. 1981). Steps in help include noticing, understanding the urgency, assuming responsibility, deciding how to help, and implementing one's decision. Like perpetrators and bystanders, rescuers evolve. Contact leads to identification, becoming aware of the human characteristics of those being killed or harmed converts bystanders from passivity to action, and gradual incremental involvement becomes an obsession to rescue. The stories of famous rescuers Oskar Schindler (Keneally 1983) and Raoul Wallenberg show this (Bandura 1999; Staub 2003:326–327).

Many Holocaust rescuers and Milgram experiment defiers were deeply connected to and identified with moral parents and families holding strong humanitarian values. Notably, they received less punitive rearing, with closer fathers and more reasoning and explanation (London 1970; Oliner and Oliner 1988; Blass 1991, 1993:40–41, cited in Berkowitz 1999:249; Tec 1986; Staub 2003:314, Baum 2008:90–91, 185). While perpetrators have over-developed social identities, rescuers were far more often emotionally mature: independent-minded, emotionally intelligent, having higher self-esteem, subscribing to universal ideals and principles (Baum 2008), and socially responsible. Rescuers differed from bystanders on locus of control, autonomy, risk taking, social responsibility, tolerance and authoritarianism, empathy, and altruistic moral reasoning (Midlarsky et al. 2005). While trait adventurousness characterized some, all rescuers showed courage when confronted with daunting risks. Some belonged to resistance groups, church groups, or nations that shaped their responses, though religion did not notably associate with rescuing. Such 'prosocial orientation' (Staub 2003) may be grounded in respect and moral standing, moral principles and identity, and in affective connections and sympathy (Staub 2003; Glover 1999).

The psychology of altruism is relevant here. Altruism is the motivation to help others or for others' welfare without regard to reward or the benefits of recognition. While the payoffs of altruism are hotly debated, helping has its own momentum: the great majority of helpers describe the experience as positive, while conversely people whose lives are more satisfying feel they have more to give others. Research shows that materialistic–competitive goals (wealth, career success, power) are inimical to helping, though not other personal goals (e.g. support and security, personal growth, competence, control) (Staub 2003:145–156).

Whole cultures of rescue confronted Nazism, for example in Denmark and Bulgaria, and Italy and Hungary before German takeovers in 1943 and 1944 respectively. National leadership prevented Bulgarian Jews being deported. The German Confessing Church, Holland's Antirevolutionary Church, and various Italian and French villages exemplify resistance. In Le Chambon-sur-Lignon, descendants of persecuted Protestant Huguenots led by their pastor and his wife, hid thousands of Jews from the Nazis (Sauvage 1989; Baum 2008:205–6). Relatives and institutions that protested killing of people with mental, physical, and intellectual disabilities acted similarly. Against German efficiency, incorruptibility, and obedience, divergent civic traditions (of freedom and equal rights in Denmark, and unpunctuality and inefficiency in Italy) may also have contributed to this outcome (Glover 1999). At a macropolitical level, realpolitik may determine whether people or nations intervene in oppression or aggression (for example, European nations deciding whether to stop Hitler before the Second World War). However, membership and memory of minority group status, prosocial orientation, and leadership all contribute to outcomes in national and whole-cultural situations.

Preventing mass human rights violations: Where is the engine-room?

As noted, the Holocaust contains individual, situational, and social determinants, and (in)humanity arises from ordinary psychological, situational, and socio-cultural processes and their evolution into extreme forms. Yet should preventive approaches to mass human rights violations target the level of individual frailty and transgression, or institutional, communal, socio-cultural, and national influences? How to address situational factors in facilitating such abuses?

It is a paradox that individuals rather than groups are generally held legally accountable for mass human rights violations, yet locating the prime cause of such violations in individual frailty and pathology seems misconceived. Moral actions while remaining the actor's personal responsibility presuppose wider influences (Bandura, 1999; Zimbardo, 2007; Staub, 2003). Research meta-analyses reveal the power of social situations on behavior is robust, yet criminal justice systems rarely address this (Zimbardo 2007:321). While individual perpetrators played key roles, the role of German society and nation was absolutely crucial, in accepting Hitler and not resisting anti-Semitic policies, for example. Virtually every German institution, occupational group, or profession contributed voluntarily (usually enthusiastically) to the Final Solution, turning their own traditional ethical protocols upside down (Higgins 2006). The effect of this inertia on further Nazi programming has been noted.

Because humans are herd animals, most will do what the herd is doing. Most will manifest as 'saints' or 'sinners' according to the health or breakdown of those communal, societal, and political forms of association with which they identify. This suggests there may be value intervening at a number of levels. Educational programmes that seek to influence the moral awareness and development of individual children and adults about racism and social inclusion are of potentially great significance, as is the preservation of the moral resources—respect, sympathy, and friendship—and cultivation of a moral identity and imagination, in promoting helping and resistance. However, pre-eminently, paying attention to these wider determinants and preventing the decline of social and national institutions that preserve civility constitutes a crucial arena for genocide prevention (Higgins 2003, 2006).

Our companion Chapter 38 considers some current measures for prevention of mass human rights violations and genocide.

Acknowledgements

Thanks to Winton Higgins and Alan Rosen for their substantive suggestions about the argument, content, and style.

References

Abrahams-Sprod, M (2006) *Life under siege: the Jews of Magdeburg under Nazi rule*. PhD thesis. Sydney: University of Sydney.

Adams, G and Balfour, D (2004) 'Human Rights, the Moral Vacuum of Modern Organisations, and Administrative Evil', in T Campbell and S Miller (eds) *Human rights and the moral responsibilities of corporate and public sector organisations*. Netherlands: Kluwer Academic, Chapter 11, 205–21.

Adorno, T (1955, reprinted 1967) *Prisms*. London: MIT Press.

Alexander, JC, with Jay, M, Giesen, B, et al. (2009) *Remembering the Holocaust: a debate*. Oxford: Oxford University Press.

Alexander, L (1948) 'War crimes; their socio-psychological aspects', *American Journal of Psychiatry*, 105, 170–77.

Alexander, L (1949) 'Medical science under dictatorship', *New England Journal of Medicine*, 241(2), 39–47.

Allport, GW (1954) *The nature of prejudice*. Reading, MA: Addison-Wesley.

Amnesty International (1980) *Testimony on secret detention camps in Argentina*. London: Amnesty International Publications.

Annas, G, and Grodin, M (eds) (1992) *The Nazi doctors and the Nuremberg Code*. New York: Oxford University Press.

Arendt, H (1963, revised edition 1968) *Eichmann in Jerusalem: A Report on the Banality of Evil*. New York: Viking.

Arendt, H (1966) 'Introduction' to B Naumann, *Auschwitz*. New York: Praeger, xxiv.

Arendt, H (1994) *Essays in understanding, 1930–1954* (J Kohn, ed) New York: Harcourt, Brace and Co.

Asch, SE (1956) 'Studies of independence and conformity: A minority of one against a unanimous majority', *Psychological Monographs*, 70 (416).

Baldwin, P (ed) (1990) *Reworking the past: Hitler, the Holocaust and the historians' debate*. Boston: Beacon Press.

Bandura, A (1999) 'Moral Disengagement in the Perpetration of Inhumanities', *Personality and Social Psychology Review*, 3(3), 193–209.

Bandura, A, Underwood, B, and Fromson, ME (1975) 'Disinhibition of aggression through diffusion of responsibility and dehumanization of the victims', *Journal of Research in Personality*, 9, 253–69.

Bankier, D (1988) 'Hitler and the policy-making process on the Jewish Question', *Holocaust and Genocide Studies*, 3(1), 1–20.

Bankier, D (1992) *The Germans and the Final Solution: Public Opinion under Nazism*. Oxford and Cambridge, MA: Blackwell.

Bauer, Y (2001) *Rethinking the Holocaust*. New Haven, CT: Yale University Press.

Baum, SK (2008) *The psychology of genocide: perpetrators, bystanders and rescuers*. New York: Cambridge University Press.

Bauman, Z (1989) *Modernity and the Holocaust*. Ithaca, NY: Cornell University Press.

Baumeister, RF, and Campbell, WK (1999) 'The intrinsic appeal of evil: sadism, sensational thrills, and threatened egotism', *Personality and Social Psychology Review*, 3(3), 210–21.

Berkowitz, L (1999) 'Evil is more than banal: situationism and the concept of evil', *Personality and Social Psychology Review*, 3(3), 246–53.

Bernard, V, Ottenberg, P, and Redl, F (1965) 'Dehumanisation: a composite psychological defense in relation to modern war', in M Schwebel (ed) *Behavioural science and human survival*. Palo Alto, CA: Science and Behavior Books, 64–82.

Bernstein, R (2002) *Radical evil: a philosophical interrogation*. Cambridge, UK: Polity Press.

Blass, T (1991) 'Understanding behavior in the Milgram obedience experiment: the role of personality, situations, and their interactions', *Journal of Personality and Social Psychology*, 60, 398–413.

Blass, T (1993) 'Psychological perspectives on perpetrators of the Holocaust: the role of situational pressures, personal dispositions, and their interactions', *Holocaust and Genocide Studies*, 7, 30–50.

Blass, T (2002) 'The man who shook the world', *Psychology Today*, March/April, 69–74.

Bloche, G and Marks, J (2005) 'When doctors go to war', *New England Journal of Medicine*, 352, 3–6.

Bock, G (1997) 'Sterilisation and 'medical' massacres in National Socialist Germany: ethics, politics and the law', in M Berg and G Cocks (eds) *Medicine and modernity: public health and medical care in nineteenth and twentieth-century Germany*. Washington DC: German Historical Institute and Cambridge University Press, 149–72.

Bond, R and Smith, PB (1996) 'Culture and Conformity: A Meta-Analysis of Studies Using Asch's (1952b, 1956) Line Judgment Task', *Psychological Bulletin*, 119(1), 111–37.

Browning, C (1998) *Ordinary men: reserve police battalion 101 and the Final Solution in Poland*. (2nd edn. with new afterword). New York: Harper Collins.

Browning, CR (2004) *The origins of the Final Solution: the evolution of Nazi Jewish policy, September 1939–March 1942*. Lincoln: University of Nebraska Press.

Bullock, A (1992) *Fanaticism and Calculation*, Hitler and Stalin: Parallel Lives. New York: Knopf.

Burleigh, M (1994) *Death and deliverance: 'euthanasia' in Germany ca. 1900–1945*. Cambridge: Cambridge University Press.

Caplan, A. (2005) 'Editorial: Misusing the Nazi analogy', *Science*, 22 July, 309, 535.

Caplan, A (2007) 'The ethics of evil: the challenge and lessons of Nazi medical experiments', in WR Lafleur, G Böhme, and S Shimazono (eds) *Dark Medicine: rationalising unethical medical research*. Bloomington: Indiana University Press, 63–72.

Card, C (2002) *The atrocity paradigm: a theory of evil*. New York/London: Oxford University Press.

Cesarani, D (2006) *Becoming Eichmann: rethinking the life, crimes, and trial of a desk murderer*. Cambridge, MA: Da Capo Press.

Cohen, S (2001) *In denial: knowing about atrocities and suffering*. Cambridge, UK: Polity/Blackwell.

Council for International Organizations of Medical Sciences and World Health Organization (1993). *International ethical guidelines for biomedical research involving human subjects*. Geneva: CIOMS.

Darley, JM and Batson, CD (1973) 'From Jerusalem to Jericho: a study of situational variables in helping behavior', *Journal of Personality and Social Psychology*, 27, 100–08.

Darley, JM and Latane, B (1968) 'Bystander intervention in emergencies: diffusion of responsibilities', *Journal of Personality and Social Psychology*, 8, 377–83.

Dawidowicz, LS (1975) *The war against the Jews: 1933–1945*. New York: Holt, Rinehart and Winston.

Dicks, H (1972) *Licensed mass murder: a socio-psychological study of some SS killers*. London: Sussex University Press.

Dudley, M and Gale, F (2002) 'Psychiatrists as a moral community?' Psychiatry under the Nazis and its contemporary relevance', *Australian and New Zealand Journal of Psychiatry*, 36, 585–94.

Ehrenfreund, N (2007) *The Nuremberg legacy: how the Nazi war crimes trials changed the course of history*. New York: Palgrave Macmillan.

Elms, A and Milgram, S (1966) 'Personality characteristics associated with obedience and defiance toward authoritative commands', *Journal of Experimental Research in Personality*, 2, 292–89.

Evans, RJ (1997) 'In search of German Social Darwinism', in M Berg and G Cocks (eds) *Medicine and modernity: public health and medical care in nineteenth and twentieth-century Germany*. Washington DC: Cambridge University Press and German Historical Institute, 55–80.

Evans, RJ (2004) *The coming of the Third Reich*. London: Penguin.

Evans, RJ (2006). *The Third Reich in power, 1933–1939*. London: Penguin.

Evans, RJ (2009). *The Third Reich at war*. London: Penguin.

Fiske, ST (2003). *Social beings*. New York: Wiley.

Fiske, ST, Harris, LT, and Cudy, ATC (2004) 'Why ordinary people torture enemy prisoners', *Science (Policy Forum)*, 3006, 1482–83.

Fogelman, E (1994) *Conscience and courage: rescuers of Jews during the Holocaust*. New York: Doubleday.

Frewer, A (2007) 'Medical research, morality, and history: the German journal 'Ethik' and the limits of human experimentation', in WR Lafleur, G Böhme, and S Shimazono (eds) *Dark Medicine: rationalising unethical medical research*. Bloomington: Indiana University Press, 30–45.

Friedlander, H (1995) *The origins of Nazi genocide: from euthanasia to the Final Solution*. Chapel Hill, NC: University of North Carolina Press.

Friedlander, S (2007) *The years of persecution: Nazi Germany and the Jews 1933–1939*. London: Phoenix (Orion). (Original edition, Weidenfeld and Nicolson, 1997).

Gaita, R (1999) *A common humanity*. Melbourne: Melbourne University Press.

Gallagher, HG (1990) *By trust betrayed: patients, physicians and the licence to kill in the Third Reich*. Revised edition. Arlington, VA: Vandermere Press.

Gibson, JT and Haritos-Fatouros, M (1986) 'The Education of a Torturer', *Psychology Today*, November, 50–8.

Gilbert, M (2002) *The righteous: the unsung heroes of the Holocaust*. Chatham, Kent: Doubleday.

Glas, G (2006) 'Elements of a phenomenology of evil and forgiveness', in NN Potter (ed) *Trauma, truth and reconciliation: healing damaged relationships*. New York: Oxford University Press, 171–202.

Glover, J (1999) *Humanity: a moral history of the twentieth century*. New Haven and London: Yale.

Goldhagen, DJ (1996) *Hitler's willing executioners: Ordinary Germans and the Holocaust*. New York: Knopf.

Graham, LR (1977) 'Science and values: the eugenics movement in Germany and Russia in the 1920s', *American Historical Review*, 82, 1133–64.

Grodin, M (1992) 'Historical origins of the Nuremberg Code', in G Annas and M Grodin (eds) *The Nazi doctors and the Nuremberg Code*. New York: Oxford University Press, 121–48.

Grodin, M and Annas, G (2007) 'Physicians and torture: lessons from the Nazi doctors', *International Review of the Red Cross*, 89(Sept), 635–54.

Grossman, D (1996) *On killing: the psychological cost of learning to kill in war and society*. Boston: Little, Brown and Co.

Gryn, H (2000) *Chasing shadows: memories of a vanished world*. London: Viking.

Hamilton, VL and Sanders, J (1999) 'The second face of evil: wrongdoing in and by the corporation', *Personality and Social Psychology Review*, 3(3), 222–33.

Hanauski-Abel, H (1996) 'Not a slippery slope or sudden subversion: German medicine and national socialism in 1933', *British Medical Journal*, 313(7 Dec), 1453–63.

Haney, C (1997) 'Violence and the capital jury: mechanisms of moral disengagement and the impulse to condemn to death', *Stanford Law Review*, 49, 1447–86.

Haney, C, Banks, WP, and Zimbardo, PG (1973) 'Interpersonal dynamics in a simulated prison', *International Journal of Criminology and Penology*, 1, 69–97.

Haslam, N, Bain, P, Douge, L, Lee, M, and Bastian, B (2005) 'More human than you: attributing humanness to self and others', *Journal of Personality and Social Psychology*, 89, 937–50.

Higgins, W (2003) *Journey into darkness*. Sydney: Brandl & Scheslinger.

Higgins, W (2006) 'Could it happen again? The Holocaust and the national dimension', in C Tatz, P Arnold, and S Tatz (eds) *Genocide Perspectives III: Essays on the Holocaust and Other Genocides*, Sydney: Brandl & Scheslinger with the Australian Institute for Holocaust and Genocide Studies, 54–77.

Hilberg, R (1961) *The destruction of the European Jews*. New York: Harper and Row.

Hudson, TL, Ruggiero, M, Conner, R, and Geis, G (1981) 'Bystander intervention into crime: a study based on naturally occurring episodes', *Social Psychology Quarterly*, 44(1), 14–23.

Johnson, E and Reuband, KH (2005). *What we knew: terror, mass murder, and everyday life of Nazi Germany*. New York: Basic Books.

Karpinski, J (2004) 'BBC Radio 4 interview with Brigadier General Janis Karpinski, June 15, 2004'.

Karpinski, J (with Strasser, S) (2005) *One woman's army: the commanding general at Abu Ghraib tells her story*. New York: Miramax Press.

Kater, M (1997) 'The Sewering scandal of 1993 and the German medical establishment', in M Berg and G Cocks (eds) *Medicine and modernity: public health and medical care in nineteenth and twentieth-century Germany*. Washington DC: Cambridge University Press and German Historical Institute, 213–34.

Keen, S (2004) *Faces of the enemy: reflections on the hostile imagination*. Original edition, 1991. San Francisco, CA: Harper San Francisco.

Kelman, HC and Hamilton, VL (1989) *Crimes of obedience: towards a social psychology of authority and responsibility*. New Haven, CT: Yale University Press.

Keneally, T (1983) *Schindler's ark*. Sevenoaks, Kent: Coronet Books.

Kershaw, I (2000) *The Nazi Dictatorship Problems and Perspectives of Interpretation*. London: Arnold Press.

Kershaw, I (2008) '"Working towards the Führer": reflections on the nature of Hitler's dictatorship', in I Kershaw (ed) *Hitler, the Germans and the Final Solution*. (Originally published 1997). Jerusalem: International Institute for Holocaust Research, Yad Vashem, and New Haven and London: Yale University Press, 29–48.

Kilham, W and Mann, L (1974) 'Level of destructive obedience as a function of transmitter and executant roles in the Milgram obedience paradigm', *Journal of Personality and Social Psychology*, 29, 696–702.

Koenigsburg, R (2009) *Hitler's ideology: embodied metaphor, fantasy and history*. Charlotte, NC: Information Age Publishing.

Kubarych, TS (2005) 'Self-deception and Peck's analysis of evil', *Philosophy, Psychiatry, & Psychology*, 12(3), 247–55.

Lafleur, WR, Böhme, G, and Shimazono, S (2007) *Dark Medicine: rationalising unethical medical research.* , Bloomington: Indiana University Press.

Lerner, M (1980) *The belief in a just world: a fundamental delusion*. New York: Plenum.

Levi, P (1987) *The drowned and the saved*. New York: Summit.

Lifton, R (1986) *The Nazi doctors: medical killing and the psychology of genocide*. New York: Basic Books.

Lie, RK, Emanuel, E, Grady, C, and Wendler, D (2004) 'The standard of care debate: the Declaration of Helsinki versus the international consensus opinion', *Journal of Medical Ethics*, 30(2), 190–3.

London, P (1970) 'The rescuers: motivational hypothesis about Christians who saved Jews from the Nazis', in J Macauley and L Berkowitz (eds), *Altruism and helping behavior*. New York: Academic Press, 241–250.

Lurie, P and Wolfe, SM (1997) 'Unethical trials of interventions to reduce perinatal transmission of the human immunodeficiency virus in developing countries', *New England Journal of Medicine*, 337(12), 853–56.

McFarland-Icke, BR (1999) *Nurses in Nazi Germany. Moral choice in history*. Princeton, NJ: Princeton.

McGovern, WM (1973) *From Luther to Hitler*. New York: Houghton Mifflin.

Macklin, R (1999) *Against Relativism*. New York, NY: Oxford University Press.

Mandler, G (2002) 'Psychologists and the Nazi socialist access to power', *History of Psychology*, 5(2), 190–200.

Markusen, E (1997). 'Professions, professionals, and genocide', in I Charny (ed) *Genocide: a critical bibliographic review*. New York/Oxford: Institute on the Holocaust and Genocide, Vol 4. Facts on File, 264–98.

Maslow, A (1987) *Motivation and personality* (3rd edn, original work published 1954). New York: Harper and Row.

Mason, T (1989) 'Intention and Explanation: A Current Controversy about the Interpretation of National Socialism', in M Marris (ed) *The Nazi Holocaust Part 3, The 'Final Solution': The Implementation of Mass Murder*. Westpoint, CT: Mecler, Volume 1, 3–20.

Merkl, P (1980) *The making of a stormtrooper*. Princeton, NJ: Princeton University Press.

Michman, D (2010) 'Despite the importance and centrality of antisemitism, it cannot serve as the exclusive explanation of murder and murderers: David Bankier's (1947–2010) path in Holocaust research'. (Translated from the Hebrew by Stephanie Nakache). Yad Vashem Studies, 38(1), 15–45. Also available at <http://www1.yadvashem.org/yv/en/about/institute/studies/issues/38-1/michman.pdf>, accessed 3 November 2011.

Midlarsky, E, Jones, SE, and Corley, RP (2005) 'Personality correlates of heroic rescue during the Holocaust', *Journal of Personality*, 73(4), (August), 907–34.

Miles, SH (2004) 'Abu Ghraib: its legacy for military medicine', *The Lancet*, 364, 725–29.

Milgram, S (1963) 'Obedience to authority', *Journal of Abnormal and Social Psychology*, 67, 371–78.

Milgram, S (1974) *Obedience to authority: an experimental view*. New York: Harper and Row.

Mommsen, H (1997) 'Cumulative radicalisation and progressive self-destruction as structural determinants of the Nazi dictatorship', in Ian Kershaw and Moshe Lewin (eds) *Stalinism and Nazism: Dictatorships in Comparison*. Cambridge: Cambridge University Press, 75–87.

Moore, B (1966) *Social Origins of Dictatorship and Democracy: Lord and Peasant in the Making of the Modern World*. Boston: Beacon Press.

Moreno, JD (2007) 'Stumbling towards bioethics: human experiments policy and the early cold war', in WR Lafleur, G Böhme, and S Shimazono (eds) *Dark Medicine: rationalising unethical medical research*. Bloomington: Indiana University Press, 138–46.

Müller-Hill, B (1988) *Murderous science: elimination by scientific selection of Jews, Gypsies and others, Germany 1933–1945*. Oxford: Oxford University Press.

Müller-Hill, B (2007) 'The Silence of the Scholars', in WR Lafleur, G Böhme, and S Shimazono (eds) *Dark Medicine: rationalising unethical medical research* . Bloomington: Indiana University Press, 57–62.

Neumann, F (1967) *Behemoth: The Structure and Practice of National Socialism 1933–44*. 2nd edn. London: Frank Cass & Co.

Noll, R (1997) *The Aryan Christ: the secret life of Carl Jung*. London: Macmillan.

Novick, P (2000) *The holocaust and collective memory: the American experience*. London: Bloomsbury.

Nuffield Council on Bioethics (2005) *The ethics of research related to healthcare in developing countries: a follow-up discussion paper*. London: Nuffield Council on Bioethics. Available at <http://www.nuffieldbioethics.org/>, accessed 26 November 2010.

Oliner, SP and Oliner, PM (1988) *The altruistic personality: rescuers of Jews in Nazi Europe*. New York: Free Press.

Paldiel, M (1988) 'The altruism of Righteous Gentiles', *Holocaust and Genocide Studies*, 3, 187–96.

Peacock, M (2009) *Killer company*. Sydney: Harper Collins.

Peck, MS (1982) *People of the lie: the hope of healing human evil*. New York: Simon and Schuster.

Perley, S, Fluss, SS, Bankowski, Z, and Simon, F (1992) 'The Nuremberg Code: an international overview', in G Annas and M Grodin (eds) *The Nazi doctors and the Nuremberg Code*. New York: Oxford University Press, 149–73.

Peters, W (1985) *A class divided then and now*. Expanded edition, original 1971. New Haven, CT: Yale University Press. See also the PBS Frontline documentary 'A Class Divided', available online at <http://www.pbs.org/wgbh/pages/frontline/shows/divided/>, accessed 4 November 2011.

Pina e Cunha, M, Rego, A, and Clegg, S (2010) 'Obedience and evil: From Milgram and Kampuchea to normal organizations', *Journal of Business Ethics*, 97(2): 291–309.

Power, S (2002) *'A problem from hell': America and the age of genocide*. New York: Basic Books.

Proctor, R (1988) *Racial hygiene: medicine under the Nazis*. Cambridge: Harvard University Press.

Proctor, R (1992) 'Nazi doctors, racial medicine and human experimentation', in G Annas and M Grodin (eds) *The Nazi doctors and the Nuremberg Code*. New York: Oxford University Press, 17–31.

Pross, C (1992) 'Nazi doctors, German medicine and historical truth', in G Annas and M Grodin (eds) *The Nazi doctors and the Nuremberg Code*. New York: Oxford University Press, 32–52.

Rennie, S (2008) 'The FDA ditches the Declaration of Helsinki', *Global Bioethics Blog*, 6 May. Available at <http://globalbioethics.blogspot.com/2008_05_01_archive.html>, accessed 4 November 2010.

Richard, FD, Bond, DF (Jnr), and Stokes-Zoota, JJ (2003) 'One hundred years of social psychology quantitatively described', *Review of General Psychology*, 7, 331–63.

Richards, H (2006) 'We knew nothing about this'. *Times Higher Education*, 8 September. Available at <http://www.timeshighereducation.co.uk/story.asp?storyCode=205253&sectioncode=26>, accessed 4 November 2011.

Robertson, G (2006) *Crimes against Humanity: the struggle for global justice*. 3rd edn. Melbourne: Penguin.

Rosen, A (2011) 'Are we letting bad guys like Gaddafi off the hook?' National Times (Fairfax Press, Sydney Morning Herald, The Age), 23 March.

Russell, N and Gregory, R (2005) 'Making the Undoable Doable: Milgram, the Holocaust, and Modern Government', *American Review of Public Administration*, 35(4) (December) 327–49.

Sauvage, P (1989) *Weapons of the spirit: the astonishing story of a unique conspiracy of goodness [film]*. Los Angeles: Friends of the Le Chambon Foundation.

Schlink, B (2009) *Guilt about the past*. St Lucia, Qld: University of Queensland Press.

Schmidt, U (2004, 2nd edn 2006) *Justice at Nuremberg: Leo Alexander and the Nazi Doctors' Trial*. Basingstoke, UK: Palgrave Macmillan.

Sereny, G (1974) *Into that darkness: from mercy killing to mass murder*. London: Pimlico.

Sereny, G (1996) *Albert Speer: his battle with truth*. London: Picador.

Sereny, G (2000) *The German trauma: experiences and reflections 1938–2001*. London: Penguin.

Sharma, DC (2004) 'India pressed to relax rules on clinical trials. Drug companies claim changes are essential, but critics fear Indian patients will become guinea pigs', *The Lancet*, 363(9420), 1528–9.

Silove, D (2000) 'A conceptual framework for mass trauma: implications for adaptation, intervention and debriefing', in B Raphael and J Wilson (eds) *Psychological debriefing: theory, practice and evidence*. Cambridge: Cambridge University Press, 337–50.

Social Medicine Portal (2008) 'FDA abandons Declaration of Helsinki for international clinical trials', June 1, 2008. Available at <http://www.socialmedicine.org/2008/06/01/ethics/fda-abandons-declaration-of-helsinki-for-international-clinical-trials/>, accessed 4 November 2011.

Soelle, D (2001) *The silent cry: mysticism and resistance*. Minneapolis: Fortress Press.

Sontag, S (2003) *Regarding the pain of others*. London: Penguin.

Staub, E (1989) *The roots of evil: the origins of genocide and other group violence*. New York: Cambridge University Press.

Staub, E (2003) 'Helping a distressed person: social, personality and stimulus determinants', in E Staub, *The psychology of good and evil: why children, adults and groups help and harm others*. Cambridge, UK: Cambridge University Press, Chapter 6, 71–99.Staub, E (2003) *The psychology of good and evil: why children, adults and groups help and harm others*. Cambridge, UK: Cambridge University Press.

Steinmetz, G (1997). 'German exceptionalism and the origins of Nazism: the career of a concept', in Ian Kershaw and Moshe Lewin (eds) *Stalinism and Nazism: Dictatorships in Comparison*. Cambridge: Cambridge University Press, 251–84.

Tec, N (1986) *When light pierced the darkness: Christian rescue of Jews in Nazi-occupied Poland*. New York: Oxford University Press.

Thomas, G, and Morgan-Witts, M (1974) *Voyage of the damned*. New York: Stein and Day.

Weindling, PJ (2006) *Nazi medicine and Nuremberg trials: from medical war crimes to informed consent*. Basingstoke, UK: Palgrave Macmillan.

Williams, JR (2008) 'The Declaration of Helsinki and public health', *Bulletin of the World Health Organization*, 86 (August), 650–652.

Winau, R (2007) 'Experimentation on humans and informed consent: how we arrived where we are', in WR Lafleur, G Böhme, and S Shimazono (eds) *Dark Medicine: rationalising unethical medical research.* Bloomington: Indiana University Press, 46–56.

Wyman, DS (1984) *The abandonment of the Jews: America and the Holocaust, 1941–1945.* New York: Pantheon.

Zimbardo, P (2007). *The Lucifer effect: how good people turn evil.* London: Rider.

Chapter 12

The Abuse of Psychiatry for Political Purposes

Robert van Voren

Introduction

For more than 40 years the issue of political abuse of psychiatry in the Soviet Union dominated the agenda of the world psychiatric community.[1] The issue has on one hand resulted in angry exchanges, yet on the other hand it has stimulated an ongoing debate on human rights and professional ethics. During those years the World Psychiatric Association (WPA), around which most of the discussions evolved, adopted an ethical code on human rights that condemns the use of psychiatry for non-medical purposes. This was updated and expanded several times, and also installed mechanisms to investigate complaints of violations of these regulations.[2] Yet at the same time, some critics believe that the WPA has not always implemented the regulations it imposed on its member societies, thereby triggering further debates on the issue.[3]

In this chapter, the case of political abuse of psychiatry in the Soviet Union is used as a main example, specifically because it was a well-documented case, because it strongly influenced the concept of medical ethics and its application internationally, and because it is generally accepted (with maybe a few exceptions) that psychiatry in the Soviet Union was abused for political purposes in a systematic manner in the course of several decades. However, beyond doubt, the Soviet Union is not the only country where political abuse of psychiatry has taken place. Over the past decades quite extensive documentation has been published on similar abuses in other countries as well. One of the countries where systematic political abuse of psychiatry took place was Romania;

---

[1] Political abuse of psychiatry refers to the misuse of psychiatric diagnosis, treatment and detention for the purposes of obstructing the fundamental human rights of certain individuals and groups in a given society. The practice is common to but not exclusive to countries governed by totalitarian regimes. In these regimes abuses of the human rights of those politically opposed to the state are often hidden under the guise of psychiatric treatment. In democratic societies 'whistle blowers' on covertly illegal practices by major corporations have been subjected to the political misuse of psychiatry.

[2] The Hawaii Declaration of 1977 had been drawn up by the Ethical Sub-Committee of the Executive Committee set up in 1973 in response to the increasing number of protests against the use of psychiatry for non-medical purposes. One of the principles stated in the declaration was that a psychiatrist must not participate in compulsory psychiatric treatment in the absence of psychiatric illness, and also there were other clauses that could be seen as having a bearing on the political abuse of psychiatry. The declaration was amended in Vienna in 1983, and in 1996 succeeded by the Madrid Declaration of 1996, which was further expanded in 1999. In addition, the organization set up Committees on Ethics and on the Review of Abuse of Psychiatry.

[3] For instance during the debate on the issue of political abuse of psychiatry in the People's Republic of China. See Van Voren, R (2002) 'The WPA World Congress in Yokohama and the issue of political abuse of psychiatry in China', *Psychiatric Bulletin of the Royal College of Psychiatrists*, December 2002.

in 1997 the International Association on the Political Use of Psychiatry (IAPUP) organized an investigative committee to research what actually happened.[4] The same organization also received information on cases in Czechoslovakia, Hungary, and Bulgaria, but all these cases were individual and there was no evidence that any systematic abuse took place. An extensive research on the situation in Eastern Germany came to the same conclusion, although in this socialist country politics and psychiatry appeared to have been very closely intermingled.[5] Later, information appeared on the political abuse of psychiatry in Cuba, which was however short-lived and never developed into a full-scale means of repression.[6] In the 1990s, the successor organization of IAPUP, the Geneva (later, Global) Initiative on Psychiatry (GIP), was involved in a case of political abuse of psychiatry in the Netherlands, in the course of which the Ministry of Defence tried to silence a social worker by falsifying several of his psychiatric diagnoses and pretending his behavior was the result of mental health problems.[7] And, finally, since the beginning of this century the issue of political abuse of psychiatry in the People's Republic of China is again high on the agenda and has caused repeated debates within the international psychiatric community.[8]

During the past decades, human rights organizations such as IAPUP were regularly approached with requests to deal with abusive situations in psychiatry in countries such as South Africa, Chile, and Argentina. In the case of South Africa, severe abuses were the result of the racially discriminatory policy of *Apartheid*, which resulted in very different conditions in mental health services for the white ruling class and the black majority. Claims that psychiatry was abused as a means of political or religious repression were never confirmed. In Argentina and Chile, the abuse concerned individual psychiatrists, who were recruited to determine which forms of torture were the most effective, not the psychiatric profession as a whole or official bodies.[9]

Admittedly, those involved in the struggle against political abuse of psychiatry, including the IAPUP and other human rights groups, never reached full consensus on what the exact boundaries were between political abuse of psychiatry and more general misuse of psychiatric practice. Over the years, many individual cases were discussed extensively, determining whether it should be considered as one of political abuse of psychiatry or not. The issue continues to be discussed, in particular because recent cases are often more complex and involve less overt government involvement.

The fact that the use of psychiatry for political purposes is reported from so many diverse countries reveals an ongoing tension between politics and psychiatry, and also that using psychiatry to stifle opponents or solve conflicts appeals not only to dictatorial regimes but to well-established democratic societies. Nevertheless, it is clear that the political use of psychiatry has been a favorite of collectivist (socialist or communist) regimes. An explanation might be that ideologies that

---

[4] (1989) *Psychiatry under Tyranny, An Assessment of the Political Abuse of Romanian Psychiatry During the Ceaucescu Years*. Amsterdam: IAPUP.

[5] Süss, S, (1998) *Politisch Missbraucht? Psychiatrie und Staatssicherheit in der DDR*. Berlin: Ch. Links Verlag.

[6] Brown, Ch A and Lago, A (1991) *The Politics of Psychiatry in Revolutionary Cuba*. New York: Transaction Publishers.

[7] For the case of Fred Spijkers, see Nijeboer, A (2006) *Een man tegen de Staat*. Breda: Papieren Tijger. The case took many years to be resolved, and although the victim was compensated and even knighted by the Dutch Queen, it is still not fully closed, and Fred Spijkers is still trying to have his false psychiatric diagnosis revoked.

[8] Munro, R (2001) *Judicial Psychiatry in China and its Political Abuses*. Amsterdam: GIP, and Munro, R (2006) *China's Psychiatric Inquisition*. London: Wildy, Simmonds & Hill.

[9] See Van Voren, R (2009) 'Political abuse of psychiatry—a historical overview', *Schizophrenia Bulletin*, November 2009.

envision ideal societies where all are equal and all will be happy often conclude that those who oppose this must be mad. This is evident especially in the Soviet Union of the 1970s, as noted under 'Soviet psychiatric abuse'. At the end of the chapter, the political abuse of psychiatry in the People's Republic of China is also discussed.

Soviet psychiatric abuse

Repressing dissent through expanding psychiatric diagnosis and interventions

The political abuse of psychiatry in the Soviet Union developed within a totalitarian environment, which greatly facilitated its growth. Professor Richard Bonnie points out that 'in retrospect, repressive use of psychiatric power in the Soviet Union seems to have been nearly inevitable. The practice of involuntary psychiatric treatment presents an unavoidable risk of mistake and abuse, even in a liberal, pluralistic society. This intrinsic risk was greatly magnified in the Soviet Union by the communist regime's intolerance for dissent, including any form of political or religious deviance, and by the corrosive effects of corruption and intimidation in all spheres of social life.'[10] It was facilitated by the belief that persons who opposed the regime were mentally ill, as there seemed to be no other logical explanation why one would oppose the best socio-political system in the world. Slovenian philosopher Slavoj Zizek succinctly wrote that 'a person had to be insane to be opposed to Communism.'[11] Soviet leader Nikita Khrushchev worded this in a speech himself: 'A crime is a deviation from the generally recognized standards of behavior frequently caused by mental disorder. Can there be diseases, nervous disorders among certain people in Communist society? Evidently yes. If that is so, then there will also be offences that are characteristic for people with abnormal minds.... To those who might start calling for opposition to Communism on this basis, we can say that... clearly the mental state of such people is not normal.'[12]

Professor Richard Bonnie, together with Soviet lawyer Svetlana Polubinskaya, who was much involved in the development of modern mental health legislation in the USSR and its successor republics, pointed out that 'repression of political and religious dissidents was only the most overt symptom of an authoritarian system of psychiatric care in which an expansive and elastic view of mental disorder encompassed all forms of unorthodox thinking, and in which psychiatric diagnosis was essentially an exercise of social power.'[13] The diagnosis of 'sluggish schizophrenia' that was developed by the Moscow School of Psychiatry and in particular by Academician Andrei Snezhnevsky, provided a handy framework to explain this behavior.[14]

---

[10] Bonnie, R (2002) 'Political Abuse of Psychiatry in the Soviet Union and in China: Complexities and Controversies', *Journal of the American Academy of Psychiatry and the Law*, 30(1), 138.

[11] Zizek, S (2008) *In Defense of Lost Causes*. London: Verso, 36.

[12] *Pravda*, 24 May 1959.

[13] Bonnie, R and Polubinskaya, S (1999) 'Unravelling Soviet Psychiatry', *Journal of Contemporary Legal Issues*, 10(279), 284–5.

[14] Andrei Vladimirovich Snezhnevsky, born in 1904 in Kostroma, graduated from the Medical Faculty in Kazan in 1925 and started working in the psychiatric hospital in his hometown. In1932–1938 he was chief doctor of this hospital and became active in the field of research. In 1938–1941 he was senior scientific associate and deputy director of the Moscow Gannushkin Psychiatric Research Institute and in 1947 he defended his dissertation on psychiatry for the elderly under the title *Senile Psychoses*. During the war he was first linked to a battalion and then became chief psychiatrist of the First Army. In 1945–1950 he worked as a lecturer at the psychiatric faculty of the Central Institute for Continued Training of Physicians and for almost two years (1950–1951) was Director of the Serbski Institute. Until 1961 he was head of the

According to the theories of Snezhnevsky and his colleagues, schizophrenia was much more prevalent than previously thought because the illness could be present with relatively mild symptoms and only progress later. And in particular sluggish schizophrenia broadened the scope, because according to Snezhnevsky patients with this diagnosis were able to function almost normally in the social sense. Their symptoms could resemble those of a neurosis or could take on a paranoid quality. The patient with paranoid symptoms retained some insight in his condition, but overvalued his own importance and might exhibit grandiose ideas of reforming society. Thus symptoms of sluggish schizophrenia could be 'reform delusions', 'struggle for the truth', and 'perseverance'.[15] However in the *World Health Organization Pilot Study on Schizophrenia,* a computer program re-assigned cases of schizophrenia from Moscow to non-psychotic categories far more frequently than in any other country, thus highlighting this aberration in classification.[16]

Several scholars analysed the concepts of sluggish schizophrenia in the USSR, and the scientific writings that focused on this diagnosis. Canadian psychiatrist Harold Merskey, together with neurology resident Bronislava Shafran, in 1986 analysed a number of scientific articles published in the *Korsakov Journal of Neuropathology and Psychiatry.* They took two sample years, 1978 and 1983, and found in total 37 and 27 articles respectively that focused on schizophrenia. In their article, they concluded that 'the notion of slowly progressive schizophrenia is clearly widely extensible and is much more variable and inclusive than our own ideas of simple schizophrenia or residual defect states. Many conditions which would probably be diagnosed elsewhere as depressive disorders, anxiety disorders, hypochondriacal or personality disorders seem liable to come under the umbrella of slowly progressive schizophrenia in Snezhnevsky's system.'[17] In addition, based on the articles they analysed, they also questioned the quality of psychiatric research in the Soviet Union. 'If the articles we are considering had been submitted in English to a Western journal, most of them would probably have been returned for radical revision. As noted above, the original writing is diffuse and cumbersome: we have attempted to make some of it more readable

psychiatric faculty of the Central Institute for Continued Training of Physicians. In 1962 he became head of the Institute for Psychiatry of the Academy of Medical Sciences of the USSR a position he held until his death on 17 July 1987. In addition, from 1951 onwards he was chief editor of the *Korsakov Journal of Neuropathology and Psychiatry.* In 1957 he became a candidate Member of the Academy of Medical Sciences, in 1962 a full member.

[15] See Bloch, S, (1989) 'Soviet Psychiatry and Snezhnevskyism', in R Van Voren (ed) *Soviet Psychiatric Abuse in the Gorbachev Era,* 55–61. In an interview with the Soviet newspaper *Komsomolskaya Pravda* two Soviet psychiatrists, Professor Marat Vartanyan and Dr Andrei Mukhin, explained in 1987 how it was possible that a person could be mentally ill while those around him did not notice it, as could happen in case of 'sluggish schizophrenia'. What did mentally ill then mean? Vartanyan: '. . . When a person is obsessively occupied with something. If you discuss another subject with him, he is a normal person who is healthy, and who may be your superior in intelligence, knowledge and eloquence. But as soon as you mention his favorite subject, his pathological obsessions flare up wildly.' Vartanyan confirmed that hundreds of persons with this diagnosis were hospitalized in the Soviet Union. According to Dr Mukhin this was because 'they disseminate their pathological reformist ideas among the masses.' A few months later the same newspaper listed a number of symptoms 'a la Snezhnevsky', including 'an exceptional interest in philosophical systems, religion and art.' The paper quoted from a 1985 *Manual on Psychiatry* of Snezhnevsky's Moscow School and subsequently concluded: 'In this way any–normally considered sane–person can be diagnosed as "sluggish schizophrenic".'

[16] WHO (1973) *The International Pilot Study on Schizophrenia.*

[17] Merskey, H and Shafran, B (1986) 'Political hazards in diagnosis of "sluggish schizophrenia"', 249. Published in the *British Journal of Psychiatry,* 148, 247–256.

in translation. At times the writing is also disturbingly incomprehensible, even to readers who grew up speaking Russian and received a Russian medical education.'[18]

Two years later, Soviet dissident and former political prisoner Semyon Gluzman carried out even more extensive research. In his analysis he quoted a large number of works by well-known associates of the Serbski Institute, and in some of these studies the political 'illness' was far from being camouflaged. In some studies patients were ill with 'excessive religiosity',[19] another study concluded that 'compulsory treatment in an ordinary psychiatric hospital may be recommended for patients with schizophrenia with delusional ideas of reform, who show a diminished level of activity and in whom we can observe a difference between their statements and behavior.' However, another patient showed an 'extreme social dangerousness and [this formed] the foundation of the recommendation for compulsory treatment in a Special Psychiatric Hospital'.[20]

Being considered 'especially dangerous criminals', many dissidents were incarcerated in these Special Psychiatric Hospitals. Often housed in former prison buildings dating back to Tsarist times, the living conditions were generally very bad. As early as 1971 Soviet Minister of Health Boris Petrovsky[21] reported to the Central Committee of the Communist Party that the living conditions in the Special Psychiatric Hospitals did not meet the standards necessary for adequate treatment of the mentally ill.[22] Petrovsky's criticism did not stand alone. In the same year, the Ministry of Health, the Ministry of Internal Affairs (MVD), and the KGB sent a plan to the Council of Ministers for improving medical assistance to persons with mental illness.[23] A few weeks later, the Central Committee received a highly critical four-page report by the Department of Science and Education of the Central Committee, addressed to the Central Committee, which provided much detail about the prevailing situation. The report mentioned that, despite special attention being paid for several years, the Central Committee was still receiving 'complaints from the population with regard to serious shortcomings in the mental health care services in the country' and that 'the state of psychiatric help continues to be unsatisfactory. According to the report, the number of people in need of psychiatric help had grown enormously: while in 1966 just over two million citizens were on the psychiatric register, the number had grown by 1971 to 3.7 million.[24] In many hospitals patients had only 2–2.5 square meters at their disposal, although the norm was 7 square meters. 'Cases in which patients are sleeping in pairs in one bed and even on the floor are not rare. In several hospitals double bunk beds have been made.'[25] The report continued: 'As a result of overcrowding of hospitals sanitary-hygienic norms are being violated,

---

[18] Merskey, H and Shafran, B (1986) 'Political hazards in diagnosis of "sluggish schizophrenia"', 251.

[19] Gluzman, S (1989) *On Soviet Totalitarian Psychiatry*. Amsterdam: IAPUP, 42.

[20] Gluzman, S (1989) *On Soviet Totalitarian Psychiatry*. Amsterdam: IAPUP, 43.

[21] Boris Vasilievich Petrovsky was a general surgeon who made several major contributions to cardiovascular surgery, transplant surgery, and oesophageal surgery. For more than 15 years (1965–80) Petrovsky was Minister of Health in the former Soviet Union.

[22] Report by B Petrovsky to the Head of the Department of Science and Education of the Central Committee of the CPSU, 25 March 1971.

[23] Excerpt from the minutes No. 31, para. 19c of the session of the Central Committee of the CPSU of 22 February 1972.

[24] In 1988 the number of persons on the psychiatric register had grown to 10.2 million. See *Ogonek* (no. 16, 15–22 April 1989, 24).

[25] (1972) *On the situation of psychiatric help in the country*, Report to the Central Committee, 18 February 1972, signed by the Head of the Department for Science and education S Trapeznikov, 1.

unacceptable conditions are created for living, diagnosing and treatment of mentally ill persons as well as for the work of the personnel. Not seldom patients are discharged prematurely.'[26]

Factors contributing to Soviet psychiatric abuse

There is ample evidence that the core group of psychiatrists that developed and implemented this system to treat dissenters as psychiatrically ill on the orders of the Party and the KGB knew very well what they were doing.[27] Yet for many Soviet psychiatrists the diagnosis of grandiose reform-ism as mental illness seemed very logical, because they could not otherwise explain to themselves why somebody would give up his career, family, and happiness for an idea or conviction that was so different from what most people believed or forced themselves to believe. In a way, the plan was also very welcome, as it excluded the need to put difficult questions to oneself and one's own behaviour. And difficult questions could lead to difficult conclusions, which in turn could have caused problems with the authorities for the psychiatrist himself.

The onset of political psychiatry can probably best be seen as the result of a combination of fac-tors that were only possible to mature under a totalitarian regime. The decision in 1950–1951 to give monopoly over psychiatry to the Pavlovian school of Professor Andrei Snezhnevsky was one crucial factor.[28] Andrei Snezhnevsky, who for almost 40 years would dominate Soviet psychiatry, was, like so many others, formed by the political reality in which he lived. His role in the political abuse of psychiatry has been subject to much debate. Some consider him as one of the main archi-tects of the political abuse, a cynical scientist who served the authorities and willingly developed a concept that could be used to declare political opponents of the regime to be mentally ill. Others have defended Snezhnevsky, pointing out that he was not the only person who believed in the concept of 'sluggish schizophrenia' and also claiming that his ideas were abused by a regime with-out his active involvement. However, Snezhnevsky himself participated in some examinations of dissidents, and thus a complete whitewashing of his role is thereby impossible.

In the mid-1990s two psychiatrists who worked in his Research Center wrote an analysis, which at their own request was never published and remained in the archives of the Geneva Initiative

---

[26] (1972) *On the situation of psychiatric help in the country*, 1.

[27] For instance, in 2001 Dr Yakov Landau of the Serbski Institute said on Polish television that 'the organs [KGB] burdened us with very responsible work. . ... They expected us to do what they asked us to do, and we knew what they expected.' There are many of such indications that leading psychiatrists knew full well what they were involved in, see the description of Andrei Snezhnevsky in this chapter and Van Voren, R (2010) *Cold War in Psychiatry*.

[28] On 11–15 October 1951, a joint session of the USSR Academy of Sciences and the USSR Academy of Medical Sciences met in compliance with an order of I. V. Stalin to institutionalize the theory of higher nervous activity of IP Pavlov. The session decreed that annual scientific conferences should be held to consider problems related to Pavlovian physiology. In response to this call, a year later a session of the Presidium of the Academy of Medical Sciences and the Board of the All-Union Society of Neuropathologists and Psychiatrists on the 'Physiological Teachings of the Academician I. P. Pavlov on Psychiatry and Neuropathology' was convened. A number of influential Soviet psychiatrists—VA Giliarovskii, MO Gurevich, and AS Shmaryan—were condemned for adhering to anti-Marxist ideology and to psychiatric theories conceived by Western psychiatrists. The named psychiatrists acknowledged the correctness of the accusations, admitted their 'errors', and promised in the future to follow Pavlov's teach-ings on psychiatry. The session's Presidium urged the development of a 'New Soviet Psychiatry' based upon experimental and clinical findings and consistent with the Pavlovian conceptualization of higher nervous activity, which considered psychiatric and neurotic syndromes in terms of the dynamic localiza-tion of the brain's functions.

on Psychiatry.[29] Fifteen years later the text is still of great interest, and provides a unique insight into Soviet psychiatry and the central role of Snezhnevsky. The authors, whose names are known to the author but who are kept anonymous for reasons of confidentiality, put the role and position of Snezhnevsky against the backdrop of a totalitarian Stalinist society, where each and every branch of society was dominated by one leader, one school, one leading force. 'We assume that [Snezhnevsky's school became the leading one] first of all because one or the other direction in Soviet psychiatry had to fulfil that role as a consequence of the general conditions [in society].'

The authors describe Snezhnevsky as a competent scientist who avoided everything that could have a negative effect on his scientific work, yet also as a person who met all the requirements imposed by the state. 'He chaired the session of the shameful "trade union meeting" in 1973 that was organized to "discuss" (as a form of harassment) Dr VG Levit, who had decided to emigrate to the United States.[30] It is hard to understand how this all could be part of the biography of one and the same person. He was a talented scientist, whose goal in life was clearly to find the scientific truth, and at the same time he was an amoral politician, who made this same truth secondary to the demands of the authorities.. . . . Such a submission was the price he had to pay for the leadership position of both himself and his school.'[31]

'We witnessed how with a sense of dependence and willingness to submit he talked with any official of the party apparatus,' the authors continue. 'Therefore we are convinced that he was not an ideologist, not an architect of psychiatric repression. He was a submissive implementer of that policy and agreed to look the other way, because he preferred to do so and not leave to do some regular job. . . . Exactly that—scientific work—was the goal in the life of Snezhnevsky and for that he paid his share all his life. That is not something new. Already doctor Faust sold his soul to the devil; there were people before him, and after him. Snezhnevsky was one of them.'[32]

On basis of the above you can conclude that the price for Snezhnevsky pursuing his scientific inquiries in the USSR was that he had to allow his science to be used politically. However, available evidence also shows that he was well aware that his science was being used for political purposes, and that he himself actively participated in it. Several diagnoses of well known dissidents were signed by him personally. On top of that Snezhnevsky was also the totalitarian leader he was expected to be. 'The atmosphere in the collective was far from ideal. In fact, in the Institute the same totalitarianism prevailed as in the rest of the country. . . . His opinion was decisive in all questions, from setting priorities in scientific work to hiring new associates, their promotion or dismissal. The scientific council. . . had no real meaning. Decisions were prepared beforehand in "the corridors of power."[33] As a result, the prevailing attitude became one of pleasing the chef, not of finding scientific results. "This excluded the development of new and original ideas."'[34]

As noted above, the key to the politicization of psychiatry was that Soviet society had become a centrally-ruled totalitarian State. Everything, even hobby clubs and sports clubs, had been politicized and nothing was possible without the will and support of the Communist Party. The purges of the 1930s, 1940s, and early 1950s, when suddenly in one night, for instance, all Esperantists in

---

[29] Initially the book, titled *Psychiatry, psychiatrists and society,* was to be published by Geneva Initiative on Psychiatry, but subsequently shelved because the authors had reason to believe that publication would be followed by repercussions that would affect their careers.

[30] Dr Vladimir Levit eventually emigrated to the United States. Such meetings of the collective to denounce those who fell out of line with the official policy were regular practice in the USSR.

[31] Anonymous. *Psychiatry, psychiatrists and society* .Unpublished manuscript, in the author's possession, 96.

[32] *Psychiatry, psychiatrists and society,* 97.

[33] *Psychiatry, psychiatrists and society,* 113.

[34] *Psychiatry, psychiatrists and society,* 114.

Leningrad would be arrested and another group or sector of society was targeted the next time, had made that perfectly clear. Doctors had to swear the Oath of the Soviet Doctor instead of the Hippocratic Oath, which made clear that the Soviet Doctor's ultimate responsibility was to the Communist Party, not to medical ethics.[35]

According to the two anonymous Soviet psychiatrists mentioned earlier, 'the main priority of the Soviet state was always itself. The interests of the individual were viewed as being secondary, and this general notion was reflected in many aspects [of psychiatric practice]. . . . The political abuse of psychiatry started much earlier than is generally assumed. It started when the State used the paternalistic tradition of Russian psychiatry and forced the psychiatrists to impose a certain way of life on their patients.'[36] For example, a doctor discharges a patient before treatment is actually completed, not because the patient can go home, but because otherwise the patient stays away from work too long. This negatively affects the statistical success-rate of the mental health institution, which in turn contravenes the 'interests of the State'.[37] In another case, one of the authors describes receiving a phone call from the local Party organs, asking to postpone the discharge of a patient for two weeks 'because we don't want to run the risk of having a Communist festivity disturbed'. The authors conclude, it is very hard for a psychiatrist not to fulfil this seemingly innocent request.

The dissident psychiatrist and former political prisoner Dr Anatoly Koryagin also mentions this pressure from judicial organs.

> At the beginning of the 1960s, working as a young psychiatrist in Siberia, I personally experienced the kind of pressure that is exerted on doctors by the KGB, by the procuracy, and by officers of the Ministry of the Interior. Lawyers and officers of the Ministry tried to impress on me many times the nature of the psychiatric illness from which this or that person was supposedly suffering—and I was a psychiatrist! They assured me that to give a psychiatric examination to such a person was a tedious formality from their point of view. In each case, in order not to become a compliant party to the official organizations, I had to refuse categorically to make individual judgements, and to demand that these 'psychiatrically ill' people be examined by a medical panel or by a panel of forensic psychiatrists.. . . Many yielded to this pressure. . . and people were placed in psychiatric hospitals without a proper forensic psychiatric examination.[38]

Soviet psychiatrists had little chance to escape the all-pervasive control by the Communist Party and its organs because of their three-fold dependency on the Soviet state: scientifically, because their research work depended on their allegiance to the Soviet authorities; politically, because they had to organize their professional life and interact with authorities so as not to lose their support; and economically, as private practice did not exist and they were all employees of the State.[39] People in leadership positions did not only need to be successful in leadership: 'that success. . . depended on other conditions; those who were able to maintain the necessary interactions with the authorities had the biggest chance of making a career. For that they had to fulfill a multitude of requirements. Next to specific personal qualities that were necessary to be able to maintain

---

[35] The Oath of the Soviet Doctor was adopted by the Presidium of the Supreme Soviet of the USSR on 26 March 1971. *Vedemosti Verkhovnogo Soveta SSSR*, 1971, 13, 145.

[36] *Psychiatry, psychiatrists and society*, 38. Both authors are known to me.

[37] *Psychiatry, psychiatrists and society*, 38.

[38] Koryagin, A (1989) 'The involvement of Soviet psychiatry in the persecution of Dissenters', *British Journal of Psychiatry*, 154, 336.

[39] *Psychiatry, psychiatrists and society*, 86.

contacts with specific party officials, there were also other demands, in particular having a character by the book.'[40]

Another factor that helped to impose political abuse of psychiatry on the psychiatric community and root out potential opposition was the fact that

> for many years there was an unchangeable yet informal hierarchy of mental health institutions. This looked more or less as follows: the highest step on the ladder formed the scientific research institutes, then the psychiatric faculties, then Moscow and Leningrad psychiatric hospitals, then oblast and city psychiatric hospitals, then oblast and city outpatient clinics and, at the lowest step, came the regional psycho-neurological outpatient clinics and cabinets. If a doctor who worked in a dispenser would change a diagnosis, it was usually considered as an 'attack' on the institution that was higher up on the hierarchical ladder. Because for many years, a diagnosis established by a 'higher institution' was obligatory to follow by a 'lower institution'.[41]

In other words, if the Serbski Institute in Moscow declared a dissident to be mentally ill, no lower-placed psychiatrist would dare to go against it.

The authors conclude: 'As a result traditional Russian paternalism combined with the traditions of Soviet bureaucracy caused a deep conflict between society and psychiatric services: patients in psychiatric institutions changed into a formal social group that was subject to discrimination; many principles of professional ethics became distorted; the stimuli to improve the professional level of psychiatrists were to a large degree lost.'[42]

And finally, one should not forget that the Soviet Union had become a closed society, a society that was cut off from the rest of the world. World psychiatric literature was unavailable, except to the politically correct psychiatric elite. 'Western psychiatric literature became rare: the number of periodicals that came was limited and a large part wound up in the "special holdings" (*spetskhran*) of the Lenin library [in Moscow] and were impossible to get access to.'[43] The power of the Party seemed endless, whether one believed in their ideals or not. And thus any person who decided to voice dissent openly ran a high risk of being considered mentally ill. As a result, the political abuse of psychiatry, that initially mostly affected intellectuals and artistic circles, grew into an important form of repression, with approximately one-third of the dissidents in the 1970s and early 1980s being sent to a psychiatric hospital, rather than to a camp, prison, or exile.[44]

Dr Koryagin, who served six years out of a total sentence of 14 years of camp and exile for having been a member of a 'Working Commission to Investigate the Political Abuse of Psychiatry', examined 17 victims or potential victims of political psychiatry. His diagnoses were used by the (potential) victims as a defense against being declared insane, or as a means to show the outside world that a hospitalized dissident had been incarcerated for non-medical reasons. On basis of his sample, Koryagin came to the interesting conclusion that the length of hospitalization seemed to correspond to the length of the sentence a political prisoner otherwise would have got. In other words, a political prisoner charged with 'slandering the Soviet state' usually stayed hospitalized for about three years (the maximum term under that Article of the USSR Criminal Code), while a

---

[40] *Psychiatry, psychiatrists and society*, 87.
[41] *Psychiatry, psychiatrists and society*, 41–42.
[42] *Psychiatry, psychiatrists and society*, 43.
[43] *Psychiatry, psychiatrists and society*, 58.
[44] This percentage is based in the files of the International Association on the Political Abuse of Psychiatry. However, as can be seen in n. 51, the KGB reported higher percentages of 'mentally ill' dissidents: 'For example, in 1973 a total of 124 persons were arrested for these crimes against 89 persons in 1974, in the context of which it is important to note that 50% of these people were mentally ill'.

person accused of anti-Soviet agitation and propaganda usually stayed in for much longer, seven years or more (again the maximum sentence under that Article). Cynically, one could say that the more crazy a person was, the more serious his damage to the Soviet state![45]

In other cases, dissidents also had the impression that mentally weaker persons were more quickly sent to camps, while the mentally strong and unbreakable faced an uncertain future in a psychiatric hospital, not having a sentence, and being tortured with neuroleptics and other means.

Historical development and practice of political abuses of psychiatry

Generally speaking, the systematic use of psychiatry to incarcerate dissidents in psychiatric hospitals started in the late 1950s and early 1960s. However, there are cases of political abuse of psychiatry known from a much earlier date. During the first years of the Soviet State some attempts to use psychiatry for political purposes took place, yet these cases can be compared to the Spijkers case in The Netherlands: applying a psychiatric diagnosis seemed to be the easiest option.

In the 1930s the political abuse of psychiatry became a more frequent phenomenon. According to a series of letters published by a Soviet psychiatrist in the *American Journal of Psychiatry*, it was a leader of the Soviet secret police, Andrei Vyshinsky, who ordered the use of psychiatry as a means of repression.[46] The author, whose name was known to the editor but otherwise remained anonymous, reported that the first Special Psychiatric Hospital in Kazan was used exclusively for political cases. Half of the cases were persons who indeed were mentally ill, but the other half were persons without any mental illness, such as the former Estonian President Paets who was held in Kazan for political reasons from 1941 to 1956.[47]

The Serbski Institute for Forensic and General Psychiatry in Moscow had a political department, headed by Professor Khaletsky. Yet, according to Soviet poet Naum Korzhavin, the Serbski was at that time a relatively humane institution with a benevolent staff.[48] However, the atmosphere changed almost overnight when in 1948 Dr Daniil Lunts was appointed head of the Fourth Department, which was later usually referred to as the Political Department. Before this, psychiatric departments had been considered a 'refuge' against being sent to the Gulag, but from that moment onwards this policy changed.[49]

---

[45] See Koryagin, A (1987) 'Unwilling Patients', in R Van Voren (ed), Koryagin: A Man Struggling for Human Dignity, Amsterdam, IAPUP, 1987 43–50. A very interesting book on the origins and scope of political abuse of psychiatry in the Soviet Union is Korotenko, A and Alkina N (2002) *Sovietskaya Psikhiatriya–Zabluzhdeniya I Umysl*. Kiev: Sphera. 2002

[46] *American Journal of Psychiatry*, 1970, vol. 126, 1327–1328; vol. 127, 842–843; 1971, vol. 127, 1575–1576, and 1974, vol. 131, 474.

[47] (1971) *Kaznimye sumasshestviem*. Frankfurt: Possev, 479.

[48] Bloch, S and Reddaway, P (1977) *Russia's Political Hospitals*. London: Gollancz, 53–54.

[49] Van Voren, R and Lunts, D (1978) *Psychiatrist of the Devil*, unpublished manuscript; Van Voren, R (1989) *Soviet Psychiatric Abuse in the Gorbachev Era*. Amsterdam: IAPUP, 16. According to Boris Shostakovich, 'D.R. Lunts was unhappy in life, with very complicated family circumstances, innerly lonely, weak, and absolutely not a bad person. Understanding of this came much later, when after the death of his wife and eldest daughter, he married S.L. Taptatova. He became completely different: more calm, soft, started to dress elegantly and thawed. Unfortunately, he was only able to live not long like this by fate. . . . His widow . . . writes, and somehow correctly, about his conviction that for those people it was better to stay in a psychiatric hospital than to be sent to prison.' Biography of DR Lunts, in *Ocherki Istorii*, published on the occasion of the 75th anniversary of the Serbski Institute, 202–204.

More cases of political abuse of psychiatry are known from the 1940s and 1950s, including that of Party official Sergei Pisarev who was arrested after criticizing the work of the Soviet secret police in connection with the so-called Doctor's Plot, an anti-Semitic campaign developed at Stalin's orders that should have led to a new wave of terror and probably to the annihilation of Jewish communities that survived the Second World War. Pisarev was hospitalized in the Special Psychiatric Hospital in Leningrad, which, together with a similar hospital in Sychevka, had been opened after the Second World War. After his release in 1955, Pisarev initiated a campaign against the political abuse of psychiatry, focusing on the Serbski Institute that he considered to be the root of all evil. As a result of his activity the Central Committee of the Communist Party established a committee that investigated and concluded that political abuse of psychiatry was indeed taking place. However, the report disappeared in a desk drawer and never resulted in any action.[50]

Until the mid-1960s, the political abuse of psychiatry in the USSR went mostly unnoticed, and also among Soviet dissidents the notion that a dangerous new form of repression threatened them remained absent. In his memoirs, Vladimir Bukovsky writes about his stay in the Serbski Institute: 'We were absolutely not afraid to be called lunatics—to the contrary, we rejoiced: let these idiots think that we are lunatics if they like or, rather, let these lunatics think we are idiots. We remembered all the stories on lunatics by Chekhov, Gogol, Akatugawa and of course also *The Good Soldier Schweik*. We roared with laughter at our doctors and ourselves.'[51] But it was only later that they realized that the old woman who cleaned the ward told everything to the doctors, who used the information to prove their mental illness. In 1974, Bukovsky wrote, together with the imprisoned psychiatrist Semyon Gluzman, a *Manual on Psychiatry for Dissenters*, in which they advised potential future victims of political psychiatry how to behave during investigation in order to avoid being diagnosed as being mentally ill.[52]

The available evidence shows that in the course of the 1960s the political abuse of psychiatry in the Soviet Union became one of the main methods of repression. By the end of that decade many well-known dissidents were diagnosed as being mentally ill. According to FV Kondratiev, an associate of the Serbski Institute, between 1961 and the date of his research (1996) 309 people were sent to the Fourth Department of the Serbski Institute for psychiatric examination after having been charged with anti-Soviet agitation and propaganda (Article 70 of the Russian Soviet Federated Socialist Republic (RSFSR) Criminal Code), and 61 on a charge of 'slandering the Soviet State' (Article 190–1 of the RSFSR Criminal Code). However, he admits that 'politicals' were also charged with other crimes, such as hooliganism, and that therefore the numbers might be higher.[53]

A report by Lieutenant-General S Smorodinski of the KGB in Krasnodarski Krai of 15 December 1969, shows that people sent to the Serbski Institute formed only the tip of the iceberg. This report, which KGB Chairman Yuri Andropov sent to the Politburo in January 1970, discussed more effective measures to register and isolate mentally ill persons, including those 'who had terrorist and other intentions dangerous to society.'[54] Among the latter, Smorodinski listed people

[50] Pisarev, S (1970) *Soviet Mental Prisons, Survey*. London, 175–180.

[51] Bukovsky, V (1978) *To Build a Castle, my Life as a Dissenter*. London: André Deutsch Publishers 199.

[52] Bloch, S and Reddaway, P (1977) *Russia's Political Hospitals*. London: Gollancz, 419–440.

[53] *Ocherki Istorii*, published on the occasion of the 75th anniversary of the Serbski Institute, 140–141.

[54] Letter of Yuri Andropov to the members of the Politburo, No. 141-A, dated 20 January 1970, 'Secret'. It is accompanied by the report by Smorodinski addressed to Yuri Andropov. The document is part of a much larger collection of documents from the Politburo, the Central Committee of the Communist Party of the Soviet Union (CPSU) and the KGB that were scanned by Vladimir Bukovsky during his research for the planned trial against the CPSU (which never took place) and which he subsequently put on the internet. See <http://www.bukovsky-archives.net>.

who tried to escape from the Fatherland, people 'fanatically trying to meet with foreigners', as well as those who tried to found new [political] parties or to suggest control mechanisms with regard to the Communist Party. According to Smorodinski one person suggested establishing a 'council to control the activities of the Politburo of the Central Committee of the CPSU and local party organs', which was considered to be an especially dangerous act; others were accused of spreading anti-Soviet leaflets. Smorodinski concluded that the Krasnodarski Krai had only 3785 beds available, while 11–12,000 persons should be hospitalized. Andropov added to Smorodinski's document: 'Similar situations occur in other parts of the country.' In other words: the number of beds in the USSR needs to be increased considerably in order to meet this urgent demand.[55]

How extensive the abuse had become in the early 1970s is also well illustrated by a report on a high-level meeting between the East German Stasi and the Soviet KGB in Berlin in April 1976, with data on the situation a few years earlier: 'The increased stability of society in the USSR is also clear from the fact that in 1974 fewer people were convicted because of slandering the state or anti-Soviet propaganda than in previous years. For example, in 1973 a total of 124 persons were arrested for these crimes against 89 persons in 1974, in the context of which it is important to note that 50% of these people were mentally ill.'[56]

Psychiatry was not only used against individuals, but sometimes also to remove larger groups of 'undesired elements' during Communist festivities or special events. In some cases they were delivered en masse, such as in 1971 in Tomsk: 'At a ceremonial meeting of the hospital staff in 1971 [in Tomsk], which I attended, [hospital director Dr Anatoly] Potapov[57] said literally the following: 'We expect to register a great number of patients on November 4–7. There'll be a special mark on their papers. They are suffering from 'paranoid schizophrenia'. We are to accept them all no matter how many there are . . .'[58] In 1980, KGB Chairman Yuri Andropov was quite explicit in a 'top secret' memorandum to the Central Committee of the Communist Party with regard to the preparations of the 1980 Olympic Games in Moscow. In his six-page report he quite explicitly wrote that 'with the goal of preventing possible provocative and anti-social actions on the part of mentally ill individuals who display aggressive intentions, measures are being taken, together with police and health authorities, to put such people in preventive isolation during the period of the 1980 Olympics.'[59] His deputy Viktor Chebrikov and Minister of Internal Affairs Nikolai Shchelokov referred to them as 'mentally ill with delusional ideas.'[60] This use of mental hospitals to separate

---

[55] The Five Year Plan of 1971–1975 included the construction of 114 psychiatric hospitals with a total capacity of 43,800 beds.

[56] MfS-HAXX, 2941, 93.
In a memorandum by KGB Chairman Yuri Andropov to the Central Committee of the Communist Party, dated 29 December 1975, more interesting figures are provided. According to Andropov, in the period 1967 until 1975 in total 1583 people were sentenced on basis of Articles 70 and 190–1 of the RSFSR Criminal Code, while in the preceding eight years (1958–1966) the total had been 3448 persons. However, later in the document he notes that during the period 1971–1974 63,108 persons had been 'profilaktizirovano' (prevented), in other words, had been convinced by various means not to continue their anti-Soviet behaviour. Memorandum by Yuri Andropov, no. 3213-A, 29 December 1975, 3.

[57] Anatoly Potapov, a psychiatrist by profession, was from 1965 to 1983 director of the psychiatric hospital in Tomsk. He would later become Minister of Health of the Russian Soviet Republic.

[58] *Moscow News* no. 37, 1990, reprinted in *Documents* 38, September 1990.

[59] *Regarding the main measures to guarantee security during the period of preparation and implementation of the XXII Olympic Games in Moscow*, signed by KGB Chairman Yuri Andropov, document 902-A, dated 12 May 1980, 3.

[60] *On the measures of the MVD of the USSR and the KGB of the USSR to guarantee security during the period of preparation and implementation of the XXII Olympic Games in Moscow*, 'top secret' memorandum to the

undesirable elements during Communist holidays and special events was not limited to the USSR, however. Similar practices have been reported from Romania under Ceausescu and in the People's Republic of China.[61]

The Soviet lesson

Looking back, the issue of Soviet political abuse of psychiatry had a lasting impact on world psychiatry. From 1971 until 1989, the issue of Soviet psychiatric abuse dominated the agenda of the World Psychiatric Association (WPA), and led to a deep rift between Western and Eastern Bloc psychiatrists and many angry exchanges. The Soviet All-Union Society of Psychiatrists and Neuropathologists was forced to withdraw from the WPA in 1983 and only returned in 1989 when most of the abusive practices had been halted after an intervention by reform-minded Soviet leaders, and in particular Soviet Foreign Minister Eduard Shevardnadze.[62] The most positive aspect is probably that the issue triggered the discussions on medical ethics and the professional responsibilities of physicians (including psychiatrists), resulting in the Declaration of Hawaii of the WPA and subsequent updated versions. Also many national psychiatric associations adopted such codes, even though adherence was often merely a formality and sanctions for violating the code remained absent. Yet at the same time, the deep conflict within the WPA during the years 1983–1989 made absolutely clear that psychiatry could easily be turned into an arena for political strife. In their attempts to keep politics out of psychiatry, the WPA leadership actually obtained the opposite: it opened the door to carefully orchestrated interventions by the political leadership in Moscow, supported by active involvement of the secret agencies Stasi and KGB. At the same time, the goal of the opponents of political abuse of psychiatry to take politics out of psychiatry was equally unsuccessful. Their work was, whether they wanted or not, an element in the Cold War between East and West, and also in their case 'higher forces' undoubtedly had their influence.[63]

With the fall of communism in Eastern Europe in the late 1980s, most of the regular practice of using psychiatry to suppress political opponents ceased to exist. Some cases surfaced in Central Asia, notably in Turkmenistan and, more recently, in Uzbekistan. Also in Russia individual cases of political abuse of psychiatry continue to take place. The ranks of the victims over the last years have included women divorcing powerful husbands, people locked in business disputes, and citizens who have become a nuisance by filing numerous legal challenges against local politicians and

---

Central Committee, signed by Nikolai Shchelokov and V Chebrikov, 2. Viktor Chebrikov was Deputy Chairman of the KGB in 1962–1982 and Chairman in 1982–8. Nikolai Shcholokov, Minister of Internal Affairs and a personal friend of Soviet leader Leonid Brezhnev, was accused of corruption in 1988 and committed suicide.

[61] For Romania see: *Psychiatry under Tyranny*, 9. In China, in preparation for the Olympic Games of 2008, the Beijing police defined a grading standard for mentally ill persons who could cause incidents and accidents and are moderately disruptive. Security brigade chiefs, civil police chiefs, and the security directors of all police branches in all the incorporated districts and county councils of Beijing were trained according to the 'Beijing City mental health ordinance'. Also a thorough investigation of basic information regarding the mentally ill of Beijing was carried out. The Beijing Police used the above-mentioned professional training and basic investigation to determine a grading standard to rate the risks posed by mentally ill persons. See <http://www.legaldaily.com.cn> 4 April 2007.

[62] For detailed information on the struggle against the political abuse of psychiatry and the WPA, as well as on how the abuse eventually came to an end, see Van Voren, R (2010) *Cold War in Psychiatry—Human Factors, Secret Actors*. Amsterdam/New York: Rodopi.

[63] Research shows that both the WPA and the International Association on the Political Use of Psychiatry were infiltrated by the Stasi. A detailed account is provided in Van Voren, R (2010) *Cold War in Psychiatry—Human Factors, Secret Actors*.

judges or lodging appeals against government agencies to uphold their rights. However, there appears to be no systematic governmental repression of dissidents through the mental health system. Instead, citizens today fall victim to regional authorities in localized disputes, or to private antagonists who have the means, as so many in Russia do, to bribe their way through the courts. Finally, many of the current leaders of Russian psychiatry, especially those who already belonged to the establishment in Soviet times, have revoked the earlier confession read at the 1989 WPA General Assembly that psychiatry in the Soviet Union had been abused systematically for political purposes. They now preferred to refer to 'individual cases of "hyper-diagnosis" or "academic differences of opinion".[64]

The case of China

Although the first reports on political abuse of psychiatry in China surfaced at the beginning of the 21st century, they concerned systematic abuse for political purposes over a large number of years. The first pack of information received by GIP was a compilation of individual cases, but also with some historical overviews. The latter documents were the most worrisome, because they indicated the existence of a systematic political abuse of psychiatry of the same format as in the Soviet Union. The individual cases mostly concerned members of Falun Gong, a national spiritual movement founded in 1992 that espoused the development of body and mind through meditation. More than 70 million Chinese, including highly placed officials and politicians, had joined it by the end of the 1990s. It was emphatically not a political movement, but when it organized a demonstration in the summer of 1999 in front of the Communist Party building in Zhongnanhai to which tens of thousands of followers flocked, the authorities reacted. Since the Communist Party did not control it, it could endanger the Party's monopoly on power. The authorities decided to ban the movement, and intervened ferociously. Thousands of followers were arrested, tortured, and beaten to death in police precincts. Others disappeared into psychiatric hospitals and were tortured there. It was a reign of terror unleashed to end the movement as quickly as possible.[65]

Other documents, obtained separately, mentioned more, however. These materials, the overwhelming majority of which came not from dissidents but from China's officially published psychiatric and legal literature from the 1950s to the present day, showed that over the past decades millions of people had become victims of political abuse of psychiatry. The abuse had started in the 1950s and 1960s of the past century, and had increased enormously during the Cultural Revolution. From 1978 onwards it had taken the form of abuse of psychiatry familiar in the Soviet Union. According to official documents, in the 1980s approximately 15 per cent of all forensic psychiatric cases had a political connotation.[66] In the beginning of the 1990s the numbers had decreased to around one-tenth of that, but with the beginning of the campaign against Falun Gong the percentage had grown again quite quickly. Also, it emerged that a sizable network of high security forensic psychiatric institutions had existed in China since the early 1950s. Moreover, in 1987 this network was systematically expanded by the central government and given the new designation of 'Ankang' (Chinese for 'Peace and Health'). As of 2009, altogether some 25 Ankang

---

64 Dmitrieva, D (2001) *Alyans Prava i Miloserdiya*. Moscow: Nauka, 2001: 116–130.

65 The most extensive work on this issue is Munro, R (2006) *China's Psychiatric Inquisition*. London: Wildy, Simmonds & Hill. Also see (2002) *Dangerous Minds*. New York: Human Rights Watch/Geneva Initiative on Psychiatry, available at <http://www.hrw.org/reports/2002/08/13/dangerous-minds>.

66 Munro, R (2006) *China's Psychiatric Inquisition*, 157–162. This includes cases in which the regular procedure for forensic psychiatric examination were bypassed, but in which judiciary agencies were involved in the arrest and forced hospitalization.

institutions, all run by the Ministry of Public Security (i.e. the police) and staffed solely by police psychiatrists, nurses, and guards, were in operation around the country. The psychiatrists who worked there were wearing white coats over their uniforms. The authorities' plan was to have at least one such institution in each of the cities with a population of over one million inhabitants.

The political abuse of psychiatry in China appeared to be mainly taking place in institutions that were under the authority of the Ministry of Public Security and the police, but not in those belonging to other governmental sectors. Mental health care in China is divided into three sectors, which hardly communicate with each other. These are the earlier mentioned Ankang institutions of the Ministry of Public Security, those that fall under the authority of the Ministry of Health, and, as a third sector (dealing with the indigent mentally-ill), those belonging to the Ministry of Civil Affairs. Information rarely escapes from the Public Security sector. Psychiatrists working in, for instance, hospitals belonging to the Ministry of Health (aside from a significant number who work part-time as police psychiatrists), have no contact with the Ankang institutions, and indeed have—in most cases—little idea of what happens there and thus can honestly claim that they were not informed about political abuse of psychiatry in their country.

Many opponents of action against the Chinese therefore point out that the majority of Chinese psychiatrists have nothing to do with these abuses, that it is only a specific different branch of psychiatry that is involved. However, many of the Falun Gong followers who fell victim to the political abuse of psychiatry were hospitalized in general psychiatric facilities rather than in Ankang institutions,[67] and also many of the 'petitioners' or whistleblowers exposing corruption, or simply persistent complainants are incarcerated in general psychiatric hospitals. Since the late 1990s the trend seems to be that fewer dissidents are hospitalized in Ankang institutions, while the use of psychiatry against petitioners seems to continue to increase. As Sinologist Robin Munro points out: 'It's a covert way to silence people . . . There is no accountability or oversight. The person disappears, effectively; and with them, whatever evidence they have compiled against officials.'[68] Indeed, part of the problem seems to be caused not so much by the wish of a totalitarian regime to use psychiatry as a tool of repression, but rather a lack of control over the psychiatric profession and the way it is being used. The absence of a uniform psychiatric training programme and the fact that there is no national mental health legislation that protects the rights of patients aggravate the situation. As a result, also many abuses occur that have no political connotation and that increasingly attract the attention of the media in China itself.[69]

How widespread the problem had become can be seen in a report from May 2010, which mentioned that on 26–27 May 2010 the Ministry of Public Security held a meeting on mental hospitals nationwide. 'The meeting concluded that hospitals with adequate conditions should center their work around: "interfering ahead of an incident, handling during an incident, admitting patients after an incident, and following up with management." According to information, since 1998, mental hospitals nationwide have admitted mental patients who caused accidents 40,000 times. Among these 30% caused serious accidents . . . The meeting emphasized: Monitoring mechanisms must be established for mental hospitals. They must resolutely prevent the giving of private favors during legal validation procedures. In the process of admitting mental patients, special attention must be paid to the gate keeping of admission procedures and objects of treatment.

---

[67] See *Dangerous Minds*, n.70.

[68] *The Guardian*, 8 December 2008

[69] See for instance <http://www.chinahearsay.com/chinas-involuntary-commitment-system-needs-to-be-changed/>: 'Farmer went to Beijing over land dispute–then spent years in psychiatric hospitals' by Raymond Li in *South China Morning Post*, 22 May 2010.

Without checking and agreement from agencies of Public Security, [mental hospitals] must not admit anyone who is not a mental patient.'[70]

The structure of forensic psychiatry in China has been modelled on the Soviet Union. Psychiatrists of the Serbski Institute, who helped develop the Soviet system of psychiatric abuse, came to Beijing in 1957 to help their Chinese 'brethren'. Diagnosis was similar, except that the Soviets preferred 'sluggish schizophrenia' while the Chinese favoured 'paranoid schizophrenia' or 'paranoia'. The consequences were however the same: lengthy psychiatric hospitalization, compulsory treatment with neuroleptics, abuse, torture. . . everything directed at breaking the will of the victim.[71]

The complexity of the political abuse of psychiatry in China prevented campaigners from making a strong case. First, it was clear that not all of Chinese psychiatry was involved, and suspension or expulsion would also hurt ethical psychiatrists. Secondly, finding support for campaigns against China proved very difficult, as China was much more an open society than the Soviet Union and nobody wanted to hurt the economic ties with this huge upcoming market. Thirdly, the absence of a well-organized dissident movement as in the Soviet Union in the 1970s, with the consequent lack of steady information on cases other than Falun Gong, meant the campaign lacked the necessary fuel. Hence, pressure on international bodies like the WPA to take action never produced the desired result.

However, thanks to monitoring work by several mainland Chinese NGOs over the past couple of years, more and more current cases of politically-abusive psychiatric detention and treatment are now coming to public light. Also, in late 2008 the official Chinese state press for the first time openly criticized the use of psychiatry to silence critics of the authorities.[72] An editorial in the official English-language newspaper *The Beijing News* labeled the practice 'barbaric' and called upon the authorities to end these practices. Although a governmental official later denied that sane people were being hospitalized and that in fact all alleged victims had been 'obsessive',[73] more articles have appeared of recent date and there seems to be a mounting pressure within China itself to bring the political abuse to an end.[74]

Conclusion

The issue of Soviet political abuse of psychiatry had a lasting impact on world psychiatry. As noted above, some leaders of Soviet psychiatry have resiled from the admission of abuses. Yet the discussions on medical and psychiatric ethics produced the Declaration of Hawaii and subsequent updates, which provide definitive guidance for similar occurrences.

The continuation of political abuse of psychiatry in the People's Republic of China, however, shows that psychiatry can still be turned into a tool of repression when the right conditions are met or created. At the same time, the issue of political abuse of psychiatry in China shows that an easy solution to the problem does not exist. In the case of the Soviet Union, the forced departure

---

[70] Ministry of Public Security: police approval required to admit 'normal' people to mental hospitals. Report from Wuhan, 27 May 2010. Reporter Qin Qianqiao available at: <http://www.shanghai-daily.com/news/china-daily-news/ministry-of-public.htm>.

[71] See for instance Munro, R. (2006) *China's Psychiatric Inquisition*, vii-viii and 117–122.

[72] *The Beijing News*, December 8, 2008.

[73] *Agence France Presse*, 10 December 2008.

[74] See for instance 'Man in mental wards for 6 years to silence him' by Raymond Li, in *South China Morning Post*, 27 April 2010; 'Four officials sacked for locking up petitioner in mental hospitals' by Raymond Li, in *South China Morning Post*, April 29, 2010.

from the World Psychiatric Association of the Soviet All-Union Society of Neuropathologists and Psychiatrists did not directly end the abuse, but it turned it into a major issue on the US–USSR agenda and eventually the abuse was ended in 1989 when it was no longer politically expedient. In the case of China, such a measure would almost certainly not have the desired effect and would have serious consequences for the majority of Chinese psychiatrists who are not involved and are dependent on international contacts. In the case of China, a long-term programme in training mental health professionals in medical ethics and the rights of patients as well as the development of legal safeguards seem to have a better chance of success. In particular a multi-disciplinary and intersectoral approach, in which lawyers join hands with ethical psychiatrists, could have the desired effect and help bring about the necessary changes.

References

Anonymous (1970/1971/1974) 'Letters', *American Journal of Psychiatry*, 1970, 126, 1327–1328; 127, 842–843; 1971, 127, 1575–1576; 1974, 131, 474.

Anonymous (1990s) *Psychiatry, psychiatrists and society* .Unpublished manuscript, in the author's possession.

Bloch, S (1989) Soviet Psychiatry and Snezhnevskyism, in R Van Voren (ed) *Soviet Psychiatric Abuse in the Gorbachev Era*. Amsterdam: IAPUP.

Bloch, S and Reddaway, P (1977) *Russia's Political Hospitals*. London: Gollancz.

Bonnie, R and Polubinskaya, S (1999) 'Unraveling Soviet Psychiatry', *The Journal of Contemporary Legal Issues*, 10, 279.

Brown, Ch A and Lago, A (1991) *The Politics of Psychiatry in Revolutionary Cuba*. New York: Transaction Publishers.

Bukovsky, V (1978) *To Build a Castle, my Life as a Dissenter*. London: André Deutsch Publishers.

Dmitrieva, D (2001) *Alyans Prava i Miloserdiya*. Moscow: Nauka.

Dmitrieva, T and Kondratiev, FV (eds) (1986) *Ocherki Istorii*. Moscow: Sersbki Institute.

Gluzman, S (1989) *On Soviet Totalitarian Psychiatry*. Amsterdam: International Association on the Political Use of Psychiatry (IAPUP).

Kaznimye sumasshestviem (1971) Frankfurt: Possev.

Koppers, A (1990) *A Biographical Dictionary on the Political Abuse of Psychiatry in the USSR*. Amsterdam: IAPUP.

Korotenko, A and Alkina, N (2002) *Sovietskaya Psikhiatriya–Zabluzhdeniya I Umysl*. Kiev: Sphera.

Koryagin, A (1987) 'Unwilling Patients', in R Van Voren (ed) *Koryagin: A Man Struggling for Human Dignity*. Amsterdam: IAPUP.

Koryagin, A (1989) 'The involvement of Soviet psychiatry in the persecution of Dissenters', *British Journal of Psychiatry*, 154, 336–40.

Li, R (2010) 'Man in mental wards for 6 years to silence him', *South China Morning Post*, 27 April 2010.

Li, R (2010) 'Four officials sacked for locking up petitioner in mental hospitals', *South China Morning Post*, April 29, 2010.

Merskey, H and Shafran, B (1986) 'Political hazards in diagnosis of 'sluggish schizophrenia', *British Journal of Psychiatry*, 148, 249.

Munro, R (2001) *Judicial Psychiatry in China and its Political Abuses*. Amsterdam: GIP.

Munro, R (2006) *China's Psychiatric Inquisition*. London: Wildy, Simmonds & Hill.

Munro, R (2008) in T Branigan, 'Psychiatric treatment used to "silence" Chinese critics', *The Guardian*, 8 December 2008.

Nijeboer, A (2006) *Een man tegen de Staat*. Breda: Papieren Tijger.

Pisarev, S (1970) *Soviet Mental Prisons*. London: Survey, 175–180.

Shostakovich, B (1996) 'Biography of D.R. Lunts', *Ocherki Istorii*, Special issue published on the occasion of the 75th anniversary of the Serbski Institute.

Süss, S (1998) *Politisch Missbraucht? Psychiatrie und Staatssicherheit in der DDR*. Berlin: Ch. Linke Verlag.

Van Voren, R (ed) (1987) *Koryagin: A Man Struggling for Human Dignity*. Amsterdam: IAPUP.

Van Voren, R (ed) (1989) *Soviet Psychiatric Abuse in the Gorbachev Era*. Amsterdam: IAPUP.

Van Voren, R (2002) 'The WPA World Congress in Yokohama and the issue of political abuse of psychiatry in China', *Psychiatric Bulletin of the Royal College of Psychiatrists*, December 2002.

Van Voren, R (2009) *On Dissidents and Madness*. Amsterdam/New York: Rodopi.

Van Voren, R (2009) 'Political abuse of psychiatry—a historical overview', *Schizophrenia Bulletin*, November 2009. Available at <http://www.ncbi.nlm.nih.gov/pmc/articles/PMC2800147/>

Van Voren, R (2010) *Cold War in Psychiatry–Human Factors, Secret Actors*. Amsterdam/New York: Rodopi.

Van Voren, R and Lunts, D (1978) Psychiatrist of the Devil. Unpublished manuscript.

Zizek, S (2008) *In Defense of Lost Causes*. London: Verso.

Documents

Adler, N, Ayat, M, and Mueller, GOW (1989) *Psychiatry under Tyranny, An Assessment of the Political Abuse of Romanian Psychiatry During the Ceaucescu Years*. Amsterdam: IAPUP.

Human Rights Watch and Geneva Initiative on Psychiatry (2002) *Dangerous Minds*. New York: Human Rights Watch. Available at <http://www.hrw.org/reports/2002/08/13/dangerous-minds>, accessed 9 October 2011.

Schizophrenia Bulletin (1989) 15(4) (Supplement).

World Health Organization (1973) *The International Pilot Study on Schizophrenia*. Geneva: WHO.

Chapter 13

Descent into the Dark Ages

Torture and its Perceived Legitimacy
in Contemporary Times

Derrick Silove, Susan Rees, and Zachary Steel

Introduction

The abolition of torture has been a central focus of and impetus to the modern human rights
movement. The belated recognition that the international community had failed to respond in a
timely manner to the Holocaust during the Second World War provided an imperative in the
post-war period to establishing effective international sanctions against gross human rights violations, exemplified by torture and genocide. In this chapter, we review briefly the development of
the international legal regime, built incrementally since the establishment of the United Nations,
which by 1984 appeared to have achieved the aim of prohibiting torture.

Against this backdrop, we consider the recent radical departure within Western democratic
states from their avowed commitment to prohibit torture under all circumstances. Attacks on the
World Trade Centre and other targets on 11 September 2001, and the consequent declaration of
the war on terror, re-opened several fundamental questions about torture, particularly whether
the practice could ever be justified and whether this form of abuse could be distinguished from
legitimate interrogation techniques. The factors promoting the participation of general and mental health personnel in this post 9/11 debacle warrants close analysis, particularly given that their
involvement occurred in a context in which international prohibitions against such practices were
well-established (Silove and Rees 2010; Polatin et al. 2010).

History of the modern movement to prohibit torture

Torture has been a ubiquitous practice throughout the pre-modern period, whether used as a
form of punishment for criminal acts or as an instrument of persecution. During the Enlightenment,
philosophers such as Voltaire outlined a vision of a secular society grounded on tolerance, respect
for diverse beliefs, and the rule of law. Torture was identified as antithetical to such a project,
a major obstacle to constructing a modern society grounded firmly on the principles of justice.
Two centuries later, the United Nations Declaration of Human Rights, forged in the wake of
the Holocaust, represented a milestone in that it unambiguously proclaimed the right of all persons to be free of the threat of torture. The Geneva Conventions had already established strong
principles governing the acceptable treatment of combatants and prisoners in times of war.
Over ensuing decades, a succession of UN and regional instruments made further progress
towards the ultimate aim of prohibiting torture although mechanisms for enforcing that principle
remained poorly developed. The underlying weakness of existing international sanctions against
torture was starkly illuminated in the 1970s, when Amnesty International published an influential

report revealing that this form of abuse continued to be used in over a third of countries worldwide (Amnesty International 1977). Public campaigns, in which medical and other health personnel were actively involved, culminated in the adoption of the UN Convention Against Torture (CAT) in 1984, a watershed in international law which explicitly aimed to institute a universal ban on torture at an international level. The CAT defined torture as:

> Any act by which severe pain or suffering, whether physical or mental, is intentionally inflicted on a person for such purposes as obtaining from him or a third person information or a confession, punishing him for an act he or a third person has committed or is suspected of having committed, or intimidating or coercing him or a third person, or for any reason based on discrimination of any kind, when such pain or suffering is inflicted by or at the instigation of or with the consent or acquiescence of a public official or other person acting in an official capacity. It does not include pain or suffering arising only from, inherent in or incidental to lawful sanctions.

Article 2 of the CAT requires parties to take effective measures to prevent torture in any territory under its jurisdiction. The prohibition is absolute and non-derogable, that is, it does not allow of any exceptional circumstances, whether they be conditions of war, threat of war, internal political instability, public emergency, terrorist acts, violent crime, or any form of armed conflict. Specifically, torture cannot be justified as a means to protect public safety or to prevent emergencies; nor can perpetrators claim immunity because they were enacting orders from superior officers or public officials. The prohibition protects all people under a nation's effective control, regardless of citizenship or how that control is exercised.

The Optional Protocol to the CAT (2002) obliges states to establish a system of regular visits by independent national and international organs to places where there are people deprived of liberty, with the intention of preventing torture or any other cruel, inhumane, or degrading treatment or punishment. (For information about signatories to the CAT and OPCAT see <http://en.wikipedia.org/wiki/United_Nations_Convention_Against_Torture>).

Research into the mental health consequences of torture

The history of research into the effects of torture and the movement to develop rehabilitation services for survivors exemplifies the synergy that can be forged between human rights advocates and mental health professionals. Following the Second World War, Eitinger pioneered this field of research by examining the neuropsychiatric consequences of concentration camp internment amongst survivors of the Nazi Holocaust (Eitinger 1961). He described what he named as the KZ or concentration syndrome which later observers, such as Allodi, referred to as the torture syndrome (Allodi 1991). Nevertheless, even as late as 1988, the scientific knowledge concerning the psychiatric consequences of torture was negligible, being based on small convenience samples of political activists (Goldfeld et al. 1988).

The adoption of the category of post-traumatic stress disorder (PTSD) in the Diagnostic and Statistical Manual Edition III of the American Psychiatric Association in 1980 represented a milestone in the field by providing a unified focus for studying the psychiatric consequences of a range of traumas, including torture. The modern trauma model proposed that traumatic events, whatever their source, triggered a final common pathway, post-traumatic stress disorder (PTSD) which was characterized by re-experiencing symptoms (nightmares, flashbacks), avoidance and emotional numbing, and hyperarousal, including sleep disturbances, physical symptoms of the flight and fight response, and concentration difficulties. Subsequent case-comparison studies, for example amongst Turkish prisoners, showed that torture indeed resulted in high rates of PTSD and related disorders such as depression (Basoglu et al. 1994). Factors such as psychological preparedness for abuse and adherence to a strong political cause could partially mitigate these adverse outcomes, however (Basoglu et al. 1994). Nevertheless, the study of torture and its consequences remains challenging given the ethical and methodological constraints that researchers confront. As a consequence, the number of studies focusing on torture survivors remains relatively small, making it difficult to ascertain with precision the impact of torture as a threat to mental health at an international level. That hiatus has been addressed by a recent meta-regression analysis drawing on the entire refugee and post-conflict mental health field (Steel et al. 2009). Of the 181 surveys identified amongst refugee and conflict affected populations from 40 national groups, 84 were found to record the prevalence of torture. This pool included 42,626 persons amongst whom the prevalence of torture was 21 per cent. The review offered strong support for the assertion that torture is a potent cause of PTSD and, to a lesser degree, depression. When methodological factors (sampling method and sample size, approach to measurement) and other substantive predictors (such as exposure to other forms of trauma) were taken into account, torture remained the strongest factor predicting risk of PTSD. The weighted average prevalence of PTSD in the studies (n=40) in which 40 per cent or more of the sample reported torture was 46 per cent (95 per cent CI, 33–60 per cent). This increased to a rate of PTSD of 53.5 per cent (95 per cent CI, 36.8–69.5 per cent) amongst the 13 studies undertaken within three years of the conflict in which the torture occured. As a broad comparison, the rates of PTSD in the general population vary between 1 and 4 per cent and amongst survivors of serious accidents approximately 10 per cent. Importantly, although the time elapsed since torture was associated with lower levels of PTSD, even in the group studied three or more years post-conflict, the absolute rates remained extremely high (44 per cent). This suggests that many torture survivors remain chronically disabled by PTSD symptoms.

In spite of progress in research in this field, several fundamental questions remain. The similar prevalence rates of depression and PTSD identified amongst torture exposed populations suggest that mental health reactions following torture are complex and not captured by any single diagnosis. The question that remains debated is whether there are substantial differences in the response to extreme forms of deliberate human rights abuses exemplified by torture as compared with fateful, single event forms of trauma such as motor vehicle accidents and natural disasters. Proponents of a complex traumatic stress disorder have pointed out that survivors of intentional human-instigated abuse manifest characteristics not fully represented by PTSD, such as uncontrollable anger attacks, pervasive hostility, social isolation and alienation, and a tendency to develop somatic complaints and dissociation (Basoglu 2009). These features have been included in the proposed category of DESNOS (Disorders of Extreme Stress Not Otherwise Specified), considered but not included in DSM IV, and to some extent in the diagnosis of EPCACE (Enduring Personality Change After Catastrophic Events), a category listed in ICD-10. As yet, the nosological status of these formulations remains to be clarified (Beltran and Silove 1999).

A parallel formulation proposed by the first author in his ADAPT model (Adaptation and Development After Persecution and Trauma) (Silove 1999; Silove and Steel, 2006) considers five key psychosocial domains that are disrupted by torture and other forms of complex, human-instigated trauma. These domains include safety and security, family and social networks, access to justice, capacity to maintain identities and roles, and ability to engage in systems of meaning, including religion and political activities. All these domains are fundamental to the principles of human rights and hence reflect an intersection point between that framework and the psychosocial matrix in which torture occurs. Such a wider formulation may have implications for interventions for torture survivors as discussed hereunder 'Treatment and rehabilitation of torture survivors'.

Treatment and rehabilitation of torture survivors

The mental health field devoted to treating torture survivors is only now emerging from its formative years. As indicated, the impetus for this movement came from the close association of health professionals with human rights organizations, for example, amongst medical groups formed under Amnesty International (Amnesty International 1977). Given the complexity of the new field of rehabilitation, which spanned the areas of human rights, transcultural mental health, psychiatric traumatology, forced displacement, and community development, it is not surprising that from the outset there was a divergence in views about the focus of interventions. Specifically there has been an ongoing debate whether the core component of treatment should involve a form of psychotherapy that focused specifically on the traumatic experiences of torture or whether refugee survivors and their families needed a broad-based, multidisciplinary psychosocial approach, focusing on issues of resettlement, acculturation, language acquisition, and building resiliency.

This debate has yet to be resolved. Critics of a multimodal approach have claimed that the field has failed to apply evidence-based treatments for PTSD that have been tested in other areas of traumatology (Basoglu 2006). Contemporary guidelines are clear that trauma-focused cognitive behavioural therapy that focuses directly on the processing of trauma memories is the treatment of choice for PTSD, although medications, such as the selective serotonin reuptake inhibitors have a demonstrated efficacy (Forbes et al. 2007). There is some evidence, for example, from refugee camps in Africa (Neuner et al. 2004) and from a clinic working with Southeast Asian refugees in the US (Hinton et al. 2005) that CBT techniques modified to the target culture and context may be effective in relieving PTSD symptoms in conflict-affected and displaced populations. In contrast, a naturalistic outcome study of refugees undertaken in a well-established service in Denmark failed to find significant changes in symptoms of disability following multi-modal interventions spanning over a year of therapy (Carlsson et al. 2006). Whereas these trends suggest that torture survivors and others exposed to extreme abuses may require a trauma-focused form of psychotherapy, many of the most experienced professionals in the field continue to caution against limiting treatment to that modality (Rudnick, 2006; Lewis, 2004). They point out that there are wide-ranging existential and psychosocial effects of torture that undermine the persons sense of integrity and trust in others, reactions that are not comparable to the psychiatric consequences of single traumas in civilian life, a perspective consistent with the ADAPT model (Silove 1999). Further, clinical experience suggests that brief therapies that focus solely on memories of torture may trigger adverse reactions including overwhelming distress, rage, and loss of control. Insufficient attention has been given to these potentially adverse outcomes. At worst, excessive pressure on torture survivors to recall past memories of abuse might represent a challenge to the rights of the patient to avoid such memories. Nevertheless, scientific study should be the final adjudication of this contentious issue. The paucity of well-designed trials amongst torture survivor leaves the question of the recommended treatment of torture survivors unresolved at present. Clearly, there is a need for the many treatment services that have been established around the world to test competing treatments by applying rigorous scientific methodologies in order to establish the evidence-base to guide future interventions.

Reversion from the Enlightenment to the Dark Ages: 'The war on terror'

During the formative period in which services for refugees were established (1970s to 1990s), there was a strong sense of common purpose amongst Western governments and mental health professionals to denounce torture and to support survivors. Consensus appeared to have been established for the two decades following the adoption of the CAT that torture was not an acceptable strategy to be pursued by state authorities. The focus of concern turned to nations in low and middle income settings, particularly those ruled by oppressive and totalitarian regimes, where governments sanctioned or turned a blind eye to torture. While not actively engaging in torture, many countries of the West, however, continued to act globally in ways that made them complicit, either covertly through links amongst intelligence agencies or by acts of omission, for example by not criticizing trading partner nations implicated in torture. This gap between stated policy and practice may have set the stage for a number of the advanced Western countries to shift position after the US Administration's declaration of a 'war on terror' in 2001. So-called enhanced interrogation techniques were instituted in US detention centres such as Abu Ghraib in Iraq, Bagram in Afghanistan, and Guantanamo Bay in Cuba. Public revelations rapidly emerged, accompanied by graphic photographs, of extreme abuses being perpetrated in these detention facilities. European and other ally countries were implicated in assisting the United States to undertake rendition of prisoners, whereby suspects captured in the war on terror were transited through European states to third countries explicitly to allow the use of extreme interrogation and torture.

It is beyond the scope of this chapter to consider the full range of international, political, and social factors that contributed to this radical policy shift. It is notable, however, that the conditions that led to this debacle cannot be attributed solely to a conservative government acting in secrecy or in opposition to the views of an enlightened public. In the immediate aftermath of September 11, some prominent academics in the US declared their qualified support for torture or, at least tacitly accepted its use under extraordinary circumstances (Dershowitz 2004). They invoked utilitarian arguments to claim justification for the use of torture against the few in order to save the lives of many. The ticking bomb scenario was widely debated even though the extreme conditions it depicted were largely hypothetical (Wolfendale 2006). It was argued that if a 'terrorist' were captured who knew the location of a bomb that was about to explode in a population-dense location, it would be justified to torture him to elicit vital information that would result in the saving of lives of thousands of innocent citizens. Critics have pointed out the inherent fallacies of the ticking bomb scenario: it depicts a rare scenario, accounting for a very small portion of persons that are tortured in the real world; it is virtually impossible to know that a bomb definitely exists until it is found; interrogators can never be sure that the person being tortured is in possession of the vital knowledge; and torture often produces false or misleading information, particularly in an emergency situation.

The case of al-Libi underscores the likelihood of eliciting misleading intelligence from torture (Thomas and Hirsh 2005). Torture was applied by the US military to detainee al-Libi who subsequently confessed that al-Qaida was working with Saddam Hussain to obtain chemical and biological weapons in order to kill Americans. The then US Secretary of State Colin Powell argued the case for war against Iraq based heavily on this confession—which he described as credible and reliable. One year later, however, al-Libi retracted his statement and the US Defense Intelligence Agency (DIA) later concurred that his original confession was made either under duress or to achieve better treatment (Thomas and Hirsh 2005). In short, in using torture, there is a substantial risk of torturing the wrong person, for the wrong reasons, and eliciting the wrong information.

The administrative steps that ultimately led to the adoption of torture in US detention centres have now been extensively documented, although further evidence continues to emerge. In 2002, the year following September 11, the US President issued a decree determining that detainees at Guantanamo Bay were not subject to the Geneva Conventions. The US Department of Justice offered expert legal advice that sanctioned interrogation methods such as waterboarding and other enhanced interrogation techniques based on the claim that these practices did not transgress the threshold for causing physical or psychological harm (Silove and Rees 2010). At the same time, the US Secretary of Defense signed a memorandum allowing the use of 15 special counter-resistance techniques including prolonged stress positions, deprivation of light and sound, hooding, forced nudity, wall slamming, and manipulation of individual phobias (Sands 2008). These practices have been deemed by leading human rights organizations to constitute torture (Lewis 2004; Physicians for Human Rights, 2005). Of interest is the recent empirical evidence that suggests that psychological forms of torture analogous to those used in so-called enhanced interrogation techniques have grave psychological sequelae (Basoglu 2009). Nevertheless, to protect the actions of the Department of Justice, the Office of Legal Counsel, the primary agency for advice to the President regarding any legal limits on his power, offered repeated advice that, in effect, allowed the Administration to circumvent the Geneva Conventions, the CAT, and the Supreme Court of the USA. One argument used was that Afghanistan under the Taliban was a 'failed state', and therefore its previous status as a signatory to the Geneva Conventions no longer applied.

There appears to be a definable set of steps that lead societies down the slippery slope to sanction the use of torture and related abuses. Political leaders may be motivated by a sense of crisis and loss of control under conditions of perceived national threat; or they may exploit periods of turmoil, seizing the opportunity to direct attention from other problems or to advance their political, social, religious, or ideological programs. Propaganda that exaggerates the immediacy and extremity of the threat provides public justification for the victimization of targeted minorities. Emotive language is used to depict these minorities as being so malevolent or inhuman that they have forfeited any right to the processes of justice owed to other citizens. Because of the exceptional circumstances, normal judicial processes are represented as inadequate, or because of their transparency to public scrutiny, as a threat to national security. Hence, strong arguments are advanced that extraordinary actions, conducted in secrecy, are needed for what are characterized as unanticipated and unusual times. It is also common for hasty quasi-legal or legal provisions to be adopted as a mechanism to provide legitimacy for governments to circumvent or exploit loopholes in state or international law. Critics who attempt to defend human rights are commonly attacked for being naive, ignorant, or acting against the interests of public safety and national security. In the aftermath, if the tide turns against the decision to use torture, as has partially occurred in the US, the responsible leaders employ a range of strategies to avoid criticism or indictment. These strategies range from claiming ignorance, blaming subordinates or superiors, and continuing to invoke the principle of necessity to justify their actions. In the US, debate continues whether torture used during the war on terror yielded information that materially contributed to overcoming terrorism, even though there is little public evidence to support this contention. The paradoxical argument commonly used is that the responsible leaders cannot reveal the evidence because it remains in the realm of classified information.

The key lesson emerging from recent history is that the extensive legal provisions that appeared to have been firmly established to prohibit torture were clearly inadequate in the face of the actions of leaders in times of state crisis. Neither Abraham Lincoln's 1863 General Order No. 100 that decreed that 'military necessity does not admit of cruelty' nor the seemingly watertight international regime of human rights instruments adopted in the decades preceding the war on terror provided immunity from the tendency to resort to torture.

Krygier (2008) argues that the only mechanism that will preserve the rule of law and due process under all circumstances is to recognise the vulnerability of the law and the potential for aberrant behaviour by governments under extreme conditions such as those that emerged in the US following 9/11. One implicit lesson may be that the legalization of human rights, a process that gained unprecedented momentum in the last 60 years, has had the unintended effect of shifting human rights activities from the grassroots, community level to the realm of legal experts. Although that trend has been essential to achieving outcomes such as the CAT, it also runs the risk of reducing the impetus to maintain and build an active and powerful human rights movement at the community level. Perhaps the greatest failure, and one that became starkly evident in the testimony given by personnel involved in torture at Abu Ghraib, was the absence of a pervasive human rights culture within society in general and the military in particular (Miller 2005). It may be that the only way that the principles of human rights can be defended in an acute situation—as opposed to providing the foundations for subsequent prosecution of offenders—is to ensure wide-ranging and effective campaigns of education in high-risk institutions such as the army, with creative strategies being implemented to promote and maintain a durable rights-based culture in these vulnerable settings.

The mental health professional's role in assessing torture

The problem of medical personnel becoming involved in torture and other cruel and inhuman activities under state direction now has an extensive contemporary history, spanning the involvement of doctors in the Nazi Holocaust, the experimentation conducted on humans by Japanese doctors during the Second World War, the direct role of doctors in administering torture during the period of the dictatorships in South America, the political misuse of psychiatry in the Soviet Union, and medical complicity with the *Apartheid* regime in South Africa (Miles 2008). In response to these abuses, the World Medical Association has acted to prohibit medical involvement in practices that may result in torture (World Medical Association 1975).

Yet, in spite of this history, Lifton identified three areas in which professionals contravened these principles during the war on terror: failure to report to higher authorities wounds that were clearly caused by torture; failure to take steps to interrupt torture when the practice was revealed by medical examination; and allowing medical records to be read (and used) by interrogators (Lifton 2004). The ethical concerns relating to this issue have been extensively debated, primarily in the recent medical and psychological literature (Seltzer 2010; Olson et al. 2008; Hall 2004; Physicians for Human Rights 2009; Bloche and Marks 2005). The issue has remained contentious both within and across discipline in mental health, with some professionals continuing to argue that mental health personnel have a role in the interrogation room (Editorial 2009; Green and Banks 2009), in spite of the broader consensus amongst psychologists and psychiatrists that they have no role in the interrogation process (Silove and Rees 2010). The matter is of such salience that in 2009, the United Nations adopted a resolution aimed at strengthening existing prohibitions against health professionals being involved in torture; and in September 2009, the American Medical Association approached the Obama administration to seek its support for the view that the participation of physicians in torture and interrogation is a violation of core ethical values.

There are cogent scientific and clinical reasons to question whether mental health professionals have the expertise to make these judgements. Pain, acute psychological trauma, and other forms of intense suffering are quintessentially subjective in nature and as yet, there are no valid behavioural indices that can quantify these experiences objectively (Silove and Rees 2010). As clinicians, we rely primarily on what the patient tells us to judge his or her level of pain, trauma, or suffering, an assessment reliant on safe, confiding, and confidential conditions that are absent in the interrogation setting. At a more general level, there is a well recognized risk of bias when professionals attempt to serve 'two masters', the patient and the organization (Physicians for Human Rights 2003). Peer support and guidelines (Physicians for Human Rights 2003; Green and Banks 2009) are not likely to be sufficient to safeguard mental health professionals from succumbing to these powerful institutional influences: there is a grave risk of a collective bias developing that becomes self-reinforcing when personnel work together in closed and secretive institutions (Silove 1990).

Mental health professionals also have a limited capacity to predict the long-term consequences of interrogation. Although there is general evidence that torture results in high rates of chronic mental disorder (Steel et al. 2009), scientific understanding of the mechanisms involved is not yet at the stage to allow accurate predictions of outcomes in individual cases. In short, mental health professions should acknowledge that there is no scientific or clinical foundation for them to claim to be able to predict adverse outcomes in the highly charged setting of interrogation in which the relationship with the prisoner is inevitably fraught.

References

Allodi, F (1991) 'Assessment and Treatment of Torture Victims: A Critical Review', *Journal of Nervous and Mental Disease*, 179, 4–11.

Amnesty International (1977) *Evidence of Torture: Studies of the Amnesty International Danish Medical Group*. London: Amnesty International Publications.

Basoglu, M (2006) 'Rehabilitation of traumatised refugees and survivors of torture', *British Medical Journal*, 333, 1230–1.

Basoglu, M. (2009) 'A multivariate contextual analysis of torture and cruel, inhuman, and degrading treatments: Implications for an evidence-based definition of torture', *American Journal of Orthopsychiatry*, 79, 135–45.

Basoglu, M, Paker, M, Paker, O, Ozmen, E et al. (1994) 'Psychological effects of torture: a comparison of tortured with nontortured political activists in Turkey', *American Journal of Psychiatry*, 151, 76–81.

Beltran, RO and Silove, D (1999) 'Expert opinions about the ICD-10 category of enduring personality change after catastrophic experience', *Comprehensive Psychiatry*, 40(5), 396–403.

Bloche, MG and Marks, JH (2005) 'Doctors and Interrogators at Guantanamo Bay', *New England Journal of Medicine*, 353, 6–8.

Carlsson, JM, Olsen, DR, Mortensen, EL, and Kastrup, M (2006) 'Mental Health and Health-Related Quality of Life: A 10-Year Follow-Up of Tortured Refugees', *Journal of Nervous & Mental Disease*, 194, 725–31.

Dershowitz, A (2004) *Tortured Reasoning*. New York: Oxford University Press.

Editorial (2009) 'Responsible interrogation. Psychologists have a moral duty to help prevent torture', *Nature*, 459, 300.

Eitinger, L (1961) 'Pathology of the Concentration Camp Syndrome', *Archives of General Psychiatry*, 5, 371–79.

Forbes, D, Creamer, M, Phelps, A et al. (2007) 'Australian guidelines for the treatment of adults with acute stress disorder and post-traumatic stress disorder', *Australian and New Zealand Journal of Psychiatry*, 41, 637–48.

Goldfeld, AE, Mollica, RF, Pesavento, BH, and Faraone, SV (1988) 'The Physical and Psychological Sequelae of Torture. Symptomatology and Diagnosis', *Journal of the American Medical Association*, 259, 2725–29.

Green, C and Banks, M (2009) 'Ethical guideline evolution in psychological support to interrogation operations', *Consulting Psychology Journal*, 61, 25–32.

Hall, P (2004) 'Doctors and the war on terrorism', *British Medical Journal*, 329, 66.

Hinton, DE, Chhean, D, Pich, V, Safren, SA, Hofmann, SG, and Pollack, MH (2005) 'A randomized controlled trial of cognitive-behavior therapy for Cambodian refugees with treatment-resistant PTSD and panic attacks: A cross-over design', *Journal of Traumatic Stress*, 18, 617–29.

Krygier, M (2008) 'War on Terror', in R Manne (ed) *Dear Mr. Rudd: Ideas for a Better Australia*. Melbourne: Black Inc. Books, 31–134.

Lewis, A (2004) 'Making Torture Legal', *The New York Review of Books*, 15 July, available at http://www. nybooks.com/articles/archives/2004/jul/15/making-torture-legal/?pagination=false (last accessed 5 April 2012).

Lifton, R (2004) 'Doctors and Torture', *New England Journal of Medicine*, 351, 415–16.

Miles, SH (2008) 'Doctors' complicity with torture: it's time for sanctions', *British Medical Journal*, 337, a1088.

Miller, DQ (2005) *Prose and cons: Essays on prison literature in the United States.* North Carolina: McFarland & Company Inc.

Neuner, F, Schauer, M, Klaschik, C, Karunakara, U, and Elbert, T (2004) 'A Comparison of Narrative Exposure Therapy, Supportive Counseling, and Psychoeducation for Treating Posttraumatic Stress Disorder in an African Refugee Settlement', *Journal of Consultant and Clinical Psychology*, 72, 579–87.

Olson, B, Soldz, S, and Davis, M (2008) 'The ethics of interrogation and the American Psychological Association: A critique of policy and process', *Philosophy, Ethics, and Humanities in Medicine*, 3, 3.

Physicians for Human Rights (2003) *Dual loyalty and human rights in health professional practice: Proposed guidelines and institutional mechanism.* Cambridge, MA: Physicians for Human Rights.

Physicians for Human Rights (2005) *Break Them Down: Systematic Use of Psychological Torture by US Forces.* Cambridge, MA: Physicians for Human Rights.

Physicians for Human Rights (2009) *Aiding Torture: Health Professionals' Ethics and Human Rights Violations Demonstrated in the May 2004 CIA Inspector General's Report.* Cambridge, MA: Physicians for Human Rights.

Polatin, PB, Modvig, J, and Rytter, T (2010) 'Helping to stop doctors becoming complicit in torture', *British Medical Journal*, 340, c973.

Rudnick, A (2006) 'Disability and PTSD—Rapid Response', *British Medical Journal*, 333.

Sands, P (2008) *Torture Team; Rumsfeld's Memo and the Betrayal of American Values.* New York: Palgrave MacMillan.

Seltzer, A (2010) 'Medical complicity, torture, and the war on terror', *The Lancet*, 375, 872–73.

Silove, D (1990) 'Doctors and the state: Lessons from the Biko case', *Social Science & Medicine*, 30, 417–29.

Silove, D (1999) 'The Psychosocial Effects of Torture, Mass Human Rights Violations, and Refugee Trauma: Toward an Integrated Conceptual Framework', *Journal of Nervous & Mental Disease*, 187, 200–07.

Silove, D and Rees, S (2010) 'Interrogating the role of mental health professionals in assessing torture', *British Medical Journal,* 340, c124.

Silove, D and Steel, Z (2006) 'Understanding community psychosocial needs after disasters: Implications for mental health services', *Journal of Postgraduate Medicine*, 52, 121–25.

Steel, Z, Chey, T, Silove, D, Marnane, C, Bryant, RA, and Van Ommeren, M (2009) 'Association of Torture and Other Potentially Traumatic Events With Mental Health Outcomes Among Populations Exposed to Mass Conflict and Displacement', *Journal of the American Medical Association*, 302, 537–49.

Thomas, E and Hirsh, M (2005) 'The Debate Over Torture', *Newsweek*, 21 November. Online publication, available at http/www.highbeam.com/doc/IGI-138720623.html.

Wolfendale, J (2006) 'Training Torturers: A Critique of the 'Ticking Bomb' Argument', *Journal of Social Theory and Practice*, 32, 269–87.

World Medical Association (1975) 'Torture & Terrorism: International Conventions Against Torture', *World Medical Association Declaration of Tokyo.*

Chapter 14

Medicine, Mental Health, and Capital Punishment

James Welsh

'. . . if one who had committed a capital offence become Non Compos before conviction, he shall not be arraigned; and if after conviction, that he shall not be executed.'

William Hawkins, English jurist, 1716 (Ferris 1997)

I am Myself Kelsey Patterson who ask that you the United States District Court Eastern District of Texas honor honor honor my rights give me my rights stop the death warrants death warrants murders stop the execution stop and remove the execution execution date execution order told to me by Major Miller on January 15 who said the execution execution punishments body health destruction disfigurement immerse iert usage scope scoap devil murder homo rape death machines death warrants death warrants. . . .

From page one of 13-page letter to Texas authorities from Kelsey Patterson, February 2004 (AI 2004a, spelling as in original).

He was executed, 18 May 2004.

This chapter discusses the death penalty as a mental health and human rights issue: the position of the death penalty in human rights law and ethics, the implementation of capital punishment, and the role of health professionals—particularly mental health professionals—in this practice.

It focuses inevitably on the US, reflecting the imbalance between the abundance of research, jurisprudence, and documentation available from that country and the paucity of information from elsewhere (though the issues discussed are relevant far beyond the US). Its starting point is the long-standing position that executing people with serious mental illness or intellectual disability is contrary to norms of justice and rational penal policy. From a human rights perspective, the death penalty is a cruel and inhuman punishment that provokes and worsens mental disorder and suffering of the condemned and his or her family, and has a brutalizing effect on those involved in carrying out the death penalty and on society in general.

Background

Executing criminals, political opponents, vanquished enemies, and people with mental illnesses has a long history. So has the involvement of medical personnel in capital punishment—as designers, participants, critics, reformers, observers, and health care managers of those condemned to die.

The French Revolution at the end of the 18th century marked the beginning of serious medical participation in state-ordered execution, if only initially in the design and refinement of the guillotine. The violent nature of this method left little place for medical tinkering, though later execution techniques would require increasing levels of medical participation.

The medical role in the death penalty for the most part of the 19th century is poorly understood and documented other than in a small number of developed countries, and that was generally restricted to examining condemned prisoners, perhaps easing their anxieties with words and medication, and then certifying their death by hanging, shooting or, in France, guillotining, when the deed was carried out.

In the late 19th century, inquiries into aspects of capital punishment were carried out on either side of the Atlantic in response to bungled hangings in New York (Report 1888) and in England (Home Office 1888).[1]

Ethics were not a concern to these inquiries; nor did the British Royal Commission on this subject in the middle of the 20th century advance significantly the ethical understanding of medical participation in execution, apart from recording a clear message from the British Medical Association (BMA) that doctors would not participate in execution by lethal injection on the grounds that it would be unethical (AI 1989). This point of principle was later overturned in the US and subsequently a number of other countries that introduced precisely that form of execution with the advice, guidance, and participation of doctors, nurses and medical technicians. The method, initially hailed as the ultimate humane execution, came under unprecedented levels of legal challenge in 2006 and 2007 (*Morales v Hickman* 2006; *Taylor v Crawford* 2006). Medical opinion also reflected scepticism regarding the humanity of the lethal injection process or executions in general and certainly the role of doctors in this process (Editorial 2007; Curfman et al. 2008). However, in May 2008 the US Supreme Court decided in the case of *Baze v Rees* (2008) that execution by lethal injection, as practised in Kentucky, was constitutional, and other states which awaited the court decision recommenced executions.

Mental health has been a key factor in capital punishment at least since the 19th century. There is a long-standing principle—established in the *M'Naghten case* in England in 1843, though articulated by English and US jurists in the 18th century (Legal Historians 2007)—that an accused 'labouring under such a defect of reason, from disease of the mind, as not to know the nature and quality of the act he was doing; or, if he did know it, that he did not know he was doing what was wrong' (House of Lords 1843) would benefit from the defence of 'insanity' and not be subject to execution (Ferris and Welsh 2004). But the role of mental health in capital punishment is far wider than solely the state of mind of the accused at the time of the crime.

---

[1] Bungled hangings in the US did not end in the 19th century. In February 1930, a 52-year-old woman was decapitated during a hanging in Arizona (Borg and Radelet 2004). Elsewhere, a decapitation was the outcome of the hanging of Barzan Ibrahim al-Tikriti, former head of the Iraqi secret police, in Baghdad on 15 January 2007 (*New York Times*, 16 January 2007).

The death penalty in human rights law

The legal standing of the death penalty in international human rights law and jurisprudence can only be given brief consideration here.[2] While capital punishment is not prohibited in international law, the desirability of its eventual disappearance 'in all countries' was acknowledged in a 1971 resolution of the United Nations General Assembly (1971) and the punishment is constrained in law by exceptions, exclusions, and limitations. For example, the International Covenant on Civil and Political Rights (adopted 1966) states that in countries that 'have not abolished the death penalty' the death penalty may only be applied 'for the most serious crimes' (Article 6(2)). This has been interpreted as ruling out execution as a punishment for a wide variety of crimes which do not result in loss of life.[3] Moreover, according to international standards the penalty cannot be applied lawfully to various kinds of offenders—children and pregnant women, for example. Resolutions of the UN Economic and Social Council (ECOSOC) stated that executions shall not be carried out on 'persons who have become insane' (ECOSOC 1984) and recommended that UN member states eliminate the death penalty for 'persons suffering from mental retardation or extremely limited mental competence, whether at the stage of sentencing or execution' (ECOSOC 1989). The UN Commission on Human Rights (1999) has urged states retaining the death penalty neither to impose the death penalty on, nor execute, 'a person suffering from any form of mental disorder'.

Regional authorities add particular details to regulation of the death penalty. The American Convention on Human Rights (Article 4(5)), for example, prohibits the execution of persons aged more than 70, and the Council of Europe requires the total abolition of the death penalty for member states as a condition of membership (Council of Europe 2004).

How do medical professionals participate in capital punishment?

Participation in capital punishment can refer to actions at any point in the process that starts with the arrest of the suspect and ends with the execution (and in some cases with an autopsy or removal of organs for transplantation). Not all such actions are contrary to accepted ethics though all might cause discomfort to some doctors who see the whole process of capital punishment as lying outside the ethical practice of medicine. The American Medical Association (AMA) has set out in its ethical review of the subject a detailed exposition of the rights and wrongs of medical participation while acknowledging the right of the individual to support or oppose the death penalty itself (AMA 2000).

The AMA analysis of ethics and the death penalty identified a number of procedures in which doctors might participate (see Table 14.1). While written with the US in mind, the issues they identify are more widely applicable. As the table shows, some of these forms of participation are regarded by the AMA as ethical and others unethical. In particular, providing health care to the death row prisoner and certifying (but not monitoring and pronouncing) the death of the prisoner by execution appear to be accepted practices. However those procedures which help bring about the death of the prisoner are regarded by the AMA as breaching ethics. Thus, providing

---

[2] For more detailed analysis see, for example, Schabas (2003), Council of Europe (2004), Hood and Hoyle (2008).

[3] See statements of the UN Human Rights Committee, Special Rapporteur on Extrajudicial, Summary or Arbitrary Executions, and the UN Commission on Human Rights, discussed in Prokosch (2004). For a detailed review of discussions on the death penalty in the UN, see Rodley and Pollard (2009), Chapter 7.

Table 14.1 Ethics and the medical role in executions (Drawn from American Medical Association (2010) *Code of Medical Ethics Opinion E-2.06, Capital Punishment*. Chicago: AMA)

Acts adjudged unethical by AMA	Acts adjudged ethical by AMA
Prescribing or administering medications that are part of the execution procedure.	Testifying as to medical history and diagnoses or mental state as they relate to competence to stand trial.
Monitoring vital signs on site or remotely and pronouncing death	Testifying as to relevant medical evidence during trial.
Attending or observing an execution as a physician.	Testifying as to medical aspects of aggravating or mitigating circumstances during the penalty phase of a capital case.
Providing technical advice regarding execution.	Testifying as to medical diagnoses as they relate to the legal assessment of competence for execution.
Selecting injection sites.	
Starting intravenous lines as a port for a lethal injection device.	Certifying death, provided that the condemned has been declared dead by another person.
Prescribing, preparing, administering, or supervising injection drugs or their doses or types.	Witnessing an execution in a totally non-professional capacity.
Inspecting, testing, or maintaining lethal injection devices.	Witnessing an execution at the specific voluntary request of the condemned person, in non-professional capacity.
Supervising lethal injection personnel.	Relieving the acute suffering of a condemned person while awaiting execution.
When a condemned prisoner has been declared incompetent to be executed, treating the prisoner for the purpose of restoring competence unless a commutation order is issued before treatment begins.	Transplantation of organs only where a prisoner has made clear his or her intention before being arraigned on a capital charge.

Source: Copyright 2010. American Medical Association. All Rights Reserved.

essential advice to the execution team, procuring lethal drugs, identifying injection sites, injecting chemicals, and being present at an execution as a physician (as opposed to as a witness) are all regarded as unacceptable by the AMA. (Not mentioned in the AMA analysis, but equally constituting participation in an execution, would be a doctor's pinning of a marker over the heart of the prisoner to provide a target for members of a firing squad.) While the US has seen a progressive reduction in the active involvement of doctors in lethal injection executions, many state laws continue to require the presence of a medical practitioner (Denno 2002, 2007) and some engage in ways which appear to breach AMA guidelines. Nevertheless, the few attempts to call doctors to account for such ethical breaches have failed.[4] The role of nurses and emergency medical technicians is under even less scrutiny and accountability. (Table 14.2 summarizes the ways in which mental health professionals can be engaged in the death penalty.)

In China, where most aspects of the death penalty are a matter of state secrecy, it is believed that the lethal injection procedure introduced in 1997 routinely involves doctors (AI 2004b). Other countries using lethal injection also have involved doctors in the practice (AI 2007a).

---

[4] Some of the ethical implications of lethal injection executions are discussed by LeGraw and Grodin (2002); Groner J (2002); and Amnesty International (2007*a*). The development of the method is discussed in detail in Human Rights Watch (2006) and Denno (2007).

Table 14.2 Participation of mental health specialists in capital cases (Ferris and Welsh 2004)

Evaluation and testimony bearing on a defendant's capacity to stand trial.
Treatment to restore or maintain a defendant's competency to stand trial.
Evaluation and testimony bearing on a defendant's criminal responsibility.
Evaluation and testimony at the sentencing stage.
Competency to assist counsel during post-conviction appeals.
Evaluation and testimony bearing on a defendant's capacity to assist counsel during post-conviction appeals including capacity to waive appeals.
Evaluation and testimony bearing on a defendant's competency to be executed.
Treatment to restore a defendant's competency to be executed.
Treatment of symptoms not relevant to the defendant's legal situation.

Reproduced from P Hodgkinson and WA Schabas, *Capital Punishment: Strategies for Abolition*, 2004 with permission from Oxford University Press.

Execution methods such as shooting, electrocution, and hanging also see doctors in attendance and playing a role which critics argue breaches medical ethics. In India, for example, it has been argued that the doctor's role in checking the heartbeat of the prisoner following hanging is unethical (Jesani 2004).

Reasons for health professional participation in executions

Given the secrecy that attends executions it is not surprising that little empirical research has been conducted on the participation of health personnel. One significant paper analysed the views of four doctors and a nurse who collectively had participated in at least 45 executions in the US. The responses of these health professionals suggested a drift into involvement rather than an ideologically driven active engagement (Gawande 2006).

Surveys suggest two potential reasons for participation by doctors. The first is lack of awareness of the current ethical guidance. Farber and colleagues, for example, found that only 3 per cent of US doctors responding to a survey knew of any applicable standards on medical participation in the death penalty (Farber et al. 2000, 2001). In a survey of doctors 20 years earlier in Denmark (a long-standing abolitionist country), 3 per cent of respondents said that they would be willing to carry out an execution. A further 10 per cent had supported the death penalty as a suitable punishment (AI 2007a: note 123). This suggests that a commitment to the notion of execution as a just punishment together with lack of awareness of current ethics as well as an opportunity could combine to provide a willing population of medical participants in executions.

Mental health professionals and capital punishment

While in some countries mental health specialists may not be involved at any stage of the capital process, it is likely that they will play some role in most countries retaining the death penalty. This immediately introduces problems. As Bonnie has noted, 'practices regarded as unproblematic elsewhere in the administration of criminal justice inevitably become controversial in capital cases' (cited in Bonnie 2005). This is certainly the case with respect to medical evidence. While there is considerable information about psychiatry and the death penalty in the US, empirical evidence globally on the role of psychiatrists and other mental health professionals is thin. One unpublished study found that the defendant's mental state at the time of the crime was the most frequent focus of specialist evidence in the countries surveyed, though psychiatrists were also involved in assessing competence to be executed, and in treating those who were found incompetent, including involuntarily, thus possibly permitting execution (Ferris and Welsh 2004).

Where mental health is weighed in the context of capital crimes, expert witnesses may be asked to provide opinion on matters relevant to the judicial process. These focus on the mental state of the accused at the time of the crime, their mental state subsequent to trial including their fitness for execution, and their intellectual capacity.

Mental state at the time of the crime

Expert opinion regarding the likely mental state of the prisoner at the time of the crime will inform the court's deliberation as to whether there was a mental or physical condition which might explain in part the behaviour of the accused. Examples of disorders tending to diminish the responsibility of the prisoner include psychotic states, behavioural or personality disorders, and even metabolic disturbances affecting behaviour.

Mental state subsequent to the crime

Changes in mental health can occur after the commission of the crime—during the investigation period, during the trial, and during post-conviction imprisonment. The current international standards urge that prisoners found to be seriously mentally impaired after their arrest, whether or not of sound mind at the time of the crime, should not be executed (ECOSOC 1989). However, there are currents of scepticism within the criminal justice system, particularly in the US, reflecting a belief that prisoners can fake symptoms of mental illness in order to increase their chances of a commutation.[5]

The phenomenon of mental illness on death row has been documented in a number of human rights reports—on the US (AI 2006a) and Japan (AI 2006b, 2008a,b; FIDH 2003) for example—as well as in the medical literature (Piasecki 2005). In addition it must be presumed that in other countries prisoners are suffering poor mental health but there is no capacity or will to assess prisoners' mental state (Hood and Hoyle 2008:214).

Human rights reports have documented the harsh conditions experienced by condemned prisoners in Japan and the fact that prisoners with mental illness are among those executed (FIDH 2003; AI 2006b, 2009). For example, on 23 August 2007 Japan executed three individuals, including Takezawa Hifumi. According to reports of his trial, doctors testifying both for the prosecution and the defence diagnosed Takezawa as mentally ill though this did not prevent his execution (AI 2008a).

Obtaining information on Japanese death row inmates is difficult in part due to the high levels of secrecy practised in capital cases in Japan. Prisoners are held isolated under strict discipline and can be held under sentence of death in such conditions for decades. Amnesty International (AI) has documented the case of man, now in his mid-70s, sentenced to death in 1968 and still on

---

[5] The scepticism regarding mental illness appears to reflect the adversarial nature of death penalty trials in the US. Occasionally a concrete critique is made, such as in the case of Christopher Newton, executed in Ohio in May 2007. The Ohio Supreme Court concluded that he had 'falsified psychiatric symptoms so as to appear to have a serious mental disorder in order to receive special treatment and psychotropic drugs' (*State v Newton*, 108 Ohio St3d 13, 2006-Ohio-81.) Newton subsequently was a 'volunteer' for execution and his lethal injection execution took nearly two hours to accomplish—so long that, according to several press reports (including Associated Press, 24 May 2007), he was permitted a toilet/bathroom break during his execution.

Box 14.1: Competence to stand trial: case study

Scott Panetti shot his parents-in-law to death in 1992. He had previously been hospitalized for mental illness, including schizophrenia and bipolar disorder, in numerous different facilities. There is compelling evidence that he was psychotic at the time of the shootings, and that he was incompetent to stand trial. However, a trial proceeded and with Panetti defending himself. He did so dressed as a cowboy, presented an often rambling narrative in his defence and tried to subpoena unlikely witnesses such as the late President John F Kennedy. Expert witnesses asserted that Panetti believed he was sentenced to death 'to stop him from preaching'. Lawyers, doctors, and family members who attended the trial variously described the proceedings as a 'circus', a 'joke', a 'farce', 'not moral', and a 'mockery', but he was convicted and sentenced to death (AI 2004c). A day before his scheduled execution in 2004, his sentence was stayed for consideration of his competence. Two further court reviews confirmed his competence before, in 2007, his appeals reached the Supreme Court which stayed the execution (*Panetti v Quarterman* 2007), arguing against too narrow an understanding of competency (AI 2007b; Bonnie 2007; Slobogin 2007) and returned the case to the US District Court for the Western District for reconsideration of the competence issue in the framework of the Supreme Court's new guidance. In March 2008, a District Court judge again found that Panetti was competent to be executed, ruling that Panetti 'has both a factual and rational understanding of his crime, his impending death, and the causal retributive connection between the two' (*Panetti v Quarterman* 2008:62). At time of writing, Scott Panetti remains on death row.

death row more than four decades later; he has shown signs of serious mental disorder since the 1980s (AI 2009). The death penalty system in Japan has been repeatedly criticized by the United Nations Human Rights Committee (AI 2009).

The execution of mentally ill prisoners has also been noted in India where 'access to mental health professionals by condemned prisoners is extremely limited' and where research on this subject is lacking (AI 2008b:116).

The psychological pressures and ill treatment to which death row prisoners are subjected have formed the basis for a number of key court judgments bearing on the length of time a prisoner can be held under sentence of death. The European Court of Human Rights ruled in the case of *Soering v UK* (1989) that the appellant, Jens Soering, a German national, whose extradition for murder the US authorities were seeking, would be likely to be subjected to an extended period of detention in harsh conditions prior to possible execution in Virginia and that such conditions would be incompatible with European law. Extradition was denied. A second ruling, by the Privy Council of the UK House of Lords in the case of *Pratt and Morgan v the Attorney General of Jamaica* (1993), held that in 'any case in which execution is to take place more than five years after sentence there will be strong grounds for believing that the delay is such as to constitute "inhuman or degrading punishment or other treatment" and that the death sentence should be commuted to life imprisonment'. This 'five year rule' now applies in countries retaining the Privy Council as final court of appeal and arguably in other Caribbean states until overturned by judicial review or constitutional amendment.[6]

---

[6] Some Caribbean states have now introduced constitutional amendments to replace the Judicial Committee of the Privy Council with the Caribbean Court of Justice (CCJ) based in Trinidad as final court of appeal. Barbados introduced an additional amendment to rule that no period under sentence of death and no

Intellectual disability

Intellectual disability (known in the diagnostic schemes of the American Psychiatric Association (2000) and World Health Organization (2007) and in US jurisprudence as 'mental retardation'), is defined by: an intelligence quotient (IQ) score below 70, significantly below average intellectual functioning, limitations in two or more areas of adaptive behaviour such as communication and self-care, and evidence that these deficits became apparent before the age of 18. It is a significant finding in the death penalty in the US (Human Rights Watch 2001; AI 2001) though little information is available in other jurisdictions (Hood 2008). The execution of people with intellectual disabilities in the US was prohibited by a Supreme Court decision in the case of *Atkins v Virginia* (2002) though implementing the ruling has been a challenge. The American Psychiatric Association subsequently recommended statutory language addressing the definition of mental retardation, procedures relating to its assessment, and qualifications of testifying experts (Bonnie 2004). This cannot resolve with scientific precision the fuzzy line between a person who is immune from execution under *Atkins* and another who is marginally above the execution threshold. Mental health professionals may find themselves evaluating an accused person and concluding that the examinee, although marginally retarded, is not sufficiently retarded to stay alive.

While mental retardation and mental illness are recognized in statute and in common law as mitigating factors, in practice there seems to be evidence that such conditions are often weighed in the opposite sense—as aggravating factors. Slobogin (2000) summarizes studies showing a positive correlation between (failed) submission of an insanity defence and subsequent execution and the prejudicial impact of a defendant history of childhood abuse, drug problems, or emotional disturbance. Dangerousness is also a factor prejudicial to the case of the defendant, even when not specified by statute as an aggravating factor (such as in Texas and Oregon).

The challenges to mental health practitioners posed by capital punishment

Mental health specialist as expert witness

Arising from long-standing prohibitions on the execution of the 'insane', the notion of mental competence can occupy a central role in some death penalty cases.

The concept of mental competence—the intellectual capacity of a person to comprehend a process to which that person is party and to participate effectively in that process—is relevant for the trial, for decision-making regarding appeals, and for 'qualifying' for being executed.

Competence to stand trial

The accused person in a capital trial must be in a fit state to appear before the court and in particular should be able to contribute to his or her own defence. Mental health professionals may contribute to an evaluation of fitness though it is a judge who will formally make the ruling on competence. There are no particular ethical barriers to this role though in some circumstances ethical challenges may arise. The US Supreme Court ruled in *Washington v Harper* (1990) that a prisoner could only be forcibly medicated when the inmate was a danger to himself or to others and when the medication was in the inmate's best interests. However the Court

---

method of execution could be adjudged cruel, unusual, or degrading. However, in 2006 the CCJ refused Barbados judicial authority to hang two men whose sentences had been commuted as a result of the five year rule.

subsequently held in *Sell v US* (2003)—a case involving a man accused of non-violent crime—that under limited circumstances in which specified criteria had been met, lower courts could order the forcible administration of antipsychotic medication to an incompetent defendant for the sole purpose of rendering him competent to stand trial provided the treatment is medically appropriate and where 'essential' or 'overriding' state interests applied. The ruling in *Sell* may provide the basis for ordering treatment to restore competence for trial in capital cases though the judgment suggested forcible treatment to restore competence for trial 'may be rare'. (*Sell v United States*, p. 12).

In an *amicus curiae* brief to the court, the American Psychological Association took a neutral stance on the substantive issue arguing that factors such as medical need, protection of fair trial rights, and exploration of non-drug-based methods of restoring competence should be given due weight by the court (American Psychological Association 2003). An *amicus curiae* brief submitted by the American Psychiatric Association supported the position eventually adopted by the court (Hausman 2003).

Competence to terminate appeals

Dropping an appeal can result in a fast track to the death chamber. An appeal delays the date of the execution and withdrawal from the appeal process is likely to result in a hastening of the execution. (Prisoners who do this are sometimes described as 'volunteers' for execution (Blume 2005)). Given the serious consequences of terminating an appeal, it is sound practice to determine if the prisoner understands the ramifications of such a decision. However, this determination has a low threshold since many prisoners will indeed understand that they are likely to be executed as a result of ending appeals—one of the objectives of this decision. Prisoners' motivations for terminating appeals range from the 'rational', such as a desire to take responsibility for their crime, and the less rational such as emotional distress, depression, or suicidal ideation. At least 90 per cent of prisoners who drop appeal procedures in capital cases in the US are permitted to do so by courts. This includes a significant number of prisoners with various mental disorders (Bonnie 2005; Blume 2005). A recommendation of the American Bar Association (ABA) Task Force (ABA 2006b) noted that, given the stakes of the decision, 'a relatively high degree of rationality ought to be required in order to find people competent to make decisions to abandon proceedings concerning the validity of a death sentence'. The argument that a death row inmate's autonomy and dignity should be respected, and that execution of a 'volunteer' should proceed as a result, seems unsustainable in the light of the circumstances facing the death row prisoner (Bonnie 2005).

Competence for execution

The concept of fitness for execution is a difficult one for critics of the death penalty to grasp. How fit does one have to be to have one's life terminated? However, international standards (as well as national laws) require that those with particular vulnerabilities such as youth, pregnancy, intellectual disability or mental illness, are spared execution and thus where this is called into question, an evaluation has to be made by a court. The test applied in the US arises from the US Supreme Court ruling in *Ford v Wainwright* (1986) in which the court determined that, in order to meet the competence threshold, a prisoner must be able to understand why he (and sometimes she) has been sentenced to death and what will happen to him when the sentence is carried out.

In practice this standard does not protect the seriously mentally ill from execution. Amnesty International (2006a) documented numerous cases in the US where seriously mentally ill prisoners whose grip on reality was very tenuous were nevertheless executed. Vuotto and Ciccone (2006) have noted that 'unlike the mentally retarded offender and the juvenile offender, the mentally ill offender is not categorically excluded from being sentenced to death'—nor from execution.[7]

Where a prisoner is found unfit for execution through lack of competence, the execution can either be commuted or the state can seek the treatment of the prisoner to allow execution at some point in the future. In the case of *Singleton v Norris* (2003), a prisoner acknowledged to have schizophrenia, Charles Singleton, appealed against forcible medication which would render him fit for execution. The Appeal Court ruled that 'Singleton's argument regarding his long-term medical interest boils down to an assertion that execution is not in his medical interest. Eligibility for execution is the only unwanted consequence of the medication.' (*Singleton v Norris*, para. 24) Singleton was medicated, was adjudged competent, and was put to death on 6 January 2004 (Stone 2004).

The evaluation of competence has divided lawyers and doctors and split the psychiatric community. Attorneys seeking a commutation for their death row client are likely to request an evaluation of competence if they believe that it will result in a positive outcome. However, the World Psychiatric Association (1996) has urged that 'Under no circumstances should psychiatrists participate in legally authorized executions nor participate in assessments of competency to be executed.' By contrast, the AMA and American Psychiatric Association have concluded that providing expert evidence bearing on competence is not incompatible with ethics since it is not the mental health specialist but rather a judge who rules on competence. These associations have decided, however, that treating a prisoner to restore competence to allow execution was unacceptable.

Future dangerousness

In two states of the US (Texas and Oregon) a prisoner qualifies for the death penalty if he or she is adjudged as likely to continue to represent a danger to society if allowed to live. This has led prosecutors in these states to introduce evidence during the sentencing phase to demonstrate the future dangerousness of the convicted prisoner. Despite an opinion submitted by the American Psychiatric Association in the case of *Barefoot v Estelle* (1983) that psychiatrists had no special expertise in making such judgements and that they were wrong more times than they were right, the Supreme Court held that psychiatric evidence on this point could be admitted in court. Subsequently one psychiatrist was reprimanded by the American Psychiatric Association for giving unscientific and prejudicial evidence in such cases (Rosenbaum 1990), and counsel for the State of Texas admitted to the US Supreme Court that a forensic psychologist's testimony that, among other things, race was a predictor of future dangerousness, had 'seriously undermined the fairness, integrity or public reputation of the judicial process' (Cited in Texas Defender Service 2004). A study in Texas showed that in a sample of more than 150 cases, predictions of future dangerousness were wrong 95 per cent of the time (Texas Defender Service 2004). As a fundamental characteristic of expert testimony is that it is based on scientific knowledge and empirical soundness, this level of error must challenge the ethical acceptability, let alone the scientific rigour, of such evidence.

Mental disability

International standards call for states to end the use of the death penalty against 'persons suffering from mental retardation or extremely limited mental competence' (ECOSOC 1989) and in the

---

[7] The mentally retarded prisoner and the juvenile offender are protected by Supreme Court rulings in the cases of *Atkins v Virginia* (2002) and *Roper v Simmons* [543 US 551(2005)] respectively.

words of the United Nations Commission on Human Rights (2001) '[n]ot to impose the death penalty on a person suffering from any form of mental disorder or to execute any such person'. The first recommendation of the American Bar Association's Task Force on Mental Disability and the Death Penalty was to recommend that defendants with significant limitations in both their intellectual functioning and their adaptive behaviour should not be sentenced to death or executed including those with dementia and traumatic brain injury, disabilities very similar to mental retardation in their impact (ABA, 2006a). Since the US Supreme Court ruling in *Atkins v Virginia* (2002) prohibiting the execution of prisoners with mental retardation, assessments of developmental status have become more critical in death penalty cases. At the same time individual states are adopting their own procedures to make evaluations, introducing variability into an already challenging area of law.

This remains a fuzzy area in which science can arguably not provide the level of precision desirable where the cost of an assessment falling on one side of a rather elastic line is the possible death of the convicted prisoner.

Involuntary treatment on death row

The desire by the state to treat convicted prisoners in order to restore them to competence with the goal of executing them has been described as an ethical dilemma with only one solution (Radelet and Barnard 1988). That solution is to commute the death sentence for those found not competent and thus remove their eligibility for execution. This is recommended by the AMA in their policy on the death penalty (American Medical Association 2000) and by the American Bar Association Task Force on Mental Disability and the Death Penalty (ABA 2006a). In the case of *Singleton*, mentioned above, treatment led directly to execution.

Attempted suicide on death row

The attempted self-killing by a condemned prisoner, sometimes just hours before he is to be put to death by the state, challenges doctors required to provide emergency care to death row prisoners. In the US, the suicide rate on death row is higher than in the general prison population which in turn is higher than that in the civil population (Lester and Tartaro 2002; Tripodi and Bender 2007). There have been at least three attempted suicides on death row in the US in which the prisoners have been rushed to intensive care for resuscitation and then returned to the prison to be put to death a matter of hours later. While it has not been suggested that the doctors resuscitating the prisoners should not have done so, this use of emergency services raises questions about the good faith of those ordering the prisoners' resuscitation and the potential ethical challenges posed by a request to resuscitate, solely in order to execute (Ferris and Welsh 2004).

Mental health on death row

Conditions on death row are usually at least as harsh as other parts of the prison system but likely to be harsher. There is much evidence in the US to suggest that prisons hold higher proportions of people with mental illness than exist in the community. This is likely to be the case in some other jurisdictions. A report by the US Department of Justice suggested that rates of mental illness in state prisons averaged around one third of inmates (Bureau of Justice Statistics 2006). Perhaps understandably there has been far less research carried out with respect to prisoners held under sentence of death though some evidence suggests significant levels of mental disorders (Lewis et al. 1986). Amnesty International (2006a) compiled a non-comprehensive but compelling sample of cases of mentally ill men held on death row, some of whom were eventually executed. Again, medical research is lacking. In Japan, prisoners are subjected to both harsh conditions but also to a policy of non-disclosure to the prisoner of the date of execution. Death row prisoners therefore have to endure the possibility that each day could be their last (AI 2006b, 2009). When this is understood in the context of prolonged periods of detention and isolation, there can be no doubt of the emotional stress prisoners live under.[8] Families of death row prisoners also share the stress of the 'structured uncertainty' (Radelet et al. 1983) of life under sentence of death—the psychological stress on the prisoner of knowing that execution awaits though not always knowing when.

The extent to which the level of mental illness in the death rows of the world constitutes grounds to apply the ECOSOC protections or common law proscriptions against execution on the grounds of mental incompetence (however that is described) is not known, and more research and legal support is needed to be able to answer that question.

Ethics and human rights

Professional ethics

The ethics of participation of doctors and mental health professionals in capital punishment has been widely discussed. At international level, medical (World Medical Association 2000), psychiatric (World Psychiatric Association 1996), and nursing (International Council of Nurses 2006)[9] associations all oppose professional participation in executions. Unsurprisingly, the most active ethical debate has occurred in the US (American College of Physicians et al. 1994; Freedman and Halpern 1996), but opinions are also heard in countries not having the death penalty. For example, Gunn (2004) has presented a viewpoint of psychiatry from a UK perspective.[10] There has also been comment in India where the death penalty is retained but used relatively infrequently (Jesani 2004; Bhan 2005). Discussion of psychiatry and the death penalty has been limited in Japan (Nakajima 2002; Yamamoto 2005) and virtually absent elsewhere.

In sum, these discussions have been framed from both a societal viewpoint and from a more traditional ethics stance. The resolution adopted by the American Psychiatric Association Board of Trustees in 1969 'oppose[d] the death penalty and call[ed] for its abolition' (West 1975). The resolution added that 'the best available scientific and expert professional opinion holds it to be anachronistic, brutalising, ineffective, and contrary to progress in penology and forensic psychiatry' (West 1975). More recent discussions have examined the challenges posed by the death penalty in scientific and in ethical terms. The concerns raised by some researchers that lethal injection may result in excruciating pain for the prisoner but can be masked by the paralyzing effects of one of the drugs used (Koniaris et al. 2005) did not persuade the US Supreme Court which ruled that lethal injection was constitutional (*Baze v Rees* 2008). In other respects, there appears to be unanimity in the US medical profession that assisting in lethal injection executions or other forms of execution is unethical. The AMA position against medical participation in executions first articulated in 1980 and regularly updated since has been supported by a wide range of other health professionals (AI 2007a).

----

[8] Nevertheless prisoners can live long lives under these conditions. Sadamichi Hirasawa died in prison in 1987 at the age of 95 after 32 years' imprisonment (Associated Press report, *New York Times* 11 May 1987).

[9] The position of the ICN is important for two reasons. The first is the real risk of a medical role in executions being transferred to nurses where medical ethics require doctors not to participate. The second is that the ICN urges nursing associations to work for the abolition of the death penalty.

[10] He acknowledges that 'it is relatively easy . . . for the Royal College [of Psychiatrists] to develop its abolitionist policy on capital punishment' [in a country without the death penalty], though adding that 'no one [in the membership] has yet written to challenge it or spoken to any of the senior members of the College about it.'

Officials of medical professional societies in Illinois felt strongly that the ethical debate had been settled and said in response to a paper sympathetic to medical participation in executions: 'we cannot recall a single professional medical association or peer-reviewed article in any major medical or nursing journal that has contradicted the position that health care professionals' participation in lethal injection execution is unethical' (Bharati and Kobler 2008).

How do these conclusions fit with human rights? While ethics and rights are two different concepts they share some important values relating to the rights of the individual. The expansion in recent years in medical literature dealing with both ethics and human rights testifies to the relatedness and relevance of these concepts to medical practice (BMA 2001). Arguably the human rights framework is increasingly being seen as the context in which ethics are situated.

The wider context

The existence of the death penalty raises questions about social and political responses to crime which reflect on a healthy understanding of social processes. To see candidates for public office extolling the virtues of capital punishment as a solution to violent crime is to witness cynicism or misguided belief triumph over rationality. To witness the suffering of families affected by the murder of a loved one seeking the death of the convicted prisoner as relief for their pain, sometimes decades after conviction, is to see the lack of resolution provided by the death penalty when it is eventually carried out. Should mental health professionals be more outspoken about capital punishment as a human rights issue? Some professional bodies believe that the debate must move beyond individual ethical decisions to a discussion within the wider society. For example, the American Public Health Association (APHA) resolved in 1986 to 'Encourage professional organizations of health workers to work for the abolition of capital punishment and to discourage their members from participating in or contributing to the carrying out of the death penalty' (APHA 1986). Some individuals have advocated for professional bodies to increase their engagement on social issues such as the death penalty (Halpern et al. 2004).

The quality and availability of mental health services is also called into question by cases which end up in capital and non-capital trials. For example, one mentally ill prisoner in Texas, Larry Robison—prior to the killings for which he was tried and convicted—had tried to obtain mental health care for paranoid schizophrenia but was neither insured himself nor covered by his parents' insurance. During Robison's trial his mental illness was cited as a mitigating factor but he was found competent on appeal and was executed in 2000. The apparent unavailability of mental health care on financial grounds is made the more disturbing when counterposed to the cost of executing a prisoner.[11]

The evolving reduction in use of the death penalty

Thirty years ago, when Amnesty International adopted its first declaration against the death penalty, only 16 countries had abolished the death penalty for all crimes. By 2007, 137 countries had abolished the death penalty in law or practice.[12] Prior to 1981 when the World Medical Association adopted a statement opposing medical participation in the death penalty, there was

---

[11] According to the *Dallas Morning News* of 8 March 1992, a death penalty case in Texas costs an average of about $2.3 million. More recent studies in other US states have put the cost much higher.

[12] Statistics do not adequately reflect the pattern of the use of the death penalty globally. For example, in Africa only seven countries executed prisoners in 2007; Belarus is the only European country that continues to use the death penalty; and the US is the sole country in the Americas to have carried out any

little international guidance on doctors and the death penalty. Since then a wide range of professional bodies have supported calls for an end to medical participation in executions or have gone further and urged an end to executions altogether—permanently (for example, the International Council of Nurses, and British and Scandinavian medical bodies but also the American Public Health Association (AI 2007a)) or at least temporarily (both the American Psychiatric Association (2000) and the American Psychological Association (2001) called for a moratorium on the death penalty).

In December 2007 the General Assembly of the United Nations voted to support a resolution calling for a worldwide moratorium on executions. The vote gave a boost to those seeking to reduce the use of the death penalty, though there was a strong resistance from states supporting the use of the death penalty—including China, Iran, Iraq, Saudi Arabia, and the US, the five countries which account for the overwhelming majority of executions worldwide in 2009 (AI 2010). Executions in these and other retentionist countries continue. China nevertheless introduced legislation in 2007 to reduce the number of offences for which the death penalty is applicable and has even spoken of working towards eventual abolition (AI 2007a). It seems likely that there will be a progressive reduction in the application of the death penalty globally. While this may reduce the extent to which doctors must make choices about involvement in this punishment, there will remain a need in the foreseeable future for the profession to speak out on the basis of clear and comprehensible principles.

The trend in the reduction of executions is visible but the imminent disappearance of the death penalty from the statute books of those countries which continue to execute is unlikely.

Conclusion

The role of physicians and subsequently mental health professionals has become entrenched in the process of capital punishment since the introduction of the guillotine in the 18th century. In a parallel evolution there has been increasing recognition that executing certain categories of person, including juveniles, pregnant women, and people with mental illness and with intellectual disability, ought to be excluded from the death penalty. International standards now call for a reduction of the scope and application of capital punishment. Since the 1980s, national and international medical bodies have debated the ethics of participation in capital punishment and strict guidelines have emerged from this process.

Despite the clarity of the emerging ethics standards, psychiatrists and psychologists continue to play a role in death penalty cases—sometimes within the existing ethical framework and sometimes in breach of it. While there is a considerable body of knowledge and debate on the death penalty in the US, in much of the rest of the world this is not the case. This is partly due to the fact that many countries no longer have the death penalty and partly because those that do can be quite secretive over their practices.

Although the use of the death penalty is diminishing, it is likely to continue to pose challenges to those committed to its abolition. Mental health professionals should continue to contribute to the understanding of the phenomena of crime and violence. But the health professions could contribute useful insights beyond merely the individual expert opinions given in particular court cases. In addition to addressing mental health aspects of the death penalty, the psychiatrist,

---

executions since 2003 (apart from the Caribbean island of St Kitts and Nevis where one man was hanged in 2008). Five countries (including the US) account for vast majority of global executions.

psychologist, and other mental health specialist has much to contribute to discussions about effective social and criminal justice responses to serious crime—responses which will break, rather than contribute to, a self-perpetuating cycle of violence.

References

ABA (2006a) *Report of the Task Force on Mental Disability and the Death Penalty*. New York: American Bar Association.

ABA (2006b) 'Recommendation and Report on the Death Penalty and Persons with Mental Disabilities', *Mental and Physical Disability Law Reporter*, 30(5), 668–76.

AMA (2000) *Policy E-2.06 Capital Punishment. Adopted June 2000 (first issued July 1980)*. Available at: <http://www.ama-assn.org/ama/pub/physician-resources/medical-ethics/code-medical-ethics/opinion206.page?>, accessed 4 November 2011.

American College of Physicians, Human Rights Watch, The National Coalition to Abolish the Death Penalty and Physicians for Human Rights (1994) *Breach of Trust: Physician Participation in Executions in the United States*. New York: Human Rights Watch.

American Psychiatric Association (2000) *Diagnostic and Statistical Manual of Mental Disorders, Fourth Edition (DSM-IV)*. Arlington: American Psychiatric Publishing.

American Psychiatric Association (2000) *Moratorium on Capital Punishment in the United States, Position Statement of the American Psychiatric Association*. APA Document Reference No. 200006. Washington, DC: APA.

American Psychological Association (2001) *Resolution: The Death Penalty in the United States*. New York: APA. Available at <http://www.apa.org/about/governance/council/policy/death-penalty.aspx>, accessed 4 November 2011.

American Psychological Association (2003) *Amicus brief in the case of Sell v US 539 U.S. 166*. Washington DC: APA. Available at <http://www.apa.org/about/offices/ogc/amicus/sell.pdf>, accessed 4 November 2011.

APHA (1986) *Policy number 8611: Abolition of the death penalty*. Available at <http://www.apha.org/advocacy/policy/policysearch/default.htm?id=1126>, accessed 4 November 2011.

AI (1977) 'Declaration of Stockholm', in Amnesty International (2009). *Codes of Ethics and Declarations Relevant to the Health Professions*. 5th revised edn. London: Amnesty International.

AI (1989) *Health professionals and the death penalty. ACT 51/003/1989*. London: Amnesty International.

AI (1999) *United States of America: Rights for all: Time for humanitarian intervention: the imminent execution of Larry Robison. AMR 51/107/1999*. London: Amnesty International. Available at <http://www.amnesty.org/en/library/info/AMR51/107/1999/en>, accessed 4 November 2011.

AI (2001). *Mental retardation and the death penalty. ACT 75/002/2001*. London: Amnesty International. Available at <http://www.amnesty.org/en/library/info/ACT75/002/2001/en>, accessed 4 November 2011.

AI (2004a) *USA. Another Texas injustice: The case of Kelsey Patterson, mentally ill man facing execution. AMR 51/047/2004*. London: Amnesty International. Available at: <http://www.amnesty.org/en/library/info/AMR51/047/2004/en>, accessed 4 November 2011.

AI (2004b) *People's Republic of China. Executed 'according to law'?—The death penalty in China. ACT 17/003/2004*. London: Amnesty International. Available at <http://www.amnesty.org/en/library/info/ASA17/003/2004/en>, accessed 4 November 2011.

AI (2004c) *USA: 'Where is the compassion?' The imminent execution of Scott Panetti, mentally ill offender. AMR 51//011/2004, January 2004*. London: Amnesty International. Available at <http://www.amnesty.org/en/library/info/AMR51/011/2004/en>, accessed 4 November 2011.

AI (2006a) *USA. The execution of mentally ill offenders. AMR 51/003/2006*. London: Amnesty International. Available at <http://www.amnesty.org/en/library/info/AMR51/003/2006/en>, accessed 4 November 2011.

AI (2006b) *Japan: 'Will this day be my last?' The death penalty in Japan. ASA 22/006/2006*. London: Amnesty International. Available at: <http://www.amnesty.org/en/library/info/ASA22/006/2006/en>, accessed 4 November 2011.

AI (2007a) *Execution by lethal injection: a quarter century of state killing. ACT 50/007/2007*. London: Amnesty International. Available at <http://www.amnesty.org/en/library/info/ACT50/007/2007/en>, accessed 4 November 2011.

AI (2007b) *USA: Supreme Court tightens standard on 'competence' for execution. AI Index: AMR 51/114/2007, June 2007*. London: Amnesty International. Available at <http://www.amnesty.org/en/library/info/AMR51/114/2007/en >, accessed 4 November 2011.

AI (2008a) *Japan: Submission to the UN Universal Periodic Review: Second session of the UPR working group, 5–16 May 2008. ASA 22/001/2008*. London: Amnesty International. Available at <http://www.amnesty.org/en/library/info/ASA22/001/2008/en>, accessed 4 November 2011.

AI (2008b) *Lethal Lottery: the Death Penalty in India*. London: Amnesty International.

AI (2008c) *The death penalty worldwide: Developments in 2007. ACT 50/002/2008*. London: Amnesty International. Available at <http://www.amnesty.org/en/library/info/ACT50/002/2008/en>, accessed 4 November 2011.

AI (2009) *Hanging by a Thread. Mental Health and the Death Penalty in Japan. ASA 22/005/2009*. London: Amnesty International. Available at <http://www.amnesty.org/en/library/info/ASA22/005/2009/en>, accessed 4 November 2011.

AI (2010) *Death sentences and executions in 2009. ACT 50/001/2010*. London: Amnesty International. Available at: <http://www.amnesty.org/en/library/info/ACT50/001/2010/en>, accessed 4 November 2011.

Atkins v Virginia (2002) 536 US 304.

Barefoot v Estelle (1983) 463 US 880.

Baze v Rees (2008) 553 US 35.

Bhan, A (2005) 'Killing for the state: death penalty and the medical profession: a call for action in India', *National Medical Journal of India*, 18(4), 205–8.

Bharati, S and Kobler, WE (2008) 'Physician participation in lethal injection execution is unethical', *Mayo Clinic Proceeding*, 83, 113–23 (responding to D Waisel (2007) 'Physician participation in capital punishment', *Mayo Clinic Proceedings*, 82(9), 1073–80).

Blume, J (2005) 'Killing the willing: "Volunteers", Suicide and Competency', *Michigan Law Review*, 103, 939–1009.

BMA (2001) *The Medical Profession and Human Rights*. London: British Medical Association.

Bonnie, RJ (2004) 'The American Psychiatric Association's Resource Document on Mental Retardation and Capital Sentencing: Implementing *Atkins v. Virginia*', Journal of the American Academy of Psychiatry and Law, 32, 304–8.

Bonnie, RJ (2005) 'Mentally ill prisoners on death row: unsolved puzzles for courts and legislatures', *Catholic University Law Review*, 54, 1169–94.

Bonnie, RJ (2007) '*Panetti v. Quarterman*: Mental Illness, the Death Penalty, and Human Dignity', *Ohio State Journal of Criminal Law*, 5, 257–83. Available at <http://moritzlaw.osu.edu/osjcl/Articles/Volume5_1/Bonnie-PDF.pdf>, accessed 4 November 2011.

Borg, MJ and Radelet, ML (2004) 'On botched executions', in P Hodgkinson and WA Schabas (eds) *Capital Punishment: Strategies for Abolition*. Cambridge: Cambridge University Press, 143–68.

Bureau of Justice Statistics/ US Department of Justice (2006). *Mental Health Problems of Prison and Jail Inmates. NCJ 213600, September 2006*. Available at <http://bjs.ojp.usdoj.gov/content/pub/pdf/mhppji.pdf>, accessed 4 November 2011.

Council of Europe (2004) *Death Penalty: Beyond Abolition*. Strasbourg: Council of Europe.

Curfman, GD, Morrissey, S, and Drazen, JM (2008) 'Physicians and execution', *New England Journal of Medicine*, 358(4), 403–4.

Denno, D (2002) 'When legislatures delegate death: the troubling paradox behind state uses of electrocution and lethal injection and what it says about us', *Ohio State Law Journal*, 63, 63–128.

Denno, D (2007) 'The lethal injection quandary: how medicine has dismantled the death penalty', *Fordham Law Review*, 76(1), 49.

ECOSOC (1984) *Safeguards guaranteeing the protection of the rights of those facing the death penalty (ECOSOC Safeguards). Resolution 1984/50, 25 May 1984.* Geneva: United Nations.

ECOSOC (1989) *Resolution 1989/64. Implementation of the safeguards guaranteeing protection of the rights of those facing the death penalty.* Geneva: United Nations.

Editorial (2007) 'Lethal injection is not humane', *PLoS Medicine*, 4(4), e171.

Farber, N, Davis, EB, Widern, J, Jordan, J, Boyer, EG, and Ubel, PA (2000) 'Physicians' attitudes about involvement in lethal injection for capital punishment', *Archives of Internal Medicine*, 160(19), 2912–16.

Farber, NJ, Aboff, BM, Weiner, J, Davis, EB, Boyer, EG, and Ubel, PA (2001) 'Physicians' willingness to participate in the process of lethal injection for capital punishment', *Annals of Internal Medicine*, 135(10), 884–8.

Ferris, R (1997) 'Psychiatry and the death penalty', *Psychiatric Bulletin*, 21, 746–8.

Ferris, R and Welsh, J (2004) 'Doctors and the death penalty—ethics and a cruel punishment', in P Hodgkinson and WA Schabas (eds) *Capital Punishment: Strategies for Abolition.* Oxford: Oxford University Press, 63–91.

FIDH (2003) *The Death Penalty in Japan: A Practice Unworthy of a Democracy.* Paris: Federation Internationale des Ligues des Droits de l'Homme. Available at <http://www.fidh.org/IMG/pdf/jp359a.pdf>, accessed 4 November 2011.

Ford v Wainwright (1986) 477 US 399.

Freedman, AM and Halpern, AL (1996) 'The erosion of ethics and morality in medicine: physician participation in legal executions in the United States', *New York Law School Law Review*, 41(1), 169–88.

Gawande, A (2006) 'When law and ethics collide—why physicians participate in executions', *New England Journal of Medicine*, 354, 1221–9.

Groner, J (2002) 'Lethal injection: a stain on the face of medicine', *British Medical Journal*, 325, 1026–8.

Gunn, J (2004) 'The Royal College of Psychiatrists and the death penalty', *Journal of the American Academy of Psychiatry and Law*, 32, 188–91.

Halpern, AL, Halpern, JH, and Freedman, AM (2004) 'Now is the time for AAPL to demonstrate leadership by advocating positions of social importance', *Journal of the American Academy of Psychiatry and the Law*, 32, 180–3.

Hausman, K (2003) 'Court sets strict criteria for medicating defendants', *Psychiatric News*, 38 (13), 2.

Home Office (1888) Findings were summarized in *Minutes of Evidence taken before the Royal Commission on Capital Punishment*, First Day, 4 August 1949. London: HMSO, 1949, para. 108, p. 15.

Hood, R and Hoyle, C (2008) *The Death Penalty: A Worldwide Perspective.* 4th edn. Oxford: Oxford University Press.

House of Lords (1843) *M'Naghten case.* UKHL J16, 8 ER 718. Available online at <http://www.bailii.org/uk/cases/UKHL/1843/J16.html>, accessed 4 November 2011.

Human Rights Watch (2001) *Beyond Reason: The Death Penalty and Offenders with Mental Retardation.* New York: Human Rights Watch. Available at <http://www.hrw.org/reports/2001/ustat/>, accessed 4 November 2011.

Human Rights Watch (2006) *So long as they die: Lethal injections in the United States.* New York: Human Rights Watch. Available at <http://hrw.org/reports/2006/us0406/>, accessed 4 November 2011.

International Council of Nurses (2006) *Torture, Death Penalty and Participation by Nurses in Executions.* Geneva: International Council of Nurses.

Jesani, A (2004) 'Medicalisation of "legal" killing: doctors' participation in the death penalty', *Indian Journal of Medical Ethics*, 1(4), 104–5.

Koniaris, LG, Zimmers, TA, Lubarsky, DA, and Sheldon, JP (2005) 'Inadequate anaesthesia in lethal injection for execution', *The Lancet*, 365, 1412–4.

Legal Historians (2007) US Supreme Court. Brief of Legal Historians, *Panetti v. Quarterman*, 127 S. Ct. 2842 (2007) (No. 06–6407). Available at <http://www.deathpenaltyinfo.org/Legal%20Historians%20Brief. pdf>, accessed 4 November 2011.

LeGraw, JM and Grodin, MA (2002) 'Health professionals and lethal injection executions in the United States', *Human Rights Quarterly*, 24, 382–483.

Lester, D and Tartaro, C (2002) 'Suicide on death row', *Journal Forensic Science*, 47(5), 1108–11.

Lewis, DO, Pincus, JH, Feldman, M, Jackson, L, and Bard, B (1986) 'Psychiatric, neurological and psychoeducational characteristics of 15 death row inmates in the United States', *American Journal of Psychiatry*, 143, 838–45.

Morales v Hickman (2006) United States District Court for the Northern District of California San Jose Division, 415 F. Supp. 2d 1037. 14 February 2006.

Nakajima, N (2002) 'Role of psychiatrists in capital punishment cases: a review', *Seishin Shinkeigaku Zasshi*, 104(3), 229–40.

Panetti v Quarterman (2007) 551 US____. Available at <http://www.supremecourt.gov/ opinions/06pdf/06-6407.pdf>, accessed 4 November 2011.

Panetti v Quarterman (2008) US District Court for the Western District of Texas, Filed 22 March 2008. Cause No. A-04-CA-042-SS, 2008 WL 2338498 (W.D. Tex. 2008).

Piasecki, M (2005) 'Death row inmates and mental health', *Journal of the American Academy of Psychiatry and Law*, 33, 406–8.

Pratt and Morgan v the Attorney General of Jamaica (1993) Privy Council Appeal No. 10 of 1993; Judgment of the Lords of the Judicial Committee of the Privy Council, Delivered 2 November 1993.

Prokosch, E (2004). 'The death penalty versus human rights', in Council of Europe (2004) *Death Penalty: Beyond Abolition*. Strasbourg: Council of Europe, 23–35.

Radelet, ML and Barnard, GW (1988) 'Treating those found incompetent for execution: ethical chaos with only one solution', *Bulletin of the American Academy of Psychiatry and Law*, 16, 297–308.

Radelet, ML, Vandiver, M, and Berardo, F (1983) 'Families, prisons, and death row inmates: the human impact of structured uncertainty', *Journal of Family Issues*, 4, 593–612.

Report (1888) *Report of the Commission to Investigate and Report the Most Humane and Practical Method of Carrying into Effect the Sentence of Death in Capital Cases*; New York, 17 January 1888; cited in A Beichman (1963) 'The first electrocution', *Commentary*, 35, 410–19.

Rodley, NS with Pollard, M (2009) *The Treatment of Prisoners under International Law*. 3rd edn. Oxford: Oxford University Press.

Roper v Simmons (2005) 543 US 551.

Rosenbaum, R (1990) 'Travels with Dr Death', *Vanity Fair,* May 1990, 141–74.

Schabas, W (2003) *The Abolition of the Death Penalty in International Law*. 3rd edn. Cambridge: Cambridge University Press.

Sell v United States (2003) 539 US 166.

Singleton v Norris (2003) US Court of Appeals for the Eighth Circuit, No. 00–1492. Available at <http://caselaw.findlaw.com/us-8th-circuit/1213175.html>, accessed 4 November 2011.

Slobogin, C (2000) 'Mental illness and the death penalty', *California Criminal Law Review*, 2, article 3.

Slobogin, C (2007) 'The Supreme Court's recent criminal mental health cases: rulings of questionable competence', *Criminal Justice*, 22(3), Fall 2007. Available at <http://www.americanbar.org/content/ dam/aba/publishing/criminal_justice_section_newsletter/crimjust_cjmag_22_3_supremecrt_ mentalhealthcases.authcheckdam.pdf>, accessed 4 October 2011.

Soering v UK (1989) (ser. A) (1989) 11 EHRR 439.

Stone, AA (2004) 'Condemned prisoner treated and executed', *Psychiatric Times*, XXI (3) March, 1–4.

Taylor v Crawford (2006) In the United States District Court Western District of Missouri Central Division, Case 2:05-cv-04173-FJG Document 76 Filed 31 January 2006.

Texas Defender Service (2004) *Deadly Speculation. Misleading Texas Capital Juries with False Predictions of Future Dangerousness*. Houston: Texas Defender Service.

Tripodi, SJ and Bender, K (2007) 'Inmate suicide: prevalence, assessment, and protocols', *Brief Treatment and Crisis Intervention*, 7, 40–54.

United Nations Commission on Human Rights (1999) *Resolution 1999/61*. Geneva: United Nations (with similar sentiments being expressed in subsequent annual resolutions).

United Nations Commission on Human Rights (2001). *Resolution 2001/68: The Question of the Death Penalty*. Geneva: United Nations.

United Nations General Assembly (1971) *Resolution 2857 (XXVI), 20 December 1971*. Geneva: United Nations.

Vuotto, AM and Ciccone, JR (2006) 'Mental illness and the death penalty: defendant's mental illness does not place him in the same protected category, preventing execution, as a mentally retarded defendant', *Journal of the American Academy of Psychiatry and the Law*, 34, 253–5.

Washington v Harper (1990) 494 US 210.

West, LJ (1975) 'Psychiatric reflections on the death penalty', *Journal of Orthopsychiatry*, 45, 689–700.

World Health Organization (2007) *International Statistical Classification of Diseases and Related Health Problems*. 10th revision (ICD-10). Online version available at <http://www.who.int/classifications/icd/en/>, accessed on 4 October 2011.

World Medical Association (2000) *Resolution on Physician Participation in Capital Punishment*. Ferney Voltaire. Available at <http://www.wma.net/en/30publications/10policies/c1/>, accessed on 4 October 2011.

World Psychiatric Association (1996) *Declaration of Madrid*. Approved by the WPA General Assembly in Madrid, Spain, on 25 August 1996. Available at <http://www.wpanet.org/detail.php?section_id=5&content_id=48> accessed 4 October 2011.

Yamamoto, M (2005) 'T he role of psychiatrists in capital punishment', *Seishin Shinkeigaku Zasshi*, 107(7), 691–5.

Chapter 15

Mental Health and Human Rights in Secure Settings

Danny H. Sullivan and Paul E. Mullen

Introduction

The treatment of those who were both mentally ill and committed criminal offences has a long and often dark history. Isolation in asylums and prisons has all too often engendered abuses of human and civil rights. To some extent the grim history of the control and exclusion of the mentally abnormal offender was mitigated by early psychiatric and penal reformers like Samuel Tuke, Philippe Pinel, John Connelly, Henry Maudsley, and John Howard. Nevertheless the threat to the rights of those doubly stigmatized as mentally disordered and criminal remains a significant issue.

This chapter will focus on the implications for human rights of current approaches to the management of the mentally abnormal offender. As offenders, they suffer a curtailment of their civil rights, potentially losing the basic right to freedom of movement together with, according to the jurisdiction, the right to vote, freedom of communication, freedom of association, freedom to indulge in consensual and otherwise legal sexual activities, and so forth. The forfeiting of some civil rights when citizens commit serious criminal offences is an accepted aspect of the criminal justice systems of all Western democracies. However rights nevertheless remain, such as not being held incommunicado or with extreme restrictions (for example being confined 18 hours a day to a small barred room with limited access to the outside world). Most apparently liberal societies also permit a similar curtailment of the civil rights of people because they are mentally ill and believed by doctors not to be able to effectively protect themselves or desist from harming others. One curiosity therefore of being both an offender and mentally ill is that the vast majority of your fellow citizens will support your rights being curtailed in the name both of justice and of therapy.

The gradual disappearance of the old asylums over the last 40 years was expected to end a psychiatric practice based on coercion and exclusion, at least within the general mental health services. Initially this hope appeared to be fulfilled. In the last decade, however, throughout most of the Western world we have seen a trend back to compulsory admissions to hospital which have once again become the norm rather than the exception. It is perhaps more troubling that many jurisdictions have embraced community treatment orders, which extend compulsion into the community. As a result the psychiatric patient's experience of compulsion is no longer restricted to episodes of admission but can characterize all their continuing care. In the Australian state of Victoria, where we work, a large number of public patients are now subjected to compulsory treatment irrespective of whether they are inpatients or in the community. This has led to practices experienced by many as equally coercive and dehumanizing when compared to the days of asylums, although now occurring in less obviously forbidding places.

Increasingly, measures of coercive control are justified not only by the patients' supposed dangerousness to themselves, but more importantly, the risk they are perceived to pose to others.

In practice such dangerousness is not confined to significant interpersonal violence but is more broadly construed to include behaviours disruptive of good social order, or disturbing to the finely-tuned sensibilities of their fellow citizens. These trends are perhaps even more obvious in forensic mental health services than in general psychiatry, for in the former, rendering the patient less dangerous is all too often equated with ensuring their good behaviour through compliance with antipsychotics.

The closure of many of the massive asylums which used to characterize psychiatric services in much of the English-speaking world has led to a dramatic decrease in the number of psychiatric beds. The beds that remain are often integrated into general hospitals or institutions of modest size, at least compared to the thousand-plus bedded asylums of the past. Alongside these changes, which should have promoted the normalization of mental health care, there has occurred a rapid escalation in secure hospital provisions. Forensic psychiatry services and secure hospitals once formed a very small and obscure area of mental health practice. Over recent decades however such services have grown exponentially.

Some of the old asylums have been reopened as secure forensic hospitals with greatly increased security, as in the Napa State Hospital, California. Units for mentally ill inmates have been opened in many prisons and jails, some of which allow compulsory psychiatric treatment. Within Chicago's Cook County Jail, for example, literally hundreds of seriously mentally ill people are housed in a prison psychiatric hospital. In the United Kingdom, private forensic hospitals have burgeoned and now provide as many secure beds as the National Health Service (NHS), and this despite a rapid growth in NHS medium secure forensic beds. In Australia, major developments and expansions of forensic secure facilities have recently occurred in Victoria, Queensland, New South Wales, and Tasmania, with the other states actively considering similar developments. Old asylums are essentially being recreated as secure forensic psychiatric facilities in prison or hospital contexts, but unlike the old asylums which at least pretended to be places of peace and protection for patients, these new hospitals are about protecting the community from the dangerous madmen.

A range of international instruments have defined (at least for signatories) minimal standards applying to those detained in prisons and other secure settings. These aspirational statements are not necessarily reflected in actual standards. Politicians may adroitly ratify such protocols, while simultaneously wishing not to appear lax on crime. Populist media responds with outrage to any efforts at humane treatment of prisoners—Christmas meals, swimming pools, and community leave for rehabilitation purposes are derided as evidence that the lunatics have taken over the asylum.

International human rights instruments generally provide for a minimum complement of rights to be claimed by those detained. In some cases, independent bodies such as the International Committee of the Red Cross (ICRC) or the Committee for the Prevention of Torture (CPT) may have rights of access to secure facilities in order to reduce the likelihood of abuses of human rights. However those jurisdictions in which most egregious abuses occur are unlikely to be signatories, or to grant such access. While human rights may signify a claim to minimum levels of treatment, asserting the claim requires a sympathetic audience, or a management which respects the claim. The weakness of human rights is its dependence upon the acceptance of the framework by those in power, and the wherewithal to assert rights-based claims. In the case of those whose stigma is defined by both mental disorder and offending behaviour, the claim to rights is perhaps most easily attenuated.

Secure mental health institutions

Secure settings are traditionally characterized by strict controls over entry and exit, and internally austere regimens of control. The patient becomes an object of constant observations on their movements and actions, often mediated by cameras attached to banks of screens in the offices of prison officers or nurses. Locked doors and barred windows constrain mobility. All too often, rigid routines strip away not just spontaneity but all novelty and change. In addition to the physical trappings of security, there also evolve processes and systems to maintain security, which also fulfil the aims of the institution: in some cases, the institution's only aim is containment, and all other aspects of existence become subsumed under that goal. Depending on the nature of the institution and its context, there can evolve a custodial culture which permeates the organization, affecting its staff as well as those held there. It is that culture which will determine how the prisoners or patients are treated. This chapter will focus then on people with mental disorders in prisons and hospitals: other secure settings, such as institutions for the intellectually disabled and immigration detention centres, are not specifically discussed as other sections in this book provide a specific focus on their special circumstances.

This chapter sometimes conflates prisons with asylums under the general rubric of secure settings. This is because prisons exist for similar purposes to forensic psychiatric units, and those detained there share much in common. The purpose of prison remains a dual one, of segregation from the community (and with that, incapacitation) and of rehabilitation (and treatment). The prevalence of mental disorder in prison (see e.g. Singleton, Meltzer, and Gatward 1998) reflects that correctional institutions exist to minister to a population which overlaps with these maintained in secure psychiatric settings.

The Penrose hypothesis (Penrose 1939) proposed that socially unacceptable behaviour is met by a response reflecting prevailing societal mores, directing people towards prison or hospital depending upon resources and social context. Penrose also suggested that the proportion of people in institutional care is relatively constant, and thus reduced access to hospital beds would result in increased incarceration, and vice versa. However, more recent analysis from 158 countries, comparing prison and hospital bed numbers, suggests that the association between numbers detained in prison or in psychiatric hospitals depends more on the relative wealth of the country: in high income countries there was little correlation (Large and Nielssen 2009).

A more recent term describing the transition from prison to hospital care is transinstitutionalization (Slovenko 2003). This term transcends the optimism of the buzzword deinstitutionalization, which suggested that closing asylums would result in increased liberty for all those detained there. The reality of transinstitutionalization is widely asserted. In Western countries a massive escalation in the number of citizens imprisoned has occurred (now topping 700 per 100,000 in the US from a base rate 20 years ago of 160 per 100,000) and there now are far more seriously mentally ill prisoners. Whether this reflects transinstitutionalization or simply an increased number—without the proportion of mentally disordered to non-mentally disordered prisoners changing—is unanswerable in the absence of adequate data. Although it was clear that institutional care had in many cases led to diminished psychosocial functioning and the loss of independent living skills (Wing and Brown 1970), numbers of those discharged to the community with the closure of many asylums in the latter half of the 20th century became homeless or resident in alternative forms of long stay accommodation (Torrey 1997); thus rather than being freed, they were in many cases simply transferred to other settings.

The sociologist Erving Goffman conceptualized the features which characterize total institutions, such as prisons and psychiatric hospitals (Goffman 1961). He described the assignation and adoption of stereotyped roles, and the severance of links with a previous (external) life through rituals and processes which emphasized difference from the 'outside.' In part, these processes are integral to any discussion on human rights in secure settings, as they mark the difference between those detained in secure settings and those without.

Michel Foucault charted the rise of secure settings to govern the lives of those detained within the 'carceral system', which he noted included not only prisons and hospitals, but also schools and military barracks (Foucault 1975). He spoke of the role of professional judgements in granting liberties to those detained, and the consequent development of 'disciplinary careers' for those who served the systems of power.

Specific populations are highly vulnerable in secure settings, and warrant special attention. Women offenders have an increased rate of mental disorder relative to males and may decompensate more rapidly when removed from relational supports such as family. Indigenous patients in post-colonial systems tend to show increased rates of mental disorder, particularly marked in offender populations. They may also respond poorly to detention, although some systems which explicitly accommodate indigenous belief systems and therapeutic experiences in service planning can have better outcomes (Tapsell and Mellsop 2007). Immigrant groups and those who share the disadvantages of relative poverty, social exclusion, poor education, and cultural alienation are also vulnerable to higher rates of both mental disorders and criminal behaviours. Those with dual diagnoses (mental heath and substance use) have higher degrees of service need which may not be met in a psychiatric setting where the focus is mental disorder alone (Ogloff, Lemphers, and Dwyer 2004). Similarly, dual disability (the combination of mental disorder and intellectual disability) and personality disorder may lead to significant problems in adaptive functioning and result in a greater burden of impairment, as well as manifesting in poor fit with the service and consequent difficulty meeting the specific needs of diagnostically complex patients.

In addition to the trappings of security apparent in prisons and hospitals, cultural differences reflect the ostensible differences in purpose between prisons and hospitals, although more secure hospitals may, unwittingly or through design, shed hospital characteristics and absorb prison features. Hospitals are intended to provide treatment in a range of modalities, and through treatment to restore health. Their purpose may be described as essentially therapeutic. Prisons may have many purposes, including treatment or rehabilitation. However their core function is custodial, correctional, or punitive. In secure hospital settings, therapeutic culture frequently clashes with custodial, and efforts to maintain a health-oriented perspective may be insidiously eroded by the intrusion of custodial attitudes and systems of 'care.' It is also noticeable that in correctional institutions, health interventions may be undermined by the custodial setting, such as the use of solitary confinement for suicide prevention or 'behaviour management.'

In recent years there have developed novel secure settings, such as post-sentence detention for sexual offenders (Mercado and Ogloff 2004) or for 'dangerous severe personality disordered' people (Tyrer 2007). These have in common that commitment is couched in therapeutic terms, but appears primarily to serve custodial aims (Sullivan, Mullen, and Pathé 2005). Detention is indeterminate in duration and the criteria for release tend to be based not upon mental health criteria but on a demonstrated reduction of risk, despite the imprecision of such prognostication (Mullen 2007).

Civil commitment

Civil commitment refers to a process of detaining people with mental disorders, usually for compulsory treatment. Commitment relies upon legislative backing to ensure that a threshold for detention is met, and includes safeguards against abuse. This is dealt with in this chapter because increasingly the justification for the use of such powers is either exclusively, or to a significant extent, based on the apprehension of a risk of violent and/or criminal behaviour.

Mental health legislation defines categories of people who may be treated, using either a diagnostic category or criteria to define disordered function. It delimits added criteria such as refusal of treatment or inability to consent, and in some cases includes treatability criteria (Maden 2007). A criterion of treatability may function as a protection against de facto detention without any opportunity for therapeutic input. Indeed such a criterion offers safeguards not only to patients, but also to treating clinicians, to prevent them becoming custodian to those whose behaviour is disordered, but who do not have a treatable mental disorder and for whom civil commitment would be essentially for warehousing purposes.

There are two other significant thresholds. The first is that of the 'least restrictive environment', a term most commonly used in the field of intellectual disability, but applicable to psychiatric treatment. The principle reflects that maximizing autonomy should be an explicit underpinning of civil commitment. The minimum incursion on liberty to provide treatment ensures that, where possible, people with mental disorders are treated voluntarily, for instance in open rather than locked facilities, and with oral rather than depot medication. However it has been argued that such a mandate does not necessarily lead to the development of community facilities or alternatives for treatment which are actually less restrictive. Like many such 'rights', the remedy is often abstract, when there exist no locations or programmes which can provide such 'less restrictive' care (Appelbaum 1999).

The second threshold is the 'harm criterion'. Led by jurisdictions in the United States, this has often been construed as an obligatory dangerousness criterion, relying upon an assessment that the person is dangerous to themselves or others to justify civil commitment. Dangerousness criteria are the hallmark of so-called police powers commitment. The moral underpinning of laws based upon this justification is that the state has a responsibility to safeguard the welfare of citizens, and may take action against those who threaten citizens. On the one hand, this provides a high threshold and may allow involuntary treatment to prevent a mentally disordered person from harming others. On the other hand, if dangerousness is a necessary criterion, this may prevent the involuntary treatment of those with less dramatic symptoms who are not dangerous, but who would benefit from treatment. This may worsen the prognosis for people by delaying treatment (Large et al. 2008).

What is lacking is the clear evidence that antipsychotic medications and current mental health systems make a significant long term impact on the patients' quality of life or even survival, rather than on medical outcomes like readmission and scores on symptom check lists. Some might happily trade mental distress for less medication, particularly when this is associated with marked side-effects: however most mental health systems rarely offer such idiosyncratic choices. Instead, coercion or compulsion appears related to the expectation that, post hoc, patients will express gratitude for their treatment and restoration to mental health. The decision not to take medication is often reformulated as lack of insight and non-compliance, stripping it of the legitimacy of a true choice.

The other moral underpinning of civil commitment is the *parens patriae* power vested in the state to look after the welfare of those incapable of looking after themselves. Such paternalism is in line with much other medical treatment, although increasingly this has been eroded by the burgeoning of protectionist mental health legislation. In addition there exist a range of alternative legal frameworks for those lacking decision-making capacity, including guardianship. Although the framing of civil commitment powers suggests the chance for the patient to benefit through circumscribed incursions on their autonomy, it is clear that removal from the general community and detention in a secure setting is not an unwelcome consequence.

Balancing the protection of the public from mentally disordered people with the rights of individual patients can be a fraught exercise. Those subject to involuntary treatment do not only have to contend with detention or restrictions on movement, medication, and the incursions of treating clinicians into their personal life; in addition a complement of other rights typically held by citizens may be diminished. These 'civil rights' can include voting, driving, owning weapons, holding some employment, access to children, reduced ability to obtain a visa for countries such as the US, life insurance, and managing finances. In general, the erosion of such rights does not flow automatically from detention, but is closely associated with commitment.

In an effort to address the discrimination which provides for some mentally disordered people to be subject to civil commitment, capacity-based (Okai et al. 2007) commitment has been put forward. Proponents of such legislation point to the disparity in justification for 'best interests' treatment between those who have mental disorder and those with physical illness, and make the strong claim that lack of decision-making capacity is the morally relevant issue which justifies involuntary treatment (Dawson and Szmukler 2006). Previous efforts at reforming the Mental Health Act 1983 (UK) led to the formation of an Expert Committee (Richardson 1999) which recommended that incapacity underpin mental health legislation, although this approach was rejected by government despite the support of patients and professionals. Moves to capacity-based legislation reflect dissatisfaction with dangerousness criteria, and a desire for 'safeguarded paternalism' (Roth 1979).

Procedures in which people are detained under common law or treated informally while lacking capacity to consent (usually due to dementia or intellectual disability) are unusual in developed countries. Detention without using mental health legislation has become known in the UK as the 'Bournewood gap' (Singhal et al. 2008) following a law suit brought against the detaining hospital by legal representatives of a man with severe autism who was held in a mental health facility, but not under mental health legislation. In the European Court of Justice it was held that this amounted to deprivation of liberty and breached his rights under the Human Rights Act 1998 (UK). The procedural safeguards of mental health legislation exist to circumscribe conditions under which psychiatric commitment is lawful, and those detained without its use may lack these protections and oversight. As a consequence the United Kingdom has developed specific legislation for those lacking capacity: the Mental Capacity Act 2005.

Opponents of civil commitment focus on its coercive nature, and the power vested in the psychiatric profession to remove from the community those labelled as mentally disordered. Moves to address the circumstances under which many were detained for long periods of time, often for spurious reasons, were associated with marked improvements in the care of the mentally disordered. The same political and social movements of the 1960s and 1970s which addressed institutionally entrenched attitudes to gender and ethnicity, also cast light onto the care of people in prisons and psychiatric hospitals. The development of robust legal frameworks has ensured that there is in theory at least independent oversight of civil commitment, and that detention is warranted by application of objective minimum standards. How robust such protections are in practice is difficult to assess, and one suspects that safeguards depend all too often on individuals as much as the legal framework. Unfortunately those mentally disordered people who are detained following offending often receive a compromised oversight, where risk can come to trump all other factors.

Some critics of involuntary commitment, such as Thomas Szasz, hail from a radical libertarian tradition and regard civil commitment as immoral, and rarely if ever justified (Szasz 1970). By this view, individual autonomy is held to be sacrosanct, and individuals, even those who are mentally disordered, should be accountable for their actions. The Szaszian position rejects psychiatric diagnoses, involuntary treatment, and the role of the state in mental health care. Although popular in the second half of the 20th century, such arguments have become increasingly marginal. They rely on an idealized notion of all humans as persistently autonomous, and fail to provide a humane response to the genuine distress and risk of self-harm or violence in some mental disorders. Moreover, weak paternalism is the hallmark of a society which respects individual autonomy and seeks both to maximize autonomy through treatment when it is diminished; and to look after those whose autonomy is severely and permanently constrained. The notion that psychiatry could only be practised as a contractual arrangement with an autonomous patient belies the effects on capacity and rational choice of some serious mental disorders, and the devastating effects for the afflicted individual and others without the option of at least limited coercive powers.

The Szaszian position is the libertarianism of the extreme right which constructs us all as totally autonomous individuals divorced from any collective, be that family, social, cultural, occupational, or economic. The libertarianism of the left accepts the reality of humans as social beings who function within specific cultural contexts but opposes authority based on position, status, or economic and social power, accepting only the persuasion of knowledge and experience. The critical question for left-leaning libertarians relates to the status of psychiatric knowledge and experience, and its persuasive power. The very existence of the coercion which pervades our mental health systems indicates a current failure to persuade sufferers of the benefits of our nostrums. The status of most knowledge in psychiatry is moderate and tentative at best. It could be, as many argue, that persuasion fails because the seriously mentally ill are incapable of reason, or even of calculating their own advantage. This is true of some. Equally, however, many who refuse to accept treatment do so on the basis of their experience of the limited utility and noxious nature of prior treatments. The more compulsion, the less the mental health professional needs to persuade. The less they persuade the less skilled they become in this all important interaction between expert and potential patient. Thus the more mental health professionals use compulsion the more they become an embodiment of a form of authority based upon threat and coercion. The mutual alienation created by our current mental health systems feeds into a focus on treatment as doing things to a sick object, irrespective of its preferences, usually first and foremost loading them up with the latest antipsychotic medication.

The situation of the mentally abnormal offender is somewhat different. These people have committed criminal offences which could have resulted in their incarceration. Their civil rights have to some extent been forfeit as a result of criminal conviction or its equivalent. Detention in a mental health facility rather than a prison might well be preferable for the individual and the wider society. Similarly, court-mandated community mental health treatment might be preferred to probation or parole supervision. The curtailing of their civil rights stems, however, from their criminal conviction, not their mental disorder; the coercion is on the authority of the court, not based on the opinions of a health professional. For those with grave reservations about the ethics and pragmatics of civil orders allowing compulsory treatment, the forensic field can paradoxically provide less challenge to their libertarian leanings than does general psychiatric practice.

In addition to constraints upon the criteria which render a person eligible for civil commitment, most jurisdictions also provide a range of other limits upon the deprivation of liberty. In the first case, different orders may exist for initial assessment, for a trial of treatment, and for ongoing treatment. Each stage of the process requires revalidation of commitment criteria, or in some cases, criteria for more protracted commitment requires a higher threshold. Procedural safeguards include oversight by a state agency, and review by independent tribunals or courts. Again, however, we face a technology of mediated control carried out in the name of the patient but against the will of the patient. The existence of such technologies of rights, however benign in intent, diminishes the need for cooperative engagement and mutual respect. In short this erodes the central element of physician as expert advisor to a patient who suffers.

Civil commitment in some jurisdictions can be a process to engage services for a mentally disordered person. Indeed, in jurisdictions such as the United Kingdom, commitment places a legally enforceable responsibility on local services to provide input. Thus commitment not only affects negative rights but may also command a complement of positive rights (e.g. housing, state benefits).

It is worth making a final point, that critics of civil commitment have at times been selective in acknowledging. The abolition of inpatient psychiatric units is not accompanied by reduced despair and enhanced mental health for those who might be affected by these processes. Rather, it moves the problem of mental disorder elsewhere—private homes, hostels, prisons, the streets—and benefits only the government, which no longer need fund these expensive services. However, the expansion of opportunities for different types of civil commitment may provide alternative populations to detain in mental health facilities, even if their problems are not traditionally thought of as psychiatric issues.

Specific issues

We spoke earlier of differences in culture and values, which may be amplified in a closed institution. Correctional culture emphasizes containment, safety, and order; therapeutic goals are trumped by the requirements of the correctional setting. Mental health staff working in correctional settings are often dependent upon correctional staff to provide security or enable access to various parts of the prison. At times they may be required to provide therapeutic consultation in the presence of correctional staff, or to prisoners who remain locked in a cell, or in some cases to prisoners who remain handcuffed or physically restrained. Clinical staff must strike a balance between maintaining practical working relationships with a correctional institution, and advocating for mentally disordered prisoners in order that they receive appropriate treatment in a humane fashion. Although a principled defence of the rights of prisoners may appear justified, the consequences might result in future loss of access or support from prison staff.

Ethical slippage may be insidious. It is noted in nomenclature, when 'patients' become 'prisoners', when 'offenders' become 'criminals', or when mentally disordered behaviour is relabelled as wilful and malicious. Indeed, the 'mad'/'bad' dichotomy may occur in therapeutic settings too. The distinction is a false one, conflating clinical description with normative values. Moreover, correctional settings may indeed engender aberrant behaviour, only realized when the person is moved to a therapeutic setting. Those working in settings providing assessment and treatment to mentally disordered offenders should monitor themselves and receive clinical supervision so as to avoid the insidious development of punitive rather than therapeutic attitudes. Ongoing off-site engagement with a health agency may provide sufficient counterbalance to negate the effect of immersion in a correctional culture.

The management of mentally disordered people in prison settings may be tendentious. It often involves the substitution of therapeutic interventions by 'management' which has as its end goal the control of unruly behaviour, and institutional smooth running rather than individual well-being. Often there are structural and systematic impediments to the relocation of mentally disordered people to therapeutic settings such as hospitals. These obstacles may include security concerns, byzantine transfer procedures and administrative obstacles, financial disincentives (prison beds cost a small fraction of secure hospital beds), and limited hospital beds.

The two predominant problems with delays in transfer to hospital relate to the principle of equivalence, and to the ethics of compulsory treatment in prison. Equivalence is the principle by which it is contended that prisoners should receive health care of a similar standard to those not detained. Sadly, this aspirational suggestion is rarely met. In addition, there are constraints upon the provision of certain treatments in prison, particular medications prone to abuse, and resource-intensive individual treatments such as psychotherapy. Thus, for mentally disordered offenders in a prison setting, transfer to a therapeutic setting is significant.

Compulsory treatment in prison is to be resisted. Even when it is permitted in emergencies, the precedent of compelling treatment is an awkward one which contravenes international treaties and reduces opportunities for the humane treatment of mental disorder. Although initially attractive through cost-effectiveness, pragmatism, and apparent necessity, in reality such compulsory treatment has marked negative consequences. The re-labelling of bad behaviour as psychiatric illness, increased reluctance to transfer to hospital, and the abuse of psychiatry for political ends are all foreseeable results when compulsory psychiatric treatment is permitted in prison. Despite the apparent humanity of treating distressed mentally disordered people, the necessity of compelling treatment only in a hospital setting provides suitable immediacy that transfer may be expedited, lest otherwise it is terminally delayed while stopgap measures occur.

It can be difficult persuading those transferred to hospital from prison that the rules have changed. Prisoners expect to serve a sentence, counting the days until their punishment has been concluded. At the expiration of this period, they may leave. In forensic units, the rules differ: periods of confinement are often indeterminate, and rely not upon the passage of time, but rather on the meeting of goals including adherence to treatment, participation in programmes, and demonstrable reduction in risk to the community. This reframing of the rules of confinement also involves a cultural shift, and may not be appreciated by those prisoners who are redefined as patients (Lindqvist and Skipworth 2000). Consequently, attempts to engage the patient in treatment may be met by surliness and passive resistance, bucking at the imposition of rules which are not initially easy to understand. Indeed, the jurisprudential system may also be uncertain about whether release is premised upon safety for the community or the passage of a sentence (Carroll, Lyall, and Forrester 2004).

Other conflicts are apparent, in the parallel existence of separate systems of behavioural control: in prison, 'management cells' may also be described as 'observation cells' but overlap with those used for 'segregation'. In hospitals, the loose equivalent is 'seclusion'. These terminologies mutually apply to isolation in a spartan cell in order variously to prevent suicide, reduce aggressive behaviour or its associated harms, or punish detained people. There are conflicts in that the use of these systems of control may not be appreciated for its purpose by those subject to such isolation. Prisoners often recount that they will not divulge suicidal ideas because they fear the consequences, being moved to a suicide-proof regime. The overlap of these multiple goals in secure settings results in difficulties in defining various interventions clearly without a blurring of the boundaries of purposes, perceptions, and punitive impact.

Sexual expression is discouraged in secure settings. Despite emphasizing normalization and return to the community as rehabilitation goals, in most psychiatric hospitals and prisons, sexual interactions, relationships, and sexual behaviour are actively prevented. In part, this attitude may reflect a discomfort with mentally disordered people expressing sexual desire, but it must also be acknowledged that issues of capacity to consent, and benign paternalism may be at play. As the staff of secure settings have a duty of care towards those detained, this duty extends to protection of those vulnerable to the predation of others. Some people with psychiatric disorders, particularly those with schizophrenia or in the manic phase of bipolar affective disorder, may be disinhibited and their judgment impaired. Others with personality disorder may be destabilized by evanescent relationships, while those with disorders of sexual preference may prey on others.

In prisons, it is often expressly denied that sexual activity occurs. There is a high price to be paid for this: seroconversion to HIV and rape are both prevalent. The denial of sexual activity leads to the reluctance of many hospitals and most prisons to provide condoms (Hellard and Aitken 2004). Refusal to consider that sexual interactions may occur between psychiatric inpatients or prisoners results in an understandable reluctance of those detained to report, discuss, or acknowledge sexual behaviours, as the response is likely to be punitive or preventative.

There has also been much discussion of the utility and sense of providing access to injecting equipment in secure settings. There is an explicit conflict between the goals of harm minimization— espoused by many treatment systems—and the security constraints which may restrict access to needles and syringes due to their use as weapons. The gross rates of infection with bloodborne viruses due to unsafe injecting and tattooing practices rarely sway decision-makers in secure settings.

Finally, the use of mental health settings or justifications to detain political dissidents or to marginalise their voice has been marked in some jurisdictions. Avoidance of the scrutiny of open court through use of mental health dispositions or commitment has occurred on occasion, particularly in totalitarian systems. However, even in apparent liberal democracies, the use of secure mental healthcare may serve valuable purposes for the criminal justice system when it enables both the re-labelling of aberrant behaviour as 'mad' rather than 'bad'; and the potentially indeterminate detention of troublesome risky individuals.

Towards providing mental health care in secure settings

The mentally abnormal offender rarely acts in a violent and/or criminal manner simply on the basis of active symptoms. They usually share with other offenders the developmental, psychological, and social vulnerabilities, often combined with substance abuse, which predispose to crime. The individual's route to offending and substance abuse always has unique elements and any effective change is only likely when those individual elements are understood and addressed. Committing more crimes is not usually a positive outcome for the mentally abnormal offender, particularly as they are rarely efficient criminals, and worse still tend to victimize those close to them, upon whom they themselves may depend to survive in the community. The mental health professional who ignores the criminogenic issues in favour of a pure focus on managing the mental disorder does their patient a gross disservice. But to engage with a patient to correct psychological and social vulnerabilities relevant to the risk of future offending is to engage with them not simply as an end in themselves in the form of their improved mental health. Rather, the patient should be regarded as a means to an end, namely community safety, to which the patient may be indifferent or antipathetic. To undertake such an engagement, ridden with contradiction, in the context of a custodial (and overtly or covertly punitive) institution may fail if the human rights of the prisoner/patient are ignored or overridden.

The role of a mental health professional in any form of custodial institution is at best conflicted, and at worse totally compromised. In correctional settings there are subtle and not so subtle pressures to suborn mental health professionals to play a role in the custodial constructions of control and containment. In the secure hospital the health needs of the patient are inevitably influenced by community perceptions about safety and retribution, or to be more precise, the evocation and exploitation of opinion by the popular press, and the political response to such pressures. In its starkest form the Guantanamo Bay experience has highlighted the ease with which mental health and other medical professionals can become drawn into playing a role in abuses of human rights, up to and including torture.

It is complex to explain the capacity of custodial institutions to capture health professionals and use their efforts and best intentions, to serve the interests of the institution above those of the patient. One element among many is the lack of a clear articulation of the theoretical and practical issues central to maintaining a balance between the twin needs for care, and of control.

Simply claiming that a health professional's responsibility begins and ends with the needs of the patient for treatment may be adequate in situations where the institution is pursuing aims which show little concern for damage inflicted psychologically, and sometimes physically, on the inmates. For example, in a maximum security prisons organized around extended, or even total 24 hour lockdowns, of inmates in isolation, a health professional can only properly adopt a stance of being totally patient-focused, and by implication actively aloof and opposed to the rest of the institution. Similarly in gulags like Guantanamo Bay, professional integrity and basic decency would demand a similar focus on the patient and alienation from the institution and its aims. The problems are increased rather than ameliorated when working in custodial institutions with regimes which at least purport and sometimes attempt to provide a more humane form of detention, with a semblance of therapy and rehabilitation. Such self-proclaimed good models of custodial care usually have the following characteristics:

1. A system of privileges for prisoners based on their perceived progress, that is, their adherence to institutional rules, in word as well as deed.

2. Moves to lower security ratings and therefore less actively restrictive environments based again upon correctional notions of progress.

3. Programmes aimed at problem behaviours such as substance abuse, anger control, and sexual offending based on a 'one size fits all' approach.

The essence of the system is the prisoner as an object of universal technologies of control and reform, imposed on all in pursuit of making them live 'good lives'. Such systems can avoid active attacks on human rights but at the price of a paternalistic objectification which aims to strip the prisoner of the capacity to resist an institutional construction of 'the good prisoner'. This is not a variant of Foucault's argument that the progress from the carceral to the therapeutic simply moved the shackles from the wrists and ankles to the mind. In these modern prisons, the drivers are numbers, and outward conformity of behaviour. There is no desire to change the prisoner's mind by having them internalize and then actively pursue the moral principles of their gaolers, if for no other reason than that their gaolers may be blind to such principles. The desire is to make sure that those detained do what they are told. Numbers are central because it is the number of programmes, the number of prisoners completing the programmes, the number of psychologists employed, the number of adverse incidents and so forth, which come to define effectiveness.

Moving from the theoretical to the practical aspects of a pure patient focus, such a noble goal has to be pursued within the context of closed institutions designed to exclude, to control, and to correct. The correctional culture is usually willing to recognize the medical needs of the 'mad'. Typically however a distinction is made between this and past and current antisocial behaviour, which is seen as a manifestation of badness. Badness requires at best correction, and at worst discipline and punishment: madness requires medication. A purely patient-focused theory can all too easily be made compatible with, or even supportive of, the crude mad/bad dichotomy and its punitive practices. The alternative to the traditional patient focus, as a defence of the patient's rights, is to develop a genuinely therapeutic practice of security and control.

An alternative approach to trying to play out a therapeutic role within a custodial framework is to attempt to perform the functions of containment, control, and correction in a manner which allows a respectful and open engagement with the patient/prisoner around these aims. This approach confronts the danger of Foucault's shift from the honest and visible constraint of the chains to the covert erosion of the confined individual's understanding of their real situation in pursuit of a self imposed oppression.

Changing names from correction to rehabilitation, from containment to setting boundaries, from control to compliance, is not entirely futile, as it may bring change in how the prisoner/patient is regarded. It also unfortunately brings the risk of even more extreme assaults on human rights. The advent of liberal democracy has not diminished the potential punishments meted out by apparently ordinary health professionals in the name of treatment. In some jurisdictions indefinite detention is reserved for the mentally ill; and post-sentence detention is reserved for those acquiring a mental health diagnosis, be it of personality disorder, paraphilia (defined as lacking volitional control over sexual appetites), or, most subjectively, Dangerous Severely Personality Disordered (DSPD).

The approach to control, if it is genuinely to incorporate human rights, requires a radical change in both goals and methods.

Table 15.1 sets out in simplified form the contrasting elements of a correctional versus a therapeutic culture. Embedded within this is a model of containment and control based on inter-action and negotiation rather than observation and incapacitation. Such a therapeutic system is vulnerable and difficult to sustain, but—we would argue—essential if incursions on the patient/prisoner's human rights are to be minimized. The therapeutic construction of security suggested here allows the possibility of integrating traditionally custodial roles of containment and control into a genuinely therapeutic interaction, which, within the constraints of what are ultimately places of exclusion, at least explicitly acknowledges both the humanity and limited autonomy of the detained.

Central to the differences in the approaches is the construction of the prisoner/patient. The custodial approach views them as a potentially troublesome object to be closely watched. The therapeutic approach positions them as a thinking, autonomous (if disordered) subject strug-gling to cope with imposed constraints and enforced contact with staff and fellow patients: that is, one who requires aid to understand and respond to these impositions in a manner that damages neither themselves nor others.

The two approaches are distinguished by their methods. The custodial relies on cameras, direct observations, routine searches, and the various technologies that track, monitor, and observe the prisoner. The therapeutic relies on the presence of staff being with and interacting with their patients. The ultimate custodial system of control reproduces the prison panopticon of Jeremy Bentham but with the guard sitting in front of banks of screens. The therapeutic manifests in staff mixing with patients. The guard is as interchangeable and anonymous as their prisoners. The health professional must be a known and trusted person who cannot be easily or quickly exchanged for a similar unit. The technologies of observation cannot be an addendum to the therapeutic

Table 15.1 Simplified major differences between security based on custodial methods and that of health professionals pursuing therapeutic goals in secure conditions

Security	
Custodial culture	**Therapeutic culture**
Observe (from office) to intervene and restrain when unauthorized behaviours are seen	Interact (in unit) to understand the patient's state of mind and situation, allowing damaging behaviours to be prevented by allowing alternative prosocial expression
Reward conformity	Reward engagement and initiative
Emphasize behaviour	Emphasize psychological adjustment
Oriented to immediate goals of institutional functioning	Oriented to long term goal of effective social functioning
Unified approach and perspective (authoritarian)	Multiple professional approaches and perspectives (negotiated)
Physical structure constrains unwanted behaviour	Therapeutic interventions, along with social and personal expectations, constrain unwanted behaviour
Ultimate goal: stopping antisocial and self-damaging behaviours during incarceration	Ultimate goal: effective autonomous functioning on return to the community.
Custodial staff	Therapeutic staff

because their use creates the identity of the observed and the observer, destroying the very possibility of prior or subsequent interactions premised on any humanistic commonalities.

The nature of secure institutions creates demands for certain types of intrusions on the privacy of inmates, irrespective of attempts to create a therapeutic culture. For example, searches of inmate's rooms and property are almost unavoidable on occasion. Searches in a custodial culture are generally conducted routinely, and to benchmarks. The custodial culture even incorporates routine body searches. The therapeutic culture does not engage in routine searches but only searches when there is a reason; and that reason is provided to those being searched. The knowledge that drugs are circulating on a unit or a series of thefts have occurred may well evoke a search of patients' rooms. Such searches occur in the patient's presence showing appropriate respect for their property.

The practicalities of establishing and maintaining a therapeutic culture are considerable. Even putting these to one side, the theoretical implications for human rights are not straightforward. The harsh reality of a prison is comprehensible, as long as one is not seduced by organizational proclamations about rehabilitation, prosocial influences, and reducing reoffending. The prisoner confronts the indifference of routine maintained by the constant threat of violence. This is a world of imposed authority where might is right and punishment if not arbitrary at least tending to the random, a world entirely familiar to many offenders. For the strong-minded well-integrated personality, such a world confirms their prejudices and strengthens their identity. The therapeutic culture can obscure the nature of the power relationships between patient/prisoner and the staff. This is not a relationship of equality, nor of choice, nor consent. The only real power available to the patient/prisoner is the power to disrupt and to refuse.

The therapeutic culture rewards and persuades rather than punishing and intimidating like the custodial culture, but they both deny their inmates a range of civil rights on the basis of their past behaviour. Foucault's accusation of moving the chains from the limbs to the very being of the patient prisoner is relevant. There is only a weak response; that the therapeutic culture neither denies nor obfuscates that it is in the business of containing and controlling the patient/prisoner. Containment and control is dictated by the perceived needs of society's agents for protection and punishment, not by the best interests of the patient/prisoner. The therapeutic culture offers more effective outcomes in terms of reduced offending and social reintegration than the custodial. It may be less damaging to the humanity and civil rights of the patient/prisoner in attaining those goals. Nevertheless, ultimately it is a method of containing and controlling those who their society fears, sometimes with good reason but often only on the basis of vengeful prejudice.

References

Appelbaum, PS (1999) 'Law & Psychiatry: Least Restrictive Alternative Revisited: Olmstead's Uncertain Mandate for Community-Based Care', *Psychiatric Services*, 50, 1271–1280.

Carroll, A, Lyall, M, and Forrester, A (2004) 'Clinical hopes and public fears in forensic mental health', *Journal of Forensic Psychiatry & Psychology*, 15(3), 407–425.

Dawson, J and Szmukler, G (2006) 'Fusion of mental health and incapacity legislation', *British Journal of Psychiatry*, 188, 504–509.

Foucault, M (1975) *Discipline and Punish: the Birth of the Prison*. New York: Random House.

Goffman, E (1961) *Asylums*. Harmondsworth: Penguin.

Hellard, ME and Aitken, CK (2004) 'HIV in prison: what are the risks and what can be done?', *Sexual Health*, 1, 107–113.

Large, MM, Nielssen, O, Ryan, CJ, and Hayes, R (2008) 'Mental health laws that require dangerousness for involuntary admission may delay the initial treatment of schizophrenia', *Social Psychiatry and Psychiatric Epidemiology*, 43, 251–256.

Large, MM and Nielssen, O (2009) 'The Penrose hypothesis in 2004: Patient and prisoner numbers are positively correlated in low-and-middle income countries but are unrelated in high-income countries', *Psychology and Psychotherapy: Theory, Research and Practice*, 82(1), 113–119.

Lindqvist, P and Skipworth, J (2000) 'Evidence-based rehabilitation in forensic psychiatry', *British Journal of Psychiatry*, 176, 320–323.

Maden, A (2007) 'Dangerous and severe personality disorder: antecedents and origins', *British Journal of Psychiatry*, 190 (supplement 49), s8–s11.

Mercado, CC and Ogloff, JRP (2007) 'Risk and the preventive detention of sex offenders in Australia and the United States', *International Journal of Law and Psychiatry*, 30(1), 49–59.

Mullen PE (2007) 'Dangerous and severe personality disorder and in need of treatment', *British Journal of Psychiatry—Supplementum*, 49, 3–7.

Ogloff, JRP, Lemphers, A, and Dwyer, C (2004) 'Dual Diagnosis in an Australian Forensic Psychiatric Hospital: Prevalence and Implications for Services', *Behavioral Sciences & the Law*, 22(4), 543–562.

Okai, D, Owen, G, McGuire, H, Singh, S, Churchill, R, and Hotopf, M (2007) 'Mental capacity in psychiatric patients: Systematic review', *British Journal of Psychiatry*, 191, 291–297.

Penrose, LS (1939) 'Mental disease and crime: outline of a comparative study of European statistics', *British Journal of Medical Psychology*, 18, 1–15.

Richardson, G (1999) *Review of the Mental Health Act 1983: Report of the Expert Committee*. London: Department of Health.

Roth, L (1979) 'A commitment law for patients, doctors, and lawyers', *American Journal of Psychiatry*, 136(9), 1121.

Singhal, A, Kumar, A, Belgamwar, RB, and Hodgson, RE (2008) 'Assessment of mental capacity: who can do it?', *Psychiatric Bulletin*, 32, 17–20.

Singleton, N, Meltzer, H, and Gatward, R (1998) *Psychiatric Morbidity among Prisoners in England and Wales*. London: Office for National Statistics.

Slovenko, R (2003) 'The Transinstitutionalization of the Mentally Ill', *Ohio North University Law Review*, 29(3), 641–60.

Sullivan, DH, Mullen, PE, and Pathé, MT (2005) 'Legislation in Victoria on sexual offenders: issues for health professionals', *Medical Journal of Australia*, 183(6), 318–20.

Szasz, T (1970) *The Manufacture of Madness: A Comparative Study of the Inquisition and the Mental Health Movement*. Syracuse, NY: Syracuse University Press.

Tapsell, R and Mellsop, G (2007) 'The contributions of culture and ethnicity to New Zealand mental health research findings', *International Journal of Social Psychiatry*, 53(4), 317–324.

Torrey, EF (1997) *Out of the shadows: Confronting America's mental illness crisis*. New York: Wiley.

Tyrer, P (2007) 'An agitation of contrary opinions', *British Journal of Psychiatry*, 190, 1–2.

Wing, JK and Brown, GW (1970) *Institutionalism and Schizophrenia*. London: Cambridge University Press.

Chapter 16

The Human Rights of People with Severe and Persistent Mental Illness

Can Conflicts between Dominant and Non-Dominant Paradigms be Reconciled?

Alan Rosen, Tully Rosen, and Patrick McGorry

Introduction

The human rights of people with disability

Historically the mental health human rights movement derived human rights for people with mental illnesses from other rights movements. The disability rights movement co-opted techniques from women's rights and black rights movements, and in turn the mental health consumer movement took many cues from the broader disability movement.

People with mental illness were relative latecomers to civil and disability rights activism. They were left out of these movements because they were still institutionalized when this movement was gathering steam, and partly because of the stigmatized views from within the movement, that individuals with psychotic disorders were too violent, volatile, or irrational, and unable to meaningfully participate in empowerment (Cook and Jonikas 2002).

There is now a clearly defined advocacy sector that is overt in trying to define disability rights. Various nations have enacted disability legislation, culminating in international disability rights conventions 'in an attempt to articulate what social justice means for people with disabilities in receipt of government funded services.' (Robin Banks—PIAC personal communication).

Whereas the old paradigm for disability viewed a disabled person who cannot function because of a particular impairment, the current paradigm assumes that, whether the disability is physical or psychiatric, the person needs some specific aid or accommodation in order to function. In this 'social model', disability is socially constructed, essentially in social and/or environmental terms (see Belfer et al. in this volume). While self-determination is an important component of the current aspirations of the recovery movement involving individuals with mental illness, claims for total self-determination seem over-idealized and unrealistic. Practical conceptions of self-determination and autonomy must allow for a balance with inter-dependence, social connectedness, and the social aspirations or will of real communities (Cook and Jonikas 2002). Consequently autonomous living with a disability becomes a dynamic interaction between the characteristics of the individual and the features of their social, cultural, natural, and built environment (Cook and Jonikas 2002). To maximize self-determination of those involved, we need to consult with individuals with psychiatric disabilities, their families, and other stakeholders regarding what this would take for each person or group.

Mental health advocacy movements

Barry (1983) identifies three distinct mental health advocacy movements that emerged from these origins in North America: Dorothea Dix's campaign for 'the humane treatment of the mentally ill' through the building of state hospitals (i.e. institutionalization as a reform), Clifford Beers' influence in establishing the mental hygiene movement leading to community mental health services, and the grass roots emergence of the mental health family and consumer empowerment movement (exemplified in the National Alliance for the Mentally Ill: NAMI). Tucker (2001) traces the origin of the consumer empowerment movement in the UK to the flattening of the authority structure inherent in the development of the then clinical therapeutic community movement, though arguably this was not so pervasive nor as long lasting as the movements just mentioned. However, it was influential in making the walls around psychiatric institutions more permeable in countries where therapeutic communities did operate. It also may have partly responsible for a shift towards community health care, and consumer voices and needs beginning to be heard by service providers.

The human rights movement in health has been enshrined in instruments such as the UN Universal Declaration of Human Rights (UDHR), which endowed every person with a claim to basic healthcare (Robertson G 2007). In mental health this has led to professional and family advocacy for the right to psychiatric treatment, which they insist should be enforceable if necessary. Mental health consumers challenge this however, denying they need compulsory treatment, whether due to their claim to having made an adequate recovery in their own terms, or to lack of insight or appreciation of the perception of others. Tucker (2001) argues that full consumer participation with greater service user–provider equity is inherent in all high quality mental health care systems, such as therapeutic communities, and that 'add-on' consumer participation is artificial and should be unnecessary. Unfortunately, not all service systems recognize the value of such integrated participation as yet, and may need to enforce consumer participation for some time to achieve satisfactory acceptance by services.

Mental health human rights and politics

Political climates, legal changes, and judicial activism have both impacted and frustrated rights advocacy for people with mental illness. From the consumer viewpoint, the rights to both obtain treatment and to refuse treatment ideally should together constitute the right to mental healthcare (Mizrahi 1992; Barrett et al. 1998), and this balance of rights was upheld judicially in parts of US from the 1960s. In the US and other Western countries, attempts by conservative politicians, such as Reagan and Thatcher, to almost simultaneously rescind the rights of and retrench services for individuals with mental illness (Sedgwick 1982) have been tempered by grass-roots local and national advocacy (Mizrahi 1992). In Italy, the emancipation of individuals with severe and persistent mental illness (SPMI) from the mental hospitals, their closure and replacement with largely community-based facilities, and the insistence on the rights of people with SPMI to full citizenship and valued membership of the community, were enshrined in the national laws of 1978 (Basaglia 1987a), and 1998 (Allison 2006; Mezzina 2007, personal communication). Hospital-based patients and staff were empowered at the same time to stand up for system-wide reforms to improve the quality of their lives and working relationships. When the arch-conservative Italian Prime Minister Berlusconi tried to reverse these reforms, the national family movement rose up against his government until it relented (Dell'Acqua 2010).

Reform agendas do not always improve human rights

Top-down imposed 'Mental Health Reforms' cannot always be guaranteed to be 'a good thing'. They are not always in the interests of individual service-users, and their misuses further down the track may be hidden, insidious, or unpredictable at the time of implementation (e.g. governmental abuse in Nazi Germany of fairly advanced psychiatric epidemiological tracking systems in the 1930s to identify mental patients for extermination) (Seeman 2007). Reorganization of services can be seen historically as cyclical, causing discontinuities of care with each turn of the wheel. So, it is important to have a mechanism such as a Mental Health Commission to consider all proposals for change carefully in advance through well-developed partnerships and regular forums among all stakeholders (Seeman 2007; Rosen et al. 2010). It is equally important to ensure that a more enabling culture (e.g. encompassing human rights, holistic, and recovery-oriented care) is nurtured and grown for endurance with any reorganization, such as a shift towards community-centred services. This is also where implementation of both squarely evidence-based and values-based practices should meet (Woodbridge and Fulford 2004; Rosen et al. 2010).

Mental health human rights and the law

Ratified legislation on unlawful detainment, torture, inhuman, or degrading treatment can and has in recent times been unreservedly over-ruled on the grounds of 'tacit medical necessity' (Hale 2007). The established principles of medicine have been decisive in such cases, on the grounds of 'medical exceptionalism'. That is, a therapeutic necessity cannot be regarded as inhumane or degrading.

The law generally takes a paternalistic view tempering the upholding of all rights to autonomy (Richardson 2007) involving three considerations: (a) the protection of the patient's health and safety; (b) the protection of others, that is public safety and keeping the peace, though it is unclear why mental disorder has been singled out for the application of special social protective powers; and (c) the right of the mentally ill person to treatment and to access to health care, which may be enforced if the person is deemed not to have decision-making competence to consent to or refuse medical treatment. This represents one of the classic dilemmas of biomedical ethics, between respect for patient autonomy and the demands of beneficence (Beauchamp and Childress 2001).

This is countered by a libertarian legal critique of involuntary commitment (McCafferty et al. 1990): that it debases fundamental rights which should not be denied on the basis of arguments for the need to protect people with mental illness and others in their orbit. Gostin (2000) argues that human rights are so basic that they should be self-evident, permanent, and widely agreed. In mental health however, that recognition has been elusive. The conflict concerning involuntary treatment provides a counter-example, where different rights are in tension with each other.

Whereas previous mental health laws had no provision for consent, more recent laws in Western countries (e.g. Hamilton 1983) have enshrined voluntary treatment, informed consent, and least restrictive care as civil rights, to be upheld whenever possible. At the same time, the 1976 landmark Tarasoff Case in California enshrines the principle that mental health professionals are legally accountable to third parties likely to be harmed by their patients. This has made mental health professionals more alert to indications that their patients may harm others, so they feel more obliged to override such rights and take measures to protect those who may be at risk of becoming victims (Elfstrom 2002).

Some have questioned the judicial verdict of not guilty and/or psychiatric commitment for criminal behaviour by reason of mental illness. Benditt (2001) considers that psychiatric commitment instead of penal incarceration is appropriate if the behaviour is criminal, if it is recurrent despite repeated detention and punishment, especially if it is associated with perceived symptoms of mental illness, and if there is some evidence that the behaviour could be ameliorated by treatment. The penal system, by contrast, presupposes offenders should be able to control or take responsibility for their behaviour, or at least be able to learn from the consequences of their behaviours. However this distinction does not safely distinguish such behaviour from the behaviours of people with mental illness. This grey area is illustrated by those mentally ill individuals who are competent to give consent to treatment when well but who do not, despite knowing they are liable to become violent when unwell (Elfstrom 2002). Arguably, they should be placed in the same legal category as the voluntarily intoxicated. That is, it is argued that they should be held responsible for their condition and legally accountable for acts performed under its influence (Elfstrom 2002).

Human rights can be seen initially as a restraint on state power over the individual, which is a precursor to the rights to provision of services and resources to ensure social, cultural, and economic justice (Akuffo 2004), Three fundamental relationships have been identified between mental health and human rights (Gostin 2000; Akuffo 2004): (a) mental health policies, programmes, and practices, through their exercise of government power to restrain, treat, and deprive people of basic citizenship rights (e.g. involuntary treatment), can violate the human rights of individuals designated mentally ill; (b) the adverse effects of severe human rights violations (e.g. incarceration, torture, genocide, sexual assault, malnutrition, starvation, intimidation, and neglect), can have on a person's mental health; (c) the mutuality which exists between mental health and human rights as both are complimentary approaches to the betterment of human beings, their well-being, and quality of life.

The UN Principles for Protection of Persons with Mental Illness and Disability Convention

In 1991, the UN adopted a resolution endorsing 'The Principles for the Protection of Persons with Mental Illness and for the Improvement of Mental Health Care' (United Nations General Assembly, 1991). These principles are sweeping in their breadth and promise concerning a wide array of rights for people with SPMI. However, they also contain some compromises regarding certain basic civil liberties, for example between the desire to treat (stating that beneficence entails the right to receive the best current mental health care), and the libertarian imperative to leave someone alone when they don't want treatment. The right to refuse treatment was removed from an earlier draft. However, it was a resolution, not a treaty, and hence not legally binding, unlike such UN declarations for other groups suffering from prejudice and discrimination, such as refugees, women, and immigrant workers (Rosenthal et al. 1993).

The UN Mental Illness Principles emphasize respect for the inherent dignity and autonomy of the human person receiving psychiatric care. They state that facilities for care, support, treatment, and rehabilitation 'should as far as possible, be provided in the community in which they live', and that hospital-based care should only occur when such community facilities are not appropriate. This preference is stated repeatedly in the principles, requiring the guarantee of vocational training and placement opportunities to assist community reintegration.

From a human rights perspective, a prime reason for prior abuse of people with SPMI in psychiatric care has been that paternalistic, albeit sometimes well-meaning, practices have over-ridden autonomy. Such a perspective must drive procedural safeguards which can serve as a brake against unwarranted coercion, because 'coercion in the name of treatment, once unleashed, is very difficult to control' (Rosenthal et al. 1993). The Drafts of the UN Principles state that they only 'represent the minimum UN standards for the protection of fundamental freedoms and human and legal rights'.

Primarily due to its non-binding nature, the UN Mental Illness Principles statement may be perceived as little more than a 'paper victory' (Perlin 2000, 2009). However, the principles were soon followed by drafting and adopting of the new Convention on the Rights of Persons with Disabilities (Perlin 2000, 2009)—a far sturdier legislative mechanism for countries with strong records on human rights, and likely to be the foundation of future legal challenges in the name of people with SPMI.

Definitions and phases of mental illness

Early stage mental illnesses

First we should consider early stage and onset issues where delays in the recognition of the 'ill health' and delays and insensitivities in engagement of individuals who are prodromal or in early stages of psychosis may result in the benefits of treatment being very compromised (Jackson and McGorry 2009). A key future strategy is to create stigma-free or 'soft entry' to care.

This means muting the psychiatric tone of the initial help seeking environment and allowing maximal patient participation and choice in the initial treatment or care options. Engagement and initial relief of distress is the immediate goal and stepwise care in relation to a clinical staging model (McGorry, 2010a,b; McGorry et al. 2006, 2007, 2010), which delicately balances benefit and risk at each stage, is a helpful approach. This is a preventive strategy which maximizes choice and the chances of recovery with minimal coercion.

What is severe and persistent mental illness?

Severe and persistent mental illness (SPMI) is not a unitary construct. It is not confined to DSM Axis I psychiatric conditions, nor should it be defined centrally in terms of diagnosis. Rather it should be defined in terms of the six Ds: Disability, Distress, Duration (and severity) of symptoms, Disorganization, Danger (to self and others), and 'De family' or Disaffiliation (lack of family support or social isolation). It can also be defined in terms of complexity including vulnerability to co-morbidities (e.g. drugs and alcohol, persistent physical health problems, intellectual disabilities, brain injury, etc) and other factors, including forensic involvement, socio-economic deprivation, psychiatric stigma, rural or remote location, and indigenous or transcultural background. For an Aboriginal person with a mental illness, a cascade of such factors can entrench disadvantage.

SPMI can also be defined in terms of the lived experience of the illness, associated disabilities, deprivations, stigma, and discrimination. Psychiatric functional impairments and disabilities include (as mentioned) social isolation and disorganization, expressed as lack of ability to adequately manage one's finances, housing, nutrition, domestic and self-care, education and training, and to find or retain a meaningful occupation. Other associated deprivations include poverty, dangerous environments, lack of protection, and neglect or abuse of one's children. All these factors contribute to stressors which exacerbate mental illness and make them persist, in those who are vulnerable. They are also consequences of such episodes. Poverty, endemic in developing countries, contributes to both higher incidence of, and poses worse outcomes for, mental illnesses in developing countries (Maingay et al. 2002; Robertson G 2007; Lancet Global Mental Health Service 2008)

The lived experience of having a severe and persistent mental illness can be wearying and fraught, and other people in the community have difficulty understanding what that experience is like: the personal and family impacts of co-morbidities, disabilities, multiple disadvantages, life disruptions and dislocations involved, and of psychiatric stigma, which many individuals with SPMI report as being much worse than the disease in its impact on their lives (Rosen et al. 2000). People with SPMI are often falsely perceived as dangerous, non-human, unapproachable, unemployable, and unmarriageable. They therefore become shunned or marginalized by the community. The organizational equivalent is 'structural stigma', an extension of the sociological concept of structural discrimination, which is the *indirect* or *unintentional* act of stigmatizing a group of people through institutional procedures, legislation, and barriers (Schomeros et al. 2007; Corrigan et al. 2004).

Finally, an area which has been increasingly scrutinized in the last five years or so is the burden of physical, including iatrogenic, illness for people with SPMI. This includes such problems as failure to seek help, diagnostic overshadowing of physical illness by having SPMI, substance (including nicotine) dependence, failure of clinicians to detect serious physical illness in individuals with SPMI and their failure to offer definitive technological solutions to such individuals, and the unwanted, enduring physical consequences (e.g. metabolic syndrome) of psychotropic medications such as anti-psychosis and mood stabilizing medications, especially in young people (Correll et al. 2009). The right in some jurisdictions to refuse medication is a related and often vexed issue, as it may prevent unwanted effects of medication, but it may also postpone recovery, sometimes indefinitely (Barrett et al. 1998).

Rights to humane care should include a holistic, well-coordinated approach which encompasses strategies to deal with all of these complexity factors (Hunt 2007).

Dominant (Western) paradigms of rights for individuals with severe and persistent mental illnesses

By 'dominant paradigms' of rights we refer to prevailing understandings and influences in international psychiatry, mental health, and rights which are mainly Western (e.g. European and/or North American) in origin, and which are frequently reflected in WHO and United Nations statements on this topic. (However it should be noted that the UDHR and the Bill of Rights were also shaped by non-Western international input). People with SPMI have internationally recognized sets of rights, and a growing expectation that they should be met. The World Health Organization (WHO) has attempted to spearhead multi-country systemic reform of mental health services, including the promotion of human rights standards and principles in mental health legislation and procedures (Arboleda-Flórez 2008; WHO 2005).

The WHO articulates ten principles that are considered basic to proper mental health systems and for the protection of the rights of the mentally ill: see Box 16.1.

Box 16.1: WHO Principles for Service Systems to protect the Rights of People with Mental Illnesses (WHO 2003, 2005; Arboleda-Flórez 2008)

   i. Promotion of mental health and prevention of mental disorders
  ii. Access to basic mental health care
 iii. Mental health assessment in accordance with internationally accepted principles
  iv. Provision of the least restrictive type of mental health care
   v. Self-determination
  vi. Right to be assisted in the exercise of self-determination
 vii. Availability of review procedures
viii. Automatic period review mechanisms
  ix. Qualified decision-makers
   x. Respect for the rule of law

The WHO document endorses the 25 principles contained in the United Nations Resolution 46/119 that covers a gamut of areas that impact the rights and care of the mentally ill, such as the following: see Box 16.2.

Box 16.2: Principles of United Nations Resolution 46/119 (United Nations 1991; Arboleda-Flórez 2008)

i. Protection of confidentiality

ii. Standards of care and treatment including involuntary admission and consent to treatment

iii. Rights of persons with mental disorders in mental health facilities

iv. Protection of minors

v. Provision of resources for mental health facilities

vi. Role of community and culture

vii. Review mechanisms providing for the protection of the rights of offenders with mental disorders

viii. Procedural safeguards to protect the rights of persons with mental disorder

ix. Obligatory notification of rights

The Declaration of Madrid of the World Psychiatric Association (WPA) specifically reminds psychiatrists and other mental health professionals that the patient should be accepted as a partner by rights in the therapeutic relationship to allow the patient to make free and informed decisions, and that when the patient is incapacitated and/or unable to exercise proper judgement because of a mental disorder, the family should be consulted and, if appropriate, legal council should be sought, to safeguard the patient's dignity and legal rights. The declaration also urges psychiatrists and other mental health professionals as members of society to advocate for fair and equal treatment of the mentally ill, for social justice, and equality for all (World Psychiatric Association 1996).

Is there a 'right to treatment'?

Treffert (1973) coined the phrase 'Dying with their rights on' to describe uncooperative individuals who are an impending danger to their own lives, yet do not meet the criteria for involuntary treatment under mental health laws that strive to uphold the rights of people with severe mental illness. He recounts instances where it was well recognized that such individuals needed commitment but did not qualify. Entirely predictably, they went to their graves with their rights intact, which could be seen as a morbid medico-legal triumph or a pseudo-heroic moral failure. Treffert (1973) states: 'persons concerned for the patient's rights to be sick and free have been more vocal and persuasive recently as the perpetual pendulum has swung from frank paternalism to frank abandonment. Both of these extremes are distasteful. There must somehow be a proper balance between these two rights to prevent the several kinds of injustices possible'.

Is there a right to self-determination for individuals with SPMI?

A related question is whether people with severe and persistent mental illness have a right to self-determination. The human right to self-determination has its roots in the right to individual freedom. Franklin D Roosevelt postulated four freedoms: of expression, of worship, from want, and from fear. However as the subsequent advent of McCarthyism showed, acceptance is not universal but contested. Human rights are rarely bestowed but rather are gained incrementally through struggle and then must be guarded vigilantly against erosion. Heron (1981a, 1981b) argues for a further all-pervasive right, of people to participate in decision-making that affects the fulfilment of their needs and interests. There are special cases of this right, or subsidiary rights. The right to information concerns any proposed treatment, the right to choose, and the right to informed consent. For example, the review (2007–10) of the Australian Mental Health Service Standards (1996) recommends that informed consent should be routinely and carefully sought from both voluntary and involuntary patients (Miller et al. 2009). Also relevant are the right to freedom of association and contract, and the right to political membership of the community as full citizens—that is the right to participate in the framing and working of political institutions. These rights—including the right to dissent, to vote, to stand for an official post, and to be a member of a jury—are often denied to individuals with mental illness in many US state jurisdictions, amounting to institutional forms of structural stigma and discrimination (Corrigan et al. 2004).

Thus in concluding this section, people with SPMI generally have the right of citizens to protection of their civil liberties. However, this exists in tension with the right to humane, least restrictive, and most effective treatment, and the furtherance of the person's economic, social, and cultural rights. For some, this right could override their civil liberties as citizens. This is related to the beliefs and responsibilities of the society in which the person with SPMI lives.

Questions nevertheless remain. In the case of physical illness, people have a responsibility to manage their own illness. Does this apply to people with SPMI even if they aren't able to manage their daily affairs? This is dubious, particularly if the person has a poor degree of insight or awareness of their condition and the actual or potential consequences of their beliefs on themselves and others. The iatrogenic consequences of treatment, as noted above, and the need for screening and treatment also complicate this question of responsibility.

Also, do the rights of the community override the rights of people with mental illness? Society has the right to protection from disturbance of peace and order, including due to mental illness. Does this override the rights of citizens who have SPMI? This is still contentious, but within the dominant paradigm, the rights of the community are usually assumed to override the rights of the individual with mental illness.

There is another related dilemma: concerns have been expressed widely for some time that the use of involuntary orders in English-speaking countries has been excessive. At the same time, research studies in these countries have indicated that more unfettered access by mental health professionals to the use of involuntary hospital admissions (Large et al. 2008) and Community (outpatient) Treatment Orders (Ajzenstadt et al. 2001; Segal and Burgess 2008, 2009) has saved lives, in terms of lessening danger to self and others, and has improved clinical outcomes. This may indicate that in present circumstances, many services have not adequately systematized the skills of developing therapeutic alliances so that they would not need to resort so much to involuntary orders. Consequently, involuntary orders in many jurisdictions have been made increasingly cumbersome to initiate because of the defensive fear by human rights advocates that they will be invoked too readily. This appears to have been a tit-for-tat symmetrical escalation. Ideally mental health professionals should be taught a more effective repertoire of negotiating skills to ensure voluntary collaboration, and therefore use involuntary orders much more sparingly. Then, when they are urgently needed, involuntary orders should not be too difficult to initiate. However, once invoked, they must have appropriate human rights checks and balances via the routine overview by independent 'umpires' or authorities that include advocates acting on behalf of individual service users (see also Introduction, pp 32–34; Chapters 3, 7, 10, 32–33; commentaries 3–5; and throughout).

Non-dominant (non-Western) paradigms

These paradigms include invoking, sometimes simultaneously, collectivist as well as individualistic, multifaceted, and even contradictory models of reality, intervention, and human rights.

Collectivist models of human rights and care

Collectivist conceptions of human rights exist as alternative and complementary viewpoints rather than as a parallel universe to more individualist models. One such 'social justice' model attempts to acknowledge and to account for the sizable unattributed gap between purely scientific or clinical conceptions of mental disorder and disability, and the experienced realities of the social world. Wakefield (1992) argues that mental disorder lies on the boundary between the 'given' natural world and the 'constructed' social world: a disorder exists when a person's internal mechanisms fails to perform their natural functions, so as to impinge harmfully on the person's well-being, as defined by social values and meanings. Wakefield cautions against falsely pathologizing social phenomena (eg: 'drapetomania', the colonially concocted affliction of slaves that run away from their masters), or conversely, accepting claims that SPMIs like schizophrenia are purely socially constructed or even do not exist.

Crow (1996) argues for a similar revision of the social model of disability to articulate more compatibility with a clinical model of impairment or disorder, so that both social and medical perspectives can interpret the range of bio-psycho-socio-cultural factors that determine social injustices and discrimination associated with psychiatric disabilities. She states that 'Disability is still socially created, still unacceptable, and still there to be changed, but by bringing impairment into our total understanding, by fully recognising our subjective experiences, we will achieve the best route to that change, the only route to the future that includes us all.'

Another leading example is that of indigenous healing systems, and the use of social integration and social support to compliment clinical interventions or in place of clinical or formally enforced treatment. There is robust evidence accumulated over more than 25 years that outcomes for schizophrenia may have been better in developing countries and traditional societies (Harrison et al. 2001; Rosen 2003; Warner 2004; Hopper et al. 2007; Hopper, 2008). This indicates the likelihood of partial or complete recovery may be improved significantly by systematically delivering both evidence-based interventions and particularly traditional cultural congenial healing practices in combination in day-to-day practice (Rosen 2006). Factors at play may include: externalization of the problem (sometimes ascribed to external sorcery); social inclusion and acceptance by the extended kinship system, rather than marginalization; the ease of finding a valued work role in a subsistence economy; and the oracular or shamanistic value placed on transmitting content of hallucinations of ancestors, particularly if your social communication is reasonably intact. These factors are at the hypothesis level, and have required a more detailed study to determine which of them may be operative. Despite cautions not to idealize these findings or minimize the associated hardships in these settings (Rosen 2003, 2006), or the significant limitations of these studies (Cohen et al. 2008) many of which had already been stated by the original authors (Hopper et al. 2007; Hopper 2008), these results have proven to be robust and enduring over many years (Harrison et al. 2001; Warner 2004). However, it may be becoming increasingly difficult to attempt to replicate these differences because of encroachment of modernity on such indigenous communities.

Complexity vs reductionism, and rights

Arguably, mental health is the discipline that most emphasizes the assessment of complexities (that is final common pathway impacts of multifactorial etiologies and precursor and precipitating factors leading to clinical disorders and dysfunctional states) and complex approaches to care (multimodal interventions and the need for coordinated service delivery systems). Contemporary approaches to medicine emphasize that, for it to function optimally, it must operate as a complex adaptive system, considering both its elements and the web of relationships between them as crucial dimensions (Institute of Medicine 2001, 2006). In some ways, we have contributed this combined biomedical-psycho-socio-cultural-ecological outlook to other clinical disciplines, largely through consultation-liaison psychiatry services to medical and surgical wards, emergency departments, and general practice. A further level of complexity is the impact and care of co-morbidities (e.g. drug and alcohol, intellectual disability, brain injury, and physical illnesses). The next level of complexity is social deprivations and the impact of social and cultural determinants on psychiatric disorders (Lancet Global Mental Health Series 2008). However, there is another overriding layer of complexity: the impact of psychiatric disorders on the assumption and exercise of human rights, and reciprocally the impact of human rights on treatment.

Too often, complexity is considered to be a burden in medicine, so every effort is sometimes made to over-simplify assessment and treatment, reducing the clinical care of people to just eliciting and treating bunches of symptoms and signs. Complexity should rather be celebrated, and psychiatry should be proud to be a discipline and a field of endeavour that unashamedly stands up for consideration of complex multi-faceted realities in all aspects of health care. We could then celebrate being a discipline that willingly combines and seeks to balance the clinical and social sciences, ethics, social justice, and human rights.

Hidden meanings and miscommunications between stakeholders

Miller (1990) demonstrates how protagonists in the ongoing discourse about the rights of people with SPMI—for example, legal and mental health professionals, consumers, and families—define key concepts and objectives differently. Though these differing assumptions may be clear to their respective advocates, they sometimes disguise different agendas.

For example, behind patient advocate groups upholding their rights to refuse treatment, is their determination to exert their right to decide what treatment they receive, and sometimes to receive no treatment or care at all, ever, under any circumstances (Treffert 1993; Barrett et al. 1998). This is not a negotiating position. Sometimes the legal insistence on the right to treatment, and clinicians' insistence on providing clinical care, may be regarded as unspoken professional attempts to retain paternalistic authority over these matters, to exert social control over deviance and to protect economic interests in dealing with persons with SPMI (Ajzenstadt et al. 2001). Patient advocate groups may suspect parents who seek to secure hospital admission, to argue against discharge, and to ensure effective financial management of their afflicted offspring affairs, of perpetuating parental control and dependency.

While this prevails, Miller (1990) argues that we will continue to speak at cross-purposes, and yet still be surprised when judicial and legislative decisions reflect misunderstanding of the often obscure motivations underlying these arguments.

Collectivist cultures and practices regarding people with SPMI

In collectivist cultures, where individual subjugation to communal will is generally internalised, some cultures habitually blame people with SPMI for their illness. For example, shame-based cultures in Asia (Rosen 2003, 2006) often discriminate against such individuals and their families on this basis. In some developing countries and cultures the cause of mental illness is externalized: for example, that it is 'sorcery' imposed by an enemy or competing clan. The upside of this is that individuals with mental illness are therefore not shunned or excluded from the community and consequently suffer less discrimination (Rosen 2003, 2006) (though some critics regard such observations as representing either a partially idealized or 'primitive' view). The downside is that the extended family or clan may focus their attention on externalized resentment and their efforts on revenge, and may ignore the need for clinical assessment, treatment, and care. Kirmayer (see Chapter 4) deals with the relevance of individual and communal human rights to collectivist cultures.

Systemic neglect and abuses of psychiatry

Countries which neglect the human rights of people with mental illness, particularly of those in psychiatric hospitals, also tend to be those where the funding and quality of mental health care are very poor, and both need simultaneous upgrading (Lancet Global Mental Health Group 2008).

In authoritarian regimes which punish most forms of political and social dissent, questionable psychiatric diagnoses may be exploited for political purposes such as social control, for example the former Soviet Union and China [see Chapter 12]. All these require examining practices concerning mental disorders and non-Western ('frontier') psychiatry within different cultural contexts, including extreme cases, conditions, and/or political changes that would challenge dominant rights perspectives.

Kingdon et al. (2004) invoke the human rights provisions of the Council of Europe against psychiatric abuses, such as psychiatric incarceration and forced medication for political purposes, electroconvulsive treatment (ECT) without anaesthetic, and excessive use of physical restraint, seclusion, and involuntary treatments. Chappell (2004) and Onken (2008) decry the frequent denial of human rights for those whom police may attempt to bring into custody for disturbing the peace or erratic behavior, police killings during such police investigations or arrests; and people with SPMI who are in correctional services custody for criminal activity. Mental health legislation and related practices must ensure that forensic patients are offered contemporary psychiatric treatment in an appropriate environment, accorded rights equivalent to other patients, possibly with the exception of leave and discharge, and decisions regarding discharge must be made by an independent body, not at a political level. Abusive practices have always haunted psychiatry, arising from ignorance, neglect, exhaustion, cruelty, or criminality. Birley (2003) specifically condemns the premeditated and purposeful intimidation and 'neutralizing' of healthy people, who are regarded to be a threat to the existing political system, by threat of and actual admission to a psychiatric hospital, and forced psychiatric medicating, thus damaging their power, autonomy, reputations, their brains, and their bodies.

Possible resolutions for people with SPMI

Current attempts to remedy possible human rights abuses

It is often argued that Westernization, democratization, or building of quasi-capitalist economies will liberalize the mental health system over some time, and will induce increased transparencies and accountability. This may then lead to exposure of the most blatant human rights abuses, and may foster communal upholding of human rights for people with psychiatric disabilities. This is questionable. The European Union has tried to place pressure upon ex-Soviet countries entering the EU to raise the access and quality of mental health care, to standardize the minimal level of services, and to eliminate human rights abuse. Political changes were followed by updated legislation (Furedi et al. 2000). So far implementation has not occurred for various reasons. Accelerating economic growth in China has not, in itself, promoted personal freedoms and the human rights agenda. However increasing media scrutiny and public access to information has raised the standards of humanitarian responses to internal national crises, such as the 2008 earthquake and infant milk contamination scandal, beyond the imperative of just saving face. These developments may provide some hope for a more humane approach to the public health scourges of suicidality and mental illness in China, which may overcome the entrenched stigma and systemic neglect associated with these conditions.

Recent advances in models of treatment/early intervention

Prevailing models of early intervention in psychosis (Jackson and McGorry 2009) are increasingly widening to include other psychiatric disorders in young people (Headspace 2007, 2008; McGorry et al. 2007; Purcell et al. 2011) and have several features conducive to upholding human rights. These include: an emphasis on low-key voluntary care wherever possible, relying on attention to establishing and sustaining engagement; shared decision making; providing choice within a range of interventions; providing extensive information and group discussions with other young people, who are further along the road to recovery; providing access via shopfront community youth-orientated centres; normative holistic general health care; involving the young person's family wherever possible; and prescribing low dose medication when necessary in the context of a step-wise or 'staged' approach (McGorry et al. 2006, 2007, 2010; McGorry 2010a, b). Such early intervention strategies are having an increasing influence on services for other phases of care (Shiers et al. 2009). Investing upstream is a best buy not only in terms of cost-effectiveness but also human rights, as much more timely and effective care can be delivered in more congenial circumstances with much less coercion (McGorry 2010a, b). This inevitably means a shift in focus to emerging adults and the creation of a missing portal and stream of care (McGorry et al. 2007).

Working harder to minimize involuntary treatment

Service systems could work much harder to minimize or dispense with involuntary treatment, locked doors, asylums, seclusion, and restraint. The Italian mental health reform movement, led by services in Gorizia and Trieste, have increasingly dispensed with psychiatric hospitals, involuntary admissions, locked doors, seclusion and restraint, over-medicating, psychosurgery and ECT, warehousing of longer term clientele, and passive dependent roles for psychiatric patients. Since even before the 1978 national mental health reform laws, these traditional methods have been progressively replaced with very small psychiatric inpatient units in general hospitals with only voluntary beds, no locked doors, no use of restraints, only very occasional use of the Mental Health Act and involuntary admissions, less emphasis on solely technical interventions and token support, 24-hour community mental health centres, community-based residential respite with ample separated facilities for men and women, more psychosocial interventions focused on recovery and regaining full citizenship, and work cooperatives or social enterprises providing real work for real pay (Basaglia 1987b; Mezzina 2005; Mezzina and Johnson, 2008; Rosen and Mezzina, 2005; Rosen et al. in press).

Advent of more recovery oriented services

There has been a gradual shift from an emphasis on 'clinical' or 'service-based' definitions of recovery to 'personal' or 'user-based' definitions (Slade et al. 2008; Burgess et al. 2011). The former are located within a medical model and relate to sustained remission, typically evidenced by reduction of symptoms and/or improvements in functioning. The latter have emerged from the ever-strengthening consumer movement in mental health, and draw on the documented 'life journeys' of people experiencing mental illness. These accounts share in common a theme which forms the basis of the alternative definition of recovery which suggests that recovery is much more than the absence of symptoms and functional impairment, and is more akin to a change in outlook that is related to leading a meaningful, purposeful life, with or without ongoing episodes of illness (Burgess et al. 2011).

Services based on similar principles as those in Italy above are now developing in centres as diverse as Madison Wisconsin, Boston, and San Francisco (US), Lille (France), Scotland and Essex (UK), Auckland (New Zealand), and Wollongong, Melbourne, and Geelong (Australia) as well as Eastern Europe, South America, and parts of the developing world.

Being subject to the same laws as everyone else

Some people with SPMI advocate being subjected to the same laws as everyone else, not special laws (e.g. Mental Health Acts). Meanwhile, more activist parts of the consumer movements and service providers shift from the emphasis particularly placed by English-speaking countries on seeking a more explicit balance between involuntary treatment provisions, and are seeking better checks and balances with more formal recognition in law of human rights of these individuals.

Humane strategies for individualistic cultures

Living wills

Some individualistic cultures that champion the primacy of individual self-determination (for example, the US) have debated the issue of 'Living wills' and sometimes with encouragement from the consumer movement, have taken tentative steps towards legislating for them. Thus, long term service users may circumvent times of diminished personal capacity, by specifying during periods of lucidity how they would like their next episode to be handled. This might include who should be contacted, what medication should be used if possible, and at what stage hospital admission or respite should be considered. Where such directives have overriding legal standing as a durable Power of Attorney, or where they are used to bolster an absolute refusal to take psychotropic medication, enthusiasm has chilled among clinicians, even as it has been stoked among patients opposed to all treatment (Appelbaum 2004). However current research indicates that most individuals who complete advanced directives do not use these directives to decline all treatment with medication, but rather to indicate a preference among alternative treatment, or to inform future treaters of particular concerns—for example, the care of their pets while they are hospitalized (Appelbaum 2004). Arguably, to achieve wider and bilateral acceptance and more practical utility, they should be framed especially in the latter two ways. Research evidence is emerging for the effectiveness of psychiatric advance directives and their variants, joint crisis plans and wellness/recovery action plans (Henderson et al. 2008). They vary to the extent they are legally binding, and as to whether health care workers and families are involved in their development, and an independent facilitator assists in their production. Different types of advance statements may co-exist and interact in complementary ways (Henderson et al. 2008).

Power of Attorney

Alternatively, or as a second-best or back-up strategy, a temporary or enduring Guardianship or Power of Attorney can be delegated or granted legally in advance by the individual with a mental illness causing mental incapacity, in some jurisdictions to a trusted confidante for transient periods during which the individual is incapacitated, though in other jurisdictions such powers are more designed for application in approaching permanent or continuous incapacity.

Shared decision-making

In applying the Institute of Medicine's (IoM 2001) bridging of the Quality Chasm to mental health services, shared decision-making has emerged as one of the top rules to guide the redesign of health care. It is defined as a collaborative process (Deegan et al. 2008) between a client and a practitioner, both of whom recognize one another as experts and work together to exchange information and clarify values in order to arrive at healthcare decisions (Deegan et al. 2008). The intervention can be computer aided, using touch-screens and peer support workers working alongside, responding to a set of questions regarding the client's concerns. The printed report is then reviewed by both client and practitioner together, entering trade-offs or negotiated solutions to concerns in the resulting joint plan. There are now high quality studies emerging, with promising preliminary evidence likely to support its systematic implementation in mental health services (Adams and Drake 2006; Deegan and Drake 2006, 2008; Patel et al 2008; Simmons et al. 2010). Ethically, such joint decision-making amounts to a Rawlsian Social Contract, which is the rational agreement struck following consultation between participants who are 'rational choosers' to not act in a manner which disadvantages others, and the submission of the participants to an overriding power to enforce the contract (Robertson M, 2007). The aim here is to actively explore ways to convert assumed 'non-rational choosers' to participants in rational joint decision-making wherever possible.

Reconciling individualistic with collectivist societal solutions

If enhanced societal value is placed by the wider society on traditional healing factors, this will favour the survival and flourishing of wider communities by synergizing the most effective of traditional and contemporary evidence-based strategies. Moreover, it will also enhance pride in and respect for traditional strategies within indigenous communities themselves (Rosen 2001, 2006). This in turn may restore the pride, curiosity, and interest of younger generations in indigenous communities in acquiring the associated traditional knowledge and skills, so that they will not be lost (Rosen et al. 2010).

These traditional strategies have an emerging evidence-base of proxy strategies in the clinical literature, e.g. the restoring of the respected role of storyteller and elder; multiple family groups as proxies for extended kinship groups (Rosen 2003, 2006). If these strategies are more widely valued, they are more likely to be studied rigorously. If these strategies are subjected to quantitative and qualitative research projects, to determine their effectiveness, they are then more likely to be resourced together with already recognized 'evidence-based' practices (Rosen et al. 2010).

Resolving seemingly contradictory approaches

How can a model that upholds human rights in the mental health sphere both encompass apparent contradictions and remain simple enough to understand and implement, so as not to create a system of unworkable complexity and/or unwieldy bureaucracy?

There are ways of lessening conflicting paradigms in mental health service policy and medico-legal systems, such as:

Integrated and wholistic approaches

For complex disorders involving multi-factorial aetiologies, and multiple clinical and functional needs, it makes sense to employ increasingly evidence based multi-modal approaches or interventions (Rosen 2001, 2006).

Pluralism—tolerating and accommodating different perspectives

'We are doomed to choose, and every choice may entail an irreparable loss' (Berlin 1988).

Despite sometimes heated ideological differences, on a day-to-day practical level professionals of different disciplines often work together cooperatively (Pilgrim and Rogers 2005). An integrative model to utilizing the synergies between social and medical frameworks has been detailed by Middleton and Shaw (2007).

Isaiah Berlin posited a 'richness of buzzing confusion (a term coined by William James in 1891) contributing to creative solutions'. Berlin's Three Level Model of Value-Pluralism rejects the foundational Western doctrine that all moral and practical dilemmas are soluble in principle through a quest for perfect co-existence or definitive resolution.

He dismisses any such quest as an appeal to divine intervention to create a perfect state of human life (Gray 1995; Berlin 1978; Berlin 1988; Berlin and Hardy 1997). The dilemma in this case is the right of the individual to live autonomously and with the dignity-of-risk (Parsons 2008) versus the right of the person's family and the community to their own peace, safety, and protection. Many desirable values such as these are rivalrous and conflictive, and their opposing pulls cannot be reconciled by applying an overarching rational standard. Arguably, most core values cause such a quandary, such as considerations of free will versus determinism.

Berlin's three-level model firstly states that conflicts will arise between codes of conduct which cannot be resolved by either theoretical or practical reasoning. Secondly, each of these values is often internally complex and inherently pluralistic, containing conflicting elements. For example, the opposite of free will contains possible elements of determinism, including fate or divine causation. It may also include communal pressures to conform, laws, and other communal constraints. Thirdly, different cultural or sub-cultural forms or traditions (e.g. individualistic vs collectivist) often develop which specify differing and incommensurable virtues. These amount to a cultural pluralism which can also be tolerated and even embraced. Hopefully we can then appreciate and learn from the richness of and creative tension between these values and traditions.

Complexity is not conflict

> Do I contradict myself?
> So I contradict myself,
> (I am large, I contain multitudes.)
> Walt Whitman, 1819–1892
> Song of Myself

The brains and minds of human beings have an enormous capacity to tolerate and accommodate apparently contradictory frameworks simultaneously without necessarily experiencing cognitive dissonance. The neologistic term 'sonance' was coined to describe this capacity, which challenges the assumptions upon which cognitive dissonance concepts and research has been based (Rosen 1975).

For pragmatism and simplicity in the face of apparent contradictions and mounting complexities, mental health service providers should integrate multi-modal, bio-psycho-socio-cultural combinations of evidence-based interventions and proxies for traditional healing factors. These should be individually planned around the needs of each individual and family. The vehicle for integration of these interventions may be the evidence based service delivery subsystem employed (eg Assertive Community Treatment Teams, Early Intervention in Psychosis Teams).

'Super Rights'

There are pervasive human 'Super Rights' (Heron 1981a, 1981b) that override contradictions between stakeholder claims to rights & responsibilities—in particular: 'the all-pervasive rights of individuals to participate in decision-making that affects the fulfilment of their needs and interests.' However, our society, while implicitly accepting this premise, is slow to adopt actions that truly address this right.

The politics of reflective practices

What appears to be lacking is a systemic and inclusive implementation of 'reflective practice' (Schon 1987, 1990). Kemmis (1985) argues that 'reflection' is not a purely individual, internal psychological process—it is a social and political process, serving human interests and shaping and shaped by ideology. It is action oriented and historically embedded. The logical development from this concept should be communities of practice, which network between teams that perform similar functions, and include all stakeholders, learning from each other's problems, mistakes, and service innovations. Regular forums for crisis teams, assertive community treatment, and rehabilitation and residential teams which occurred during the development of more rigorous community-based components of service in Australia, all exemplify this.

Ways forward

In a system that demands a balance between upholding the rights of people with SPMI and the rights of the community, what are the keys to satisfying both? There are two main ways. One, and initially the easiest to implement, is to systemize ways of minimizing involuntary care. The second and more enduring way is to make key changes to allow full participation by consumer and family groups in the governance, structure, and function of services, and to provide them with formal regular input into mental health law reform and challenging of public and governmental discrimination, as they affect individuals with SPMI. Simultaneously the power imbalance in services must be addressed.

Systematized strategies to decrease involuntary treatment

This can be done by optimizing practices which foster therapeutic alliances and which favour consultative and collaborative care with consumers and their families. These should include early detection and intervention strategies, convenient access, and mobile, flexible, respectful, welcoming, and age appropriate engagement practices, joint decision-making strategies, jointly constructed individual treatment and recovery plans, early warning sign/relapse signature plans, and living wills, involving routine and regular consultation with individual consumers and their families.

Social inclusion as the key to upholding human rights in mental health services

Social inclusion in this context involves ensuring that every stakeholder group is seen and experiences belonging the community, has its voice heard, seriously considered, and acknowledged as legitimate (Huxley 2007). Social inclusion can form a strong bridge between the older and newer paradigms of human rights for people with SPMI. Practically this means having an open and continuing discourse within service and policy arenas with all constituencies represented. In research, this intermittently exists, informing decisions and actions. It attempts to be representative and purports to protect the interests of the least powerful stakeholders (e.g. standing ethics committees).

All stakeholders (including consumers, carers, and local community) need to be represented in legitimate positions with direct influence on the executive authorities of mental health systems. This means positions on executive management and boards, leadership of clinical teams, service provider roles in clinical teams, and service commitment to genuine and regular consultation with stakeholder groups.

Service-wide consumer and community participation

Such a widening of service participation models could be fostered by shifting our perspectives to joint service provider, consumer, and carer collaborative initiatives, such as shifting ownership from artificially narrow silos of responsibility (e.g. health department) to a consultative-all-of-government and all-of-community endeavour. This is beginning to happen in a number of

Western states and countries to mixed critical response (e.g. Mental Health Commissions of Canada, New Zealand, and Western Australia (Rosen et al. 2010)). The obstacles that must be overcome with such initiatives are the lack of consensus between interest groups, lack of co-operation and/or coordination, and lack of will and resources to enact and roll out integrative systemic changes in service delivery organizations.

Harmonize mental health and legal perspectives

Policy changes must be coordinated with legal change. As new mental health policy evolves, we must eliminate any gaping chasms between the clinical and legal spheres—e.g. in the US, in the same jurisdiction there are mental health service system policies which are rights-based and recovery orientated, while archaic laws remain on the statutes which contradict these policies and restrict civil liberties (Corrigan et al. 2004)—for example, incompetence laws whereby individuals with SPMI can lose the right to vote, to marry, and to serve on a jury. Laws affecting such individuals are often based on prejudice, being overtly weighted towards stereotypes of people with mental illness being universally dangerous and irrational, and protection of the community. They result in undue discrimination and denial of full citizenship.

Holistic mental health service models

We also need to adopt a genuine holistic or multi-faceted bio-psycho-socio-cultural approach to psychiatric interventions, rather than the prevailing dominance of a narrow bio-medical model. The medical model can be a powerful tool and metaphor for constructive action (Beels 1989), and individuals and families are entitled to accurate clinical information, as long as it is not allowed to eclipse all other considerations. It should not be allowed to overwhelm the other approaches needed to achieve recovery (for example, social justice, social action, individual and collective empowerment perspectives). Such multi-modal approaches underline the shifting of the balance of power from medical dominance towards more interdisciplinary and collaborative decision-making and care (Rosen and Callaly 2005).

Squarely address the power imbalance

How do we avoid managerial tokenism, gestural consultation, or the co-opting and assimilation of official or employed consumer advocates into the pre-existing power elites? In indigenous relations with colonizing populations, indigenous negotiators are often viewed with suspicion by both the less and more powerful groups, and sometimes are accused of being 'double agents' by both groups. Such suspicions will always prevail while there is a strong power imbalance in the management arrangements. Joint decision-making in management and service planning requires movement towards equalization of power between stakeholder groups. Most of the possible resolutions that we have advocated work towards equalizing of such power relations.

Conclusion

The modern mental health rights movement had its roots in the Western disability movements. De-institutionalization was both a product of the movement and the instigator of a now established international advocacy sector. It was instrumental to the beginning of serious consideration of the social model of disability in psychiatric circles.

As human rights in mental health have become codified both within and between countries there has been a global push for meaningful consumer participation in mental health service delivery.

There have at times been political and ideological counter-movements to rescind newer rights. Sovereign protection of the newer rights since de-institutionalization has not always been whole-hearted.

Top-down reforms have historically been erratic in their guiding principles. Unfortunately there have been times when people with SPMI and their rights have fallen through the cracks during larger mental health service and mental health law restructures.

The law has been at the heart of many social, political, and medical human rights battles. Laws have both validated freedoms of and legitimized abuses towards people with SPMI. On the whole, in most democracies the focus has been on balancing the individual's rights with the community's interests, though some major legacies of bygone attitudes remain in legislation, e.g. structural stigma enshrined in some voting and jury exclusions of individuals with a mental illness.

Proponents of strands of law across the world have seen a mandate grow around least-restrictive forms of care, while the increased litigiousness of the Western world has pushed mental health services to adopt more conservative policies to manage risk, thus demonstrating the knots that mental health law can find itself in.

Recent UN principles and conventions have concentrated on individual rights. While the latest convention, the Convention on the Rights of Persons with Disabilities, is the strongest yet, little of this work has filtered down so far to significant change in national laws.

SPMI is a functional description recognizing the full bio-psycho-socio-cultural influences on the aetiology of mental illness. The lived experience is central to such a view, and this approach allows for structural links to be observed so that both explicit and tacit systems of discrimination can be addressed.

An inherent 'right to treatment' may be debatable, but a right to access treatment on an equitable basis is becoming generally accepted. A right to self-determination is the most fiercely debated issue. This right is widely applied and upheld with the amount of passion and rigour attributed to upholding other similar individual rights provided within a jurisdiction.

In countries where newer restraints on autonomy are put into policy (e.g. CTOs), governments and general populations are yet to settle on the level of autonomy that satisfies all stakeholders.

What many models of mental health human rights provisions lack is the flexibility to question the individualistic paradigm within which most issues are assessed. More collectivist societies seem to offer drastically different solutions to the 'self-determinism dilemma', albeit the evidence-base is still ambiguous regarding differential outcomes, and their political rhetorics can be antagonistic to Western policy reform processes.

Regardless of paradigm, stakeholders are the key to harmonizing theoretical and popular human rights concerns. Most stakeholder groups are naturally biased towards their own interests, though just as vast complexity need not be a barrier to solutions, bias can be factored for in seeking optimal benefit.

There appears to have been a symmetrical escalation between those who are concerned about how Western countries are escalating their uses of involuntary orders and want to raise the bar to make them harder to initiate, and those who demonstrate that involuntary orders can save lives, who want to make them easier to implement. Ideally, mental health professionals should be taught a more effective repertoire of negotiating skills to ensure voluntary collaboration, and therefore use involuntary orders much more sparingly. Then, when they are urgently needed, involuntary orders should not be too difficult to initiate. However, once invoked, they must have appropriate human rights checks and balances via the routine overview by independent 'umpires' or authorities that include advocates acting on behalf of individual service users.

So what can be done to enhance and ensure the more consistent exercise the human rights of people with SPMI, partly by decreasing the need for resorting to involuntary orders?

- Implement more consultative and recovery-oriented service models, including wholistic bio-psycho-socio-cultural aspects of care, with some aspects borrowed from traditional cultures, such as assisting individuals to complete their psychosocial life transitions (or rites of passage) and involving the support of an extended kinship network or proxies for it.

- Early intervention and other methods of timely engagement in more congenial settings ('meeting people on their own turf') to prevent delays which increase severity and toxicity, and to minimize involuntary treatment.

- Review and reform of mental health related laws will reduce barriers to equal citizenship due to structural stigma.

- Living wills and shared decision-making are processes that would work especially well in individualistic societies.

Perhaps the most important method of progressing human rights for people with SPMI is to move beyond the notion that individual rights and community interests are necessarily dichotomous, whenever friction occurs due to multiple and complicated needs, and apparently competing interests.

Pluralism and pragmatism and the routine implementation of 'super rights' may crystallize common-ground solutions if emerging models of early intervention, recovery and social inclusion become systematized as regular ingredients of service delivery and mental health law.

Acknowledgements

This chapter has been informed by discussions and site visits organized by Dr Roberto Mezzina and Dr Peppe Del'Acqua, Trieste, Italy; Professors Ron Diamond and Len Stein, Madison, Wisconsin; and Professor Steven Segal, Berkeley, USA; and by conversations with Mr Douglas Holmes, Ms Leonie Manns, Ms Paula Hanlon, Ms Janet Meagher, Mr Ron Coleman, Mr John Jenkins, Ms Jenna Bateman, Ms Vivienne Miller, Dr Ken Thompson, Dr David Shiers, Professor John Strauss, Dr Kalysanandarum, Dr Courtenay Harding, Ms Marianne Farkas, Dr Jean-Luc Rolande, Dr George Witte, Dr Michael Dudley, and Dr Fran Gale.

References

Adams, JR and Drake, RE (2006) 'Shared Decision-Making and Evidence-Based Practice', *Community Mental Health Journal*, 42(1), 87–105.

Ajzenstadt, M, Aviram, U, Kalian, M, and Kanter, A (2001) 'Involuntary outpatient commitment in Israel: Treatment or control?', *International Journal of Law and Psychiatry*, 24, 637–57.

Akuffo, K (2004) 'The involuntary detention of persons with mental disorder in England and Wales— A human rights critique', *International Journal of Law and Psychiatry*, 27, 109–33.

Allison, L, Chair, Senate Select Committee on Mental Health (2006) Report of site visits and meetings in Trieste, Italy, with Dr Roberto Mezzina, Dr Peppe Dell'Acqua, Dr, Franco Rotelli and others related to the deinstitutionalisation of people with mental illness in the region. Appendix to Report by Senate Select Committee on Mental Health Services, Commonwealth Government of Australia, 2006. Available at <http://www.democrats.org.au/campaigns/mental_health_services_report/>.

Appelbaum, PS (2004) 'Law and psychiatry: psychiatric advance directives and the treatment of committed patients', *Psychiatric Services*, Jul;55(7): 751–2, 763.

Arboleda-Flórez, J (2008) 'Mental Illness and Human Rights', *Current Opinion in Psychiatry*, 21, 479–84.

Barrett, KE, Taylor, DW, Pullo, RE, and Dunlap, DA (1998) 'The right to refuse medication: Navigating the ambiguity', *Psychiatric Rehabilitation Journal*, 21(3) Health Module, 241.

Barry, A (1983) 'The importance of Mental Health Advocacy', *Psychosocial Rehabilitation Journal*, VI(4), 35–41.

Basaglia, F (1987a) 'Problems of Law and Psychiatry', in N Scheper-Hughes and AM Lovell (eds) *Psychiatry Inside Out: Selected Writings of Franco Basaglia*. New York: Columbia University Press, 271–98.

Basaglia, F (1987b) 'Critical Psychiatry After the Law 180', in N Scheper-Hughes and AM Lovell (eds) *Psychiatry Inside Out: Selected Writings of Franco Basaglia*. New York: Columbia University Press, 299–304.

Beauchamp, T and Childress, J (2001) *Principles of Biomedical Ethics*. New York: Oxford University Press.

Beels, CC (1989) 'The Invisible Village', in CC Beels and LL Bachrach (eds) *Survival Strategies for Public pstychiatry, New Directions for Mental Health Services, 42*. San Francisco: Jossey-Bass.

Benditt, T (2001) 'Mental Illness and Commitment', in J Humber and R Almeder (eds) *Biomedical Ethics Reviews: Mental Illness and Public Health Care*. Totowa, NJ: Humana Press Inc, 3–24.

Berlin, I (1978) *Concepts and Categories: Philosophical Essays*. London: Hogarth Press.

Berlin, I (1988) 'On the Pursuit of the Ideal', *The New York Review of Books*, March 17, 1988.

Berlin, I and Hardy, H (ed) (1997) *The Sense of Reality: Studies in Ideas and Their History*. London: Farrar, Straus & Giroux.

Birley, J (2003) 'Political Abuse of Psychiatry', *Psychiatry*, 3(3), 22–25.

Burgess, P, Pirkis, J, Coombs, T, and Rosen, A (2011) 'Assessing the value of Existing Recovery Measures for routine Use in Australian Mental Health Services', *Australian & New Zealand Journal of Psychiatry*, 45(4), 267–80.

Chappell, D (2004) 'Protecting the Human Rights of the Mentally Ill: Contemporary challenges for the Australian Criminal Justice System', *Psychiatry, Psychology and Law*, 11(1), 13–22.

Cohen, A, Patel, V, Thara, R, and Gureje, O (2008) 'Questioning an Axiom: Better prognosis for Schizophrenia in the Developing World', *Schizophrenia Bulletin*, 34(2), 229–44.

Cook, JA, and Jonikas, JA (2002) 'Self-Determination Among Mental Health Consumers/Survivors: Using lessons from the past to guide the future', *Journal of Disability Policy Studies*, 13(2), 87–95.

Correll, CU, Manu, P, Olshanskiy, V, Napolitano, B, Kane, JM, and Malhotra, AK (2009) 'Cardio-metabolic risk of second generation antipsychotic medications during first-time use in children and adolescents', *JAMA*, 302 (16) (Oct 28), 1765–73.

Corrigan, PW, Markowitz, FE, and Watson, AC (2004) 'Structural Levels of Mental Illness Stigma and Discrimination', *Schizophrenia Bulletin*, 30(3), 381–490.

Crow, L (1996) 'Including all of our lives: Renewing the social model of disability', in Colin Barnes and Geof Mercer *Exploring the Divide*. Leeds: The Disability Press, Chapter 4, 55–72.

Deegan, P, Rapp, C, Holter, M, and Reifer, M (2008) 'A Program to Support Shared Decision Making in an Outpatient Psychiatric Medication Clinic', *Psychiatric Services*, 59(6), 603–605.

Deegan, PE and Drake, RE (2006) 'Shared Decision Making and Medication Management in the Recovery Process', *Psychiatric Services*, 57(11), 1636–39.

Dell'Acqua, G (2010) *Public Lecture, The Future of Italian National Mental Health Reforms: The legacy of Franco Basaglia and beyond*. The Mental Health Conference of Australia & New Zealand, The Transcultural Mental Health Conference Of NSW, and the Italian Institute of Australia, Sydney September 2010.

Elfstrom, G (2002) 'Involuntary Outpatient Commitment', in J Humber and R Almeder (eds) *Biomedical Ethics Reviews: Mental Illness and Public Health Care*. Totowa, NJ: Humana Press Inc, 27–54.

Furedi, J, Mohr, P, Swingler, D, Gheorghe, MD, Hotujac, L, Svesleak, M, Kocmur, M, Koychev, GI, Mosolov, SN, Pekenak, J, Rybakowski, J, Svestleak, K, and Sartorius, N (2000) 'Psychiatry in selected countries of Central & Eastern Europa: an overview of the current situation', *Acta Psychiatrica Scandinavia*, 114(4), 223–31.

Gostin, LO (2000) 'Human Rights of Persons with Mental Disabilities', *International Journal of Psychiatry*, 23(2), 127–28.

Gray, J (1995) *Isaiah Berlin*. London: Harper-Collins.

Hale, B (2007) 'Justice and equality in mental health law: The European experience', *International Journal of Law and Psychiatry*, 30, 18–28.

Hamilton, JR (1983) 'Observations on the Mental Health Act 1983', *International Journal of Law and Psychiatry*, 6, 371–80.

Harrison, G, Hopper, K, Craig, T et al. (2001) 'Recovery from psychotic illness: a 15- and 25-year international follow-up study', *British Journal of Psychiatry*, 178, 506–17.

Headspace: National Youth Mental Health Foundation. Establishment report. Melbourne: Australian Government Promoting Better Mental Health – Youth Mental Health Initiative, 2007. Available at <www.headspace.org.au>.

Headspace: Australian Youth Mental Health Network, 2008. Available at <http://www.headspace.org.au>

Henderson, C, Swanson, JW, Szmukler, G, Thornicroft, G, and Zinkler, M (2008) 'A Typology of Advance Statements in Mental Health Care', *Psychiatric Services*, 59(1), 63–71.

Heron, J (1981a) 'Philosophical Basis for a New Paradigm', in P Reason and J Rowan (eds) *Human Inquiry: A Sourcebook of New Paradigm Research*. Chichester: Wiley, 18–30. Available at <http://www.human-inquiry.com/Experiential%20Research.pdf>, accessed 20 January 2012.

Heron, J (1981b) *Paradigm Papers*. British Postgraduate Medical Federation, University of London, with Human Potential Research Project, University of Surrey.

Hopper, K (2008) 'Outcomes elsewhere: course of psychosis in "other cultures"', in C Morgan, M Kwame, and P Fearon (eds) *Society and Psychosis*. Cambridge: Cambridge University Press.

Hopper, K, Harrison, G Janca, A, and Sartorius, N (2007) *Recovery from Schizophrenia: An International Perspective: A Report from the WHO Collaborative Project, the International Study of Schizophrenia*. Oxford: Oxford University Press.

Hunt, P (2007) 'Right to the highest attainable standard of health', *The Lancet*, 370 (Aug 4), 369–71.

Huxley, P (2007) *Looking toward excellence: the measurement of social inclusion in mental health services*, 18th Themhs Conference Melbourne, 2007.

Institute of Medicine of the National Academies (2001) *Crossing the Quality Chasm: A New Health System for the Twenty-first Century*. Washington: National Academies Press.

Institute of Medicine of the National Academies (2006) *Improving the Quality of Health Care for Mental and Substance-Use Conditions, Committee on Crossing the Quality Chasm: Adaptation to Mental Health and Addictive Disorders, Board on Health Care Services*. Washington, DC: The National Academies Press.

Jackson, HJ and McGorry, PD (2009) *The Recognition and Management of Early Psychosis*. 2nd edn. Cambridge: Cambridge University Press.

Kemmis, S (1985) 'Action Research and the Politics of Reflection', in D Boud, R Keogh, and D Walker (eds) *Reflection: Turning experience into learning*. London: Routledge.

Kingdon, R, Jones, R, and Lonnqvist, J (2004) 'Protecting the human rights of people with mental disorder: new recommendations emerging from the Council of Europe', *British Journal of Psychiatry*, 185, 277–79.

Lancet Global Mental Health Series (2008) 'Scale up services for mental disorders: a call for action', *The Lancet*, 370, 1241–52.

Large, MM, Nielssen, O, Ryan, CJ, Hayes, R (2008) 'Mental health laws that require dangerousness for involuntary admission may delay the initial treatment of schizophrenia', *Social Psychiatry & Psychiatric Epidemiology*, 43, 251–56.

Maingay, S, Thornicroft, G, Huxley, P, Jenkins, R, and Szmukler, G (2002) 'Mental health and human rights: the MI Principles—turning rhetoric into action', *International Review of Psychiatry*, 14, 19–25.

McCafferty, G and Dooley, J (1990) 'Involuntary Outpatient Commitment: An Update', *Mental and Physical Disability Law Reporter*, 14(3), 277–86.

McGorry, PD, Tanti, C, Stokes R et al. (2007) Headspace: Australia's National Youth Mental Health Foundation—where young minds come first. *Medical Journal of Australia*, 187(Suppl. 7), 68–70.

McGorry, P (2010a) 'Risk syndromes, clinical staging and DSM V: new diagnostic infrastructure for early intervention in psychiatry schizophrenia', *Schizophrenia Research*, 120, 49–53.

McGorry, PD (2010b) 'Staging in neuropsychiatry: a heuristic model for understanding prevention and treatment', *Neurotoxicity Research*, 18(3–4), 244–55.

McGorry, PD, Hickie, IB, Yung, AR, Pantelis, C, and Jackson, HJ (2006) 'Clinical staging of psychiatric disorders: a heuristic framework for choosing earlier, safer and more effective interventions', *The Australian and New Zealand Journal of Psychiatry*, 40(8), 616–22.

McGorry, PD, Purcell, R, Hickie, IB, Yung, AR, Pantelis, C, and Jackson, HJ (2007) 'Clinical staging; a heuristic model for psychiatry and youth mental health', *Medical Journal of Australia*, 187(7 sup ll), S40–42.

McGorry, PD, Nelson, B, Goldstone, S, Yung, R (2010) 'Clinical staging: a heuristic and practical strategy for new research and better health and social outcomes for psychotic and related mood disorders', *Canadian Journal of Psychiatry*, 55(8), 486–97.

Mezzina, R (2005) *The Italian Mental Health Reforms, Keynote address*, The Mental Health Service Conference of Australia and New Zealand, Adelaide, 2005.

Mezzina, R, Johnson, S (2008) 'Home Treatment and "Hospitality" within a Comprehensive Community Mental Health Centre', in S Johnson, J Needle, JP Bindman, G Thornicroft (eds) *Crisis Resolution and Home Treatment in Mental Health*. Cambridge: Cambridge University Press, 251–266.

Middleton, H and Shaw, I (2007) 'A Utilitarian Perspective of Social and Medical Contributions to three Illustrative Conditions, and recent UK-NHS Policy Initiatives', *Journal of Mental Health*, 16(3), 291–305.

Miller, RD (1990) 'Hidden agendas at the law-psychiatry interface', *The Journal of Psychiatry & Law*, 18(1), 35–38.

Miller, V, Rosen, A, Gianfrancesco, P, and Hanlon, P (2009) 'Australian *National Standards for Mental Health Services*: a blueprint for improvement', *International Journal of Leadership in Public Services*, 5(3), 25–42.

Mizrahi, T (1992) 'The right to treatment and the treatment of mentally ill people', *Health and Social Work*, 17(1), 7–11.

Onken, SJ (2008) *One Can Learn From Many Sources: Honoring the First Territory, keynote paper*, The Mental Health Services Conference of Australia and New Zealand, Auckland 2008.

Parsons, C (2008) 'The Dignity of Risk: Challenges in Moving On', *Australian Nursing Journal*, 15(9), 28.

Patel, SR, Bakken, S, and Ruland, C (2008) 'Recent Advances in shared decision making for mental health', *Current Opinion in Psychiatry*, 21, 606–12.

Perlin, ML (2000) *The Hidden Prejudice: Mental Disability on Trial*. Washington DC: American Psychological Association, 175–204.

Perlin, ML (2009) '"A Change is Gonna Come": The Implications of the United Nations Convention on the Rights of Persons with Disabilities for the Domestic Practice of Constitutional Mental Disability Law', NYLS Legal Studies Research Paper No. 08/09 #21, *North Illinois University Law Review*, 29, 483–98.

Pilgrim, D and Rogers, A (2005) 'The Troubled Relationship between Psychiatry and Sociology', *International Journal of Social Psychiatry*, 51(3), 228–41.

Purcell, R, Goldstone, S, Moran, J et al. (2011) Toward a Twenty-First Century Approach to Youth Mental Health Care: Some Australian Initiatives, *International Mental Health Journal*, 40(2), 72–87.

Richardson, G (2007) 'Balancing autonomy and risk: A failure of nerve in England and Wales?', *International Journal of Law and Psychiatry*, 30, 71–80.

Robertson, G (2007) 'Health and human rights series', *The Lancet*, 370(Aug 4), 368–69.

Robertson, M (2007) 'Psychiatrists and Social Justice, Part 1: The Concept of Justice and Part 2: When the Social Contract Fails', *Journal of Ethics in Mental Health*, 2(2), 1–9.

Rosen, A (1975) *Medical Sociology Research Proposal*, via Dr. Muriel Baxter, Department of Sociology, University of Aberdeen, Scotland.

Rosen, A (2001) 'New Roles for Old: The role of the psychiatrist in the Interdisciplinary Team', *Australasia Psychiatry*, 9(2), 133–137.

Rosen, A (2003) 'What developed countries can learn from developing countries in challenging psychiatric stigma', *Australian Psychiatry*, 11, 579–85.

Rosen, A (2006) 'Destigmatizing day-to-day practices: what developed countries can learn from developing countries', *World Psychiatry*, 5(1), 21–24.

Rosen, A and Callaly, T (2005) 'Interdisciplinary Teamwork and Leadership', *Australasian Psychiatry*, 13(3), 234–40.

Rosen, A, Goldbloom, D, and McGeorge, P (2010) 'Mental Health Commissions—making the critical difference to the development and reform of mental health services', *Current Opinion in Psychiatry*, 23, 593–603.

Rosen, A and Mezzina, R (2005) *Mental Health Reforms in Italy Vs English Speaking Countries*, 17th Annual TheMHS (The Mental Health Service) Conference, of Australia & New Zealand, September, Adelaide, South Australia.

Rosen, A and Mezzina, R (2007) *Mental Health Reforms in Italy Vs English Speaking Countries*, National Conference on adapting Italian national mental health reforms for general health and social services, May, Trieste, Italy.

Rosen, A, O'Halloran, P, Mezzina, R (in press) International Trends in Community Mental Health Services, in HL McQuiston, JM Feldman, JM Ranz, WE Sowers (eds) *Handbook of Community Psychiatry*. New York: Springer.

Rosen, A, Rigby, CW, Berry, H, Hart, C, Long, I, Fanning, P, Kelly, B, Tonna, A, and Wannan, J (2010) *Impact of drought on Indigenous Communities, Report on Drought Mental Health Assistance Project, report 2008–2009*, Centre for Rural & Remote Mental Health, University of Newcastle, and NSW Health.

Rosen, A, Walter, G, Casey, D, and Hocking, B (2000) 'Combating psychiatric stigma: An overview of contemporary initiatives', *Australasian Psychiatry*, 8(1), 19–26.

Rosenthal, E and Rubenstein, LR (1993) 'International Human Rights Advocacy under the "Principles for the Protection of Persons with Mental Illness"', *International Journal of Law and Psychiatry*, 16, 257–300.

Schomeros, G, Matschinger, H, and Angermeyer, MC (2007) 'Familiarity with Mental Illness and Approval of Structural Discrimination Against Psychiatric Patients in Germany', *Journal of Nervous and Mental Disease*, 195(1), 89–92.

Schon, DA (1987, 1990) *Educating the Reflective Practitioner*. San Francisco: Jossey Bass.

Sedgwick, P (1982) *PsychoPolitics*. London: Harper Collins.

Seeman, MV (2007) 'Mental health reform not always beneficial', *Psychiatry*, 70(3), 252–9.

Segal, S and Burgess, PS (2008) 'Use of community treatment orders to prevent psychiatric hospitalization', *Australia and New Zealand Journal of Psychiatry*, 42(8), 732–9.

Segal, S and Burgess, PS (2009) 'Preventing Psychiatric Hospitalisation and Involuntary Outpatient Commitment', *Social Work in Health Care*, 48(3), 232–42.

Shiers, D, Rosen, A, and Shiers, A (2009) 'Beyond Early Intervention: can we adopt alternative narratives like 'Woodshedding' as Pathways to Recovery in Schizophrenia', *Early Intervention in Psychiatry*, 3(3), 163–171.

Simmons, M, Hetrick, S, and Jorm, A (2010) 'Shared decision-making: benefits, barriers and current opportunities for application', *Australasian Psychiatry*, 18(5), 394–397.

Slade, M, Amering, M, and Oades, L (2008) 'Recovery: An international perspective', *Epidemiologia e Psichiatria Sociale*, 17, 128–37.

Treffert, D (1973) '"Dying With Their Rights On", Letters to the editor', *American Journal Of Psychiatry*, 130(9), 1041.

Tucker, S (2001) 'Psychosis and the Therapeutic Community: Beyond the user movement?', *Therapeutic Communities*, 22(3), 233–47.

United Nations General Assembly (1991) *Principles for the Protection of Persons with Mental Illness and for the Improvement of Mental Health Care*, Resolution 119, 46th Session, Meeting 75, December 17 Report A/46/721.

Wakefield, JC (1992) 'The Concept of Mental Disorder: On the boundary between biological facts and social values', *American Psychologist*, 47(3), 373–88.

Warner, R (2004) *Recovery from schizophrenia: psychiatry and political economy.* 3rd edn. Hove: Brunner-Routledge.

Woodbridge, K and Fulford, W (2004) *Whose Values? A Workbook for Values-Based Practice in Mental Health Care.* London: The Sainsbury Centre for Mental Health.

World Health Organization (2003) *Mental Health Legislation and Human Rights.* Geneva: WHO.

World Health Organization (2005) *WHO resource book on mental health, human rights and legislation: stop exclusion, dare to care.* Geneva: World Health Organization. Available at <http://www.who.int/mental_health/policy/legislation/policy/en/>, accessed 3 April 2012.

World Psychiatric Association (1996) Madrid Declaration on Ethical Standards for Psychiatric Practice. Available at < http://www.wpanet.org/detail.php?section_id=5&content_id=48 >, accessed 5 November 2011.

Chapter 17

Survival, Evasion, Resistance, and Escape

A Framework Proposal for the Comprehension and Prevention of Health Professionals' Complicity in Detainee Abuse

Jonathan H. Marks

Of all the revelations about the G. W. Bush administration's 'war on terror', some of the most troubling relate to the involvement of health professionals. Psychologists were the principal 'grand architects' of aggressive detention and interrogation regimes operated by both the Defense Department and the Central Intelligence Agency (CIA)—regimes that incorporated a variety of coercive techniques including sleep deprivation, exposure to temperature extremes and loud noise, stress positions, and, in the case of the CIA, dousing with cold water and waterboarding, a procedure that induces a desperate feeling of suffocation.[1] Mounting evidence shows psychologists and physicians provided psychological and medical assessments of detainees prior to abusive interrogations, advised interrogators how to ramp up interrogation stressors, monitored aggressive interrogations—ostensibly with the power to intervene—and recorded the effects of aggressive interrogation techniques on detainees.[2]

Memoranda released by the Obama administration (in response to Freedom of Information Act requests made by the American Civil Liberties Union) emphasize from the outset the critical dependence on the participation of health professionals—especially physicians and psychologists—in legal endorsements of so-called 'enhanced interrogation techniques' by the Office of Legal Counsel in the Department of Justice. For example, when Jay Bybee affirmed the legality of ten aggressive interrogation tactics for Abu Zubaydah in August 2002 (including waterboarding),

---

[1] See the Senate Armed Services Committee (SASC) Report of December 2008, available at <http://documents.nytimes.com/report-by-the-senate-armed-services-committee-on-detainee-treatment#p=1>, accessed 21 January 2010. See also the CIA Inspector General's Report of May 2004 available at <http://media.luxmedia.com/aclu/IG_Report.pdf>, accessed 6 November 2011. See also Jane Mayer (2008) *The Dark Side*, especially Chapter 7.

[2] These claims are discussed in further detail elsewhere—see, for example, JH Marks (2007) 'Doctors as Pawns? Law and Medical Ethics at Guantanamo Bay', 37 Seton Hall L. Rev. 711–731; JH Marks (2005) 'Doctors of Interrogation', Hastings Center Report, 35(4), 17–22; Bloche, MG and Marks, JH (2005) 'Doctors and Interrogators at Guantanamo Bay', *New Engl. J. Med.*, 353(1), 6–8; Bloche, MG and Marks, JH (2005) 'When Doctors Go To War', *New Engl. J. Med.*, 352(1), 3–6. See also Steve Miles (2009) *Oath Betrayed: America's Torture Doctors*. 2nd ed. In Defense Department interrogations, psychologists and psychiatrists attached to the interrogation mission were designated 'behavioral science consultants' and assigned to teams known colloquially as 'Biscuits:' see, for example, Jane Mayer, supra n. 32.

the advice was expressly premised on the condition that 'a medical expert . . . will be present throughout . . . and . . . the procedures will be stopped if deemed medically necessary to prevent serious mental or physical harm.'[3] Another legal memo penned in 2005 by Steven Bradbury contains more than 80 references to the CIA's Office of Medical Services (OMS); medical professionals, staff, or personnel; medical advice or judgment; medical screening; medical safeguards; medical monitoring; medical intervention; medical evaluation; medical contraindications and medical literature.[4] Among the most disturbing references are those to advice from the OMS that waterboarding was 'medically acceptable' subject to limitations on the duration and number of repetitions, physician monitoring, and the concealed presence of emergency tracheotomy equipment in case the detainee was unable to resume breathing afterwards.[5]

Although medical personnel may have occasionally intervened during the course of interrogations,[6] there is also substantial evidence that they stood by and permitted some extreme abuses, thus seriously risking the physical and mental health of detainees, and violating their fundamental rights, as conferred by human rights law and the laws of war.[7] Consider, for example, the Defense Department's aggressive interrogation of Mohamed Al Qahtani at Guantanamo Bay. Lasting up to 20 hours per day for 48 of 54 days in late 2002 and early 2003, it was not only humiliating, but resulted in Qahtani's pulse dropping to 35 beats per minute, and on two occasions his temperature falling to 95 degrees.[8] The CIA waterboarded Abu Zubaydah

---

[3] See <http://dspace.wrlc.org/doc/bitstream/2041/70967/00355_020801_004display.pdf>. The advice also notes that Zubaydah had been injured during capture and records that the OLC has been informed that 'steps will be taken to ensure that this injury is not in any way exacerbated by the use of these [interrogation] methods and that adequate medical attention will be given to ensure that it will heal properly.' Id. p. 4. The opinion relies on the advice, presence and intervention of medical personnel throughout: see pp. 3, 4, 11, 15, and 16.

[4] See 10 May 2005 Memorandum for John Rizzo. *Re Application of 18 U.S.C. 2340–2340A to Certain Techniques That May Be Used in the Interrogation of a High Value al Qaeda Detainee.* Available at <http://www.justice. gov/olc/docs/memo-warcrimesact.pdf>, accessed 6 November 2011. For a searchable copy, see <http:// www.globalsecurity.org/intell/library/policy/national/olc_050510_bradbury_20pg.htm>, accessed 6 November 2011. For a recent collection of several core 'torture memos,' see David Cole (ed) (2009) *The Torture Memos: Rationalizing the Unthinkable.* A discussion of some of these memos occurs in Sheri Fink, *Bush Memos Suggest Abuse Isn't Torture If a Doctor Is There,* Propublica.com, at <http://www.propublica. org/article/memos-suggest-abuse-isnt-torture-if-a-doctor-is-there-417>, accessed 6 November 2011.

[5] Id. at p. 16. The legal memo refers here to the OMS Guidelines on Medical and Psychological Support to Detainee Rendition, Interrogation and Detention, December 2004. However, in the version of that document released to the ACLU, the relevant portions of the OMS Guidelines have been redacted.

[6] See International Committee of the Red Cross (ICRC). 2007. *Report on the Treatment of Fourteen 'High-Value Detainees' in C.I.A. Custody.* 14 February. Available at <http://www.nybooks.com/icrc-report.pdf>, accessed 6 November 2011.

[7] For the rights of detainees in more detail, see Jonathan H Marks (2006) '9/11 + 3/11 + 7/7 =? What Counts in Counterterrorism?', 37 Colum. Hum. Rts L. Rev. 559, and Jonathan H Marks, *Doctors as Pawns,* supra n. 2.

[8] See Adam Zagorin and Michael Duffy, 'Inside the Interrogation of Detainee 063', *TIME,* 12 June 2005, available at <http://www.time.com/time/magazine/article/0,9171,1071284,00.html>, accessed 6 November 2011; see also Interrogation Log Detainee 063, 23 November 2002, <http://www.time.com/time/2006/log/ log.pdf>, accessed 6 November 2011; presenting a partially-redacted copy of the interrogation log. For a discussion of the medical ethical implications of this interrogation, see also Steven Miles, 'Medical Ethics and the Interrogation of Detainee 063', 7 *Am. J. Bioethics* 3, and Steven Miles, *Oath Betrayed,* supra n. 2 at Appendix I. For the role of lawyers in approving this interrogation: see Philippe Sands (2008, revised 2009) *Torture Team: Rumsfeld's Memo and the Betrayal of American Values.* As Sands notes at p. 224, Al Qahtani had been captive for a year before these interrogations began.

and Khalid Sheikh Mohammed 83 and 183 times respectively in a month (in addition to other aggressive interrogation tactics).[9] Zubaydah later told the Red Cross: 'I struggled without success to breathe. I thought I was going to die. I lost control of my urine. Since then I still lose control of my urine when under stress.'[10]

Limitations of space preclude comprehensive examination of the complicity of health professionals in detainee abuse, and the manner in which lawyers, psychologists, and physicians were central to constructing and supporting the Bush administration's regime of aggressive detention and interrogation. Legal and ethical critiques of health professionals' participation in these interrogations have been addressed elsewhere,[11] as have experts' criticisms of the efficacy of these techniques and their impact on the moral legitimacy of the US.[12] Instead, two practical questions—how did this happen, and how might its recurrence be avoided?—are addressed and tentatively answered. The frame used is that of human rights law and bioethics, to which scholars of psychology, sociology, and anthropology (among others) may provide further substance. While a few psychologists were instrumental in creating aggressive interrogation regimes,[13] psychology may offer much to help prevent the recurrence of those regimes.[14] If, as this author contends, the complicity of health professionals was pivotal to the systematic abuse of detainees, then the answers will have far-reaching implications for counterterrorism policy and practice.

Looking back: some retrospective reflections

The focus on individual health professionals and the ethics of purportedly discrete decision-making in health care settings is sometimes described as 'quandary bioethics' or 'micro-bioethics.' However, to understand how health professionals could have been complicit in detainee abuse,[15] the *micro* level of analysis, focusing on individuals, must be broadened to encompass *meso* and *macro* levels. The latter refers to the broad socio-cultural and political factors that shaped the United States' 'war on terror' after 9/11.[16] The former refers to organizational and community

---

[9] See Central Intelligence Agency (CIA) Inspector General. 2004. *Counterterrorism, Detention and Interrogation Activities (September 2001–September 2003)*. Available at <http://media.washingtonpost.com/wp-srv/nation/documents/cia_report.pdf>, accessed 6 November 2011 (pp. 90–91).

[10] ICRC Report, supra n. 6.

[11] See, for example, Jonathan H Marks, *Doctors as Pawns?*, supra n. 2.

[12] I discuss these issues in Jonathan H Marks (2010) 'A Neuroskeptic's Guide to Neuroethics and National Security', Am. J. Bioethics, 1(2), 4–12, and Jonathan H Marks, 'The Language and Logic of Torture', 9(1) Comparative Literature and Culture, available at <http://docs.lib.purdue.edu/clcweb/vol9/iss1/11>, accessed 6 November 2011.

[13] Id.

[14] Although a new administration has brought new policies and approaches, it would be naïve to assume that we need no longer be concerned about the potential for repressive responses to the threat of international terrorism. While that threat continues (or is perceived to continue), the risk that we will take repressive measures in response remains, whether or not such measures are as extreme or widespread as before.

[15] In this essay, the term 'health professionals' is used broadly to include physicians, psychologists, physician assistants and nurses.

[16] The term 'mezzo' was employed in Jonathan H Marks (2010) 'Looking Back, Thinking Ahead: The Complicity of Health Professionals in Detainee Abuse' in R Goodman and M Roseman (eds) *Interrogations, Forced Feedings, and the Role of Health Professionals: New Perspectives on International Human Rights, Humanitarian Law, and Ethics* (Harvard). However, the term 'meso' is used and preferred here since it shares Greek etymology with 'macro' and 'micro', and it is already familiar to scholars in the social and natural sciences.

perspectives, including situational and systemic factors that influence behaviour. A number of intersecting communities are relevant, such as the military, intelligence services, health professionals, and legal professionals.[17] Understanding incentives for both ethical and unethical behaviours at the meso and macro levels is essential to any comprehensive critique of misconduct, and to the formulation of preventive measures.

Macro perspectives

Macro level factors contributing to the development of aggressive interrogation strategies in the war on terror have been elaborated elsewhere,[18] and are summarized here.

There is some evidence that responses to terrorism after 9/11 were fuelled by emotion, which exacerbated cognitive biases and skewed deliberative processes within government and wider society. George Tenet, former director of the CIA, repeatedly acknowledged that after 9/11 there was 'palpable fear' within government because there was so much that was unknown.[19] A number of psychological studies have demonstrated the effect of fear on policy choices.[20] Post-9/11, the resulting cognitive biases appeared to give moral salience to claims favoring aggressive treatment of detainees. These included assertions by administration officials that detainees at Guantanamo Bay were 'the worst of the worst' and that Mohamed al Qahtani, presumably worst of all, was 'the 20th hijacker'.[21]

At the same time, other considerations were ignored—for example, that hundreds of detainees at Guantanamo Bay had been handed over to US forces by the Northern Alliance in return for the promise of 'wealth and power beyond your dreams'.[22] When many detainees produced no intelligence whatsoever, this was interpreted as resistance, rather than innocence or ignorance. Al Qahtani's '20th hijacker' label ensured he was the first Guantanamo Bay detainee whose mistreatment was prescribed by a 'special interrogation plan.' But the plan's architects may have suppressed the fact that the US government also identified another prisoner, Zacarias Moussaoui, as the 20th hijacker.[23] As Philip Zimbardo—the principal investigator of the famous Stanford Prison

---

[17] For a discussion of the ethics of the lawyers in the Office of Legal Counsel in the Department of Justice, see for example David Luban (2007) *Legal Ethics and Human Dignity*, David Cole (ed) (2009) *The Torture Memos: Rationalizing the Unthinkable*, and W Bradley Wendel (2009) *The Torture Memos and the Demands of Legality*, Cornell Law School Research Paper 09–019 (reviewing several books by Harold Bruff, Jack Goldsmith, Jane Mayer, Philippe Sands, and John Yoo that touch on this issue.) For a more detailed discussion of the role of lawyers in the Department of Defense, see Philippe Sands, *Torture Team*, supra n. 8.

[18] Jonathan H Marks, *9/11 + 3/11 + 7/7 =?* supra n. 7.

[19] George Tenet, Interview with Scott Pelley. *60 Minutes* (29 April 2007), available at <http://www.cbsnews.com/stories/2007/04/25/60minutes/main2728375_page3.shtml>, accessed 6 November 2011.

[20] Jennifer S Lerner et al. (2003) 'Effects of Fear and Anger on Perceived Risks of Terrorism: A National Field Experiment', 14 *Psychol. Sci.* 144, 146. On the effects of moral emotions—including moral outrage—see Sabrina Pagano and Yuen Huo (2007) 'The Role of Moral Emotions in Predicting Support for Political Actions in Post-War Iraq', 28(2) *Political Psychology*. On the impact of 'feeling threatened' on policy decisions, see Carol Gordon and Asher Arian (2001) 'Threat and Decision Making', 45(2) *J. Conflict Resolution* 196–215.

[21] I discuss this further in Jonathan H Marks (2007) 'The Language and Logic of Torture', 9(1) *Comparative Literature and Culture*, available at <http://docs.lib.purdue.edu/clcweb/vol9/iss1/11>, accessed 6 November 2011.

[22] Id.

[23] Id.

Experiment—notes, substantial empirical evidence demonstrates the power of labelling to dehumanize people subjected to punitive conditions.[24]

How labels, in conjunction with cognitive biases, may have affected military personnel in high-pressure interrogation environments, is further discussed in this chapter. The designation that Moussaoui and al Qahtani shared exemplifies a *narrative construct* that fuelled aggressive counter-terrorism policies. At the macro level, additional narratives operated—most notably, 'ticking bombs', Al Qaeda affiliates armed with nuclear devices that could destroy an entire American city.[25] This narrative was reinforced when the administration prepared the case for the invasion of Iraq by claiming that Saddam Hussein had *both* weapons of mass destruction and links to Al Qaeda, and that we could not 'wait for the final proof—the smoking gun—that could come in the form of a mushroom cloud.'[26]

These factors—emotional responses, cognitive biases, and narrative constructs—powerfully coalesced so that broad sections of the public became an internal 'coalition of the willing', supporting torture as a necessary evil.[27] This was exacerbated by what might be called 'the false promise of force'.

Faced with threats described as exceptional and unparalleled in magnitude—a suspect claim, given the threat of 'mutually assured destruction' in the Cold War—officials said 'the gloves' had to 'come off'.[28] In particular, this meant using what were euphemistically dubbed 'enhanced inter-rogation techniques', which, it was assumed, would enhance public safety. A perilous trade-off was presented—that fundamental detainee rights (including freedom from torture, and from cruel, inhuman, and degrading treatment) must be sacrificed to guarantee security.[29] Although experts have long asserted that force is not a reliable method for the extraction of intelligence,[30] its use may have offered short-term emotional rewards for those who deployed it, providing a release from the grip of fear. Experts in interrogation recognize the false promise torture offers,[31] but this is not so obvious to the public or to young trainee interrogators exposed to Hollywood confections such as *24*—a television series the dean of the US Military Academy at West Point criticized for its 'toxic effect', promoting a torture-tolerant culture and undermining the training and

---

[24] Philip Zimbardo (2007) *The Lucifer Effect: Understanding How Good People Turn Evil*, 308–310.

[25] This analysis is extended in Jonathan H Marks, *The Language and Logic of Torture*, supra n. 21.

[26] Office of the Press Secretary of the White House, President Bush Outlines Iraqi Threat (7 October 2002) available at <http://georgewbush-whitehouse.archives.gov/news/releases/2002/10/20021007-8.html>, accessed 6 November 2011.

[27] See, for example, Steven Kull et al. (2004) *Program on International Policy Attitudes/Knowledge Networks, Americans on Detention, Torture and the War on Terrorism*, <http://www.pipa.org/OnlineReports/Terrorism/Torture_Jul04/Torture_Jul04_rpt.pdf>, accessed 6 November 2011.

[28] Cofer Black, former director of the CIA Counterterrorism Center. Congressional Testimony, 26 September 2002, available at <http://www.fas.org/irp/congress/2002_hr/092602black.pdf>, accessed 6 November 2011.

[29] For a powerful critique of the relationship between liberty and security, see Jeremy Waldron (2003) 'Security and Liberty: The Image of Balance', 11 *J. Pol. Phil.* 191, 195. The administration continued to deny that it was involved in torture and engaged lawyers to narrow the definition of the term: see Jonathan H Marks, *The Language and Logic of Torture*, supra n. 21.

[30] See, for example, S Budiansky (June 2005) 'Truth Extraction', *Atlantic Monthly*, 32–35; (2007) '"Torture is for Amateurs": A Meeting of Psychologists and Military Interrogators', *Peace and Conflict: Journal of Peace Psychology*, 13(4); Ali Soufan (5 September 2009) 'What Torture Never Told Us', *New York Times*,. Available at <http://www.nytimes.com/2009/09/06/opinion/06soufan.html?_r=2>, accessed 6 November 2011.

[31] Id.

performance of US military personnel.[32] The purported elimination of legal constraints (discussed more fully elsewhere),[33] the dehumanization of detainees, and the extreme pressure to obtain actionable intelligence, created a potent cocktail, greatly increasing the likelihood that abuses would take place, and that detainee deaths would result.

Meso perspectives

To understand the systemic and structural factors contributing to unethical and illegal behaviours of health professionals, a number of communities and sub-communities need to be understood. Three clusters of communities are mentioned here. The first comprises national security and military communities involved in counterterrorism: in particular, the CIA, the National Security Agency, the Federal Bureau of Investigation (FBI) and the Department of Defense. Within the Defense Department, distinctions should also be drawn between the civilian and military leadership, and among the departments' various agencies. These communities have different cultures and often disagree—most famously, the FBI repudiated aggressive interrogation approaches favoured by the civilian leadership in the Defense Department.[34]

The second cluster comprises health professionals, such as physicians, psychologists, physician assistants and nurses, and their professional bodies. Again, there are important distinctions here—among different categories of health professional and the responses of their professional associations.[35] The third cluster is smaller, its members being at the intersection of the first two clusters: health professionals who contract with, consult for, or are employed by defence and national security agencies. At its core are psychologists who played a significant role in formulating the new aggressive interrogation tactics and were also—despite the conflict of interest—key architects of the American Psychological Association's policy on interrogation (in particular, the 2005 Report of its Presidential Task Force on Psychological Ethics and National Security) formulated in the wake of revelations of detainee abuses.[36]

Since limitations of space preclude considering each of these clusters exhaustively; the focus is narrowed to military health professionals and their related communities. Looking broadly first at the military, a number of key organizational and structural factors can be identified.[37] First, experienced interrogators did not occupy sufficiently senior positions in the military hierarchy, so they could not bring their expertise or authority to bear on the Army's development of new aggressive

---

[32] Jane Mayer (19–26 February 2007) 'Whatever It Takes: The Politics of the Man Behind 24', *New Yorker*, 66–82.

[33] See, for example, Jonathan H Marks, *What Counts?*, supra n. 7.

[34] In the author's view, understanding pockets of resistance to aggressive interrogation strategies (for example, in the FBI, the US Naval Criminal Investigation Service, and the military judge-advocates general) is vital to help understand how others might similarly be motivated to resist. This is discussed briefly in Philippe Sands, *Torture Team*, supra n. 8, at pp. 239–240.

[35] For a critique of a variety of professional associations and their respective positions and responses, see for example Jonathan H Marks, *Doctors as Pawns?*, supra n. 2. Compare M.G. Bloche (2011) 'Doctors as Warriors II' in MG Bloche, *The Hippocratic Myth* (Palgrave).

[36] For a discussion of the 2005 PENS Task Force Report and its sequelae, see, for example, Amy Goodman and David Goodman (2007) 'Psychologists in Denial', in Amy Goodman and David Goodman, *Standing Up to the Madness: Ordinary Heroes in Extraordinary Times*.

[37] Jean Maria Arrigo and Ray Bennett (2007) 'Organizational Supports for Abusive Interrogations in the "War on Terror"', 13(4) *Peace and Conflict: Journal of Peace Psychology*, 411–421; see also Stephanie Erin Brewer and Jean Maria Arrigo (2009) 'Places That Medical Ethics Can't Find' in R Goodman and M Roseman (eds) *Interrogations, Forced Feedings, and the Role of Health Professionals* (Harvard).

interrogation strategies. If they had, they would have challenged the claim that so-called 'enhanced interrogation techniques' were really enhanced (as several of them have recently done publicly).[38] Second, from the late 1980s, the Department of Defense gave greater priority to imagery and signals intelligence than to human intelligence. As a result, after 9/11 (and, in particular, following the invasion of Iraq in 2003), experienced interrogators were in extremely short supply. This led to lower standards for the selection, training, and placement of new military interrogators. The Army even instructed 19-year-old novices to interrogate detainees who did not respond to direct questioning—a task that, in previous conflicts, had been reserved for only the most experienced interrogators.

When health professionals were introduced into this troubled detention and interrogation environment, most were tasked with providing health care to detainees. Although many delivered the best care they could with the available resources, some evidently did not report abuses, and others may even have colluded in suppressing them.[39] A relatively small number of psychologists and psychiatrists were assigned to the intelligence-gathering mission and charged with ramping up physical and psychological stressors, purportedly to aid interrogations. This was irrespective of whether they had a desire to do so, or any experience of interrogation, or potentially relevant professional skills.[40]

A number of other factors may have impaired the ability of health professionals to act ethically in these environments. First, military health professionals often have financial constraints. Many entered the health professions via the military because they had no other way to pay for their medical education.[41] Speaking out against detainee abuses could entail not just social costs but serious financial implications. If forced to leave the military, these health professionals would likely face the prospect of having to repay the cost of their professional education.[42] Second, even without such concerns, they might perceive that they have a limited capacity to intervene. Believing that they can only protest so many times before being dismissed as unpatriotic or accused of 'crying wolf',[43] they might reasonably fear that such characterizations could—at the very least—adversely affect their future assignments, deployments, and promotion. However, saving their objections for the most egregious cases and remaining silent in others might then be interpreted as acquiescence in the use of aggressive tactics.

In addition to these *inhibitory* factors, a third factor may have contributed to the more enthusiastic embrace of unethical behaviours. As more than one experienced interrogator has explained to the author, some health professionals in the interrogation environment suffer from *wannabe-ism*![44] Military health professionals are often perceived by their non-medical colleagues as 'not real soldiers.' Doctors ordinarily wear a caduceus (the staff entwined by two snakes and topped with wings) that marks them out as different; when they act as health care providers, they are non-combatants under the Geneva Conventions, with the concomitant privileges and protections

---

[38] See the articles cited in n. 30 supra.

[39] See, for example, Steve Miles (2009) *Oath Betrayed: America's Torture Doctors* (UC Press).

[40] See Bloche and Marks, *Doctors and Interrogators*, supra n. 2. See also M.G. Bloche, 'Doctors as Warriors I' in M.G. Bloche (2011) *The Hippocratic Myth* (Palgrave).

[41] Marks, *Doctors as Pawns?*, supra n. 2 at 729.

[42] Id.

[43] I discuss this further in Jonathan H Marks (2005) 'Doctors of Interrogation', 35(4) Hastings Center Report 17–22.

[44] See, similarly, Katherine Eban (17 July 2007) 'Rorschach and Awe', *Vanity Fair*, available at <http://www.vanityfair.com/politics/features/2007/07/torture200707>, accessed 6 November 2011.

afforded by the laws of war.[45] However, health professionals attached to the intelligence mission as behavioural science consultants surrender their non-combatant status under international law. Their new assignment somewhat compensates the loss of this *legally* privileged status through the acquisition of a *socially* privileged status within the military: their association with and potential entry into the inner sanctum of the intelligence community. This prospect of belonging and acceptance can generate in behavioural science consultants more than willingness to assist their intelligence colleagues; they may wish to become 'one of them.' CS Lewis identified the hazards created by the unbridled desire to gain admission to a privileged inner circle or 'ring,' when he observed that '[o]f all the passions, the passion for the Inner Ring is most skillful in making a man who is not yet a very bad man do very bad things.'[46]

These factors may well have contributed to the complicity of health professionals in systemic abuses of detainees at Abu Ghraib and elsewhere. Different theorists have accounted for this phenomenon in slightly different ways. For Robert Lifton, the concept of the 'atrocity-producing situation'—which he fashioned to explain the conduct of Nazi doctors—had explanatory power for detainee abuses in the war on terror.[47] Another concept, 'behavioural drift,' denotes the slide into unprofessional and ultimately illegal behaviours.[48] Psychologists have used this term defensively to describe the activities of wayward interrogators, while elevating the potential role of psychologists attached to the intelligence mission in detecting and counteracting this tendency.[49] However, considerable evidence suggests that psychologists assigned to advise interrogators may equally be subject to behavioural drift. For example, the interrogation log of Mohamed al Qahtani records the intermittent presence of a psychologist during his life-threatening and profoundly humiliating interrogation.[50] This psychologist, who advised on the content of al Qahtani's aggressive interrogation plan, chaired a behavioural science consultation team at Guantanamo Bay, and publicly available documents suggest he had a larger role as one of the architects of the overarching aggressive interrogation strategy.[51] Another related concept is '*moral seduction*.' Forged in the context of conflicts of interest, this excludes 'the most Machiavellian fringes of professional communities,' and focuses on 'the majority of professionals [who] are unaware of the gradual accumulation of pressures on them to slant their conclusions.'[52] Like behavioural drift, this concept recognizes the

[45] First Geneva Convention for the Amelioration of the Condition of the Wounded and Sick in Armed Forces in the Field (12 August 1949, in effect from 1950). Art. 24. Available at <http://icrc.org/ihl.nsf/FULL/365?OpenDocument>, accessed 6 November 2011.

[46] CS Lewis (1944) *The Inner Ring*, available at <http://www.lewissociety.org/innerring.php>, accessed 6 November 2011. The author is extremely grateful to David Luban for bringing this essay to his attention.

[47] Robert Jay Lifton (2004) 'Doctors and Torture', 351 *New Eng. J. Med.* 415–416, available at <http://www.nejm.org/doi/full/10.1056/NEJMp048065>, accessed 6 November 2011.

[48] See Gerald P Koocher (2006) 'Varied and Valued Roles', *Monitor on Psychol.*, July-Aug. 2006, at 5, available at <http://www.apa.org/monitor/julaug06/pc.html>, accessed 6 November 2011, and Stephen Behnke (2006) 'Ethics and Interrogations: Comparing and Contrasting the American Psychological, American Medical and American Psychiatric Association Positions', *Monitor on Psychol.*, July-Aug. 2006, at 66, available at <http://www.apa.org/monitor/julaug06/interrogations.html>, accessed 6 November 2011.

[49] Id.

[50] Bloche and Marks, *Doctors and Interrogators*, supra n. 2. For a book length discussion of the evolution of this aggressive interrogation plan, see Philippe Sands, *Torture Team*, supra n. 8.

[51] This psychologist participated in a 'Counter Resistance Strategy Meeting' held on 2 October 2002. See pages 14–17 of a PDF file of documents recently made public by Senator Levin's office: <http://levin.senate.gov/download/?id=20d5eeec-4892-4d34-9b15-c32ee31f8245>, accessed 6 November 2011.

[52] Don Moore et al. (2006) 'Conflicts of Interest and the Case of Auditor Independence: Moral Seduction and Strategic Issue Cycling', 31(1) *Academy of Management Review* 1–20, available at <http://faculty.haas.

often gradual nature of the process, while serving to emphasize that it does not take place in a vacuum—other people and the systems they put in place may advance or hinder the process.

Individual perspectives

In addition to the macro and meso perspectives described above, many strands from research in cognitive psychology may offer additional perspectives. This research has been used to explain why doctors make clinical mistakes,[53] and it might equally explain the behaviours of those attached to interrogation units—especially, health professionals and young novice interrogators with little or no experience of interrogation. For example, *fundamental attribution error* describes the tendency to attribute behaviours to disposition or personality, rather than situational factors.[54] In a medical context, a physician might attribute the symptoms of a poorly-dressed, unshaven man in the emergency room with alcohol on his breath to alcoholic cirrhosis, therefore missing a different chronic condition that left untreated, would be potentially very serious.[55] At Guantanamo Bay, detainees' failure to provide intelligence apparently was attributed to the grim determination of hardened terrorists not to reveal anything. As noted above, the detainees' label 'worst of the worst'[56] solidified this perception, so that an alternative explanation (that many detainees had no terrorist involvement and no information to impart) was neglected.[57]

Labelling may also have fueled *confirmation bias,* which leads people to focus on information that corroborates their initial judgment and to ignore information that contradicts it.[58] In medicine, *confirmation bias* can lead to *diagnosis momentum.*[59] Once a diagnosis is reached, despite incomplete or inconsistent evidence, the physician may be reluctant to revisit it—as may his colleagues, particularly if they occupy more junior physicians in the medical hierarchy. Consequently, a series of ineffective therapies may be deployed, sometimes for years. Similarly, the 'diagnosis' of a detainee as a terrorist may be difficult for intelligence operatives to revisit, particularly since military culture emphasizes obedience to authority and tends to heighten the forces of conformity and compliance operating within groups. Consequently, one set of aggressive (but unsuccessful) interrogation techniques may be swiftly followed by another. The alternative explanation, that a detainee does not have intelligence, will be arrived at with the greatest reluctance.

---

berkeley.edu/tetlock/Vita/Philip%20Tetlock/Phil%20Tetlock/2004_Current/2005%20Conflicts%20of%20 interest%20and%20auditor%20independencepageproofs.pdf>, accessed 6 November 2011.

[53] Jerome Groopman (2007) *How Doctors Think* at 44–46. Much of the research in cognitive psychology on which Groopman relies is discussed in far more detail elsewhere. See, for example, D Kahneman, P Slovic, and A Tversky (eds) (1982) *Judgment under Uncertainty: Heuristics and Biases,* D Kahneman and A Tversky (eds) (2000) *Choices, Values, and Frames,* T Gilovich, D Griffin, and D Kahneman (eds) (2002) *Heuristics and Biases: The Psychology of Intuitive Judgment,* C Camerer, G Loewenstein, and M Rabin (eds) (2004) *Advances in Behavioral Economics.*

[54] Jerome Groopman (2007) *How Doctors Think* at 44–46.

[55] Id.

[56] Eric Saar and V Novak (2005) *Inside the Wire: A Military Intelligence Soldier's Eyewitness Account of Life at Guantanamo* at 193.

[57] For a critique of the allegations made against detainees based solely on the government's documents, see Mark P Denbeaux, et al. (2006) *Second Report on the Guantanamo Detainees: Inter- and Intra-Departmental Disagreements About Who Is Our Enemy,* available at <http://law.shu.edu/news/second_report_guantanamo_detainees_3_20_final.pdf>, accessed 6 November 2011. This does not suggest, of course, that none of the detainees had intelligence value.

[58] *See,* e.g. Groopman, supra, n. 54 at 65–66.

[59] Id. at 128.

Commission bias creates a preference for doing something rather than nothing,[60] and a rapport-building interview might seem like 'nothing' when compared to an aggressive interrogation—particularly in the eyes of novices. It has also been suggested that inexperienced interrogators erroneously assumed that information from cruel, bad, harsh enemies can only be produced by similarly cruel, bad, harsh techniques.[61] Fictional examples of torturous interrogations, whether from the US television series *24* or elsewhere, would certainly have reinforced this view. An important mechanism for this reinforcement is the *availability heuristic,* a form of mental shortcut in which the probability of an event is assessed by reference to the ease with which an example comes to mind.[62] Heroes torture hardened terrorists, producing vital nuggets of actionable intelligence at the last possible moment, and saving innocent lives. Writers and movie directors overlook gentler, more prolonged rapport-building interviews that do not have the same dramatic impact, but that nonetheless generate more complex less time-sensitive intelligence. Consequently, these approaches are less available to the public, and to inexperienced interrogators.

These cognitive pitfalls can be exacerbated by emotional responses, such as anger and fear. Such emotions may have been especially acute at both Guantanamo Bay and Abu Ghraib. At Guantanamo Bay, there was a widespread belief (particularly in 2002–3) that another attack on the US mainland was imminent and that al Qahtani and other so-called 'high value detainees' possessed information that could be used to prevent such an attack. At Abu Ghraib, daily mortar assaults and improvised explosive devices (IEDs) frequently killed or maimed US military personnel. The distorting effect of anger and fear on cognition is known as *affective bias.* Although emotion can be vital in shaping goals and focusing attention, it can be a 'terrible advisor'.[63] Here it may have contributed to interrogators and health professionals more highly valuing information that confirmed their emotional needs and desires.[64]

Thinking ahead: preliminary reflections on prophylaxis

Situational and systemic challenges to the ethical behaviours of health professionals in detention and interrogation environments are substantial. There is no single solution. A suite of measures will be required. Although there is a body of cognitive and behavioural research that can help policy makers fashion these measures,[65] there is a need for further empirical research, both qualitative and quantitative, in the field as well as in the lab, and for concomitant funding—for example from the National Institutes of Health and the National Science Foundation. This research

---

[60] Id. at 169.

[61] See Ronnie Janoff-Bulman (2007) 'Erroneous Assumptions: Popular Belief in the Effectiveness of Torture Interrogation', 13 (4) *Peace and Conflict: Journal of Peace Psychology* 429–435 at 432, describing this as an example of 'resemblance criterion' and as a 'crude form' of the mental shortcut know as the *representativeness heuristic.*

[62] Amos Tversky and Daniel Kahneman, 'Judgment Under Uncertainty: Heuristics and Biases', in *Judgment Under Uncertainty,* supra n. 53 at 465; see also Groopman, supra n. 54 at 64.

[63] Antonio Damasio (2003) *Looking for Spinoza: Joy, Sorrow and the Feeling Brain* at 40. I discuss the relationship between emotion and cognition in more detail in Jonathan H Marks, *What Counts,* supra n. 7.

[64] See, for example, Pat Kroskerry, *Diagnostic Failure: A Cognitive and Affective Approach,* available at <http://www.ahrq.gov/downloads/pub/advances/vol2/Croskerry.pdf>, accessed 6 November 2011.

[65] Much empirical ethics-related research appears in the business ethics literature, and is framed for business ethics scholars and managers: see, for example, the following summaries of empirical research: Robert C Ford and Woodrow D Richardson (1994) 'Ethical Decision-Making: A Review of the Empirical Literature', *Journal of Business Ethics,* 13, 205–221 and Terry W Loe, Linda Ferrell, and Phylis Mansfield (2000) 'A Review of Studies Assessing Ethical Decision Making in Business', *Journal of Business Ethics,* 25, 185–204.

can help determine and refine the kinds of intervention might increase the likelihood of ethical behaviours in such unusually charged environments.[66] In the meantime, some tentative, non-exhaustive recommendations can be made. An instructive analogy might help demonstrate why this problem merits serious consideration, and how it could be addressed.

From a SERE-modelled problem to a SERE-modelled solution

For the purpose of this analogy, the origins of the aggressive interrogation regimes used by the CIA and the Defense Department, described in more detail elsewhere,[67] are briefly reviewed. During the Korean War, 36 US airmen signed false confessions describing a US plot to aerial-bomb civilian targets in North Korea.[68] The alleged bomb plot, although untrue, seriously embarrassed the US government which, after the war, determined to explore how the airmen could have been made to act in this way. Psychologists, commissioned to interview the men and provide explanations of their behaviour,[69] found that the airmen had 'broken' following their exposure to stress positions and other psychological pressures. This led to two enterprises: one defensive, the other offensive.[70]

In particular, the defensive enterprise was to create the SERE training programme for US military personnel, to help them when they fell behind enemy lines or into the custody of enemy captors. SERE is an acronym: 'S' stands for 'survival' (for example, how to rely on local flora and fauna as sources of food); the first 'E' stands for evasion (of the enemy, avoiding being taken captive); the 'R' is for 'resistance' (to interrogation once captured); the second 'E' stands for 'escape' (from captivity). The theory behind the 'R' component is that inoculating US personnel against enemy interrogation tactics was best achieved by exposing them to those tactics. Thus a significant part of SERE involves exposure to psychological stressors including sleep deprivation, exposure to temperature extremes and loud noises (among others) and, until 2007, waterboarding.[71] The Bush

....

[66] The author recognizes but cannot explore here the epistemological, methodological, and normative issues presented by the interpretation, synthesis, and application of a variety of sources of empirical data (from the simplified lab experiment to the more complex oral history).

[67] See, for example, Jonathan H Marks (2010) 'A Neuroskeptic's Guide to Neuroethics and National Security', *Am. J. Bioethics: Neuroscience* 1(2), 4–12. See also the SASC Report, supra n. 1 and Jane Mayer, supra n. 1.

[68] J Margulies (2 October 2006) The More Subtle Kind of Torment. *Washington Post.* A19, available at <http://www.washingtonpost.com/wp-dyn/content/article/2006/10/01/AR2006100100873.html>, accessed 6 November 2011.

[69] AD Biderman (1957) 'Communist Attempts to Elicit Confessions from Air Force Prisoners of War', *Bull. N.Y. Acad. Med.* 33(9), 616–625, at <http://www.ncbi.nlm.nih.gov/pmc/articles/PMC1806204/pdf/bullnyacadmed00378-0046.pdf>, accessed 6 November 2011. See also LE Hinkle and HG Wolff (1957) 'The methods of interrogation and indoctrination used by the Communist state police', *Bull. N.Y. Acad. Med.* 33(9), 600–15, at <http://www.ncbi.nlm.nih.gov/pmc/articles/PMC1806200/pdf/bullnyacadmed00378-0030.pdf>, accessed 6 November 2011.

[70] The author does not consider the offensive application here, in particular, the CIA's exploration of psychological stressors that led to the KUBARK interrogation manual in 1963. A copy of the KUBARK Counterintelligence Interrogation Manual (1963) is available at <http://www.gwu.edu/~nsarchiv/NSAEBB/NSAEBB122/#kubark>, accessed 6 November 2011.

[71] Senate Armed Services Committee Inquiry into the Treatment of Detainees in U.S. Custody, December 12, 2008 Available at <http://documents.nytimes.com/report-by-the-senate-armed-services-committee-on-detainee-treatment#p=1>, accessed 6 November 2011. Unlike detainees, when SERE cadets were waterboarded, they were given a code word they could use to make it stop. There were, of course, numerous other distinctions that would have made the procedure all the more gruelling for detainees—among them, prolonged detention and isolation, and the frequency and intensity with which the waterboard was used.

administration turned to these techniques when it was looking for a sourcebook for aggressive interrogations.[72] But the analogy offered here draws on the SERE model to prevent rather than promote abuse.

The power of the analogy does not turn on the effectiveness of the SERE programme at inoculating US servicemen and women. Rather, it is the determination of the US government, so disturbed by its airmen's false confessions, to address the problem, that they commissioned research to understand the problem and then established a training programme to address it. Taking seriously the complicity of health professionals in detainee abuse similarly calls for a systematic research programme to shed further light on the mechanisms discussed, coupled with a training programme that aims to address the problem and prevent its recurrence.[73] As well as studying those who succumbed to pressure, those who dissented should be considered—including, for example, a psychologist in the US Naval Criminal Investigation Service who refused to participate in the design of aggressive interrogations,[74] and a small number of Navy physicians who refused to get involved in force-feeding detainees.[75] The research would require significant funding (and peer reviewed publication), while the training programme would need to be supplemented by institutional structures that support its graduates.

The new training programme might be called *HealthSERE* to distinguish it from its more troubled analog. 'S' would be for survival, but this time: how a health professional can survive (and thrive) in a military environment given the competing pressures and institutional cultures. The first 'E' again stands for evasion—how health professionals can evade 'capture' by the military mission or those tasked with the discharge of that mission. The 'R' is similarly for resistance: how health professionals can learn to resist the social pressures to act unethically when, despite their best efforts to the contrary, they find themselves attached to problematic military missions. The final 'E' is again for escape: how professionals can escape from situations in which these pressures become intolerable. The source of the psychological stressors would come not from being exposed to temperature extremes and the like that traditional SERE trainees endure, but from facing simulated assignments that create tensions with the trainees' ethical obligations as health professionals.

Training on its own will, of course, not be sufficient. Each of the components will require additional supporting structures. For example, in extreme cases, whistleblowing may be the only means of escape. For this reason, greater protections and rewards for whistleblowers will be required. Building on this framework, several additional measures are discussed below. However, it is likely that the proposed multi-disciplinary research will lead to a richer understanding of the problems and to the further refinement of these measures.

----

[72] Id.

[73] Factors other than explicit pressure may come into play, including subtle influences and obligations of reciprocity—particularly in environments like Abu Ghraib prison, where health professionals depended on their military colleagues to defend them from repeated mortar attacks. Although such research and training might be relevant for other kinds of professionals and for other kinds of military personnel too, this is not explored here.

[74] Jane Mayer (2008) *The Dark Side* at pp. 195–6.

[75] See Susan Okie (2005) 'Glimpses of Guantanamo: Medical Ethics and the War on Terror', *N. Engl. J. Med.*, 353, 2529–2534. There is also value in exploring the extent and efficacy of pockets of resistance in other professions, e.g. judge-advocates general (military lawyers).

Counternarratives

A potentially valuable tool to minimize detainee abuse is the promulgation of *counternarratives*—
stories (often personal stories) that challenge dominant cultural narratives,[76] including those
described above. Counternarratives can help combat dehumanization by debunking simplistic
notions of 'them' and 'us'. One of the core responsibilities of a free and informed press is to help
craft and communicate counternarratives for society at large. Though there is much evidence that
the media often failed in this regard in the 'war on terror',[77] a number of human rights groups[78]
and a few independent film-makers have begun to fill the gap: see, for example, 'The Road to
Guantanamo' (2006),[79] which tells the story of three British detainees at Guantanamo Bay ('The
Tipton Three') and 'Taxi to the Dark Side' (2007),[80] a film about the Afghan taxi driver, Dilawar,
who died in US custody at Bagram Air Base in December 2002.

   Although films with first-hand testimony from former detainees and their families can provide
powerful counternarratives, their reach is limited and audiences are self-selecting. Truth and reconciliation commissions (TRC) can help create official counternarratives that may reverse (or at
least erode) dominant cultural narratives. Over the last four decades, there have been dozens of
TRCs, most famously in South Africa. There is only one precedent for such a commission in the
US, which was informal and confined to exploring a single event.[81] A TRC with a comprehensive
mandate to explore detainee abuses would be a massive endeavor. It would confront considerable
geographical challenges (given the many countries of origin of detainees in the war on terror and
their families), and would raise thorny questions about whether immunity from prosecution
should be granted in return for cooperation. Following the November 2008 election, the incoming
Obama administration was reportedly considering some kind of non-partisan commission with
subpoena power to investigate detainee abuses in the Bush administration's war on terror.[82] Such
a commission had the potential to establish widespread social counternarratives, but the proposal
was abandoned, overtaken by other events and policy priorities. The absence of some kind
of commission intensifies the need for and urgency that counternarratives be developed and

---

[76] Compare William Casebeer and James Russell (2005) 'Storytelling and Terrorism: Towards a Comprehensive
    "Counter-Narrative Strategy"', *Strategic Insights*, IV(3) (March 2005), available at <http://www.nps.edu/
    Academics/centers/CCC/publications/OnlineJournal/2005/Mar/casebeerMar05.html>, accessed 6
    November 2011 arguing for the use of counternarratives to dissuade terrorists and potential insurgents
    from violent behaviours. The argument here is for *self*-directed use of counternarratives to minimize the
    temptation to develop abusive detention and interrogation policies and practices, and to defuse public sup-
    port for such policies and practices.

[77] Jonathan H Marks (2008) 'The Fourth Estate and the Case for War in Iraq' in Mark Gibney et al. *The Age
    of Apology: Facing Up to the Past* at 298–314. See also Eric Umansky (2006) 'Failures of Imagination:
    American Journalists and the Coverage of American Torture', *Columbia Journalism Rev.*, 45(3), 16–31.

[78] See, for example, Physicians for Human Rights (2008) *Broken Laws, Broken Lives: Medical Evidence of
    Torture by the US Personnel and its Impact,* available at <http://physiciansforhumanrights.org/library/
    reports/broken-laws-torture-report-2008.html>, accessed 6 November 2011. See also Almerindo Ojeda
    (2008) *The Trauma of Psychological Torture* for affidavit evidence of detainee abuse.

[79] See <http://en.wikipedia.org/wiki/The_Road_to_Guantanamo, accessed 6 November 2011.

[80] See <http://en.wikipedia.org/wiki/Taxi_to_the_Dark_Side>, accessed 6 November 2011.

[81] For further information regarding the Greenshoro Truth and Reconciliation Commission, see <http://
    www.greensborotrc.org>, accessed 6 November 2011.

[82] Mark Benjamin (13 November 2008) *Obama's Plans for Probing Bush Torture,* available at <http://www.
    salon.com/2008/11/13/torture_commission/>, accessed 6 November 2011. The non-partisan commission
    would build on and go beyond the investigation conducted by the Senate Armed Services Committee
    under the leadership of Senator Carl Levin: see supra n. 51.

acculturated in military and health professional communities. The value of this approach becomes even more apparent when confronting systemic cognitive biases.

Debiasing

There is a substantial literature addressing debiasing and its challenges,[83] and illuminating the role counternarratives might play in counteracting cognitive biases. Jolls and Sunstein contend that an important antidote to bounded rationality—as manifested by cognitive biases and resultant errors in judgment—is to deploy the law as a debiasing tool.[84] In their view, the law can and should be used to restructure the environment to alter not individuals' motivations but their perception of the world around them. For example, *optimism bias*—people's tendency to underestimate their probability of facing a bad outcome—is often evident in relation to consumer goods. But this may be counteracted by providing concrete, narrative information, which tends to be more effective than general statistics.[85] Smokers are more likely to believe that cigarettes will harm their health if they are given specific examples—stories of individual patients who have suffered—than if provided with cancer statistics.[86] As Jolls and Sunstein argue, the law could 'require the real-life story of an accident or injury to be printed in large type and displayed prominently so that consumers would be reasonably likely to see and read it before using the product.'[87] Because images may run an especially high risk of manipulation, these authors prefer narrative.[88] This approach, they argue, occupies a 'middle ground between inaction or naïve informational strategies, and "insulating" strategies of heightened liability standards or outright bans'.[89] However, debiasing strategies used *in conjunction with* legal bans, may also be effective at increasing compliance, particularly when legal prohibitions are being devalued or undermined by social practices. The Army Interrogation Field Manual in force on 11 September 2001 made some small effort at debiasing. It went beyond stating that certain interrogation approaches were unlawful, and tried to counteract the tendency to use them, arising from the kinds of biases articulated above. The manual states that the use of coercion (including intimidation, threats, and insults) is 'not necessary to gain the cooperation of sources for interrogation . . ., is a poor technique that yields unreliable results, may damage subsequent collection efforts, and can induce the source to say what he thinks the interrogator wants to hear'.[90] That caution—which fell far short of the thick counternarratives proposed above—was far from effective in the Bush administration's war on terror. Given the administration's official policies and the related social pressures, this is hardly surprising.

---

[83] For a thoughtful example, see G. Keren (1990) 'Cognitive aids and debiasing methods: can cognitive pills cure cognitive ills?' in JP Caverni, JM Fabre, and M Gonzales (eds) *Cognitive biases*, 523–52.

[84] Christine Jolls and Cass Sunstein (2006) 'Debiasing through Law', 35 *Journal of Legal Studie* 199–241.

[85] Id. at 210, citing Richard E Nisbett et al., 'Popular Induction: Information Is Not Necessarily Informative' in *Judgment under Uncertainty: Heuristics and Biases*, supra n. 53 at 101–116.

[86] Id. at 212

[87] Id. at 213

[88] Id. at 215. In a recent co-authored book, Cass Sunstein reiterates the view that images may be manipulative, but he does not rule them out entirely: see Richard Thaler and Cass Sunstein (2008, revised 2009) *Nudge* at p. 145.

[89] Id. at 216

[90] Army Field Manual 34–52 Intelligence Interrogation (1992), available at <http://www.loc.gov/rr/frd/Military_Law/pdf/intel_interrrogation_sept-1992.pdf >, accessed 6 November 2011. The new field manual is FM 2–22.3 (FM 34–52) Human Intelligence Collector Operations 2006, available at <http://www.marines.mil/news/publications/Documents/FM%202-22.3%20%20Human%20Intelligence%20Collector%20Operations_1.pdf>, accessed 6 November 2011.

Powerful counternarratives—cautionary tales placed in text boxes that interrupt documentary flow and capture attention—might form the subject of future manuals and pedagogical materials. Stories could be recounted of innocent detainees who were abused and, in some cases, died of injuries they received while in US custody. (The death of Afghan taxi driver, Dilawar, is one of numerous lamentable examples.) Despite Jolls and Sunstein's concern about images, it may sometimes be appropriate and instructive to supplement these stories with still or moving images (in training videos, for example) in addition to audio recordings of oral testimony or interviews.

Other stories might demonstrate how an aggressive interrogation produced no actionable intelligence or spectacularly unreliable results—including 'information' that was clearly fabricated or subsequently retracted once interrogations were stopped. A notable case is that of Ibn al-Shaykh al-Libi, rendered by the United States to Egyptian authorities who tortured him.[91] As a result, al-Libi claimed there were links between Saddam Hussein and al Qaeda. These were used to bolster the case for war in Iraq. After al-Libi was freed, he retracted his claims, stating he had fabricated them to end his torture. Another potential example is the so-called '20th hijacker' Mohammed al-Qahtani, whose humiliating and life-threatening interrogation was discussed above; he has subsequently retracted much of what he said during that interrogation.[92]

Contrasting with these cautionary tales, narratives of effective rapport-building strategies abound in recent and more distant history. Hanns Scharff, the famous Luftwaffe interrogator, was renowned for his effectiveness using rapport-building techniques.[93] Similar techniques were used in the United States by PO Box 1142, a secret interrogation installation operating during the Second World War in Fairfax, Virginia. As one former member of that unit recently explained, they 'got more information out of a German general with a game of chess or Ping-Pong than they do today, with their torture'.[94] Recent examples are equally powerful. Mark Bowden, the journalist who wrote a provocative article in 2003 endorsing the aggressive interrogation of Khalid Sheik Mohammed,[95] recently appeared to have had a change of heart, in a piece giving details of rapport-building interrogation tactics that led US forces to Abu Musab al-Zarqawi in Iraq.[96] These stories, which can help debunk urban myths about the utility of coercion, should be told and retold, not just during training programmes but also in the wake of any attack that is likely to provoke abuses.

Social and institutional acculturation of human rights

Counternarratives are likely to work best when they complement measures designed to achieve the acculturation of human rights.[97] In the United States, commentators in mainstream media

---

[91] Douglas Jehl (9 December 2005) 'Qaeda-Iraq Link U.S. Cited Is Tied to Coercion Claim', *N.Y. Times*.

[92] Adam Zagorin (3 March 2006) '"20th Hijacker" Claims That Torture Made Him Lie', *Time Magazine*, available at <http://www.time.com/time/nation/article/0,8599,1169322,00.html>, accessed 6 November 2011. Other examples are given in JH Marks (2010) 'A Neuroskeptic's Guide to Neuroethics and National Security', *Am. J. Bioethics: Neuroscience*, 1(2), 4–12.

[93] Raymond F Toliver (1978) *The Interrogator: the Story of Hanns Scharff, Luftwaffe's Master Interrogator*.

[94] Petula Dvorak (6 October 2007) 'Fort Hunt's Quiet Men Break Silence on WWII: Interrogators Fought "Battle of Wits"', *Washington Post*, p. A01, available at <http://www.washingtonpost.com/wp-dyn/content/article/2007/10/05/AR2007100502492.html>, accessed 6 November 2011.

[95] Mark Bowden (October 2003) 'The Dark Art of Interrogation', *The Atlantic*, available at <http://www.theatlantic.com/magazine/archive/2003/10/the-dark-art-of-interrogation/2791/>, accessed 6 November 2011.

[96] Mark Bowden (May 2007) 'The Ploy', *The Atlantic*, available at <http://www.theatlantic.com/magazine/archive/2007/05/the-ploy/5773/>, accessed 6 November 2011.

[97] See Jonathan H Marks, *What Counts,* supra n. 7.

rarely use the phrase 'human rights violation' to describe detainee abuses occurring at home or at the hands of US forces, although the State Department readily uses human rights language to describe comparable abuses occurring abroad.[98] The general public might take human rights more seriously if branches of government did the same.[99] As this author has argued elsewhere, proposed counterterrorism legislation and policies should receive a human rights impact assessment (the accuracy of which should be revisited periodically).[100] But to acculturate human rights among professional communities, including military health professionals, additional measures are required. These include reforming qualifying and continuing education. Education reforms should be part of a suite of measures that works towards two related goals: first, that military health professionals are better prepared to face challenging ethical decisions and, second, that they are empowered to make courageous decisions on the ground.[101] To achieve this, the situational and systemic factors discussed above must also be addressed. Taking the high road in a stressful interrogation environment can be hard. But, as the philosopher and legal ethicist David Luban has noted, 'situational changes alter the relative gradient of both the high road and the low road', and even 'minor manipulations of the environment can cause astonishingly large changes in the ease or difficulty of action'.[102]

Ethics and policy guidelines

For military personnel, health professionals, and military health professionals, it is vital that ethics guidelines should be as clear as possible. Clarity does not remove the need for ethical analysis by individual health professionals, but its absence may create confusion, mischief or both. Clear ethical statements from professional associations can practically and legally empower health professionals working for the military or national security agencies to say no when they are asked to do something they believe to be unethical.[103]

Ethical guidelines should be clear about what roles are impermissible for health professionals and, in this author's view, should also incorporate human rights norms.[104] When health professional organizations adopt ethical policies after due deliberation and consultation, and those

---

[98] For the US State Department's recent human rights country reports, see <http://www.state.gov/g/drl/rls/hrrpt/>, accessed 6 November 2011. There are a number of city and state human rights commissions in the United States: see, for example, the New York City Commission on Human Rights <http://www.nyc.gov/html/cchr/>, the San Francisco Human Rights Commission <http://www.sf-hrc.org/>, and the Illinois Human Rights Commission <http://www2.illinois.gov/ihrc/Pages/default.aspx>. However, their remit tends to be confined to addressing complaints of discrimination in employment, real property transactions, access to financial credit, and public accommodations.

[99] See Jonathan H Marks, *What Counts,* supra n. 7.

[100] Id.

[101] In the formulation of some of the measures proposed in this section, the author is indebted to M Gregg Bloche (2001) 'Caretakers and Collaborators', 10 *Cambridge Q. Healthcare Ethics* 275 at 283, emphasizing—months before 9/11—the need for the training of health professionals in both ethics and international human rights norms, for institutional mechanisms to nurture professional autonomy, and for international support from (among others) professional bodies.

[102] David Luban(2007) *Legal Ethics and Human Dignity* at 284. See also Thaler and Sunstein, *Nudge*, supra n. 88.

[103] This is further discussed in Jonathan H Marks, *Doctors as Pawns?*, supra, n. 2.

[104] For a more detailed critique of the relevant professional associations and their codes ethics, see Jonathan H Marks, *Doctors as Pawns?*, supra n. 2 and Jonathan H Marks, *Looking Back, Thinking Ahead*, supra n. 16. Compare MG Bloche (2011) 'Doctors as Warriors II' in MG Bloche, *The Hippocratic Myth*.

policies prohibit health professionals from acting in certain ways, the military should respect them—especially when it has been consulted and has communicated that it will respect them. Sometimes this has not happened. Efforts to circumvent or undermine the policies adopted by professional associations—most notably, the Army memo encouraging psychiatrists to participate in designing and monitoring interrogations, despite the contrary positions of the World Medical Association, the American Medical Association, and the American Psychiatric Association[105]— can create doubts about the meaning and significance of those policies. This increases the likelihood of unethical behaviours occurring, particularly given the stressful nature of detention and interrogation environments.

Education and mentorship

To better prepare them for challenges they may face in the future, military personnel, health professionals, and—most importantly here—military health professionals should receive better training in international humanitarian law and human rights law. These fundamental legal norms should undergird health professionals' ethical obligations,[106] and health professionals should be well-informed about them. In two recent studies of US medical schools and medical students respectively, less than a third of medical schools reported offering any curriculum on health and human rights, and 94 per cent of students reported receiving less than one hour's instruction on the Geneva Conventions.[107] Little more than a third of student respondents knew that the conventions required them to treat the sickest first, irrespective of nationality. A similar percentage could not say when they were required to disobey an unethical order. Some even thought they could inject a fearful prisoner with saline solution knowing the prisoner had been led to believe he was receiving a lethal injection.[108] This profound lack of training leaves them poorly equipped to address or counteract the prevailing views of their combatant colleagues. When the Pentagon surveyed 1700 soldiers in Iraq between August and October 2006, less than half thought Iraqi civilians should be treated with dignity and respect, and more than a third believed torture was acceptable if it might save a comrade's life or procure information about insurgents.[109]

Education in human rights and international humanitarian law should enrich and supplement basic ethics training for health professionals. This education need not impart a comprehensive knowledge of international human rights jurisprudence, nor generate the capacity to undertake complex assessments of when interference with qualified human rights may be justifiable. However, human rights education should equip health professionals in at least three ways. First, they should have a basic but solid grounding in human rights law and the laws of war. They should be familiar with core international human rights and humanitarian law treaties, and appreciate the nature of states' associated obligations. They should also know that international law does not just prohibit torture, but lesser forms of abuse that constitute cruel, inhuman, and degrading

---

[105] See Jonathan H Marks and M Gregg Bloche (2008) 'The Ethics of Interrogation', *N. Engl. J. Med.* 359, 1090–1092. See also Nada L Stotland (2008) 'Letter to the Editor', *N. Engl. J. Med.* 359, 2728–2729.

[106] See Jonathan H Marks, *Doctors as Pawns?*, supra n. 2.

[107] See, respectively, LE Cotter et al. (2009) 'Health and Human Rights Education in U.S. Schools of Medicine and Public Health', *PLoSONE* 4(3), e4916 and Wesley Boyd et al. (2007) 'US Medical Students Knowledge About the Military Draft, the Geneva Conventions and Military Medical Ethics', 37(4) *International Journal of Health Services* 634–650.

[108] Id.

[109] Humphrey Hawksley (4 May 2007) *US Iraq troops 'condone torture'*, BBC News, <http://news.bbc.co.uk/1/hi/world/middle_east/6627055.stm>, accessed 6 November 2011.

treatment, and that there is also a positive obligation to treat detainees humanely.[110] They should know that interference with qualified human rights cannot be justified if it violates the prohibition on discrimination.[111] Second, human rights education should sensitize health professionals to the circumstances and ways in which exercising their professional skills may raise human rights issues or potentially facilitate human rights violations. Third, they should learn about how they might use their professional expertise, access to resources, and social status to protect and promote human rights.[112]

Two additional points about ethics training should be noted. First, ethics education must do more than merely create familiarity with codes of ethics. Comprehensive ethics education should develop ethical sensitivity (particularly, the ability to identify ethical issues), improve ethical reasoning skills, and foster the kind of moral imagination that can generate creative solutions to complex problems.[113] Second, ethics education alone is not sufficient.[114] Mentorship by experienced health professionals who encourage junior colleagues to take ethical obligations seriously, may increase the likelihood that they and their colleagues will behave ethically.[115]

Structural reforms

Structural incentives are also required if military health professionals are to act ethically despite the countervailing situational pressures. Making these changes requires input and support from both military institutions and health professional organizations. An expert panel, comprising members with knowledge of military and medical structures, should formulate the requisite changes after broad public consultation and careful deliberation. Among the potential measures, the panel would need to consider hotlines (or help lines) connecting isolated health professionals (whether in forward operating bases, detention centres, or elsewhere) with colleagues who have experience in practical ethics consultations and who are insulated from the military mission. It seems likely that if these systems were put in place and well publicized—both within the military and relevant professional organizations—they would offer vital assistance to health professionals who believe they are being asked to act unethically.[116] Moreover, while not a first resort, whistle-blowing may be permissible and, in some cases, required when internal mechanisms for dissent

---

[110] These requirements are discussed further in Jonathan H Marks, *What Counts*, supra n. 7 and in Jonathan H Marks, *Doctors as Pawns?*, supra n. 2.

[111] Id.

[112] For a more detailed discussion of the relationship between professional ethics and human rights, and its practical implications, see Jonathan H Marks (2011) 'Toward a Unified Theory of Professional Ethics and Human Rights', *Mich. J. Internat'l Law* (forthcoming).

[113] Nancy Tuana (2007) 'Conceptualizing Moral Literacy', 45(4) *Journal of Educational Administration* 364–378.

[114] M Anderson et al. (2007) 'What do mentoring and training in the responsible conduct of research have to do with scientists' misbehavior? Findings from a national survey of NIH-funded scientists', 82(9) *Academic Medicine* 853–860.

[115] Jean Maria Arrigo and Ray Bennett, supra n. 37, advocate similar mentorship for interrogators to ensure the communication and acculturation of ethical norms.

[116] For similar recommendations designed to address a distinct (but not entirely unrelated) source of social pressure and ethical challenges for health professionals, see Jonathan H Marks (2008) 'Expedited Industry-Sponsored Translational Research: A Seductive but Hazardous Cocktail?', 8(3) *American Journal of Bioethics* 56–58.

have been exhausted.[117] In such cases, whistleblowing must be encouraged and rewarded.[118] At the very least, measures to limit the potential adverse career and financial consequences of *bona fide* whistleblowing should be introduced, as should communication strategies to publicize these measures and to assure potential beneficiaries of their efficacy. Other measures include a reassessment of the chains of command and reporting structures for health professionals,[119] as well as the manner in which health professionals are assessed and promoted in the military, and the role that medical personnel and professional ethical considerations should play in that process. Such measures (and others like them that cannot be considered in detail here) should serve to enhance the role of military health professionals as guardians of human rights.

Accountability

Taking measures to hold serious wrongdoers accountable can send important signals to others. If speaking out is the only course of action that entails social and other costs, military health professionals are more likely to remain silent. But if complicity or acquiescence is perceived as having serious costs, these professionals may be more likely to stand up and speak out. In the most extreme cases, health professionals may find themselves subject to court-martial or criminal prosecution (if not in the US, then potentially in other countries exercising universal jurisdiction for torture, which is a serious international crime).[120] In most cases, however, accountability is more likely to involve disciplinary action by licensing bodies—in the United States, the state licensing boards. To date, no military health professionals have been prosecuted for complicity in detainee abuses in the war on terror. There have been several calls for disciplinary accountability on both sides of the Atlantic, and numerous complaints have been lodged with health professional associations, as well as licensing boards.[121] However, almost all the complaints have been dismissed for procedural reasons, and none of them has led to any sanctions to date.[122] Unless cases are formally investigated, it is likely that complainants and human rights activists will take measures to achieve informal or social accountability—such as building public databases that collate documentary and affidavit evidence of the alleged involvement of named health professionals in the abuse of detainees.[123]

---

[117] In the space provided, I cannot provide a comprehensive review of the whistleblowing literature. Nor can I offer an independent theory. But see, for example, C Fred Alford (2001) *Whistleblowers: Broken Lives and Organizational Power*.

[118] This does not mean 'outing' a whistleblower or otherwise exposing him to potential harm. Although Joseph Darby, the whistleblower at Abu Ghraib, had been promised anonymity, his identity was disclosed on national television by then Secretary of Defense Donald Rumsfeld who ostensibly thanked him. At the time, Derby was sitting in a crowded canteen in Iraq with hundreds of his fellow soldiers; as a result, he had to be whisked away for his own safety. See Dawn Bryan (5 August 2007) *Abu Ghraib whistleblower's ordeal*, available at <http://news.bbc.co.uk/1/hi/world/middle_east/6930197.stm>, accessed 6 November 2011.

[119] See MG Bloche, 'Doctors as Warriors I' in MG Bloche, The Hippocratic Myth, supra n. 35.

[120] The exercise of universal jurisdiction is discussed more fully elsewhere: see Jonathan H Marks (2004) 'Mending the Web: Universal Jurisdiction, Humanitarian Intervention and the Abrogation of Immunity by the Security Council', 42 *Colum. J. Transnat'l Law* 445–490.

[121] For a more detailed discussion of accountability, see George Annas (2007) 'Human Rights Outlaws: Nuremberg, Geneva and the Global War on Terror', 87(2) *Boston U. Law Rev.* 427–466.

[122] Id. The author does not intend to pre-judge the merits of any individual complaint.

[123] Id. For an example of such an enterprise, see *When Healers Harm*, a web-based database that links to documents supporting claims that health professionals were complicit in detainee abuse, available at <http://whenhealersharm.org/>, accessed 6 November 2011.

Conclusion

At the time of writing, there has not been another successful terrorist attack in the mainland United States since 11 September 2001. In the event of such an attack, the temptation to deploy aggressive detention and interrogation regimes is likely to recur—perhaps with even greater force. The outcome depends, in part, on whether the measures described above are explored. Although some measures may need to be targeted at other populations, the focus here has been on military health professionals. These professionals are a vital resource if we wish to avoid the recurrence of some of the most serious excesses of the Bush administration's 'war on terror'. There is no guarantee that such excesses can be completely prevented in the event of a national security crisis. Nor is it suggested that we engineer all professional training to address such crises. However, the kinds of measures discussed here and the cognitive and behavioural research that should inform them are also likely to shed light on and enhance the more quotidian activities of health professionals, whether they possess military training or not. Wherever they exercise professional skill and judgment, health professionals should be educated, mentored, and empowered to be guardians of human rights, and to speak out against any practice or environment that violates these fundamental norms. This is important for the rights and well-being of detainees, the integrity of the health professions, and the legitimacy of the state in whose name human rights violations so often occur.

Acknowledgements

This article revises and expands on the views set out in Jonathan H Marks (2009) 'Looking Back, Thinking Ahead: The Complicity of Health Professionals in Detainee Abuse' in R Goodman and M Roseman (eds), Interrogations, Forced Feedings, and the Role of Health Professionals: New Perspectives on International Human Rights, Humanitarian Law, and Ethics (Harvard). The author is grateful to M Gregg Bloche and also to the following for feedback on an earlier draft provided during a faculty fellows' seminar at the Edmond J Safra Center for Ethics at Harvard: Lawrence Lessig, Tommie Shelby, Moshe Cohen-Eliya, Nir Eyal, Eric Beerbohm, and Daniel Viehoff.

Coercive Treatment in Psychiatry

A Human Rights Issue?

Thomas Wilhelm Kallert

Introduction

In the last few years there has been an increasing interest in the issue of coercion in psychiatry, as was particularly demonstrated at the 2007 WPA Thematic Conference 'Coercive treatment in psychiatry: a comprehensive review' (Kallert et al. 2007a). This may have been the first international scientific event dedicated to a critically important, highly sensitive, and hotly debated issue in psychiatry. The conference largely realized the aim to explore most of the clinical, legal, and ethical aspects of coercive treatment, to facilitate the presentation of the views of both users and professionals on the event theme, and to present recent research results and initiatives on mental health related human rights. Human rights organizations, such as the Global Initiative on Psychiatry and the European Committee for the Prevention of Torture and Inhuman or Degrading Treatment or Punishment (CPT) of the Council of Europe, were officially represented at the conference.

Conferences such as the above highlight the importance of human rights in coercive treatment. The issue itself, however, does not receive the necessary attention—neither in the legal context nor in the field of clinical psychiatry—as will be demonstrated in this brief comment.

Human rights and mental health legislation

Some recent, mostly European, research initiatives demonstrated wide variations in mental health laws. This makes consistency difficult and fails to emphasize human rights issues that could arise as a consequence.

An analysis of civil law issues associated with involuntary hospitalization in psychiatric establishments of 12 European countries (Kallert et al. 2007b) revealed major cross-national differences. They included basic conditions, as well as additional criteria for involuntary admission, time periods for making decisions, the association between involuntary placement and treatment, patients' rights to register complaints, roles of relatives, and safeguarding procedures of these processes. With the aim of protecting justice and equality, the most important consequences for cross-national harmonization might be to simplify the legal decision process, and to establish a transparency of regulations to lodge appeals.

The latter issue must be urgently addressed, as demonstrated in a review of the European Court of Human Rights (ECtHR) case law concerning psychiatric commitment. Of the almost 118,000 decisions taken by the ECHR in a 50-year period, only 108 dealt with situations concerning psychiatric commitment (Niveau and Materi 2007). The most worrying conclusion was that the possibility of an individual gaining access to the ECtHR depends on the degree of democracy in his country and on the access to legal assistance through non-governmental organizations or individual intervening parties.

Further, an analysis of the potential of the European Convention of Human Rights to secure the human rights of people with mental disorders and disabilities concluded (Hale 2007) that the convention is better at protecting them from unwanted or unnecessary treatment or care than it is at securing for them equal access to the treatment and care they want or need.

Psychiatrists themselves seem to be increasingly interested in clarifying the legal conditions for involuntarily treating people with mental disorders. One example for this is the task force of the Turkish Psychiatric Association having drafted a proposed mental health law (Arikan et al. 2007) which suggests a model emphasizing the right to psychiatric treatment, but also recommending close judicial oversight to prevent potential abuses of discretion by the system. The other recent example is the suggestion (Szmukler et al. 2010) to construct a legal framework combining the particular and complementary strengths of both incapacity and civil commitment schemes. Such legislation would be an important step in reducing unjustified legal discrimination against mentally disordered persons and in providing a sound basis for 'coercive' treatments.

Human rights and selected clinical issues from the field of coercive treatment

As concerns involuntary stays in psychiatric establishments, patients report restrictions on movement, forced medication, patronizing communication, confiscation of property, and other intrusive measures (Kuosmanen et al. 2007). A substantial proportion of these patients do not know their legal status.

Further, in several European countries there is a clear link in the mental health laws between commitment and involuntary treatment measures (Kallert and Torres-Gonzalez 2006). This failure to distinguish commitment from involuntary treatment means that decisions regarding patients' rights of freedom to move may damage those patients' rights to consent to or reject treatment measures.

At the level of the individual clinical unit, such issues currently can only be counterbalanced by following guidelines on the use of coercive measures, the establishment of which is an ongoing process (mostly carried out by national professional associations) in many countries, and by improving elements of good clinical practice itself, like training the clinical behavior of key workers (Sorgaad 2007) or providing information on patients' rights in a standardized way (Johnsen et al. 2007).

Initiatives on a regional or state level to improve the situation, in the sense that it could be one of the health care political aims to minimize the overall use of coercive measures, are rare. Two (research) projects from the US (LeBel et al. 2004; Smith et al. 2005) have clearly shown that it would need several ingredients at different levels of decision and implementation to stimulate such general changes in clinical practice. They identified the following elements that contributed to substantial changes regarding the use of restraint and seclusion in hospitals within a decade. *Leadership* was stimulated by several staff and user-representatives' activities in the way that some very important high-ranking health political activities were defined: seclusion and restraint were announced as representing 'treatment failure', data collection and comparison across hospitals was improved, and staff training programmes were emphasized. *Independent (patient) advocates* were assigned to each hospital. *Further state policy changes* comprised, e.g., the definition of procedures for patient and staff debriefing sessions after the use of seclusion or restraint, and that orders for restraint and seclusion were limited to no more than 60 minutes. *Psychiatric emergency response teams* were implemented in each hospital. *Unit sizes* were decreased and *patient-to-staff ratios* improved. The implementation of an *incident management system* contained 35 indicators (e.g. details of each forced medication): data were aggregated on a monthly basis and shared with the hospitals as benchmarking, available at each ward as a report. Further, *second-generation antipsychosis medications* were used more frequently, and the quantity and quality of *active non-pharmacologic patient treatment* increased. In the opinion of the author, these examples clearly demonstrate that only really comprehensive and long-lasting efforts would be adequate to bring about sustainable changes in attitudes and clinical practice that might have some impact on the divergence between coercive measures and human rights.

Selected recent initiatives and unsolved issues in the field

Whether the development of the legislation of human rights might also contribute is an open question, not only because of all the national differences regarding the mental health laws. The focus of the mental health laws themselves on reducing coercive treatment is probably not as clear as it should be (Kallert and Torres-Gonzalez 2006), and the inclusion of human rights in these texts is not as pronounced as it should be. Further, the example of recent discussions (e.g. in Germany) on the ratification of the UN Disability Convention (13 December 2006) demonstrated that there are huge differences in the views of several stakeholder groups to whom general terms like 'being disabled' apply. These ranged from not applicable to mentally ill persons, to clearly applicable with the consequence that all coercive measures stand in contradiction to the convention and mental health laws should be changed accordingly.

Whether the current practice and organization in national mental health care systems is compatible with a rights-based approach regarding coercive treatment seems more than questionable. In an era of European reinstitutionalization (Priebe et al. 2005), with increasing figures of forensic beds and long-stay places in homes and rising figures of involuntary admissions to hospitals, the potential infringement of patients' rights should be clearly monitored. However, the general impression from 12 European countries is that activities of supervision authorities are largely performed as formal routine (Kallert and Torres-Gonzalez 2006). Supervision refers to checking duly filled-in and signed paperwork, but does not stimulate or demand practical changes. Despite the complexity of the regulations, or perhaps because of it, the face-to-face interview between the person with the mental illness and the supervising authority is exceptional. Changes to the patient's legal status dictated by an authority and not previously suggested by the health professionals are extremely rare. Although appeal proceedings of the patients are foreseen by most of the laws, they rarely occur. Most of the regulations do not contemplate other coercive measures by which the patient might be affected while staying in hospital. It seems that once the patient is placed in the hospital, the authority delegates the responsibility to the health professionals, assuming that they will always act in the best interests of the patient.

Further, there are no standardized instruments available assessing the standards of care provided in long-stay psychiatric and social care institutions. A currently ongoing European research project ('Development of a European model of best practice for people with long-term mental illness in institutional care'—DEMoBinc) aims to develop a toolkit assessing this issue. As a result of a huge literature search and a Delphi exercise involving four expert panels (service users, mental health professionals, carers, and advocates), one area of this toolkit will assess how the human rights of the residents are respected.

Patients in hospitals and related settings, intellectually disabled people in homes and institutions, physically disabled patients, minors, and people with acute psychosis are subgroups bearing a special risk for being treated coercively or experiencing hidden coercion. These deserve greater attention in clinical practice and research (Kallert 2008).

The currently available database is too small to provide an empirically well-founded comment on the global situation of coercive treatment in psychiatry. We need more detailed and systematic information from (research) projects on this general issue in regions like Africa or in regions characterized by non-Christian religions as well as in regions governed by totalitarian political systems. In my opinion, global organizations like the World Health Organization or the World Psychiatric Association could play a leading role in stimulating greater attention for this issue, e.g. by founding specific sections dealing with the issue from a global perspective.

Conclusions

The mental health response to all of these problematic issues associated with human rights must be a comprehensive one. First steps may be to lower the threshold for open discussions in the field, and to define better standards and procedures on how to deal with the challenges of this theme. All parties and disciplines interested in this theme, even if their interests are different from each other, must be involved in further discussions. And the psychiatric profession must further reduce resistance from various circles to dealing with issues related to coercive treatment because this might damage the discipline's image vis-à-vis competing fields and taint recent successes in diagnostic and therapeutic methods. The author closes this commentary by referring the reader to a recent book publication addressing the issue of coercive treatment in psychiatry (Kallert et al. 2011). This volume could be seen as an example of needed comprehensive initiatives. By exploring important clinical, legal, and ethical aspects of coercive treatment the editors and contributing authors give a crystal clear signal that it is absolutely essential, for all clinical and research work in this sensitive human rights field, to act according to highest ethical standards in the best interest of our patients.

References

Arikan, R, Appelbaum, PS, Sercan, M, Turkcan, S, Satmis, N, and Polat, A (2007) 'Civil commitment in Turkey: reflections on a bill drafted by psychiatrists', *International Journal of Law and Psychiatry*, 30, 29–35.

Convention on the Rights of Persons with Disabilities (adopted on 13 December 2006 at the United Nations Headquarters in New York).

Hale, B (2007) 'Justice and equality in mental health law: the European experience', *International Journal of Law and Psychiatry*, 30, 18–28.

Johnsen, L, Oysaed, H, Bornes, K, Moe, TJ and Haavik, J (2007) 'A systematic intervention to improve patient information routines and satisfaction in a psychiatric emergency unit', *Nordic Journal of Psychiatry*, 61, 213–18.

Kallert, TW (2008) 'Coercion in psychiatry', *Current Opinion in Psychiatry*, 21, 485–89.

Kallert, TW and Torres-Gonzalez, F (eds) (2006) *Legislation on coercive mental health care in Europe. Legal documents and comparative assessment of twelve European countries.* Berlin, Bern, Bruxelles, Frankfurt/M, New York, Oxford, Wien: Peter Lang Europäischer Verlag der Wissenschaften.

Kallert, TW, Mezzich, J and Monahan, J (eds) (2011) *Coercive treatment in psychiatry-Clinical, legal and ethical aspects.* Chichester, UK: Wiley-Blackwell.

Kallert, TW, Monahan, J, and Mezzich, J (2007a) 'World Psychiatric Association (WPA) Thematic Conference. Coercive treatment in psychiatry: a comprehensive review', *BMC Psychiatry* 2007, 7, Suppl 1 (entire supplement).

Kallert, TW, Rymaszewska, J, and Torres-Gonzalez, F (2007b) 'Differences of legal regulations concerning involuntary psychiatric hospitalization in twelve European countries: implications for clinical practice', *International Journal of Forensic Mental Health*, 6, 197–207.

Kuosmanen, L, Hätönen, H, Malkavaara, H, Kylmä, J, and Välimäki, M (2007) 'Deprivation of liberty in psychiatric hospital care: the patient's perspective', *Nursing Ethics*, 14, 597–607.

LeBel, J, Stromberg, N, Duckworth, K et al. (2004) 'Child and adolescent inpatient restraint reduction: a state initiative to promote strength-based care', *Journal of the American Academy of Child and Adolescent Psychiatry*, 43, 37–45.

Niveau, G and Materi, J (2007) 'Psychiatric commitment: over 50 years of case law from the European Court of Human Rights', *European Psychiatry*, 22, 59–67.

Priebe, S, Badesconyi, A, Fioritti, A et al. (2005) 'Reinstitutionalisation in mental health care: comparison of data on service provision from six European countries', *British Medical Journal*, 330, 123–26.

Smith, GM, Davis, RH, Bixler, EO et al. (2005) 'Pennsylvania state hospital system's seclusion and restraint reduction program', *Psychiatric Services*, 56, 1115–22.

Sorgaad, KW (2007) 'Satisfaction and coercion among voluntary, persuaded/pressured and committed patients in acute psychiatric treatment', *Scandinavian Journal of Caring Sciences*, 21, 214–19.

Szmukler, G, Daw, R, and Dawson, J (2010) 'A model law fusing incapacity and mental health legislation', *Journal of Mental Health Law*, Special Issue, 11–24.

Chapter 18

Psychiatrists and the Pharmaceutical Industry

On the Ethics of a Complex Relationship

Philip B. Mitchell

A problem of unheralded proportions

Psychiatry—and academic psychiatry in particular—is facing a credibility problem of unheralded proportions that is being played out publicly in the pages of 'The New York Times' and 'The Wall Street Journal' and in the US House of Congress.

The issue is the relationship between psychiatry and the pharmaceutical industry. While the spotlight of public disapprobation has focused upon a small number of leading figures, it is an issue for all psychiatrists. Furthermore, though certainly an issue for the entire medical profession, it would appear that psychiatry has become particularly enmeshed, despite claims of an unreasonable focus on this discipline.

The stakes are high. Psychiatry has always been on tenuous scientific ground because of the limited understanding of the aetiological processes underlying mental illnesses, leading to debates over theories and therapies that are often based largely on polemic rather than reason or evidence. It has been vulnerable to the influential, persuasive, and mellifluous voices—be they of pharmacological or psychological bent. For a discipline whose repute has been under attack from various quarters, it is essential that it gets its house in order—not only for the sake of patients and their families, but also for the credibility of the profession. This is a timely wake-up call for psychiatry worldwide (Freedman et al. 2009).

Public and media concern about this relationship

The recent highly publicized 'outing' of the details of the relationship between medical practitioners and the pharmaceutical industry has largely arisen from two sources: US Senator Charles Grassley (Republican of Iowa), and a series of articles in the medical press, particularly the British Medical Journal and Nature, with frequent communications by the Australian medical journalist Ray Moynihan (amongst others).

Grassley's senatorial enquiries have claimed exorbitant and opaque relations between some senior US psychiatrists and industry. Some of the high-profile clinicians implicated include Charles Nemeroff of Emory University (Harris 2008b, a; Wadman2008), Joseph Biederman of Harvard (Editorial 2008; Biederman, 2008), Frederick Goodwin (Harris 2008a), and Alan Schatzberg, the president-elect of the American Psychiatric Association (Carey and Harris 2009). The allegations against Nemeroff and Biederman relate to failure to accurately disclose to their respective universities their amount of earnings from the pharmaceutical industry; the allegations against Nemeroff have led to his standing down as Chair of the Department of Psychiatry at Emory. The allegation against Goodwin related to transparency of disclosure of industry funding for programmes on his US radio show 'The Infinite Mind'. For Schatzberg, the issue has been transparency over his financial holdings in a company that has developed a therapeutic compound upon which he has researched and reported.

In March 2008, Grassley and another US Senator (Kohn) introduced the 'Grassley-Kohn Physician Payments Sunshine Act of 2008' to mandate disclosure of remuneration to doctors. This has yet to be passed. It should be noted though, that such disclosure is already legislated in the US states of Maine, Minnesota, Vermont, and West Virginia.

Ray Moynihan is a journalist who had worked with the Australian Broadcasting Commission where he initiated investigative reporting into the relationship between the medical profession and the pharmaceutical industry. Receiving a Harkness Fellowship to pursue this line of work based at Harvard, Moynihan has published both formal research (Moynihan et al. 2000; Moynihan and Sweet 2000) and commentaries (Moynihan 2003a; Moynihan et al. 2000) on this topic. In late 2008, he was interviewed on this matter in *Nature Neuroscience* (Bjorn 2008). One of Moynihan's areas of focus has been on 'disease mongering', i.e., the creation of new poorly-defined concepts of illness that are in the commercial interests of industry. Furthermore, he was a key player in recent legal action in Australia which compelled the pharmaceutical industry in that country to register on-line details of all pharmaceutical industry sponsored educational events (<http://www.medicinesaustralia.com.au/pages/page136.as>). Other targets for Moynihan have included industry sponsorship of professional scientific meetings such as that of the Royal Australian and New Zealand College of Psychiatrists (Moynihan 2008a), and the 'independence' of so-called 'opinion leaders' (Moynihan 2008b).

Institutional concern: The example of the National Institutes of Health

Even prior to the Grassley inquiries, there had been major concerns at the US National Institutes of Health (NIH). In the most highly publicized individual case (Bhattacharjee 2007), Trey Sunderland, once chief of the geriatric psychiatry branch at the National Institute of Mental Health in Bethesda, Maryland, was found guilty of failing to report more than US$600,000 in consulting fees from Pfizer while providing spinal fluid samples to the company for Alzheimer's studies. In late 2006, he was convicted of violating US federal conflict-of-interest laws and sentenced to two years of probation, 400 hours of community service, and an obligation to repay US$300,000 of his earnings. The broader concern at NIH led to a formal Conflict-of-Interest Inquiry being instigated by the NIH Director Elias Zerhouni, which found that 44 current and former employees had violated conflict-of-interest rules (Steinbrook 2004; Weiss, 2005). This inquiry resulted in changes in NIH rules related to financial interests in pharmaceutical companies, with senior NIH staff being required to divest all stocks in relevant companies, and (for all staff) a blanket prohibition on both consulting and other activities with medical and pharmaceutical companies (Hooper 2005).

Aims of this chapter

This chapter will explore the nature of, and reasons for, the growing aberrations in this relationship, focusing both on the broader relationship between medicine and the pharmaceutical industry, and on the relationship with psychiatry in particular. It will examine recent proposals—from academia, professional bodies, and the pharmaceutical industry itself—for 'normalizing' and regulating this relationship. This chapter will work to the premise that it is not the relationship *per se* that is the problem, but how that is enacted at both high and low levels within psychiatry. Whilst some argue that the medical community should divorce itself completely from industry, this is unrealistic. Very few effective compounds have been developed without private industry. Even the introduction of lithium into clinical practice required the expertise of private industry to finally gain FDA approval (Johnson and Gershon 1999). There is no doubting, however, that the relationship between the medical profession and industry is currently dysfunctional. The challenge is how this association can become one based on integrity and transparency.

The nature of the relationship between the medical profession and the pharmaceutical industry

There are few, if any, analogies for the relationship between the medical profession and the pharmaceutical industry. Industry develops medicines to be used by patients, but (in most cases) is unable to directly advertise or sell to these patients, rather marketing via 'intermediaries'—the doctors who prescribe and the pharmacists who dispense.

Moynihan (2003a, b) provides the analogy of: 'Twisted together like the snake and the staff, doctors and drug companies have become entangled in a web of interactions as controversial as they are ubiquitous'. He argues forcefully for recognition of such 'entanglement' and the imperative for 'disentanglement'. Somewhat more extreme and polemical, the UK academic psychiatrist Moncrieff (2006) has argued in ideological terms. She contends that the 'politics of neoliberalism' underlie the drive to formulate anxiety and inadequacy in terms of disrupted biochemistry requiring psychotropic therapies, thereby driving individuals to become more accepting of 'pressured working conditions' and more likely to 'inhibit social and political responses'.

However, as thoughtfully discussed by Komesaroff (Komesaroff and Kerridge 2002): 'medical practitioners and the pharmaceutical industry serve interests that sometimes overlap and sometimes conflict'. In other words, there are substantial (in their terms) 'dualities of interests' between the profession and industry, as well as the potential for major conflict of interests, which have led to the current parlous situation.

There is a critical need to develop guidelines for developing a healthy adult relationship between the profession and industry. The major 'duality of interest' is the need to develop improved treatments that will reduce morbidity and mortality rates for the many medical conditions for which current therapies are either inadequate or non-existent. The challenge is how to do this without compromising the integrity of the professional bodies themselves (Moynihan et al. 2008).

General literature on the relationship of doctors to industry

Contact between the medical profession and the pharmaceutical industry is extensive (Blumenthal 2004). In the US, Campbell et al. (2007) reported on doctor–industry relationships in a survey of 1,662 physicians conducted by the Institute of Medicine as a Profession (IMAP). Most physicians (94 per cent) reported some type of relationship with industry, most commonly receiving food in the workplace or drug samples. More than one third received reimbursement for costs associated with professional meetings or continuing medical education (CME), while more than one quarter received payments for consulting, giving lectures, or enrolling patients in trials. Cardiologists were much more likely to receive payments than family practitioners.

In a highly-cited review of studies on the relationship between the pharmaceutical industry and the medical professional (subtitled 'Is a gift ever a gift?'), Wazana (2000) examined all relevant publications that had been published since 1993, identifying 29 suitable data-based reports. These studies found that physicians generally endorsed the propriety of having relationships with industry.

Such contacts usually began during medical school, and continued at a rate of about four times per month. Wazana found that having meetings with pharmaceutical representatives was significantly associated with both requests from physicians for adding drugs to hospital formularies, and to changes in their own prescribing practice. Drug company-sponsored CME activities preferentially highlighted the sponsor's products compared to other CME programmes. Attending sponsored CME events and accepting funding for travel or lodging for educational symposia was associated with increased prescription rates of the sponsor's medication. Attending presentations given by pharmaceutical representative speakers was also associated with such prescribing. Wazana recommended that this clear evidence of the impact of such contacts on prescribing and professional behaviour needed to be addressed at the level of policy and education.

In the same year as Wazana's review, Angell (2000) wrote an editorial in the *New England Journal of Medicine*, raising major concerns about the growing links of academia with industry. She commented: 'Academic institutions and their clinical faculty members must take care not to be open to the charge that they are for sale'. Further, in an aside of pertinence to this current chapter focusing on psychiatry, she stated: ' . . . as we spoke with research psychiatrists about writing an editorial on the treatment of depression, we found very few who did not have financial ties to drug companies that make antidepressants'.

Research on the various types of clinician relationships with industry

In the only qualitative study of this relationship, Doran et al. (2006) reported on the outcome of in-depth interviews with 50 Australian medical specialists. The authors categorized medical specialists into three types: confident engagers, ambivalent engagers, and avoiders. 'Confident engagers' (the majority of those interviewed) described themselves as engaging with industry in the belief that the relationship between themselves and the pharmaceutical industry was essentially sound and beneficial and could be effectively managed to maintain benefits to both parties. 'Ambivalent engagers' (the next largest group) included specialists who described engaging with industry but felt uneasy in this engagement. They described an interaction coloured by wariness of having their autonomy compromised and creating a conflict of interest. 'Avoiders' (the minority) described a tendency to avoid contact with industry as much as possible, though they found this difficult in light of the proliferation of industry promotional objects and advertisements.

Specific 'points of contact' between the profession and industry

Gifts

'Gifts' may vary from the simple (pens, pads, or cheap meals such as pizza), to provision of educational books and equipment (such as stethoscopes or weighing machines), to tickets for sporting or cultural events, through to sponsorship to attend major national or international meetings (usually involving at least business-class travel and accommodation at five-star hotels). As reviewed by Wazana (2000), meals are more an issue for junior staff, whereas sponsorship to attend meetings or payment for speaking at industry-sponsored events (honoraria) is more likely to be offered to specialists. Furthermore, such offers to consultants are more likely to be given to those with research links to industry, or to those on industry advisory panels.

In one of the few studies to document the extent and nature of the giving and receipt of gifts, McNeill et al. (2006) surveyed 823 Australian medical specialists. They found that a high proportion of specialists received offers of food (96 per cent), items for the office (94 per cent), personal gifts (51 per cent) and journals or textbooks (50 per cent). Most were invited to product launches, symposia, or educational events (75–84 per cent) and 52 per cent received offers of travel to conferences. A high proportion of offers were accepted (over 65 per cent), excepting for lower acceptance rates for invitations to product launches (49 per cent), sponsored symposia (53%), and offers of travel including partners (27 per cent). Fifteen percent of specialists had requested financial support, for example to attend conferences. Most gifts and requests complied with national professional and industry guidelines, but some did not, including personal gifts, tickets to sporting events, entertainment, and travel expenses for partners.

Brennan et al. (2006) in a broad discussion on the relationship between industry and US academic centres, emphasized the impact of receipt of even small gifts. Drawing from social science research (Dana and Loewenstein 2003), he commented on the general human impulse to 'reciprocate' for even small gifts, and that those receiving such gifts are often unable to remain objective as they 'reweigh information and choices in light of the gift'. Further, he stated that '. . . the expectation of reciprocity may be the primary motive for gift-giving'. In the Taskforce Report of the Association of American Medical Colleges in 2008 (AAMC 2008) this issue is expanded upon: 'Thus, although strong motivation and altruistic intent exist in most physician-industry interactions, the interaction may be unwittingly undermined when innate reciprocity mechanisms are engaged'.

Key opinion / thought leaders

Key opinion leaders are senior doctors (usually academics) whose opinions are considered influential in determining both diagnostic and therapeutic practice. As quoted by a retired industry sales representative in a confronting commentary by Moynihan (2008b): 'Key opinion leaders were salespeople for us, and we would routinely measure the return on our investment, by tracking prescriptions before and after their presentations'. Undoubtedly, significant resources are lavished on this group, and those targeted by Grassley's inquiries would be considered within this category. This has led to calls for public disclosure of earnings received from industry, a call currently not headed by professional guidelines, but ironically a call that recently has been acceded to by industry itself, with Eli Lilly, GSK, Merck, and Pfizer promising in late 2008 and early 2009 to disclose all remuneration to medical practitioners. Healy (2006) has also discussed the potential influential role of such opinion leaders in the development of so-called 'independent' clinical practice guidelines.

Moynihan et al. (2000) have found that in media reports on new medications in which an expert was cited, 50 per cent of such experts had financial ties to industry, and in only one-third of these cases were those ties acknowledged. This blurring of roles by some opinion leaders (in Moynihan's provocative terms, 'Independent experts or drug representatives in disguise?' (Moynihan et al. 2008)) coincides with reduced budgets for quality health journalism by many media outlets, meaning less scrutiny by journalists of press releases from industry and their associated public relations companies. Furthermore, there have been calls for registries of 'untied' experts and the publication of such a list in the *BMJ* (Lenzer and Brownlee 2008). The interested reader is referred to the *BMJ* 'Head to Head' commentary on the pros and cons of the industry utilization of key opinion leaders (Buckwell 2008). These disturbing revelations highlight the need for senior clinicians to be transparent about any potential conflicts of interest in media releases or in contributions to clinical practice guidelines.

Advisory boards / speakers bureaux

Industry advisory boards may be national or international. Little has been written about these, as they are somewhat opaque to the outside world. While ostensibly established to provide independent scientific advice to industry, they vary enormously in actual practice. In my own experience, many do act with integrity and professional independence, providing helpful 'sounding boards' to industry, even to the point of frank and skeptical responses to in-house industry research or marketing programmes. Others are almost obsequious in their relationship with the companies, focusing largely on marketing strategies and the provision of 'friendly' speakers for new product launches—be they speaking on specific products or on relevant clinical issues—thereby providing 'academic credibility' to the company and product.

There has been considerable recent debate about the acceptability of company speaker bureaux, with the Association of American Medical Colleges (AAMC 2008) recently proscribing this practice for US academics—a stance not accepted by a number of industry representatives on that guideline panel. While many speakers use such opportunities for quality product-independent continuing education, others are less scrupulous, sometimes unquestioningly using company-developed presentation material with minimal alteration, or agreeing to edit material to be consistent with the 'company line' (a form of 'ghostwriting'—see below). Remuneration may be considerable, particularly for those involved in company-sponsored 'satellite' symposia linked to major conferences, or those on international speaking 'tours'. In the US, this has led to a formal regulated distinction between meetings supported by 'untied educational grants' over which industry has no editorial control, and those for which the 'educational' content is are clearly product-related.

These circumstances highlight the need for open disclosure of earnings by the clinician speakers, especially in view of the considerable potential influence of eminent academic figures. A related, and not unreasonable concern, is the time distraction of such speaker bureau activities for academics and senior clinicians from their primary research, teaching, administrative, and clinical responsibilities.

The related broader issue is that of industry involvement in continuing medical education (Moynihan et al. 2008). At present it is believed that 80–90 per cent of CME activities are currently funded and/or organized by industry. Certainly, there has been a concomitant major decline over recent decades in CME auspiced by professional and academic bodies.

Trainees, medical students, nurses, and consumers

Industry contact with these groups has increased in recent years. A number of academics (Rogers et al. 2004; Mohl2005) and media commentators (Moynihan 2003b) have written on the relationship between industry and trainees or medical students. All emphasize the need for training and awareness of these vulnerable groups on how to relate to industry. There is a curious contradiction in student and trainee attitudes. In general, they are worried about others (such as consultants) accepting gifts, but are themselves unconcerned about the effect of (and may even feel entitled to) gifts such as meals or pens. Some student groups, such as the American Medical Student Association have actively campaigned about these issues (e.g. the student organization 'PharmFree'). More recently, students at Harvard organized major demonstrations on the influence of industry on academics at that institution (Wilson 2009), and have published a 'report' on various medical schools, with those (such as Harvard) who receive large amounts of industry sponsorship being given an 'F' (for failure) (Kluger 2009).

An important issue in the training of students and trainees is the 'hidden medical curriculum', i.e. the 'true' attitudes and behaviour of consultants towards industry that are observed by junior staff, rather than the rhetoric the senior staff espouse. Other vulnerable (and currently more naïve) groups include non-medical clinicians (particularly nurses) and consumer or carer organizations.

Sponsorship of major national and international scientific conferences

This is a fraught and complex area (Moynihan et al. 2008). There was a recent public furor related to the 2008 annual conference of the Royal Australian and New Zealand College of Psychiatrists, whereby the chair of the scientific committee resigned over that College's refusal to reject industry sponsorship. In the UK, at least one major college conference has declined any industry sponsorship (Moncrieff et al. 2008). However, the issue is not straightforward, as many national and international conferences would require prohibitive registration fees if no industry sponsorship was available. There have been calls for the provision of industry sponsorship of such meetings untied to advertising or exhibition space. While such calls are commendable, it is unrealistic to expect substantial industry commitments without the *quid pro quo* of such opportunities for marketing. In this light, the announcement in early 2009 by the American Psychiatric Association (Steenhuysen 2009) of a cessation to the practice of allowing industry-sponsored symposia as a major means of earnings for the APA annual scientific conference is striking, and very likely to be seen as a precedent for other major national and international meetings. Furthermore, the APA has decided to phase out industry-sponsored meals at those conferences.

International psychiatric organizations and their relationship to industry

Over the last few decades there have been *sotto voce* concerns about a lack of probity in the relations between some international clinical organizations and industry, with the worries mainly focusing on the ethics of the bodies themselves, rather than industry. Such concerns appear to have resulted in improved governance of these bodies, tighter financial control, independent auditing procedures, and the reduction in influence of some individuals.

Industry-sponsored research

It is important to reiterate that few innovative compounds which have been developed by the public sector have progressed to the point of marketing approval by regulatory authorities. However, it should also be acknowledged that (particularly in recent years) many novel compounds and/or basic mechanisms have been discovered by universities or research institutes, with subsequent licensing of intellectual property rights for drug development to industry.

Related to this, there has been growing concern (Turner et al. 2008; Mathew and Charney 2009) about the high rates of failure (or at the least, excessive delays) in publishing negative trial results. Examples in psychiatry include the prolonged delays in acknowledging some of the negative outcomes of trials in bipolar disorder of topiramate and lamotrigine, and the distortion of the literature on antidepressant efficacy by the failure to publish negative trials. The recent mandatory prior registration of clinical trials should minimize this is as an issue.

Involvement in pharmaceutical industry-sponsored research is not uncommon. Henry et al. (2005b), surveying a large number of Australian specialists, found that participation in such research was more common for those in hospital and/or university (49 per cent) practice than in private practice (33 per cent). The major concerns of the specialists involved in such research were delay in publication or non-publication of key negative findings (5–7 per cent), and concealment of results (2 per cent). About 9 per cent reported at least one event that could represent a breach of research integrity. In a related paper, Henry et al. (2005a) reported that clinicians involved in sponsored research were more likely to have broader involvement with industry. They were significantly more likely to have been offered industry-sponsored items or activities valued at more than AU$500 and support for attending international conferences. Furthermore, they were more likely to be a paid consultant for industry and to be a member of an advisory board.

Acknowledgment of potential financial conflicts of interest in reporting of clinical trials

In 1984, the *New England Journal of Medicine* became the first of the major medical journals to require authors of original research to disclose any financial ties with companies making products discussed in submitted papers (Angell 2000). Since then, this has become standard practice for most refereed journals. In 2005, Perlis et al. (2005) reported on the first study of the relationship between industry funding and the outcomes of clinical trials in psychiatry. Sixty per cent of trials reported receiving industry sponsorship, and 47 per cent had at least one author with a financial conflict of interest. Of 162 identified randomized controlled trials in major journals, those which reported conflicts of interest were 4.9 times more likely to report positive results.

The issue of appropriate disclosure of conflict of interests remains contentious, as indicated by a recent editorial in *JAMA* (DeAngelis and Fontanarosa 2009) which commented on controversy over an apparent failure by an author to declare financial relations with industry (by involvement in an industry speakers bureau) in a published report of a NIH-sponsored trial of escitalopram and cognitive therapy.

In one of the few commentaries in this literature by industry-employed psychiatrists, Paul and Tohen of Eli Lilly (2007) spoke on the need for full disclosure of potential conflicts of interest and the requirement for independent verification of research results. They stated: '. . . we too are concerned that the problem of financial [conflict of interest], if not adequately addressed may completely erode the credibility of psychiatric research and thus undermine the essential trust that patients have in their physicians and in the treatments they prescribe'.

Authorship of industry-sponsored trial reports and review articles

There has been recent concern about the apparently common practices of 'ghostwriting' and guest authorship. In one of the first reports to raise this issue in psychiatry, Healy and Cattell (2003) examined articles on the antidepressant sertraline published in the late 1990s. They compared publications coordinated by a medical writing agency with articles not coordinated by such agencies. They found that articles linked to these agencies involved more authors and were cited more frequently. Healy and Cattell raised concern about the apparent limited access of the academic authors to the raw data of these trials, and the common failure of these publications to acknowledge the actual, but 'non-academic', writers. Similar concerns have been raised about the engagement of physicians, including involvement in the production of ghost-written articles, in promoting off-label indications for gabapentin (Steinman et al. 2006) which included its use in neuropathic pain and bipolar disorder. (It should be noted, however, that some employees of the company involved did courageously publish negative findings; one example of this was the report of Pande et al. (2000)).

In a more recent paper, Ross et al. (2008) used documentation from legal proceedings concerning the anti-inflammatory agent rofecoxib to provide the hitherto best-documented 'case history' of the relationship between the pharmaceutical industry, medical publishing companies, and academic clinicians. In a damning exposé, this data- and document-based report detailed pharmaceutical company (in this case, Merck) employees working either independently or in collaboration with medical publishing companies in preparing manuscripts on clinical trials, and subsequently recruiting external academically-affiliated investigators to be the publication 'authors'. These recruited academic authors were frequently given first or second authorship positions. For scientific review articles, similar processes were documented, with the academic recruits frequently being the sole authors, and moreover being offered honoraria for their participation. While industry financial support was acknowledged in most of the clinical trial reports, this was reported in only half of the review articles. As discussed by the authors, it is unlikely that such practices differ from those of other companies and other products. This report led to robust editorial commentary in *JAMA* (DeAngelis and Fontanarosa 2008). The continued practice of ghost-written articles has also been raised in the investigations of US Senator Grassley, in this instance involving Wyeth.

A related issue is the reporting of pharmaco-economic analyses, an increasingly important area of research, as such data is now routinely demanded by government agencies responsible for deciding upon subsidization of medications, at either national, regional, or institutional levels. In a report focusing on economic studies of antidepressants, Baker et al. (2003) quantitatively analyzed all articles with original comparative cost or cost-effectiveness outcomes for antidepressants. They found that studies sponsored by manufacturers of newer antidepressants favoured these drugs more than did non-industry studies. Moreover, industry-sponsored modeling studies were more likely to favour industry than were non-industry sponsored studies.

'Disease mongering'

Moynihan and others (Moynihan and Henry 2006) have espoused the concept of 'disease mongering'—'the selling of sickness that widens the boundaries of illness in order to grow markets for those who sell and deliver treatments'. According to Moynihan, examples of this disease mongering include the medicalization of the menopause and the portrayal of 'minor' problems such as irritable bowel syndrome, high cholesterol, and osteoporosis as serious medical disorders. Healy (2006) has described the major increase in the rates of diagnosis of bipolar disorder as an example of this phenomenon, occurring in response to the growing availability of new mood stabilizers. One concrete outcome of this debate has been the 2004 decision of the European drug regulator to withdraw its approval of premenstrual dysphoric disorder (PMDD) as an indication for the SSRI Prozac, citing that 'the condition was not a well-established disease entity' (Moynihan 2004). While many would accept there is some validity to this concept of disease mongering, it is naïve to believe that it is the product of the pharmaceutical industry alone, as there is an equally self-serving academic research industry for many conditions that have been either newly described, or for which there has been a resurgence of interest.

'Untied' industry sponsorship of medical school/academic department research

Recent press reports have highlighted the extensive amounts of industry funding of university research programmes, particularly at prestigious institutions such as Harvard. There has been a growing disquiet about the potential influence of such funding, for example on the focus of academic research agendas being on conditions of primary interest to industry drug development programmes. In Australia, there has been vigorous debate about the academic value and propriety of funding by Eli Lilly of a collaborative research programme (Lilly MAP) with the department of psychiatry at the University of Melbourne (Singh et al. 2004; Raven 2004; Malhi 2004).

Why are psychiatrists in the (dubious) 'lead'?

Despite ripostes from the American Psychiatric Association that there has been an unreasonable focus on psychiatrists in recent US media commentaries, the large number of senior psychiatrists allegedly exposed in these recent reports demands some serious reflection by the profession.

In many ways, a strong industry focus on psychiatry would not be unsurprising. Psychotropics are among the most widely prescribed agents, particularly the antidepressants, for which prescribing rates have increased dramatically worldwide since the early 1990s (McManus et al. 2000). The new antipsychotic agents have also been heavily prescribed. Psychotropics have been responsible for a major proportion of profits for a number of companies. Furthermore, the limited distinction between the various new antidepressants and antipsychotics has led to aggressive marketing competition between the responsible companies. Indeed, Moynihan has reported that psychiatrists receive more industry-funded CME than other specialists in Australia (data as yet unpublished). A further factor may be that psychiatrists are among the lowest earning specialty groups, perhaps making them more vulnerable to financial inducements such as travel to overseas conferences or other gifts.

Industry-sponsored events now account for about 90 per cent of all CME activities across medicine. The attraction of educational events with national and international colleagues in expensive hotels locally or overseas is not difficult to appreciate. Furthermore, for academic psychiatrists and other clinical disciplines, research funding through competitive government funding schemes (such as NIH in the US, or MRC in the UK) is increasingly difficult to obtain. Academics also often have few sources of funding other than that offered by industry to attend international scientific meetings.

How are the various bodies responding to this issue?

Professional organizations

The ethical guidelines of the *American Psychiatric Association* (APA 2008), 'APA Principles of Medical Ethics with Annotations especially Applicable to Psychiatry')—derived from those of the parent American Medical Association—are virtually silent on the issue of relationships with the pharmaceutical industry. As detailed above, very recently (Steenhuysen 2009) the APA has announced a gradual cessation of industry-sponsored symposia at their annual scientific conference, and a phasing out of industry-sponsored meals.

In contrast to the APA, the UK *Royal College of Psychiatrists* (RCPsych 2008) has produced a specific publication focusing on this issue: 'Good Psychiatric Practice: Relationships with Pharmaceutical and other Commercial Organizations' (Royal College of Psychiatrists Report CR148). This report details guidance on the relationship between individuals, researchers, and the UK College administration itself with industry. It delineates three central principles: transparency, full declaration of relationships, and the need to educate trainees. It does not proscribe relations with industry, rather encouraging transparency and open disclosure. For example, it does not proscribe industry-sponsorship of conference travel or accommodation, nor does it prohibit industry sponsorship of conferences.

In Australia, the *Royal Australian and New Zealand College of Psychiatrists* has adapted the ethical guidelines of the *Royal Australasian College of Physicians* (Komesaroff 2005) in the development of the 'RANZCP Ethical Guideline on The Relationship Between Psychiatrists and the Health Care Industry' (RANZCP 2008). This ethical guideline provides specific recommendations on clinical trials, sponsorship of conference attendance, support for organization of meetings, receipt of gifts and entertainment, drug samples, remuneration of services, involvement in advisory boards, and involvement of industry with students and CME. As a specific example, these guidelines proscribe receipt of support to attend conferences unless the individual is a speaker or chair. In practice, this recommendation is rarely adhered to, being routinely flouted with respect to both national and international meetings.

University medical schools

In 2006, the *American Board of Internal Medicine Foundation* (ABIM) and the *Institute on Medicine as a Profession* (IMAP) published the ABIM-IMAP taskforce policy recommendations on conflicts of interest (Brennan et al. 2006). These recommendations argue that self-regulation has been unsuccessful and that more stringent regulation is necessary. That group proposed the elimination or modification of common practices related to small gifts, pharmaceutical medical samples, continuing medical education, funds for physician travel, speakers bureaus, ghostwriting, and consulting and research contacts. They called for academic medical centres to take the lead in eliminating conflicts of interest between physicians and the healthcare industry.

In 2008, the Association of American Medical Colleges released a formal report on 'Industry Funding of Medical Education' (AAMC 2008). This thoughtful, balanced, and robust report began with an acknowledgement of the appropriateness of a partnership with industry, yet the need to manage this:

> An effective and principled partnership between academic medical centers and various health industries is critical in order to realize fully the benefits of biomedical research and ensure continued advances in the prevention, diagnosis, and treatment of disease. Appropriate management of this partnership by both academic medical centers and industry is crucial to ensure that it remains principled, thereby sustaining public trust in the proposition that both partners are fundamentally dedicated to the welfare of patients and the improvement of public health.

The AAMC report described the 'core principles of medical professionalism' as autonomy, objectivity, and altruism. It commented further upon the relationship with industry: 'The fault lies not only with industry; the acceptance, indeed the expectation of such financial incentives by academic professionals and their institutions has encouraged these practices', and 'In their educational interactions, academic medical institutions and industry are mutually accountable for maintaining a principled partnership based on the primary goal of providing the highest quality of care for patients'.

Specifically the AAMC Report recommends clarity about the extent to which interactions with industry are prohibited, and commends the necessity for educational programmes on the relationship with industry for students, trainees, and teaching faculty. It proscribes receipt of gifts, cautions on the distribution of samples, restricts access of pharmaceutical representatives, and recommends auditing industry-sponsored CME activities (particularly with regard to content and meals). Strikingly, the report strongly discourages involvement of faculty in industry-sponsored speakers bureaus (it should be noted that the industry representatives on the Taskforce declined support of this particular proposal), and proscribes payment for attendance at industry-sponsored meetings and acceptance of gifts at such events. Furthermore, it states that industry-supplied food and meals should be considered as gifts and therefore not accepted. Acceptance of travel funds is proscribed, as is allowing written or oral presentations to be ghost-written. Those involved in decisions about purchases of pharmaceuticals or devices should declare all conflicts of interest. The taskforce also commended convening an expert panel comprised of academic and industry representatives to explore new opportunities and best practice in information exchange between those two groups.

What has been the impact of these ABIM-IMAP and AAMC reports? In a recent commentary, Rothman and Chimonas (2008) describe a surprisingly widespread acceptance of these major shifts in US practice. Contrary to the fears of many, the authors observed no significant movement of academic faculty out of those medical colleges with strong conflict-of-interest policies. Furthermore, they noted 'an increasing number of accounts of physicians taking personal pride in turning down speakers bureau invitations'. In Australia, a qualitative study of internal medicine physicians has indicated a polarization of responses to ethical guidelines on relations to industry (Osborn 2009).

Medical journals

In an editorial in *JAMA*, DeAngelis and Fontanarosa (2008), made the following proposals: all clinical trials must be prospectively registered; the contributions of all proposed authors must be detailed and any compensation reported; all funding sources must be acknowledged; financial conflicts of interest must be provided and considered by editors prior to agreement to publish; analysis of data and preparation of the manuscript must have been undertaken by the named authors; statistics must have been conducted by a person not employed by industry; authors not complying with these guidelines must be reported to appropriate authorities; peer reviewers must not divulge details to third parties; industry should have no input into medical education programmes; and physicians should not serve on speakers bureaux or accept gifts from industry. They conclude: 'Ensuring, maintaining, and strengthening the integrity of medical science must be a priority for everyone'.

Pharmaceutical industry organizations

In late 2008, the *Pharmaceutical Research and Manufacturers of America* (PhRMA)—the umbrella representative industry group in the US—published an update of its voluntary code of conduct, the 'Code of Interactions with Healthcare Professionals' (PhRMA 2008). This differed from previous editions in proscribing gifts such as pens, pads, and mugs, as well as entertainment and recreational benefits such as tickets to the theatre or sporting events. It did, however, allow for provision of starter packs and engagement of clinicians in speakers bureaux.

In Australia, the analogous body—*Medicines Australia*—published the 15th Edition of its 'Code of Conduct' in March 2007 (Medicines Australia 2007). For the first time, and under the direction of the Australian Competition Tribunal, this code detailed mandated web disclosure of all industry-sponsored educational and marketing activities in Australia and the associated costs, though at this stage not disclosure of the names of clinicians receiving remuneration. This would appear to be the first national mandated detailing of such activities, and has revealed that approximately 30,000 such events occur each year, involving at least 800,000 attendances, costing about AU$32 million p.a. In a recent article in the *Weekend Australian* (Cresswell 2009), there was reported concern over the number of 'educational events for doctors that include weekends costing more than AU$300,000 at five-star hotels'.

Recommendations and remaining areas of uncertainty

Where do these developments leave psychiatry and the broader medical community? There is clearly a need for the medical profession to get its own house in order. Self-regulation has not worked, despite the best of intents. This is a problem for both industry and the profession. Psychiatrists now have a major credibility problem with the public; it is an issue of trust.

The central principles of the relationship must be integrity and transparency. Inadequacies in disclosure have been at the centre of recent scandals in the US. Should there be full disclosure, as proposed by Grassley? The ground is already moving rapidly under our feet. A number of US companies have recently decided to publicly detail all remuneration to clinicians. In Australia, all promotional and educational events are disclosed by court order, though clinician payments are not, as yet, required to be reported.

We have no alternative but to drastically improve the transparency of the relationship, both in terms of remuneration received and disclosure of any potential conflicts of interest (in all publications, media statements, and guidelines). However, if we go down the route of disclosure of earnings from industry, questions remain. First, should this be in broad terms (such as a generic declaration of remuneration from activities such as advisory boards, consultancies, honoraria for speaking engagements, sponsored travel and/or accommodation to meetings, involvement in industry-sponsored trials, payment for publications written with industry, retainers, or shares in pharmaceutical companies) or should actual dollar earnings be disclosed? I believe that we will inevitably need to declare actual earnings, and should do so soon, but I accept that this may be too great a demand for the medical profession at this point in time. Second, to whom should such details be provided? To the public via websites, such as that of *Medicines Australia*? For clinicians, to the relevant professional bodies? For academics, to university administrators?

While the details of such disclosure will need to be determined, it is clear that we must expeditiously formalize a relationship of integrity and transparency between the medical profession and the pharmaceutical industry. Furthermore, universities and other medical bodies, such as the professional colleges, should seriously consider developing detailed recommendations such as those of the AAMC (Greenland 2009).

The credibility and destiny of medicine are in our hands. We must not fumble the ball at this critical juncture.

Potential conflicts of interest

In the financial year 2007–2008, Philip Mitchell was paid a total of AU$6,500 for lecture honoraria, consultancies, and advisory board membership from pharmaceutical companies that manufacture and market psychotropic agents (AstraZeneca, Eli Lilly, and Pfizer). He also received travel support to attend an international scientific forum at which he gave an invited lecture in a symposium in the main programme of the meeting. He has not been a member of a pharmaceutical company advisory board since early 2008. Since the beginning of 2009, he has donated all remuneration from industry to charitable organizations. He has never owned stocks in pharmaceutical companies, nor received retainers. He has been a site investigator for a number of industry-sponsored trials, the most recent being in 2004. Mitchell has also received remuneration from state and federal health departments for various committee memberships, including three years serving on the Australian Drug Evaluation Committee (the advisory committee to the Australian drug regulator, the Therapeutic Goods Administration).

References

AAMC (2008) *Industry funding of medical education: Report of an AAMC Task Force*, 1–34.

Angell, M (2000) 'Is academic medicine for sale?', *New England Journal of Medicine*, 342, 1516–8.

APA (2008) *The principles of medical ethics*. Arlington, VA: American Psychiatric Association, 1–39.

Baker, CB, Johnsrud, MT, Crismon, ML, Rosenheck, RA, and Woods, SW (2003) 'Quantitative analysis of sponsorship bias in economic studies of antidepressants', *British Journal of Psychiatry*, 183, 498–506.

Bhattacharjee, Y (2007) 'Inside Government Going Private', *Science*, 316(5827), May 18, 2007.

Biederman, J (2008) 'Credibility crisis in pediatric psychiatry', *Nature Neuroscience*, 11, 1233.

Bjorn, G (2008) 'Straight talk with. . . Ray Moynihan', *Nature Medicine*, 14, 1142–3.

Blumenthal, D (2004) 'Doctors and drug companies', *New England Journal of Medicine*, 351, 1885–90.

Brennan, TA, Rothman, DJ, Blank, L, et al. (2006) 'Health industry practices that create conflicts of interest: a policy proposal for academic medical centers', *JAMA*, 295, 429–33.

Buckwell, C (2008) 'Should the drug industry work with key opinion leaders? Yes', *British Medical Journal*, 336, 1404.

Campbell, EG, Gruen, RL, Mountford, J, Miller, LG, Cleary, PD, and Blumenthal, D (2007) 'A national survey of physician-industry relationships', *New England Journal of Medicine*, 356, 1742–50.

Carey, N and Harris, G (2009) 'Psychiatric group faces scrutiny over drug industry ties', *The New York Times*, 26 March 2009.

Cresswell, A (2009) 'Drug companies censured over lavish doctors seminars', *Weekend Australian*.

Dana, J and Loewenstein, G (2003) 'A social science perspective on gifts to physicians from industry', *JAMA*, 290, 252–5.

Deangelis, CD, and Fontanarosa, PB (2008) 'Impugning the integrity of medical science: the adverse effects of industry influence', *JAMA*, 299, 1833–5.

Deangelis, CD and Fontanarosa, PB (2009) 'Resolving unreported Conflicts of Interest', *JAMA*, 302, 198–199.

Doran, E, Kerridge, I, Mcneill, P, and Henry, D (2006) 'Empirical uncertainty and moral contest: a qualitative analysis of the relationship between medical specialists and the pharmaceutical industry in Australia', *Social Science & Medicine*, 62, 1510–9.

Editorial (2008) 'Credibility crisis in pediatric psychiatry', *Nature Neuroscience*, 11, 983.

Freedman, R, Lewis, DA, Michels, R, Pine, DS, Schultz, SK, Tamminga, CA, Andreasen, NC, Brady, KT, Brent, DA, Brzustowicz, L, Carter, CS, Eisenberg, L, Goldman, H, Javitt, DC, Leibenluft, E, Lieberman, JA, Milrod, B, Oquendo, MA, Rosenbaum, JF, Rush, AJ, Siever, LJ, Suppes, P, Weissman, MM, Roy, MD, Scully, JH, Jr, and Yager, J (2009) 'Conflict of interest—an issue for every psychiatrist', *American Journal of Psychiatry*, 166, 274.

Greenland, P (2009) 'Time for the medical profession to act: new policies needed now on interactions between pharmaceutical companies and physicians', *Archives of Internal Medicine*, 169(9), 829–31.

Harris, G (2008a) 'Radio Host Has Drug Company Ties', *The New York Times*.

Harris, G (2008b) 'Top Psychiatrist Didn't Report Drug Makers' Pay'. *The New York Times*.

Healy, D (2006) 'Manufacturing consensus', *Culture, Medicine & Psychiatry*, 30, 135–56.

Healy, D and Cattell, D (2003) 'Interface between authorship, industry and science in the domain of therapeutics', *British Journal of Psychiatry*, 183, 22–7.

Henry, D, Doran, E, Kerridge, I, Hill, S, Mcneill, PM, and Day, R (2005a) 'Ties that bind: multiple relationships between clinical researchers and the pharmaceutical industry', *Archives of Internal Medicine*, 165, 2493–6.

Henry, DA, Kerridge, IH, Hill, SR, McNeill, PM, Doran, E, Newby, DA, Henderson, KM, Maguire, J, Stokes, BJ, Macdonald, GJ, and Day, RO (2005b) 'Medical specialists and pharmaceutical industry-sponsored research: a survey of the Australian experience', *Medical Journal of Australia*, 182, 557–60.

Hooper, C (2005) 'Conflict-of-interest regulations for NIH employees finalized: The changes', *The NIH Catalyst*. Available at <http://www.nih.gov/catalyst/2005/05.09.01/page4.html>.

Johnson, G and Gershon, S (1999) 'Early North American research on lithium', *Australia and New Zealand Journal of Psychiatry*, 33 Suppl, S48–53.

Kluger, J (2009) 'Is Drug-Company Money Tainting Medical Education?' *TIME*.

Komesaroff, PA (2005) 'Ethical issues in the relationships with industry: an ongoing challenge. New Guidelines open for public comment', *Journal of Paediatrics and Child Health*, 41, 558–60.

Komesaroff, PA and Kerridge, IH (2002) 'Ethical issues concerning the relationships between medical practitioners and the pharmaceutical industry', *Medical Journal of Australia*, 176, 118–21.

Lenzer, J and Brownlee, S (2008) 'Naming names: is there an (unbiased) doctor in the house?', *British Medical Journal*, 337, a930.

Malhi, G (2004) 'Partnerships between academic psychiatry and the pharmaceutical industry', *Australasian Psychiatry*, 12, 225–26.

Mathew, SJ and Charney, DS (2009) 'Publication bias and the efficacy of antidepressants', *American Journal of Psychiatry*, 166, 140–5.

McManus, P, Mant, A, Mitchell, PB, Montgomery, WS, Marley, J and Auland, ME (2000) 'Recent trends in the use of antidepressant drugs in Australia, 1990–1998', *Medical Journal of Australia*, 173, 458–61.

McNeill, PM, Kerridge, IH, Henry, DA, Stokes, B, Hill, SR, Newby, D, Macdonald, GJ, Day, RO, Maguire, J and Henderson, KM (2006) 'Giving and receiving of gifts between pharmaceutical companies and medical specialists in Australia', *Internal Medicine Journal*, 36, 571–8.

Medicines Australia (2007) *Code of Conduct*. 15th edn. Deakin, ACT: Medicines Australia,1–215.

Mohl, PC (2005) 'Psychiatric training program engagement with the pharmaceutical industry: an educational issue, not strictly an ethical one', *Academic Psychiatry*, 29, 215–21.

Moncrieff, J (2006) 'Psychiatric drug promotion and the politics of neoliberalism', *British Journal of Psychiatry*, 188, 301–302.

Moncrieff, J, Thomas, P, and Huws, R (2008) 'Some progress in UK psychiatry', *British Medical Journal*, 337, a1780.

Moynihan, R (2003a) 'Who pays for the pizza? Redefining the relationships between doctors and drug companies. 1: Entanglement', *British Medical Journal*, 326, 1189–92.

Moynihan, R (2003b) Who pays for the pizza? Redefining the relationships between doctors and drug companies. 2: Disentanglement', *British Medical Journal*, 326, 1193–6.

Moynihan, R (2004) 'Controversial disease dropped from Prozac product information', *British Medical Journal*, 328, 365.

Moynihan, R (2008a) 'Is the relationship between pharma and medical education on the rocks?', *British Medical Journal*, 337, a925.

Moynihan, R (2008b) 'Key opinion leaders: independent experts or drug representatives in disguise?', *British Medical Journal*, 336, 1402–3.

Moynihan, R and Henry, D (2006) 'The fight against disease mongering: generating knowledge for action', *PLoS Medicine*, 3, e191.

Moynihan, R and Sweet, M (2000) 'Medicine, the media and monetary interests: the need for transparency and professionalism', *Medical Journal of Australia*, 173, 631–4.

Moynihan, R, Bero, L, Ross-Degnan, D, Henry, D, Lee, K, Watkins, J, Mah, C, and Soumerai, SB (2000) 'Coverage by the news media of the benefits and risks of medications', *New England Journal of Medicine*, 342, 1645–50.

Moynihan, R, Doran, E, and Henry, D (2008) Disease mongering is now part of the global health debate. *PLoS Med*, 5, e106.

Osborn, M, Day, R, Komesaroff, P, and Mant, A (2009) 'Do ethical guidelines make a difference to decision making?' *Internal Medicine Journal*, 39(12), 800–805.

Pande, AC, Crockatt, JG, Janney, CA, Werth, JL, and Tsaroucha, G (2000) 'Gabapentin in bipolar disorder: a placebo-controlled trial of adjunctive therapy. Gabapentin Bipolar Disorder Study Group', *Bipolar Disorder*, 2, 249–55.

Paul, SM and Tohen, M (2007) 'Conflicts of interest and the credibility of psychiatric research', *World Psychiatry*, 6, 33–4.

Perlis, RH., Perlis, CS, Wu, Y, Hwang, C, Joseph, M, and Nierenberg, AA (2005) 'Industry sponsorship and financial conflict of interest in the reporting of clinical trials in psychiatry', *American Journal of Psychiatry*, 162, 1957–60.

PhRMA (2008) *Code of interactions with healthcare professionals*.

RANZCP (2008) *Ethical Guideline #5: The Relationship Between Psychiatrists and the Health Care Industry*. Melbourne, Australia: Royal Australian and New Zealand College of Psychiatrists, 1–17.

Raven, M, Rogers, W, and Jureidini, J (2004) 'Partnerships between academic psychiatry and the pharmaceutical industry', *Australasian Psychiatry*, 12, 83–84.

RCPSYCH (2008) *Good psychiatric practice: Relationship with pharmaceutical and other commercial organisations*. London: Royal College of Psychiatrists, 1–23.

Rogers, WA, Mansfield, PR, Braunack-Mayer, AJ, and Jureidini, JN (2004) 'The ethics of pharmaceutical industry relationships with medical students', *Medical Journal of Australia*, 180, 411–4.

Ross, JS, Hill, KP, Egilman, DS, and Krumholz, HM (2008) 'Guest authorship and ghostwriting in publications related to rofecoxib: a case study of industry documents from rofecoxib litigation', *JAMA*, 299, 1800–12.

Rothman, DJ and Chimonas, S (2008) 'New developments in managing physician-industry relationships', *JAMA*, 300, 1067–9.

Singh, B, Copolov, D, Grainger, D, and Goh, J (2004) 'Partnerships between academic psychiatry and the pharmaceutical industry: the Lilly MAP Initiative', *Australasian Psychiatry*, 12, 220–4; discussion 25–6.

Steenhuysen, J (2009) 'U.S. psychiatrists to end drug company seminars', *Reuters*.

Steinbrook, R (2004) 'Financial conflicts of interest and the NIH', *New England Journal of Medicine*, 350, 327–30.

Steinman, MA, Bero, LA, Chren, MM, and Landefeld, CS (2006) 'Narrative review: the promotion of gabapentin: an analysis of internal industry documents', *Annals of Internal Medicine*, 145, 284–93.

Turner, EH, Matthews, AM, Linardatos, E, Tell, RA, and Rosenthal, R (2008) 'Selective publication of antidepressant trials and its influence on apparent efficacy', *New England Journal of Medicine*, 358, 252–60.

Wadman, M (2008) 'Pharma payment probe widens its net', *Nature*, 455, 1017.

Wazana, A (2000) 'Physicians and the pharmaceutical industry: is a gift ever just a gift?', *JAMA*, 283, 373–80.

Weiss, R (2005) '44 Violated Ethics Rules, NIH Director Tells Panel', *The Washington Post*.

Wilson, D (2009) 'Pfizer Worker Photographed Protesters at Harvard', *New York Times*.

Commentary 4

Protecting the Human Rights of People with Mental Illnesses: A Call to Action for Global Mental Health

Vikram Patel, Arthur Kleinman,
and Benedetto Saraceno

Introduction

People with mental illnesses (a term we use to include people with mental disabilities) have historically been subjected to abuses of human rights in all spheres of their lives, not least when they have been incarcerated in mental hospitals. However, programmes to challenge the stigma against people with mental illnesses, user-led advocacy, and the emergence of community mental health care have addressed some of the worst forms of abuse in many developed countries. We have assembled selected photographs in this article, derived mainly from news and civil society organizations, depicting the conditions of care of people with mental illnesses in some developing countries. These include horrifying conditions in mental hospitals, as well as instances of abuse in communities. We admit at the outset that these images do not constitute an 'epidemiology' of human rights abuses; neither does such representative data exist, nor do we think it is feasible to carry out such an investigation. Notwithstanding this limitation, we believe that the images we have selected demonstrate that the situation is far too prevalent, and that the abuse of even a single person with a mental illness is one too many. Indeed, we argue that these extreme forms of abuse represent the tip of the iceberg of abuses faced by people with mental illnesses; thus, the frequent experience of violence, lack of access to evidence based psychosocial interventions, and the inappropriate use of physical and chemical restraints occur, to varying degrees, in all countries. We argue that these abuses are due to several factors, notably the stigma attached to mental illnesses, the culture of institutions, the lack of community mental healthcare, and the silence of the global health community including, most disturbingly, the mental health community. We contend that combating this shameful situation is the single most important priority for global mental health. We draw inspiration from the efforts of those who have attempted to reform mental healthcare institutions and produce tangible benefits in protecting the human rights of people with mental illnesses. We call for action by stakeholders in mental health, in particular mental health practitioners working in partnership with users and civil society groups, to bring this outrage to an end.

Using images in public health

Images of persons facing abuse and human rights violations have been utilized, with great effect, by activists and advocates for a number of causes (Sontag 2003). Images bring a crucial tool to public health scholarship and to advance the cause of public health (Sember 2003); the images of dying children, through HIV/AIDS or hunger, are examples of such effective use of disturbing images. Yet, in preparing this chapter, where we had access to scores of disturbing photos of the condition of people with mental illness, we felt it necessary to elicit independent views of ethicists and mental health professionals about their use. As Sember has noted, 'the power of images lies in their capacity both to convey information and to evoke reaction, often in the form of a feeling or an impulse' (Sember 2003) and we were conscious that the images we use were likely to arouse anger about the abuse of people with mental illnesses (the desired goal of this article) but also potentially anger about the misuse of images (Kleinman and Kleinman 1996). Without these images our article would not have the evidence needed to make our case. But, we were equally aware that using them, without the explicit permission of the individuals depicted (as would be the case for most such images) raises ethical concerns which might overwhelm the purpose of our article. A critical concern is regarding the ethics of violating the confidentiality of the victims. However, we wondered why such ethical principles should apply to these photos but not to the images of children dying of malnutrition or people dying of HIV/AIDS. We haven't found a satisfactory answer as yet to this apparent dissonance and, in the end, the photos we have chosen do not disclose the identity of an individual or have been suitably modified to obscure their identity. Another concern is that there is likely to be another side to the story we see in the images—no doubt, there are explanations for each of these images which may attenuate our outrage. However, they cannot ever justify what we can see. There is no justification for the kinds of practices we are criticizing based on cultural relativism because ethical relativism is simply unsustainable in the area of human suffering and caregiving. Furthermore, there is evidence that advocating for the human rights of the mentally ill is an effective tool in their defence to improve services (Caldas de Almeida 2007). There might be concern that such images might damage the work of psychiatrists in developing countries but our goal is not to undermine psychiatry (indeed, all three authors are psychiatrists); instead, we seek to demonstrate that an evidence- and rights-based psychiatry is, in fact, part of the solution, just as it is starting to be in developed countries. Yet another concern could be that our article would abet those who, with varying political motives, seek to undermine medical and psychiatric services that people with mental illnesses need: our response would be exactly the opposite, for humane and evidence-based services are a major component of the solution to these abuses. Some may be concerned that such images of 'sub-human' care may perpetuate stigma against people with mental illnesses; this is, in fact, the central tenet of our article, i.e. these appalling conditions of care are in themselves one of the causes of stigma against people with mental illnesses.

The abuse of people living with mental illnesses

Consider the first set of images which show people living in institutions for persons with mental illnesses (Figures 1 and 2). These are images of possibly the last community on Earth whose grotesque maltreatment can continue to arouse little reaction from the global health communities: people living with mental illnesses. Unsurprisingly, the WHO declared that there was a 'global emergency in human right violations for people suffering from mental illnesses' and, in 2006, released the Denied Citizens Photo Context (<http://www.who.int/features/galleries/2005/mental_health/01_en.html>).

In spite of these efforts, countless persons with mental illnesses continue to remain, as the newsmagazine *Time* labels them on its cover issue of its Asia edition on 23 November 2003, 'the forgotten' (<http://www.time.com/time/magazine/article/0,9171,536274,00.html> and <http://www.time.com/time/asia/photoessays/mental_illness/index.html>). This issue of the magazine chronicles many deeply distressing photographs of the conditions of care in mental hospitals in South-East Asia. People with mental illnesses in these hospitals have simply been forgotten by their

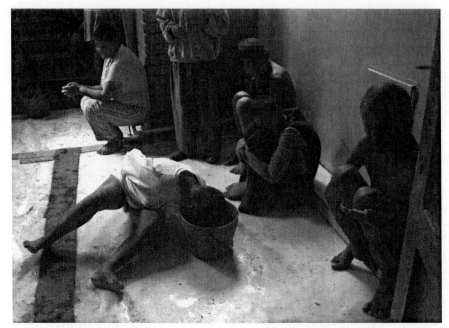

Figure 1 A scene from the male ward of a mental hospital showing a patient drinking water out of a pail. © Copyright AFP.

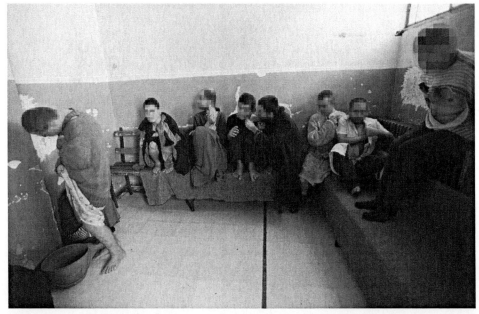

Figure 2 A scene from the male ward of a mental hospital showing a man urinating in front of other patients. © Copyright AFP.

families, by those who are supposedly caring for them, by the medical practitioners in the countries where they live, by most human rights organizations, by the global health community. These abuses are, in our view, the greatest blemish on the conscience of global health today. But perhaps an even greater blemish is the resounding silence of the response from the global community, in particular the professional mental health community. These images represent what health systems mete out to people whose sicknesses are not only denied basic care, but which tragically may rob them of the ability to articulate their grievances. The images show, at the very least, the literal and metaphorical stripping of all rights and dignity of persons with mental illnesses (Figure 3).

These images may represent an extreme scenario of abuse—but they are by no means uncommon. There are few representative investigations of conditions of care in mental hospitals; one such example is the National Human Rights Commission report of 1999 which chronicles the state of the mental hospitals of India, most of which date from the colonial period and between them are home to over 80 per cent of all psychiatric beds in that country (National Human Rights Commission 1999). The report concludes that human rights violations are the rule, rather than the exception, in these hospitals. Reassuringly, a recent review of mental hospitals in India revealed significant improvements in the quality of care of many institutions, but also revealed inadequate progress in many others (Murthy and Sekar 2008). Several anecdotal reports, illustrated in some of the images in this article, show that chaining, or other forms of inhuman restraints, is common practice in mental hospitals and traditional healing centres, in many parts of the world (Figures 4 and 5).

In hospitals, the restraints are not always physical—the inappropriate use of sedative medications and unmodified electroconvulsive therapy represent other examples of abuse. Psychiatric institutions tend to be more like human warehouses than places of care and treatment; the buildings are more often than not decrepit and filthy and people lack proper clothes, clean water, and decent food. There is a fundamental lack of respect for the dignity of persons with mental illnesses.

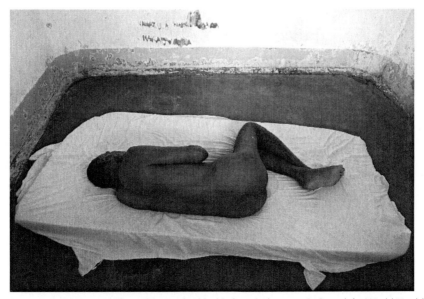

Figure 3 A man with mental illness lying naked in his hospital room. © Copyright World Health Organization (WHO), 2011. WHO/A. S. Kochar.

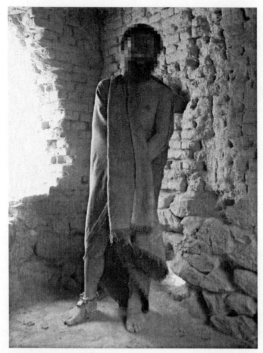

Figure 4 A man with mental illness, chained in a healing shrine. © Copyright World Health Organization (WHO), 2011. PAHO/A. Waak.

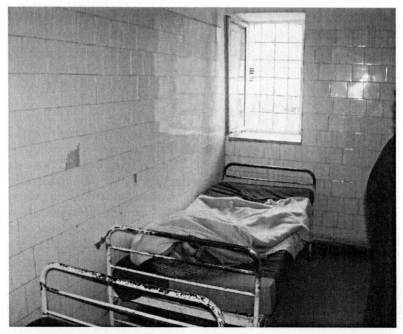

Figure 5 A man with mental illness chained to his hospital bed. © copyright Global Initiative on Psychiatry, Netherlands. © Copyright Global Initiative on Psychiatry, Netherlands.

Too often, people are placed in seclusion for long periods of time with no human contact, sometimes in small, prison-like rooms, at other times confined in cage beds. Seclusion and restraints are used for convenience and for punishment. Adults and children can be subject to horrific violence and rape—by staff or fellow patients—and these practices often go unreported and unpunished, leaving the perpetrators free to continue the abuse (Figure 6). Even when psychiatric facilities are decent and no physical violence is perpetrated, too many people—and this is true of some facilities in developed countries as well—receive no form of stimulation, and spend days, months, and even years living in excruciating boredom, watching TV with a cigarette in hand or lying listlessly in bed or engaged in a recreation more akin to school arts and crafts rather than a real engagement in meaningful adult activities that will ultimately lead to integration into the community. This aimlessness, inactivity, and social isolation is inhuman and degrading and, it seems to us, far from being conducive to recovery or good mental health.

Abuse takes place also in homes and in communities—some families, simply unable to cope, tie up their mentally ill relatives to the bed so that they can go about their daily existence in the comfort of knowing that their relative will not come to any harm (Figures 7 and 8). Others are left on the streets where they are at risk of more abuse (Figures 9, 10, and 11). Still others may be left to the mercy of informal healing systems. The tragedy of Erwaddi in 2001 in South India where over 20 persons with mental illnesses died when a fire swept through their healing temple—because they were chained to their beds and there was no one to unchain them when the fire broke out at night—is only exceptional because there was a fire. These harrowing narratives are a reflection of the desperate measures undertaken largely to help families cope with difficult behaviour, in places where there is virtually no community mental health system (Minas and Diatri 2008). As other authors have remarked, 'in some communities, people with mental illness are chained to trees or posts simply to prevent them from assaulting family members, from wandering, or from being attacked by neighbours or strangers. Having to care for a person with chronic mental illness may

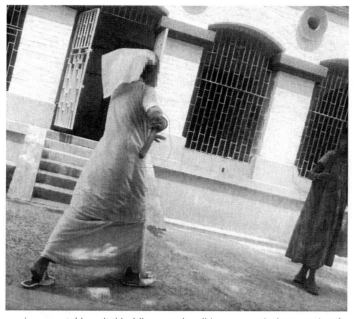

Figure 6 A nurse in a mental hospital holding a rod walking aggressively towards a female patient.
© Copyright Forum for Mental Health Movement, India.

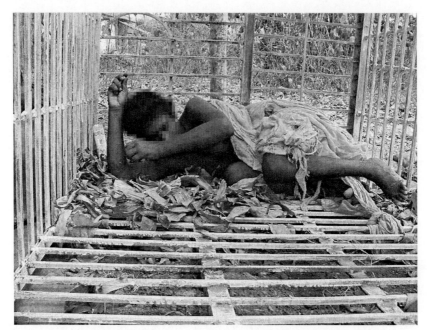

Figure 7 A man with mental illness in a homemade cage constructed by his family.
© Copyright AFP.

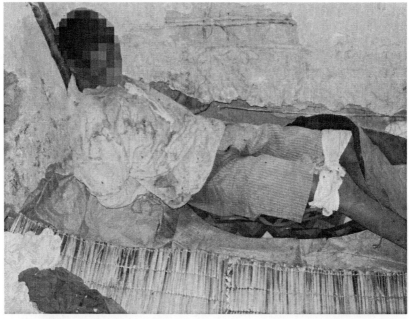

Figure 8 A young man with a mental disability physically restrained in his home. © Copyright World Health Organization (WHO), 2011. WHO/Pierre Virot.

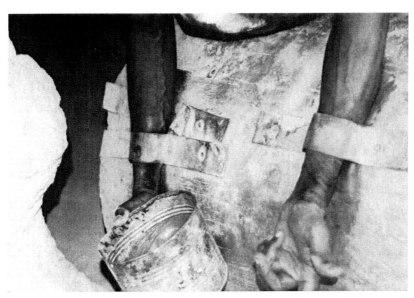

Figure 9 A woman with mental illness with arms shackled to a log of wood and begging.
© Copyright World Health Organization (WHO).

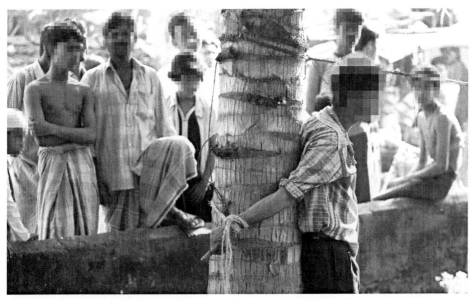

Figure 10 A young man with mental illness tied to coconut tree in his village for having stolen food. © Copyright Vikram Patel, 2011.

be the critical element that prevents a family unit from achieving some degree of self-sufficiency under already precarious conditions' (Silove et al. 2000). We place the primary responsibility for these abuses in the community at the door of the public health care system which has failed to provide humane, affordable, evidence-based care which, in turn, directly serve to protect the human rights of people with mental illnesses (Silove et al. 2000; Minas and Diatri 2008).

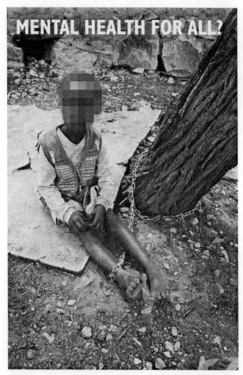

Figure 11 A child with a mental disability chained to tree. © Copyright H. Timmermans, The Global Initiative on Psychiatry.

Barriers to reforms

Throughout history, the mentally ill or disabled have suffered appalling abuse in all societies. Much of this abuse stemmed from a belief that mental illnesses represented a spiritual, moral, or supernatural disturbance which could inspire fear or, at the very least, lack of empathy. The iconic image of Pinel unchaining patients in a Paris asylum in the 18th century is a poignant reminder of the history of mental health care reforms in Western Europe (Figure 12). In some societies, the mentally ill were treated as dissidents—and vice versa—and dispatched to labour camps masquerading as mental hospitals. Although our chapter only contains photographs of human rights violations in developing countries for the explicit reason that we wish to highlight the grave need for community mental health services in these countries, we acknowledge that such violations also occur in psychiatric hospitals in more developed countries despite their much stronger human rights standards. While people may not be in chains or naked, they may be kept in crowded rooms and inhumane conditions. Toilets may be dirty, physical restraints are not an uncommon practice, overuse of sedative medication is not uncommon, and physical health needs of people with mental illnesses are often ignored leading to higher mortality (Prince et al. 2007). The de facto psychiatric system for many chronically mentally ill persons in many countries is the prison system. In this context, the problem of human rights violations of people with mental illnesses represents a global emergency. However, the community psychiatry movement, led by champions from Europe, Australia, and the Americas, has made considerable progress in ensuring that the rights of the mentally ill and disabled are enshrined in public health legislation and practice. The large mental hospitals where some of the worst abuses occurred are now a distant memory in many of

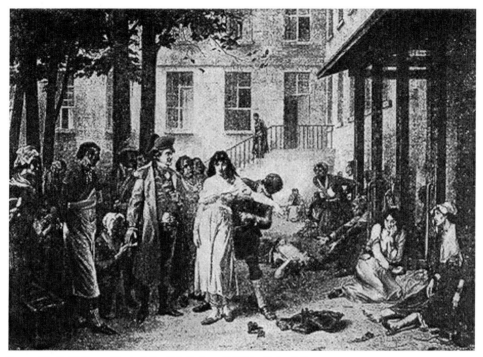

Figure 12 Dr Philippe Pinel at the Salpêtrière, 1795 by Robert Fleury.

those countries, new mental health legislation protects most patients from being coerced into taking treatments, families and patients now receive options of care which include community housing and disability benefits, and consumers receive representation in policy making and advocacy.

Not so for the 85 per cent of the world's people with mental illnesses who live in developing countries. As the images in this article and elsewhere attest, the worst abuses of human rights continue unchecked in many countries. Even for those who may not experience the misfortune to being shackled naked, the vast majority receive no medical care, even though there is now good evidence in support of efficacious and cost-effective treatments for many mental illnesses (Patel et al. 2007). Despite the enormous increase in global health resources in the past decade, the overwhelming majority of initiatives explicitly exclude those with mental illnesses from their generosity. It seems as if the suffering of people with mental illnesses, their indignities and their abuse, is less important to the global health community than the other forms of suffering chosen as a 'priority'. Who makes these decisions, and on what basis, one might ask? We may only speculate about this, but surely stigma—precisely the same type of stigma which afflicted those with HIV/AIDS—must play a central role in explaining the stunning silence in the face of this moral outrage. But, unlike persons with HIV/AIDS whose fortunes in terms of access to care have transformed in the past five years, those with mental illnesses have been severely failed by two critical factors.

The first is the very nature of mental illnesses. Apart from their very wide variety and characteristics, which make a coherent activist campaign difficult, there is the real problem that the severe disorders which are typically associated with the most extreme abuses, are precisely those which impair the ability of persons to articulate their grievances and needs effectively, and which lead to people being marginalized and excluded by their own fellow community members. Thus, the cognitive impairments associated with chronic schizophrenia or severe intellectual disabilities are likely to pose considerable impediments to activism and advocacy by affected persons. Not only is it difficult to advocate from such a weakened position, it is even more difficult to get global celebrities to hug you and share a podium with you. Put bluntly, people with mental illnesses are simply not an attractive human commodity for philanthropy.

The second, and potentially much graver obstacle, is the collusion of the psychiatric and other specialist mental health professional groups with the silence of the global health community. We think that part of this has to do with the nature of all large institutions accommodating a population that for different reasons may be vulnerable. Analyses of the nature of large institutions by Irving Goffman in the 60s or Michel Foucault and Franco Basaglia in the 70s have become classic references showing the intrinsic and perverse risks of all institutions. Another major factor which allows these relics from the past to continue is the lack of resources from governments and donors to build sustainable community mental health systems, offering few alternatives to these institutions. In addition, some psychiatrists may serve their own interests and privileges in adhering to large institutions; indeed, a recent compilation of case studies in psychiatric reform in Latin America which emphasized de-institutionalization identified lack of support and frank opposition from some sections of the psychiatric profession as one of the critical barriers to mental health reforms (Caldas de Almeida 2007). Despite these constraints, there have been a number of inspiring initiatives, led by mental health professionals often working in concert with civil society groups, to reform mental health systems, focusing on improving the rights-perspectives in mental hospitals and strengthening community care options—but these are drops in the ocean of the scandal being played out each day (see Box 1).

Box 1: Addressing human rights of people with mental illnesses through building community mental health care

There are numerous examples of mental health professionals working towards promoting the human rights of people with mental illnesses, often against great odds and with very scarce resources. Just as our selection of photographs is aimed to highlight the crisis of human rights abuses, without claiming to be representative of the quality of care for people with mental illnesses, we have selected four examples of innovative programmes to illustrate that such abuses can be tackled through committed efforts to scale up evidence based, affordable, and community oriented mental health services.

The St Camille Association (<www.amis-st-camille.org>) provides shelter, medical treatment, and follow up to people with mental illnesses, and promotes their social reintegration and rehabilitation through work. Several farms and centres have been created where people with mental illnesses can cultivate manioc and other local products, as well as breed chicken, pigs, and rabbits. The Association currently runs 12 centres in Côte d'Ivoire and Benin and has helped 2500 people, of whom 1800 have successfully reintegrated into their village of origin. The Association currently serves about 70,000 meals a day with the financial help of European non-governmental organizations.

In 1989 the City of Santos in Brazil initiated a radical reform of the city health system. The basic assumption of the reform was that health is not just a right for the citizens but also a duty for government. It was in this framework that the Santos Psychiatric Hospital was brought under the authority of the City government. A group of mental health professionals

> **Box 1: Addressing human rights of people with mental illnesses through building community mental health care** (*continued*)
>
> initiated a radical reform of the inhumane care practices in the hospital. An intensive programme aimed at changing the attitudes of the personnel, decreasing the stigma and discrimination of the patients, and inaugurating an open door policy, led in the end to a progressive shift of psychiatric care from hospital to the community. The rights of the patients were at the centre of every type of intervention and the word '*ciudadania*' (citizenship) became the paradigm of reference of any medical, psychological, and social intervention. The example of Santos became a reference for Brazil and a movement for the rights of people with mental illnesses was initiated and led finally to the Santos innovation becoming federal government policy (Coelho et al. 1996).
>
> The Chain-Free Initiative in the Eastern Mediterranean Region of the WHO (<http://www.who.int/topics/mental_health/en/>) was launched as a pilot project in Afghanistan and Somalia with the overall objective of contributing to the quality of mental health services. This involved combating existing stigma associated with mental illnesses and providing people with mental illnesses with equal opportunities to access basic humanitarian treatment in hospitals, homes, and the environments in which they live. Specific strategies included hospital reform (chain-free hospitals); the enablement of families and communities to provide improved domestic conditions for people with mental illness (chain-free homes); and the development of community care programmes, raising mental health literacy in the community and among health workers, and ensuring that basic rights are monitored and guaranteed (chain-free environment).
>
> In Indonesia the term *pasung* refers to the physical restraint or confinement of 'criminals, crazy and dangerously aggressive people'. (Minas and Diatri 2008) In 2006, the only psychiatrist on Samosir Island in North Sumatra, an island with a population of approximately 130,000, became aware of cases of *pasung* in this small but widely dispersed community. Such individuals were systematically identified as part of a new community mental health initiative. Most of the 15 persons identified suffered from schizophrenia, and had been restrained in iron or wooden shackles for between two to 21 years. More than half of the ill people had had previous psychiatric treatment that had been discontinued, almost always because of the unavailability of affordable treatment. When affordable treatment was offered almost all patients and families accepted the treatment. Despite the fact that many of the people had been in *pasung* for many years, all except two of the 13 who were released were still free at follow-up. (Minas and Diatri 2008)

A call to action

The continuing neglect of the health and human rights needs of people with mental illnesses worldwide, but especially so in developing countries, is one of the greatest public health scandals of our times, which one of has recently described as a 'failure of humanity' (Kleinman 2009), on par with the unacceptably high rates of child and maternal mortality and the lack of access to life-saving treatments for HIV/AIDS until recently. We have drawn attention to this outrage in a recent editorial in a leading psychiatric journal (Patel et al. 2006). More recently, the *Lancet* launched a series of articles on global mental health, culminating in a call for action demanding an evidence- and rights-based approach to addressing mental illnesses (Lancet Global Mental Health Group 2007). The series has led to the new Movement for Global Mental Health, launched on 10 October 2008, which seeks to create a coalition of individuals and institutions representing all those who are concerned about the right for people with mental illnesses to receive evidence-based care (<www.globalmentalhealth.org>) (Patel et al. 2011). The Movement seeks to build a common platform for the diverse stakeholder communities concerned with global mental health, to stand shoulder to shoulder, in solidarity to promote the rights of people with mental illnesses to receive care and live a life with dignity.

We call upon the mental health professional communities and human rights advocates to name and shame those health systems and hospitals which continue to allow such abuses and, at the same time, to celebrate the work of those who have challenged discrimination and promoted the human rights of people with mental illnesses. We exhort donors to invest in the scaling up of innovative community programmes which promote social inclusion and evidence-based treatments. It is obvious to us that a range of strategies will be needed to drive the process of reformation of the mental healthcare system with the goal of protection of human rights of people with mental illnesses, including increasing the coverage of affordable and evidence-based care, especially in rural and underserved areas (Lancet Global Mental Health Group 2007), public health education, legislative reform and enforcement, reform of the culture of institutions, and the training of health professionals (Silove et al. 2000).

Global mental health is now acknowledged as a dynamic and relevant field of global health (Patel and Prince 2010). This is an opportune time to act. We call upon our colleagues in the global and mental health professions to make the human rights of people with mental illnesses the most important priority for mental health care reform globally; until such abuses are not addressed comprehensively, the stigma against people with mental illnesses and, indeed, against the mental health professions themselves, will not be eradicated.

Acknowledgements

We are grateful to Alex Cohen, Diana Samarasan, RS Murthy, Michael Schwartz, and anonymous reviewers for comments on an earlier draft of this article. We are also grateful to the individual photographers and agencies who made their photos available for use in this article at no charge: HealthNet TPO (Peter Ventvogel), the World Health Organization, and the Global Initiative of Psychiatry (photographer Harrie Timmermans). We are grateful to Agence France Presse for discounting the purchase of their photos.

References

Caldas De Almeida, JM (2007) 'What can we learn from mental health services reform in Latin America & the Caribbean?', in JM Caldas De Almeida and A Cohen (eds) *Innovative mental health services in Latin America and the Caribbean.* Washington, DC: Pan American Health Organization, iv–xi.

Coelho, F, Campos, B, Maierovitch, C, and Henriques, P (1996) *Contra a mare à Beira-Mar: A experiencia do Sistema Unico de Saude em Santos.* Sao Paulo: Editora Pagina Aberta Ltda.

Kleinman, A (2009) 'Global mental health: a failure of humanity', *The Lancet,* 374, 603–4.

Kleinman, A and Kleinman, J (1996) 'The appeal of experience, the dismay of images: Cultural appropriations of suffering in our times', *Daedalus Journal of the American Academy of Arts and Sciences,* 125, 1–23.

Lancet Global Mental Health Group (2007) 'Scaling up services for mental illnesses—a call for action', *The Lancet,* 370, 1241–52.

Minas, H and Diatri, H (2008) 'Pasung: Physical restraint and confinement of the mentally ill in the community', *International Journal of the Mental Health Systems,* 2, 8.

Murthy, P and Sekar, K (2008) 'A decade after the NHRC quality assurance initiative: current status of government psychiatric hospitals in India', in D Nagaraja and P Murthy (eds.) *Mental Health Care and Human Rights.* Bangalore: National Human Rights Commission and NIMHANS, 101–141.

National Human Rights Commission (1999) *Quality Assurance in Mental Health*. New Delhi: NHRC.

Patel, V, Araya, R, Chatterjee, S, Chisholm, D, Cohen, A, De Silva, M, Hosman, C, Mcguire, H, Rojas, G, and Van Ommeren, M (2007) 'Treatment and prevention of mental illnesses in low-income and middle-income countries', *The Lancet*, 370, 991–1005.

Patel, V, Collins, PY, Copeland, J, Kakuma, R, Katontoka, S, Lamichhane, J, Naik, S, and Skeen, S (2011) 'The movement for global mental health', *British Journal of Psychiatry*, 198, 88–90.

Patel, V, Kleinman, A, and Saraceno, B (2006) 'Beyond evidence: the moral case for international mental health', *American Journal of Psychiatry*, 163, 1312–5.

Patel, V and Prince, M (2010) 'Global Mental Health: a new global health field comes of age', *JAMA*, 303, 1976–7.

Prince, M, Patel, Saxena, S, Maj, M, Maselko, J, Phillips, MR, and Rahman, A (2007) 'No health without mental health', *The Lancet*, 370, 859–77.

Sember, R (2003) 'Images in public health', *American Journal of Public Health*, 93, 1626–9.

Silove, D, Ekblad, S, and Mollica, R (2000) 'The rights of the severely mentally ill in post-conflict societies', *The Lancet*, 355, 1548–9.

Sontag, S (2003) *Regarding the pain of others*. New York: Farrar, Strauss & Giroux.

Commentary 5

Detained, Diagnosed, and Discharged

Human Rights and the Lived Experience of Mental Illness in New South Wales, Australia

Meg Smith

In most jurisdictions, detention in hospital on health grounds applies to people who have a contagious infection or who have a mental illness. In both instances, the aim of detention is, first, to protect the public. Management of the illness or the rights of the person are secondary.

Voluntary admission to psychiatric care implies that you have a problem and that you wish to seek treatment for that problem. My first admission to a psychiatric hospital was voluntary and was the longest—three months. It was voluntary only in that I agreed to stay there. Once I had admitted myself to the hospital I really did not have many options. I was, in effect, homeless, unemployed, and alone in a strange city. I had run out of options to cope with an increasingly severe episode of depressive illness. Being a psychiatric patient at least put a roof over my head and I got three meals a day. But in the absence of discharge planning or any support to help me to re-establish myself in the community I was unable to leave the hospital. The criteria for discharge seemed to be to get well enough to organize and plan one's own discharge.

The second admission was during an acute psychotic episode. I started off as a voluntary patient when my partner took me to the hospital after seven weeks of psychosis. I was made an involuntary patient after I walked out because I didn't understand what the hospital was, how it could help me, and why I had to stay there. The committal process was under the 1958 NSW Mental Health Act. You were mentally ill if you had a mental illness. This was not defined in the legislation and it was up to the admitting psychiatrist to make the diagnosis. The diagnosis was manic phase of manic-depressive psychosis and I was automatically given a six-month order. In 1981 this meant compulsory treatment and detention against my will until the hospital decided I was well enough to be discharged. There were no rights that I was to be protected from assault or exploitation or neglect in the hospital. I walked out of the hospital after another patient assaulted me. The assault was not recorded in my hospital file. Nor were the incidents of over-medication and serious side effects that I had experienced. The committal to care in a psychiatric institution assumed that care and treatment would be provided. It did not guarantee that such care and treatment would be provided. Committal also meant that my assets and financial affairs were put under the Office of the Protective Commissioner without any investigation into my circumstances with my family or my employment or assets. There were no clear guidelines or processes about how to regain control of my financial affairs once I was discharged from hospital.

1981 in Australia was an interesting time to become a psychiatric patient. The magistrate before whom I appeared during this stay in hospital was one of the legal advocates who challenged the adequacy of the mental health legislation and the arbitrary way in which hospital staff made many people involuntary patients. At the time, mental health staff did not have to provide evidence of mental illness or what treatment was proposed to the magistrate. Relatives and carers were not included in the process of admission and discharge. Doctors and mental health staff who had made the recommendation to detain the person did not attend the hearings. There was no-one at the magistrate's hearing to legally represent the person or to offer alternative ways of managing the circumstances of the person. The six-month involuntary detention order I received was standard at that time and was often not necessary—many patients recovered their capacity to understand and consent to medical treatment long before the six-month period elapsed.

By the late 1970s, a social movement had begun around the issues of psychiatric care. A number of inquiries and reports highlighted the urgent need for change in psychiatric services in NSW. These reports included: the inquiry chaired by David Richmond in 1983; the Ministerial Implementation Committee chaired by William Barclay in 1988; the Steering Committee on Mental Health chaired by Ann Deveson, 1988; the Report of the Mental Health Services Policy Consultancy by Peter Eisen and Kevin Wolfenden to the Australian Health Ministers' Advisory Council in 1988; and the Royal Commission into Deep Sleep Therapy and Mental Health Services chaired by Justice Slattery, 1991. All identified serious issues in the care of people living with mental illness and the inadequacies of a psychiatric system based on large institutions to house patients indefinitely rather than resources to enable recovery in the community.

The two hospital admissions I experienced were very different. The first was voluntary to a clinic which had no more than 25 patients and which took people with 'neurotic' or 'personality' disorders. In other words, articulate people who could gain insight into their disorder and respond to therapy that would change their thoughts, feelings, and attitudes. All thoughts, feelings, and attitudes were scrutinized in group therapy—sexual, moral, philosophical, religious, and political, as well as the emotional. I came away from the experience feeling that my whole personality was sick and that there was no hope for recovery. The people interviewed by McGuinness and Wadsworth (1991) at Royal Park Hospital reported similar experiences: they had come to hospital to understand what was happening to them. Instead, they found themselves being given drugs with little or no explanation about how the drugs could help. Most came away from the experience traumatized by the hospital experience and with little or no understanding of the problems that had brought them to the hospital in the first place (McGuinness and Wadsworth 1991).

The freedom to manage one's financial affairs

Since the 1878 Lunacy Act in New South Wales, the financial affairs of the mentally infirm were committed to the Master of Lunacy. The Lunacy Act 'empowered the Master to sell or otherwise dispose of the property of an insane person to meet the cost of his care, the maintenance of his dependants or payment of his debts or to make other arrangements for the management of his property'. This office continued until 1972 when the Office of the Protective Commissioner was established to deal with the estates of people committed as lunatics. While ostensibly this was to protect the person from financial exploitation, the reason was often to ensure that the person's assets could be used to pay for the hospital fees. Kate Millett draws the analogy that the assets of involuntary patients, like Jews in Germany during the Holocaust, were used by the state to pay for their detention and oppression (Millett 1990, 1994). In Australia, Medicare rebates for psychiatric care were not introduced until after my second admission to psychiatric hospital. For both of my admissions I got a number of free days of hospital but after that I had to pay—or if I could not afford to pay, my family would pay.

By 1990, the automatic process of taking away a patient's financial independence was also being challenged. The law had been changed to require the process of taking away one's financial independence during episodes of mental illness to include real risk of financial exploitation. Lifestyle choices and management of one's finances that were at odds with societal norms could therefore not be used to take away a person's financial independence.

Between 1958 and 1983 when the Act was repealed, many psychiatric 'diagnoses' were used to admit people with a range of social and emotional issues as well as victims of economic circumstances and those who professed unpopular moral, religious, or political ideologies. During my first admission to a psychiatric unit in 1972 about half of the patients were women and young people who were victims of domestic violence and/or sexual abuse. One quarter of the patients were people addicted to alcohol or other drugs who were there for rehabilitation or by court order as an alternative to prison. The few remaining patients were young people like me who were experiencing an acute episode of mental ill health.

It was an interesting time to have a mental illness in the early 1970s when I had my first contact with the world of psychiatry. In the 1970s in NSW, consumer movements in health and psychiatry began to challenge the quality of treatments in psychiatry and the real outcomes for victims of mental illness. Early writings of the women's movement offered a critical analysis of the medicalization of emotional, economic, and mental health issues (Hanisch 1969; Matthews 1984).

Were my human rights abused? In effect—yes. The right to one's own thoughts, the right to one's own philosophy of life, and the right to assert one's sense of self. I am not my mental illness. My symptoms of mental ill health are not necessarily caused by my lifestyle, my political, religious, or ethical beliefs, or my sexual identity.

From the hospital to the community

Community care instead of hospital treatment of people with mental illness had begun to remove some of the stigma of admission to a mental hospital. Community health centres were established in the mid 1970s and these eventually took on the role of support and care for people disabled by mental illness who were living in the community. Severe mental illnesses, such as manic depressive illness (now known as bipolar disorder) and schizophrenia, were starting to be seen as biochemically based and, more importantly, treatable disorders from which one could recover. The rights of people affected by mental illness to appropriate care and treatment were highlighted in a number of inquiries into mental health legislation, the operation of psychiatric facilities, access to services for people with disabilities, and the rights of people detained under mental health legislation (Richmond 1983; Slattery 1991).

Mental illness or life sickness?

The issues of human rights in mental health care were beginning to be discussed in the 1970s when I completed my clinical psychology training. Rosenhan and other community psychologists were questioning the authority of mental health professionals to determine who was mentally ill and the validity of psychiatric diagnosis and compulsory psychiatric treatment (Rosenhan 1973; Rappaport and Seidman 1986). Students in my postgraduate psychology class admitted themselves to psychiatric hospitals with fictitious symptoms of 'mental illness' and then observed what happened when they behaved normally. I did not do this class exercise because I got academic credit for having been a real psychiatric patient. But, having been a real psychiatric patient, I was intrigued by the experiences of my fellow students. I had experienced much scrutiny of my behaviour, feelings, and attitudes during my first hospital admission. Most of it, I inferred or was told, was evidence of my sickness. My fellow students, in similar situations and behaving as they normally would, were also told that their behaviour, attitudes, and feelings were evidence of sickness. The experiences matched those of Rosenhan's pseudo patients in his classic 1973 study (Rosenhan 1973). A patient who is taking notes, approaching staff to talk, engaging with other patients, or questioning hospital rules was analysed and the behaviour interpreted in ways that were negative—demonstrating paranoia, challenging authority, being intrusive (Rosenhan 1973). Being discharged from hospital did not mean having a clean bill of health. Discharge summaries included terms such as 'schizophrenia in remission', 'resolution of manic phase of manic depressive illness', or 'personality disorder'. The effect of the experience on my fellow students was profound. Most found it a traumatizing experience. The few days they spent on a ward as a patient was stressful and dehumanizing. Being clinical psychology students, they expected to receive counselling or at least some individual counselling. It most cases this was brief or did not happen in the first few days after admission.

For me, coming to terms with living with a mental illness has also meant coming to terms with having an illness that has the potential to leave me subject to treatment against my will by the state. Contagious diseases and mental illness are the only medical conditions that can be treated involuntarily by the state. Containment of people with contagious diseases protects others and prevents the spread of the infection. The containment of people with mental illness serves two functions: to protect the community or the person from harm and to treat the illness if the person cannot make his or her own decisions about care and treatment. In both situations, the priority has been to protect the community from the behaviour of the person.

Chelmsford and the beginnings of change

Chelmsford Hospital in NSW was a private hospital where those who could afford it could go as a voluntary patient to recover from episodes of mental ill health. By the time Chelmsford was investigated over its psychiatric care, over thirty people had died and many others were left with permanent brain damage from the treatments administered at the hospital.

The Chelmsford Hospital tragedy precipitated a wide-ranging scrutiny of the mental health system in NSW. The Chelmsford patients were like me in many ways. We had admitted ourselves voluntarily to a clinic to get help for depression or anxiety or other mental health issues. I got psychoanalytic group treatment. The Chelmsford patients got electroconvulsive treatment and deep sleep therapy induced by barbiturates and other psychotropic drugs. Individual treatment plans and a cooperative approach to therapy was not available in most treatment regimes. The diagnosis determined the treatment not the individual circumstances of the person. In the case of Chelmsford, a psychologist determined that the person was 'depressed' and needed deep sleep therapy (Slattery 1991).

Is there a better way to work with people who are living with a mental illness?

No matter what careful thought goes into legislation, the lived experience of people with mental illness is linked to social, economic, and community circumstances. Mental states cannot be seen separately from the society in which one lives. In NSW, the 1878 Lunacy Act gave doctors more power in determining 'lunacy' and management of people in asylums. Although as mentioned above, the Master of Lunacy was established to determine protection of the detained person's property and estate and to collect fees for the care of detained persons, the main aim of the legislation was to manage those judged to be lunatic and to remove them from public hospitals and prisons.

One laudable aim of current mental health legislation is to minimize the effects of mental illness and treatment on the lives of people living with mental illness. However, definitions of mental illness are often linked only indirectly to social and economic circumstances. Treatment of mental illness—particularly compulsory treatment—is more often linked to psychological processes such as lack of insight or denial (Quadrio 1988). Such psychological rationales for detention and involuntary treatment have replaced the moral guidelines of the early lunacy laws which institutionalized the destitute, the victims of economic circumstance, and those who failed to conform to societal standards of behaviour (Matthews 1984).

The slowness of systems to change can never keep up with new discoveries in medical science and social factors. The 1958 Act in NSW became law just before the phenothiazine tranquillisers and new antidepressant drugs became widespread in psychiatric hospitals in the Western world. The benign intent of the 1958 Act to care for people in medical clinics under the supervision of medical staff was a radical departure from the 1878 Lunacy Act that it replaced. The assumption was that medical staff would help not harm patients under their care and that medical treatment was safe. The Chelmsford tragedy illustrates how good intentions can result in tragedy where vulnerable people are exposed to unregulated power structures, lack of supervision of medical staff, and treatments not based on evidence that they work (Slattery 1991).

Guardianship legislation: disability, impairment, and capacity

The movement to reform mental health legislation and service delivery in NSW also examined the issues for people with developmental disability and dementia. The inquiry into mental health services chaired by David Richmond in 1983 examined the population of psychiatric hospitals in NSW and found that there were many people who were inappropriately placed in psychiatric institutions (Richmond 1983). Richmond identified five groups that needed very different services: people with acute mental illness; people with chronic mental illness; people with developmental disability; people with alcohol or other drug problems; and people with dementia. In many cases, these groups of people were treated inappropriately with psychotropic drugs and had little or no access to community care and support if they were discharged from psychiatric institutions.

Disability, handicap, impairment, incapacity, and need

People with disabilities began to lobby about their rights and access to community services in the 1970s and early 1980s. The movement was led by people with sensory disabilities and physical disabilities who perceived themselves as people first and their disability as peripheral to their sense of identity. They did not see that their disability should interfere with their rights as citizens and access to community resources, employment, protection against discrimination, and social acceptance. They were articulate and effective lobbyists. The Anti Discrimination Act of 1976 did not include discrimination against people with physical or intellectual disability until 1981. However, when I enquired about whether or not it included mental illness after I was employed as a lecturer at the Milperra College of Advanced Education in 1982, the legislation did not include mental illness. The only way I could take action about discrimination in employment was to say that I had an intellectual disability. It was not until 1991 that the Commonwealth Disability Discrimination Act included mental illness and other brain impairments. The development of legislative frameworks for people living with a disability occurred in parallel with the reform of mental health legislation in the 1980s and 1990s. The impetus for the reforms came largely from incentives from the Australian government. Funding by the Australian government for disability services prompted mental health reform groups to redefine mental illness as 'psychiatric disability' in order to gain the benefits of funding for rehabilitation, supported employment, accommodation, and support programmes for people living with mental illness.

While this was a political ploy to access government funding for psychiatric care, the change in focus from mental illness to disability opened up changes in thinking about the place of people living with mental illness in the community. I found myself on committees with other people with a disability who did not share the shattered identity and community dislocation of people with mental illness. I became a community member of the Guardianship Board when it commenced in 1989. The guardianship legislation provided a number of protections for people with a disability. Having a disability did not necessarily mean that a person needed any intervention. A guardian could only be appointed for a person with a disability if, because of the disability, a person had the incapacity to make decisions about their lives and then only if there was a decision that needed to be made. The guardian, if appointed, could not coerce the person and had to take into account the stated wishes of the person.

But what about people with mental illness who needed to be coerced and given treatment against their will in some situations? Debate about the legislative changes needed for people with disability and people with mental illness began to diverge. The 1989 Guardianship Act in NSW included provisions about the rights of a person with a disability: the wishes of the person needed to be considered; the order made had to be the least restrictive option; mediation was offered before the hearing to determine if informal arrangements could solve the issues before an order was made. The guardian, if appointed, could advocate on behalf of the person, and refuse medical treatment or services if this was considered not in the best interests of the person. The new Mental Health Act of 1990 did include the option of 'least restrictive' alternative. Legal representation was now required at hearings at which involuntary treatment was being considered. The definition of mental illness was restricted to treatable mental illnesses—in effect, schizophrenia, depressive illness, and bipolar disorder. Being 'mentally ill' under this definition was not enough to be committed to involuntary care. There had to be a danger to the person or to other people.

But many people who were victims of mental illness did not pose a danger to themselves or other people. They were however at risk from social factors. Advocacy groups such as The Depressive and Manic Depressive Association in NSW lobbied for 'damage to reputation' to be included in this section, arguing that the personal and social consequences of untreated manic illness could lead to loss of employment, social relationships and social status, and self esteem. The treatment proposed by the hospital had to be a programme that would lead to recovery from the episode of mental illness.

Would I admit myself to a psychiatric unit now given all the social and legislative changes that have occurred since my last admission in the 1980s? As a person living with a mental illness, I do have more rights now than I had in 1980. The range of services is much broader. The protections against illegal detention and negligent treatment are much stronger. I am much more informed about what can happen during an episode of mental ill health and can access effective treatment much more quickly.

But there will always be people experiencing a first serious episode of mental ill health who do not have the personal resources that I have built over the years. In the area of mental health there will always be a need for strong advocates and vigilance about the current treatments and services that are offered to people experiencing mental ill health. Legislating for human rights is only part of the solution. Empowering people through education, advocacy, and support will always be an essential part of ensuring that the human rights of people living with mental ill health are protected.

References

Andrews, G, Hall, W, Teeson, M, and Henderson, S (1999) *The Mental Health of Australians.* Canberra: Mental Health Branch, Commonwealth Department of Health and Aged Care.

Eisen, P, Wolfenden, K, Australia Department of Community Services and Health, and Australian Health Ministers' Advisory Council (1988) *A National mental health services policy: report of the Consultancy to advise Commonwealth, State and Territory health ministers*: Canberra: Dept. of Community Services and Health and Australian Health Ministers' Advisory Council.

Errington, M (1987) '"Mental illness" in Australian legislation', *Australian Law Journal*, 61, 182–91.

Hanisch, C (1969) 'The Personal is Political', in *The Redstockings Collection: Feminist Revolution*, March 1969, 204–205.

Joyce, PR (1987) 'Changing trends in first admissions and readmissions for mania and schizophrenia in New Zealand, 1974–1984', *Australian and New Zealand Journal of Psychiatry*, 21, 82–86.

Matthews, JJ (1984) *Good and mad women: the historical construction of femininity in twentieth-century Australia*. Sydney: George Allen and Unwin.

McGuinness, M and Wadsworth, Y (1991) *Understanding, Anytime—A consumer evaluation of an acute psychiatric hospital*. Melbourne, Victoria: Victorian Mental Illness Awareness Council.

Millett, K (1990) *The Loony Bin Trip*. New York: Simon and Schuster.

Millett, K (1994) *The Politics of Cruelty: An Essay on the Literature of Political Imprisonment*. New York: W.W Norton & Co.

Quadrio, C (1988) 'Re-medicalisation and regression in psychiatry', *Australian and New Zealand Journal of Psychiatry*, 22, 242–45.

Rappaport, J and Seidman, E (1986) *Self help and serious psychopathology*. Preliminary and Interim Report #NIMH37390. Urbana-Champaign: University of Illinois.

Richmond, D (1983) *Inquiry into health services for the psychiatrically ill and developmentally disabled: Summary of recommendations*. Sydney: Health Commission NSW.

Rosenhan, DL (1973) 'On Being Sane in Insane Places', *Science*, New Series, 179(4070), 250–58.

Slattery, J (1991) *Report to the NSW Government: Report of the Royal Commission into Deep Sleep Therapy and the Former Chelmsford Private Hospital*. Sydney: Parliament of NSW.

Part 3

Some Vulnerable Groups

This section, while not purporting to be comprehensive, concerns a range of vulnerable groups.

Sarah Mares and Jon Jureidini review the impact of harsh policies of deterrence, and in particular indefinite mandatory detention, on asylum seekers including children arriving in Australia from 2000 until late 2007. They consider the ethical and human rights implications of policies which wilfully exposed children to abuse and neglect and negative developmental and mental health outcomes. They undertake an examination of various consequentialist arguments that seek to justify indefinite mandatory detention or contest it. They also consider the ethical demands on health professionals who assess and attempt to treat children and their families who are harmed by immigration policy and practice.

Zachary Steel, Catherine R. Bateman Steel, and Derrick Silove recapitulate the history of advances in understanding trauma (in which PTSD was central), concurrent with advances in human rights, especially regarding the issue of torture. The fusion of human rights and mental health concerns saw the advent of trauma-focused psychiatric epidemiology, with Western governments as willing funders of services for asylum-seekers. However, this consensus ended from the early 1990s, when governments aimed at stemming refugee flows by adopting new policies of deterrence: for example restricting the rights to work, welfare, housing, healthcare, and legal support for those gaining entry to host countries. These policies violate asylum-seekers' civil-political rights (through mandatory detention, inappropriate decision outcomes based on systematic misreading of evidence etc) and exclude them from economic and socio-cultural rights, including those to which states are often signatories. Those working with asylum-seekers observe the mental health consequences. The authors also highlight debates about how well Western based trauma models account for and address cultural and indigenous mental health issues and rights, and how to enable these explanatory approaches to work together in research and practice.

In the light of the relevant conventions and legislation, Beverley Raphael and colleagues survey the impact of rights violations and failure of rights instruments on the mental health of women in general and that of women with mental disorders and their carers in particular. Violence and abuse, health and sexuality, roles, ethnicity, indigenous status, and the situations and needs of female children are considered. The preponderance and antecedents of post-traumatic stress, anxiety, depression and eating disorders among women, women's particular vulnerabilities if suffering from schizophrenia and other psychoses, the challenges of substance abuse problems and co-morbidities, and the problems of misdiagnosis, stigma, and resultant lost opportunities for prevention and treatment, are all crucially related to rights. The authors raise broad questions about how to educate and effect broad cultural change for women.

While acknowledging other forms of trafficking, Kathleen Maltzahn and Louella Villadiego use trafficked women's firsthand accounts to illuminate the plight of women trafficked for prostitution. They consider the United Nations 2000 protocol against trafficking, noting the resurgence of concern in conjunction with growing attention to women's rights internationally, and therefore pressure to extend rights into what had been hitherto regarded as the 'private' sphere. They note the linkage to gender-based violence, and the linkage to and lineage with the ancient practice of slavery. The horrors encountered and their impacts on these women's physical and mental health are outlined. The debate about links of trafficking to prostitution is also reviewed, and the human rights violations inherent in both. The importance of not suggesting that these women are the sum of their negative experiences or that they are crippled by the violence is vital. Growing awareness of human rights frameworks, trafficking, prostitution, and the experiences of these women, is crucial to change. Providing specific information from Turkey about women's mental health and human rights, Şahika Yüksel, Dilek Cindoğlu, and Ufuk Sezgin discuss the social regulation, coercion, and control of women's sexualities (including non-mainstream sexualities), physical and sexual violence against women and consequent trauma-related disorders, and the rights-related context for and implications of these violations. They consider sexual abuse, partner and marital rape, date rape, and honour killings as internationally neglected crimes and human rights violations. The authors also tackle rights and mental health issues associated with sexual violence in war, sexual torture, sexual trafficking, and sexual health STDs. They foreshadow the need for substantial operational and legal measures to be undertaken through national and supra-national bodies to address some of these problems.

Ernest Hunter, Helen Milroy, Ngiare Brown, and Tom Calma address indigenous mental health and rights particularly in Australia, where wealth and advantage fail to overcome escalating social problems and profound disadvantage on all parameters. Remembering the historical and international quest for indigenous rights and the 'Great Australian Silence' that until recently erased indigenous Australians from wider Australian consciousness, the authors delineate the struggle for their rights. Reforming and repealing racist or discriminatory legislation without challenging barriers to participation (education, employment, political representation) has reinforced cultural exclusion. Recently, privileging certain rights ('law and order' in Northern Territory Indigenous communities) undermined other rights: the rule of law and equity with other Australians. Paternalism and ambivalence produced misguided proposals. Globally, health rights, non-discrimination, equality, and other rights are interdependent. 'Risk factors' are inadequate and medical solutions and treatment programmes do not suffice: rather, causal risk processes need analysis and response using holistic approaches to health and human rights frameworks. Indigenous minorities are often invisible: ensuring indigenous agency is imperative to any lasting gains. Racism in society, institutions and sectors promulgating policy—including health—needs identification and action. Bridging the gap between policy and implementation requires setting commitments in achievable time frames, matched with necessary funds and programme support.

Ian Hall and Evan Yacoub offer a brief historical account of human rights violations experienced by people with intellectual disabilities, including segregation, sterilization, and euthanasia. With reference to the UK and the European Convention on Human Rights, they observe how diagnostic overshadowing and problems with accessing health care diminish the right to life, and the prohibition of torture and degrading treatment is not infrequently breached through excessive restraint, punishment, and/or abuse, sometimes for years. Those accused of offences may be denied a fair trial while victims of crime and abuse are also at a disadvantage. Children may be denied access to parents and families, parents denied their children and/or support with raising them, and adolescents and adults denied the right to a sexual life and to procreate. Problems with ignorance, prejudice, and discrimination remain widespread. Countering such violations are recent inclusive policy developments, including normalization and social role valorization. Potential solutions include enshrining the Convention on the Rights of Persons with Disabilities (CRPD) into national law, reforming national law to cover private providers, developing specific standards and individualizing support (including financial support) across settings, maximizing capacity and avoiding overly risk-averse approaches to key decisions, exposing abuses, and improving professional standards and training.

Myron Belfer and Diana Samarasan note that the contract model of Western justice produces outliers, including people with severe disabilities and children with disabilities. Noting the increasing proportion of children with disabilities, they comment how although children's needs, development, and rights have been appreciated more clearly in recent history, the potential of children with disabilities continues to be ignored and they are often regarded as sources of shame or blame. Often institutionalized, isolated, and exploited, the approach to their clinical care is frequently conceived on a deficit model rather than one which emphasizes and enables participation. The authors note the direction within the WHO's International Classification of Impairments, Disabilities and Handicaps, the UN Convention of the Rights of the Child, and particularly the UN CRPD, to progressively mandate the participation of people (including children) with disabilities. They examine two prominent examples of initiatives to address the lack of voice for the rights of children with disabilities: the Guardianship Councils in Brazil and the Social Charter of the European Union. Child health and related clinicians at all levels of training should embrace a paradigm shift towards inclusion of children with disabilities.

In the light of the question 'What constitutes a life worth living as an ageing member of our society?' and related human rights frameworks for older persons, Carmelle Peisah, Henry Brodaty, and Nick O'Neill note the impacts of ageism and discrimination, disability and dependency, and mental disorders. They consider the challenge of realizing rights for disabled, marginalized, and/ or mentally ill older people. They reflect on the domains of independence/autonomy, safety and dignity, and care. Independence/autonomy is examined in relation to healthcare (e.g. obtaining consent for psychotropic drug use), personal care and accommodation, relationships and sexuality, and end of life decisions. Safety and dignity includes freedom from all types of abuse, especially in residential settings and in these settings' use of physical and chemical restraints for mentally ill and dementing older people. Care includes the right to health and community care (both often constrained by family and community resources), and is complicated by questions about the person's decision-making capacity. The involuntary detention and care of older people outside mental health settings is a vexed issue. The impact of the CRPD for older people with mental disorders is yet to be seen.

Louise Newman explores how psychiatry through classifications and treatments has regarded essentialist, fixed, conformist understandings of gender roles and heteronormative sexual preference as intrinsic to mental health: sexual minorities are therefore deemed to require treatment. Thus biology determines psychology and social gender roles, rather than culture and meaning having a role in shaping gender identity and sexual orientation. The chapter especially tracks psychiatry, the 'natural gender' account, and 'Gender Identity Disorder'. While diverse non-Western cultures accept sex roles and fluid gender identity, Western culture tolerates sexual ambiguity less well. Where sex reassignment (only to the opposite sex) surgery is available, the applicant's mental health and competency is assessed and the professional regulates treatment access. Individuals with gender dysphoria and their loved ones suffer considerable psychosocial and mental health consequences. Pressures to conform and treat intensely affect families, schools, and society, reassignment treatments are scarce, (mental) health professionals often are anxious and have negative attitudes, and services remain non-specific and culturally unaware. Persecution remains widespread internationally. Yet gender expression and sexuality are fundamental in international rights conventions. Newman promotes social reform encompassing increasing tolerance of gender diversity, culturally competent health services, and inclusive medicine that facilitates understanding and insight for self-determination.

Adrian Carter and Wayne Hall discuss the competing aims of addiction policies, balancing user freedoms, user obligations not to harm, and state obligations to protect others from harms. Given strong social disapproval, the overlaps with criminality and the need to protect society, treating debilitating and chronic addictions often receives a low priority. Assessing rights violations therefore depends on one's viewpoint: is addiction a wilful, immoral act requiring full responsibility, or a mental illness requiring treatment? Against punitive and total abstinence responses, the authors advocate medical treatment (based on sufferers' marginality and difficulty with accessing healthcare), maintenance therapies, harm minimization and treatment for other conditions (e.g. HIV), based on the risk to health and life of not doing so. They discuss rights in prisons and during pregnancy, when treating under legal coercion, when undertaking unevaluated, invasive and risky treatments, for co-morbid populations, and in decriminalizing currently illicit drugs for adult use. States largely ignore such rights, particularly within criminal populations, despite clear UN and WHO guidelines. Human rights law suggests the treatment of addiction should be recognized as a health issue, not simply a criminal justice one, and should not remove rights (e.g. liberty) without out due legal process.

In their commentary, Lakshmi Vijayakumar and Lillian Craig Harris discuss the size of the problem of suicide, its underreporting, the stigma of suicide, and ambivalence towards it. They note areas of particular vulnerability and concern, including refugees, prisoners, arranged marriages and 'love failure', the frequency of suicide pacts especially in the developing world, domestic violence, and child sexual abuse. The authors speak about the need for social change, the need for services, and an increasing role for the voices of suicide attempt survivors and families of those who have died, in advocating for new legal and educational remedies to enhance suicide prevention. They emphasize that suicide prevention is everyone's business.

Chapter 19

Civilian Populations Affected by Conflict and Displacement

Mental Health and the Human Rights Imperative

Zachary Steel, Catherine R. Bateman Steel, and Derrick Silove

The mental health impact of trauma on conflict affected societies is now an issue of major concern to the global community. Mental health professionals have played a prominent role in this, drawing in particular on the modern model of traumatic stress (Steel et al. 2009). There has been a convergence between research documenting the mental health effects of organized violence and the establishment of clinical services for traumatic stress. The genesis of much of the recent international work on conflict and mental health stems from the early work by mental health professionals in the global rights-based campaign to abolish torture and other forms of abuse. As a consequence, dedicated centres to provide care for survivors of political violence have been established in most high income countries (HICs) with initiatives by international aid organizations to develop psychosocial programmes to address mental health concerns in conflict-affected countries. In all these endeavours, a model of traumatic stress coalescing around the psychiatric diagnosis of post-traumatic stress disorder (American Psychiatric Association 1980) become a pivotal tool to advocate for both the mental health needs of affected populations and the upholding of human rights.

These developments have sparked debate about the potential dangers of extending Western notions of trauma to diverse cultural contexts. Critics have warned of the 'medicalization' of experiences that are quintessentially human rights violations; and of the risk to local cultural healing mechanisms when the trauma model is extended beyond the context in which it was first developed (Breslau 2005; Kleinman 1995). Hence, a rights-based understanding of the development of mental health initiatives and research with displaced and conflict-affected populations could provide an important framework to critically appraise the contribution of mental health professionals to this field, to understand the controversies that have arisen about the trauma model, and to provide a heuristic model in order to advance work in this area.

Mental health and human rights

Violent conflict, mental health, and civil and political rights

The modern trauma model, in which post-traumatic stress disorder (PTSD) was central, emerged during a period when there were major advances at the international level in the human rights field, particularly in the promotion of civil and political or first generation rights that restrain the power of the state over the individual. Specifically, the two fields converged in relation to the issue of torture. From a mental health perspective, there was increased momentum in the late 1970s to document the psychiatric consequences of torture. In parallel, and drawing on these mental health concerns, the UN established the Declaration on the Protection of All Persons from Torture in 1975, which explicitly prohibited the use of this practice under any circumstances, an instrument that prepared the way to the ratification of the UN Convention Against Torture in 1984. During this period, the World Medical Association adopted the Declaration of Tokyo (1975) explicitly proscribing doctors from participating in torture.

Systematic documentation of the medical and psychological consequences of torture and forced displacement began soon after the Declaration in 1975 (Amnesty International 1977). Reports of the psychological effects of torture appeared in the psychiatric literature in the late 1970s with a survey of available data being published by the Danish Medical Group in 1980 (Rasmussen and Lunde 1980). The Indochinese conflict and the concurrent political instability in South and Latin America during the mid to late 1970s proved to be historical watersheds in this movement. Allodi's work with Latin American refugees in Toronto gave further momentum to combining a focus on human rights documentation with research and clinical care in the mental health field (Allodi 1979; Allodi and Rojas 1985; Allodi 1980). Threats to their own safety in Chile obliged Lira and Weinstein to adopt pseudonyms when publishing their seminal work describing the effectiveness of testimony therapy offered to torture survivors in that country (Cienfuegos and Monelli 1983). Amongst Indochinese refugees, Murphy (1977) identified high levels of war related mental health problems in a sample of 102 displaced Vietnamese in Binh Duong Province in 1972. The author noted that the psychological damage tended to be persistent, with evidence that evacuees continued to manifest psychological symptoms five years subsequent to the original survey.

The introduction of PTSD in the American Psychiatric Association's Diagnostic and Statistical Manual of Mental Disorders, 3rd ed. (DSM-III) (American Psychiatric Association 1980) provided a psychiatric focus for researchers and clinicians working with trauma survivors. In relation to the human rights field, the adoption of PTSD provided a tool to identify the psychological consequences associated with exposure to human rights abuse and organized violence. By the mid 1980s, detailed descriptions of the post-traumatic symptom presentations of Indochinese refugees began to appear in the literature based particularly on the experiences of Cambodian survivors of the Pol Pot genocide (Kinzie et al. 1984; Mollica et al. 1987). In parallel, clinical surveys amongst torture survivors supported the expectation that PTSD-like syndromes followed exposure to extreme stress across diverse cultural and ethnic backgrounds (Goldfeld et al. 1988; Petersen 1989; Weisaeth 1989).

This early research established what Miller and colleagues (2006a) subsequently have identified as a model of 'trauma-focused psychiatric epidemiology', a framework that has come to dominate the mental health field in the area of mass conflict, human rights abuse, and displacement. This fusion of human rights and mental health concerns transformed notions of trauma, PTSD, and other post-traumatic psychiatric outcomes such as depression, beyond the boundaries of psychiatry to incorporate a broader humanitarian arena (Breslau 2004). Steel and colleagues (2009) have undertaken a comprehensive review of the field, identifying 161 publications since 1980 documenting the findings of 181 surveys amongst displaced and conflict-affected populations from 40 source countries. The research often has been undertaken in collaboration with key human rights organizations, international agencies and NGOs, including Médecins Sans Frontières (Kaz de Jong et al. 2002); Physicians for Human Rights (Keller et al. 2003); World Vision (Bolton et al. 2002); the International Rehabilitation Council for Torture Victims (Modvig et al. 2000); the Transcultural Psychosocial Organization (TPO) (Joop de Jong et al. 2001); and the World Health Organization (Joop de Jong et al. 2003; Joop de Jong et al. 2001). The results of trauma-focused psychiatric epidemiological surveys have been published in some of the highest ranking medical journals such as The Lancet and the Journal of the American Medical Association, the latter devoting an annual edition to violence and human rights (Cole and Flanagin, 2009). Although the humanitarian focus behind this body of research has at times been implicit, the science of traumatic stress and its measurement has taken centre stage, and the overall body of research has been pivotal in advancing the human rights imperative.

It is noteworthy that the application and use of the new trauma model remained uncontroversial in the Western countries in which the lead researchers were based, most probably because the focus was on human rights violations in low- and middle-income countries, or amongst refugees from these regions. In parallel with the research, Western governments were willing funders of specialist services for the care and resettlement of refugees and survivors of organized violence in refugee camps and in other post-conflict settings. The early to mid 1990s marked a change in the consensus between government, researchers, and service developers as HICs increasingly began to pursue policies aimed at limiting the flow of refugees and other displaced persons from conflict-affected populations (UNHCR 1997, 2000). This complicated the position of mental health researchers, some of whom began applying psychiatric epidemiological approaches to measure the impact of policies of deterrence on displaced populations within their own countries, and, as a consequence, found themselves increasingly in conflict with the policies of their own governments.

Asylum seekers, policies of deterrence, and economic, social, and cultural rights

These new policies of 'humane deterrence' aimed to restrict the flow of asylum seekers by implementing several measures: attempting to prevent arrivals; implementing stringent refugee determination procedures; and limiting the rights of those who gained entry to the host country (Silove et al. 2000). Conditions in the host country have attracted most research attention. Asylum seekers living in the community commonly have limited, if any, access to a range of rights enshrined in UN conventions: to work, welfare support, housing, health care, and legal support. As a consequence, asylum seekers commonly find themselves destitute or highly dependent on charitable organizations for their daily living needs. In Australia, for instance, it has not been uncommon for asylum seekers to be denied work rights and welfare support during the full refugee determination procedure, a process that can take two or more years to be finalized (Silove et al. 2006; Steel and Silove 2001a). These policies exclude asylum seekers from second generation rights, that is, the rights enshrined in the International Covenant on Economic Social and Cultural Rights, the convention that places governments under specific obligations to ensure that all persons, without discrimination, have access to an adequate standard of living, including the right to work, healthcare, food, security, housing and family life (Hall 2006). Clinicians and other professionals working with asylum seekers noted from the outset the harmful consequences of harsh asylum policies on the mental health of their clients (Aron 1992; Baker 1992; Silove et al. 1993).

It has only been in recent years, however, that a sufficient evidence base has accumulated to support these clinical observations. In the first systematic study involving 40 consecutive asylum seekers attending a community assistance centre in Sydney, Silove and colleagues found a strong association with the severity of post-traumatic stress symptoms and post-migration stresses, most of which were directly related to the restriction imposed policies of deterrence (Silove et al. 1997). Although cross-sectional in design, this research provided evidence for a possible link between harsh government policies and poor mental health. Salient ongoing stressors included delays in processing refugee applications, being interviewed by or experiencing conflict with immigration officials, being denied a work permit, unemployment, and loneliness and boredom. In a second study, Steel et al. (1999) confirmed the association between post-migratory stress and PTSD amongst a sample of 196 Tamil asylum seekers, refugees, and immigrants living in Sydney. In addition there was evidence that trauma-affected individuals showed greater vulnerability to the effects of asylum induced post-migration difficulties, suggesting that pre- and post-migration adversity tended to compound the risk. There was also an association between length of time in the asylum process and PTSD symptoms (Steel and Silove 2000). More recently our research group examined prospectively the impact of the refugee decision on a cohort of 62 asylum seekers making the first refugee application in Sydney, Australia (Silove et al. 2007b). At post-decision, those granted refugee protection showed substantial improvements in post-traumatic stress disorder, anxiety, depression, and mental health functioning, whereas those who had to appeal negative refugee decisions maintained high levels of symptoms on all psychiatric indices. This suggested that establishing secure residency status for asylum seekers may be critical to their recovery from trauma-related psychiatric symptoms.

These findings have been replicated and extended by research undertaken in other countries. In Sweden, Sondergaard and colleagues (2001) reported the findings of a longitudinal mental health survey amongst 86 Iraqi and Kurdish refugees and asylum seekers followed up over the first year of resettlement. Higher exposure to negative events in the post-migration setting was associated with greater levels of psychological distress. Laban and colleagues (2005) found that difficulties related to the asylum procedure, work restrictions, and family separation were cumulative in increasing risk to psychiatric disorder in a sample of 294 Iraqi asylum seekers in the Netherlands. The authors also found that asylum seekers resident for two years or longer had twice the risk of psychiatric disorder compared to those who had been resident for six months or less (Laban et al. 2004). A second study from the Netherlands found that post-migration stress was associated with higher levels of depression and PTSD in a sample of 178 refugees and 232 asylum seekers, with the latter group reporting significantly more exposure to stressors than the refugee sample (Gerritsen et al. 2006). In Ireland, Begley et al. (1999) found that, amongst 43 asylum seekers, high levels of post-migration stress were directly related to the immigration procedures and living restrictions they encountered, with over 75 per cent of the sample experiencing difficulties in visiting their home country, delays in processing refugee applications, not being allowed to work, fear of deportation, and loneliness, boredom, and discrimination. More recently, Ryan and colleagues (Ryan, Benson, and Dooley 2008) found a strong association between post-migration stress and psychological distress amongst 172 asylum seekers resident in Ireland. A two-year follow-up of the sample demonstrated a persistent impact of post-migration stress on mental health, with those receiving a positive refugee outcome showing improvement in symptoms.

These findings amongst asylum seekers are supported by the larger body of refugee and post-conflict studies that have revealed a consistent relationship between the conditions of the recovery environment and mental health functioning. In a meta-analysis, Porter and Haslam (2005) examined the role of post-displacement factors in 59 studies covering a total population of 22,221 refugees in studies that compared displaced populations with 45,073 non-refugee groups. Factors associated with poorer psychological outcomes amongst refugees included institutional or insecure accommodation, restricted economic opportunity, being repatriated, internal (as opposed to external) displacement, and exposure to ongoing conflict. In a secondary analysis of the data, Porter (2007) showed a compounding pattern of post-displacement factors. For instance, insecure residency was associated with poorer mental health when the source conflict was ongoing and weaker when it was resolved. In the aforementioned meta-regression analysis of 181 epidemiological surveys involving displaced and conflict-affected populations, Steel et al. (2009) found that populations with insecure residency had higher rates of depression than populations permanently resettled to a safe country.

This collective body of research identifies the importance of the post-migration recovery environment in mediating psychosocial recovery for refugee and asylum-seeking populations. As such, the combined data indicate the importance of second generation human rights and the policies that shape mental health outcomes. In particular, policies of so-called 'humane deterrence' in fact have led to an abrogation by recipient countries of key second generation economic, social, and cultural rights of asylum seekers. Research, in turn, has shown the close link between the loss of these rights and adverse mental health outcomes. The body of research has helped advance not only an understanding of the factors needed for recovery in refugee populations, but also provides an evidence base that supports advocacy for human rights based policies in relation to the processing of asylum seekers. Although we have drawn on this research to illustrate the mental health consequences of denying second generation rights, other issues facing asylum seekers such as the application of stringent refugee determination procedures (Bogner et al. 2007; Herlihy et al. 2002; Rousseau et al. 2002) and the effects of mandatory detention (Robjant et al. 2009; Silove et al. 2007a) involve civil and political or first generation rights.

Transgressions of first generation rights in relation to asylum seekers

For close to two decades, there have been concerns that assessors of refugee applications may misunderstand and misinterpret manifestations of traumatic stress amongst asylum seekers, resulting in inappropriate refugee decision outcomes (Aron 1992; Baker 1992). In 2002, Rousseau and colleagues systematically reviewed 40 cases considered by the Canadian Immigration and Refugee Board, finding that certain symptoms of post-traumatic distress particularly those of confusion, avoidance, or delayed disclosure of events, were systematically interpreted by decision-makers as bringing into question an applicant's credibility. Herlihy and colleagues (Herlihy et al. 2002) have found that inconsistencies in testimony in trauma narratives increase with greater severity of traumatic stress symptoms, yet the identification of inconsistency is a major factor influencing rejection of refugee claims (Millbank 2009). These observations have prompted several studies (Bogner et al. 2007; Moradi et al. 2008; Rousseau et al. 2002) and commentaries (Herlihy and Turner 2006, 2007; Steel et al. 2004a) that together add to the concern that current procedural shortcomings in testing refugee claims may lead to the *refoulement* of bona fide refugees, an outcome of serious human rights concern. Distinct from other asylum research which has examined the effects of economic and social exclusion, this emerging body of research examines issues of procedural fairness in administrative decision-making, rights that relate to first generation civil and political rights.

Another major human rights issue relates to the detention of asylum seekers. This controversy has been particularly prominent in the Australian context, although the practice of detention is common in other parts of the world including the United States, the United Kingdom, European countries, and parts of Asia (UNHCR, 2006). In Australia, mandatory detention for all unauthorized entrants to Australia including women and children was introduced in 1992. Despite mental health professionals being quick to point out the mental health risks associated with this policy (Silove et al. 1993), the government's overriding concern was to ensure border protection; hence, the mental health concerns tended to be ignored or dismissed. From a human rights perspective, the policy was highly controversial since it appeared to result in multiple breaches of international law affecting both first and second generation rights. Based on protections enshrined under the International Covenant on Civil and Political Rights, the human rights committee of the UN have identified repeated breaches by Australia in relation to the asylum detention policy (see Box 19.1). Similarly, within Australia, the Human Rights and Equal Opportunities Commission (HREOC) has found multiple breaches in relation to detention with reference to the Convention on the

Rights of the Child (CROC). The reports of the Commission are noteworthy given that many of the provisions of the CROC are drawn from the body of second generation rights (see Box 19.2). In the controversy that was provoked by this detention policy, mental health professionals increasingly found themselves in the frontline of the ensuing debate, prompted by their direct experience of the psychological consequences of detention in their daily practice. Yet, the government of the time continued to deny that there were any adverse mental health consequences arising from detention (Silove, et al. 2007a). The need for systematic evidence therefore became a pressing issue. A series of studies commencing in 2001 addressed this concern, in spite of the formidable logistic and ethical obstacles in mounting scientific studies in this area. All studies documented extraordinarily high levels of psychiatric impairment amongst detainees (Mares and Jureidini 2004; Momartin et al. 2006; Steel et al. 2004b; Steel et al. 2006; Steel and Silove 2001b; Sultan and O'Sullivan 2001). This evidence base along with the testimony of health professionals working within the centres proved to be pivotal in generating a strong coalition amongst the health community in Australia advocating that immigration detention was particularly harmful to children and that the policy needed comprehensive review (Professional Alliance for the Health of Asylum Seekers and their Children 2002). The impetus gained by this issue led to the formation of the largest alliance of health professionals in Australian history. Ultimately, the government's resolve to resist the pressure from medical and other groups was overcome by repeated high-profile scandals such as that the wrongful detention and neglect of Cornelia Rau, an Australian citizen suffering from schizophrenia who was mistakenly held in immigration detention for nine months. A process of substantive policy reform followed with the removal of children and their families from detention and the establishment of time limits and review for adults on mainland Australia. However, the practice of detention for asylum seekers continues for boat arrivals, who are interdicted at sea and held in off-shore detention facilities, indicating continued need for advocacy in this area which remains highly politicized.

These related areas of research amongst asylum seekers offer important examples of the need for mental health professionals to consider both first and second generation rights, with the latter being of particular importance to marginalized and vulnerable communities. In some settings, it is possible to trace a pattern in which the denial of economic, social, and cultural rights appears to progressively result in the subsequent erosion of civil and political rights. This pattern has been particularly evident for asylum seekers in the US, UK, and throughout many European states (Malloch and Stanley 2005; Welch and Schuster 2005). In these settings, challenges to the right to protection against state-sponsored abuses have been extended to the curtailment of basic freedoms and economic and social rights, based on claims that asylum seekers are a burden on the host society.

The trauma model and cultural rights

The previous sections have reviewed the development and expansion of the trauma model into research with displaced and conflict-affected populations over the previous three decades. We have argued that a concern for the protection of human rights has motivated research in this field from the outset, at first by providing researchers with a tool to document the mental health consequences of conflict and organized violence, and more recently to assess the effects of economic and social exclusion and other policies implemented by governments to deter asylum seekers. Nevertheless, the pre-eminence and globalization of the trauma model as a foundation for research has also led to a growing critique of the underlying constructs. Commentators have raised concern that, rather than promoting the rights of conflict-affected populations, the universal trauma model may have a corrosive impact on the societies in which it is applied (Bracken et al. 1995; Kagee and

Naidoo 2004; Kleinman 1995; Pupavac 2006; Summerfield 1999). The central tenet of this critique is the observation that many non-Western societies have strong collective cultural identities, as compared to Western populations where there is a tendency to privilege notions of identity based on the individual. As such, it is argued that mental health models based on a predominantly individualistic notion of trauma and suffering may not be fully applicable, and indeed may be damaging when applied to non-Western populations (Kleinman 1995).

The notion of 'category fallacy', one of the corollaries of this central critique, questions the validity of applying categories such as PTSD across diverse cultural domains (Summerfield 2001). The weight of concern relates to whether adequate critical appraisal has been given to the cultural relevance and value of the category to the local cultural setting (Breslau 2004; Kleinman 1995; Summerfield 1999). Underpinning the ongoing controversy about the trauma model and its applicability to diverse cultures is a fundamental human rights issue that relates to the identification of rights of the third generation, namely collective and cultural rights and, in particular, the rights of indigenous societies to their own cultural heritage and self-determination.

Concerns over the condition of indigenous peoples worldwide has long been recognized and raised repeatedly within the United Nations and its predecessor, the League of Nations. As such, the UN Declaration on the Rights of Indigenous Peoples was the outcome of a long and laborious process (Iyall Smith 2008). In 1970, Special Rapporteur Martinez Cobo was commissioned by the United Nations Economic and Social Council (ECOSOC) to investigate the problem of discrimination against indigenous populations. A series of detailed reports published between 1981 and 1987 identified an extensive array of problems facing indigenous peoples throughout the world. In many instances, it was found that national governments simply denied the existence of indigenous peoples within their borders, hence ignoring widespread discrimination which was clearly present. In response, the UN ECOSOC established the Working Group on Indigenous issues to (i) review developments pertaining to the human rights of indigenous peoples and (ii) elaborate international standards to protect those rights.

The first draft of a declaration on the rights of indigenous peoples was approved by the UN Sub-Commission on the Prevention of Discrimination and Protection of Minorities in 1994. After some 12 years of negotiation, a draft Declaration on the Rights of Indigenous Peoples was adopted by the Human Rights Council and Ratified by the UN General Assembly on 13 September 2007.

From the principles embedded in the Declaration, it is implicit that there may be legitimate concerns about imposing health models and practices (including mental health) on indigenous cultures. In particular the Declaration enshrines the principles of self-direction in relation to strategies for developing health programmes and the need to respect traditional healing practices (see Box 19.2).

Indigenous healing systems may operate through models that differ greatly from those in which posttraumatic reactions have been documented and researched. Although PTSD has been recorded across a wide range of cultures, some doubt remains as to how the construct relates to local mental health models and belief systems. In 2003 our group undertook research in Timor Leste (East Timor) four years after national independence. This followed a prolonged period of Indonesian rule associated with extensive human rights abuses. Ethnographic work with the East Timorese community identified a comprehensive range of terms used to describe mental illness, terms that did not clearly map onto western diagnostic categories including PTSD (Silove et al. 2008). While it appears that the Timorese, like many indigenous communities, do not have a concept that matches that of PTSD, members of the community readily endorse the constituent symptoms, and recognize that their presence is associated with functional impairment (Silove et al. 2008). These findings therefore present a complex picture, suggesting it is important to

Box 19.1: Breaches of international humanitarian law found against the use and implementation of mandatory immigration detention within the Australian context

The United Nations Human Rights Committee has found that Australia has variously breached the fundamental human rights of immigration detainees with respect to the protections offered under the International Covenant on Civil and Political Rights (ICCPR)

Article 7
No one shall be subjected to torture or to cruel, inhuman or degrading treatment or punishment. In particular, no one shall be subjected without his free consent to medical or scientific experimentation.

Article 9(1)
Everyone has the right to liberty and security of person. No one shall be subjected to arbitrary arrest or detention. No one shall be deprived of his liberty except on such grounds and in accordance with such procedure as are established by law.

Article 9(4)
Anyone who is deprived of his liberty by arrest or detention shall be entitled to take proceedings before a court, in order that that court may decide without delay on the lawfulness of his detention and order his release if the detention is not lawful.

Article 10
All persons deprived of their liberty shall be treated with humanity and with respect for the inherent dignity of the human person.

Article 17(1)
No one shall be subjected to arbitrary or unlawful interference with his privacy, family, or correspondence, nor to unlawful attacks on his honour and reputation.

Article 23(1)
The family is the natural and fundamental group unit of society and is entitled to protection by society and the State.

Article 24(1)
Every child shall have, without any discrimination as to race, colour, sex, language, religion, national or social origin, property or birth, the right to such measures of protection as are required by his status as a minor, on the part of his family, society and the State.

The Human Rights and Equal Opportunity Commission has found that Australia has multiple breaches of the human rights of children: Convention on the Rights of the Child (CROC)

Article 3(1)
The best interests of the child are a primary consideration in all actions concerning children.

Article 6(2)
To enjoy, 'to the maximum extent possible' their right to development.

Breaches of international humanitarian law found against the use and implementation of mandatory immigration detention within the Australian context *(continued)*

Article 19(1)
The right to be protected from all forms of physical or mental violence.

Article 20(1)
The right of unaccompanied children to receive special protection and assistance to ensure the enjoyment of all rights under the CROC.

Article 22(1)
Children seeking asylum receive appropriate assistance.

Article 23(1)
The right of children with disabilities to 'enjoy a full and decent life, in conditions which ensure dignity, promote self-reliance and facilitate the child's active participation in the community.

Article 24(1)
The right to enjoy the highest attainable standard of physical and mental health.

Article 28(1)
The right to an appropriate education on the basis of equal opportunity.

Article 37(c)
Children are treated with humanity and respect for their inherent dignity.

Article 39(1)
Right to live in 'an environment which fosters the health, self-respect and dignity' of children in order to ensure recovery from past torture and trauma.

---

examine more fully the overlap and interaction of international constructs of mental disorder with culture-specific notions, with the aim of achieving a comprehensive and coherent account of mental suffering in each setting.

Anthropological observations have also repeatedly found that traditional non-Western cultures tend to adopt illness models that differ to varying degrees from Western notions (Murphy 1976). For example, traditional models tend to be holistic, integrating physical and psychological aspects of illness without making the dualistic distinctions typical of Western systems (Phan and Silove 1999). Symptoms identified by Western-derived diagnoses may have particular meaning in a different cultural context, an issue of importance in relation to attributions and interventions. For instance, ethnographic work undertaken by Grayman and colleagues (2009) amongst conflict-affected Acehnese communities identified a popular belief regarding the activities of mischievous spirits in producing some of the nightmares experienced by trauma-affected individuals. This field work presented demonstrates how incorporating an understanding of indigenous explanations of different types of nightmares is critical to interpreting traumatic symptoms in this population. A sole focus on specific constellations of symptoms delineated by psychiatric diagnostic systems (such as DSM), without simultaneous attention to the local cultural meanings, may obscure indigenous models and belief systems in a way that separates sufferers from traditional healing mechanisms.

These considerations also need to be extended to include the importance of workers in the trauma field being cognizant of the broader cultural, human rights, and political context in which they operate. To illustrate some of the dangers of a narrowly focused trauma treatment approach, the editors of the journal *Culture, Medicine and Psychiatry* devoted an edition to case studies identifying the unintended consequences of extending notions of PTSD and other traumatic responses across a range of complex socio-political environments (Breslau 2004). For instance, based on ethnographic observations in Haiti between 1995 and 2000, James (2004) described the consequences of establishing treatment services for trauma survivors in that country. These services were developed following a long period of state sponsored terror in Haiti. Access to development aid and specialist treatment service were made available to existing victim organizations that had been advocating for the rights of the dispossessed. These organizations, however, were organized on sectarian lines, each advocating for selective groups. Notions of traumatic suffering used by aid organizations as indicators of individual and community need became highly politicized, leading to the development of a secondary economy whereby excluded communities could purchase acceptable 'trauma portfolios' that granted them access to the assistance and development aid including access to counselling. The study illustrates that the highly complex nature of post-conflict settings may be poorly understood by 'imported' programmes of care that that run the risk of creating structures that lead to further victimization for vulnerable communities. In a separate case study amongst Somali refugees displaced to Ethiopia, Zarowsky (2004) identified a deep reluctance to speak about the psychological symptoms associated with violence. Instead trauma narratives covered topics of survival, anger, and loss. Zarowsky observed that expressions of personal distress were predominantly incorporated within the framework of politics. These observations suggest that recovery from mass trauma within this setting required a social rather than an individual focus. A risk evident in these and other examples is that indigenous healing mechanisms and the confidence of local systems to mobilize traditional problem-solving approaches may be undermined unless Western models are combined with ethnographic work to understand the socio-cultural setting. In addition, in all contexts, complex human rights and political influences need to be carefully evaluated to ensure that services and interventions do not inadvertently add to problems such as discrimination and exploitation.

The issue of the differential in resources and power between expatriate clinicians and researchers and the local community is an additional issue of great importance. The principles enshrined in the Declaration on the Rights of Indigenous Peoples necessitate that mental health researchers and clinicians approach work with refugee and conflict-affected populations in a manner which is fundamentally rooted in a local cultural context and respectful of the rights of participant communities to direct and have ownership of research and therapeutic activities. In order to achieve these outcomes, mental health practitioners need to be mindful of the immense power differentials between well resourced evidence-based models available to Western researchers and forms of traditional knowledge which may be vulnerable due to the impact of conflict on supporting social structures. The aim to safeguard and promote indigenous rights in such settings confers a positive obligation on the practitioner to act as an enabler in a process that values local worlds, cultural knowledge, and indigenous healing systems. This does not *ipso facto* disqualify the thoughtful introduction of some elements of Western developed psychiatric models in such contexts. It calls for a process of identifying and incorporating local understandings and approaches that allow these insights to be situated within a broader historical, cultural, and political context. The form that this will take will depend in part on each social context. Miller and colleagues provide examples of how this might be reflected in practice (Miller et al. 2006a; Miller and Rasco 2004). These authors urge researchers to go beyond questions of morbidity in order to consider broader questions that increase value to communities and services, and where possible strengthen local healing worlds. Important components in this process may include seeking to understand and document local idioms of distress and explanatory illness models (Groleau et al. 2006; Miller et al. 2006b; Patel et al. 1995). Also important are local definitions of functioning and impairment and how these relate to illness models (Bolton and Tang 2002; Bolton et al. 2004). In considering models of service delivery it is valuable to incorporate investigations of culturally specific patterns that shape help-seeking behaviour, and to identify local resources that people access to address problems with their social and emotional well-being. Many of these essentially ethnographic strategies build on a long tradition of anthropological methods that privilege and value the lived experiences of each cultural context. In addition to the benefits associated with generating a more accurate and culturally relevant assessment of need, these approaches assist in the fulfilment of the indigenous right to self-determination, in maintaining cultural medical heritage, and to having a voice in the development of programme of assistance.

The lack of clear methodological models and the many practical limitations within unstable post-conflict settings may limit the capacity of researchers to integrate anthropological and epidemiological methods. Nevertheless, if research and practice endeavour to engage creatively with both traditions, there is a greater possibility that mental health professionals and researchers will identify more accurately the relevant forms and expressions of suffering, enabling them to advocate effectively, and in a manner that prioritizes and respects the broader issue of protecting the fragile social and cultural fabric, a process that ultimately is vital for recovery after conflict. Engagement in the complicated arena of promoting this combined approach will have the additional benefit of ensuring that multiple levels of human rights considerations will be promoted and protected. In both research and practice, a growing number of clinicians and researchers

Box 19.2: Articles from the Declaration on the Rights of Indigenous Peoples of particular relevance to mental health researchers and practitioners

- *Article 1* Indigenous peoples have the right to the full enjoyment, as a collective or as individuals, of all human rights and fundamental freedoms as recognized in the Charter of the United Nations, the Universal Declaration of Human Rights and international human rights law.

- *Article 8* Indigenous peoples and individuals have the right not to be subjected to forced assimilation or destruction of their culture.

- *Article 15* Indigenous peoples have the right to the dignity and diversity of their cultures, traditions, histories and aspirations which shall be appropriately reflected in education and public information.

- *Article 23* Indigenous peoples have the right to determine and develop priorities and strategies for exercising their right to development. In particular, indigenous peoples have the right to be actively involved in developing and determining health, housing and other economic and social programmes affecting them and, as far as possible, to administer such programmes through their own institutions.

- *Article 24* Indigenous peoples have the right to their traditional medicines and to maintain their health practices, including the conservation of their vital medicinal plants, animals and minerals. Indigenous individuals also have the right to access, without any discrimination, to all social and health services.

have begun to find ways to address the complex task of reconciling the trauma model with third generation rights. In the aforementioned epidemiological study of mental health needs in East Timor, Silove et al. (2008) utilized indigenous terms for mental illness to identify cases, alongside a 'Western' derived set of psychiatric screening tools. Hinton and colleagues have looked at culturally specific conditions such as 'hit by the wind' experienced by Vietnamese refugees (Hinton et al. 2003), and 'weak heart' syndrome amongst the Khmer (Hinton et al. 2002). Miller and colleagues (Miller et al. 2006b, 2008) identified a traumatic grief syndrome amongst conflict-affected Afghans that appeared to have more cultural salience than a diagnosis of PTSD (Miller et al. 2009).

Conclusion

The debates surrounding mental health models of traumatic stress have, in effect, uncovered many key issues relevant to human rights principles and practice in conflict-affected and refugee communities. The inclusion of the diagnosis of PTSD in DSM-III in 1980 and the development of an associated focus on the mental health consequences of exposure to traumatic stress appears to have provided an important and powerful tool in identifying some of the harm associated with abuses of civil and political rights, and, more recently, the domains of economic, social, and cultural rights. The counterweight to this development has been the concern (Bracken et al. 1995; Breslau 2004; Kagee and Naidoo 2004; Kleinman 1995; Pupavac 2006; Summerfield 1999) about the potential threat that universal application of the psychiatric model poses to indigenous collective rights. Lack of careful consideration of the socio-cultural context may inadvertently risk violating the cultural and collective rights of those we purport to help. An approach that integrates anthropological, epidemiological, and psychiatric approaches will have the benefit of ensuring that multiple levels of human rights considerations are promoted and protected.

References

Allodi, F (1979) *Psychiatric effects of torture: A Canadian Study*. Paper presented at the Annual meeting of the Canadian Psychiatric Association (Sept. 26–28): Vancouver, BC.

Allodi, F and Rojas, A (1985) 'The health and adaptation of victims of political violence in Latin America' (Psychiatry effects of torture and disappearance) in *Drug Dependence and Alcoholism, Forensic Psychiatry, Military Psychiatry*, 27. New York: Plenum Press, 243–48.

Allodi, FA (1980) 'The psychiatric effects in children and families of victims of political persecution and torture', *Danish Medical Bulletin*, 27(5), 229–32.

American Psychiatric Association (1980) *Diagnostic and Statistical Manual of Mental Disorders*. 3rd edn. Washington, DC: American Psychiatric Association Press.

Amnesty International (1977) *Evidence of Torture: Studies of the Amnesty International Danish Medical Group* (No. PUB 72/00/77). London: Amnesty International Publications.

Aron, A (1992) 'Applications of psychology to the assessment of refugees seeking political asylum', *Applied Psychology An International Review*, 41, 77–91.

Baker, R (1992) 'Psychosocial consequences for tortured refugees seeking asylum and refugee status in Europe', in M Basoglu (ed) *Torture and Its Consequences: Current Treatment Approaches*. New York, NY: Cambridge University Press, 83–106.

Begley, M, Garavan, C, Condon, M, Kelly, I, Holland, K, and Staines, A (1999) *Asylum in Ireland: A Public Health Perspective*. Dublin: Department of Public Health Medicine and Epidemiology, UCD.

Bogner, D, Herlihy, J, and Brewin, CR (2007) 'Impact of sexual violence on disclosure during Home Office interviews', *British Journal of Psychiatry*, 191, 75–81.

Bolton, P, and Tang, AM (2002) 'An alternative approach to cross-cultural function assessment', *Social Psychiatry & Psychiatric Epidemiology*, 37(11), 537–43.

Bolton, P, Wilk, CM, and Ndogoni, L (2004) 'Assessment of depression prevalence in rural Uganda using symptom and function criteria', *Social Psychiatry & Psychiatric Epidemiology*, 39(6), 442–47.

Bracken, PJ, Giller, JE, and Summerfield, D (1995) 'Psychological responses to war and atrocity: the limitations of current concepts', *Social Science & Medicine*, 40(8), 1073–82.

Breslau, J (2004) 'Cultures of trauma: Anthropological views of posttraumatic stress disorder in international health'. *Culture, Medicine & Psychiatry*, 28(2), 113–26.

Breslau, J (2005) 'Response: deconstructing critiques on the internationalization of PTSD', *Culture, Medicine & Psychiatry*, 29(3), 361–70.

Cienfuegos, AJ, and Monelli, C (1983) 'Testimony of political repression as a therapeutic instrument', *American Journal of Orthopsychiatry*, 53, 43–51.

Cole, TB, and Flanagin, A (2009) '2010 Theme Issue on Violence and Human Rights Call for Papers', *JAMA*, 302(22), 2487–87.

de Jong, K, Mulhern, M, Ford, N, Simpson, I, Swan, A, and Van der Kam, S (2002) 'Psychological trauma of the civil war in Sri Lanka', *Lancet*, 359(9316), 1517–18.

de Jong, JT, Komproe, IH, Van Ommeren, M, et al. (2001) 'Lifetime events and posttraumatic stress disorder in 4 postconflict settings', *JAMA*, 286(5), 555–62.

de Jong, JT, Komproe, IH, and Van Ommeren, M (2003) 'Common mental disorders in postconflict settings', *Lancet*, 361(9375), 2128–30.

Gerritsen, AA, Bramsen, I, Deville, W, van Willigen, LH, Hovens, JE, and van der Ploeg, HM (2006) 'Physical and mental health of Afghan, Iranian and Somali asylum seekers and refugees living in the Netherlands', *Social Psychiatry and Psychiatric Epidemiology*, 41(1), 18–26.

Goldfeld, AE, Mollica, RF, Pesavento, B H, and Faraone, SV (1988) 'The physical and psychological sequelae of torture: Symptomatology and diagnosis', *JAMA*, 259(18), 2725–29.

Grayman, JH, Good, M -J D, and Good, BJ (2009) 'Conflict nightmares and trauma in Aceh', *Transcultural Psychiatry*, 33, 290–312.

Groleau, D, Young, A, and Kirmayer, LJ (2006) 'The McGill Illness Narrative Interview (MINI): an interview schedule to elicit meanings and modes of reasoning related to illness experience', *Transcultural Psychiatry*, 43(4), 671–91.

Hall, P (2006) 'Failed asylum seekers and health care: Current regulations flout international law', *British Medical Journal*, 333, 109–110.

Herlihy, J, and Turner, S (2006) 'Should discrepant accounts given by asylum seekers be taken as proof of deceit?', *Torture*, 16(2), 81–92.

Herlihy, J, and Turner, SW (2007) 'Asylum claims and memory of trauma: sharing our knowledge', *British Journal of Psychiatry*, 191, 3–4.

Herlihy, J, Scragg, P, and Turner, S (2002) 'Discrepancies in autobiographical memories—implications for the assessment of asylum seekers: repeated interviews study', *British Medical Journal*, 324(Feb 9), 324–27.

Hinton, D, Hinton, S, Pham, T, Chau, H, and Tran, M (2003) '"Hit by the Wind" and Temperature-Shift Panic among Vietnamese Refugees', *Transcultural Psychiatry*, 40(3), 342–76.

Hinton, D, Hinton, S, Um, K, Chea, A, and Sak, S (2002) 'The Khmer "Weak Heart" Syndrome: Fear of Death from Palpitations', *Transcultural Psychiatry*, 39(3), 323–44.

Iyall Smith, KE (2008) 'Comparing state and international protections of indigenous peoples' human rights', *American Behavioral Scientist*, 51(12), 1817–35.

James, EC (2004) 'The political economy of 'trauma' in Haiti in the democratic era of insecurity', *Culture, Medicine & Psychiatry*, 28(2), 127–49.

Kagee, A and Naidoo, AV (2004) 'Reconceptualizing the sequelae of political torture: Limitations of a psychiatric paradigm', *Transcultural Psychiatry*, 41(1), 46–61.

Keller, AS, Rosenfeld, B, Trinh-Shevrin, C, et al. (2003) 'Mental health of detained asylum seekers', *Lancet*, 362(9397), 1721–23.

Kinzie, JD, Fredrickson, RH, Ben, R, Fleck, J, and Karls, W (1984) 'Posttraumatic Stress Disorder among Survivors of Cambodian Concentration-Camps', *American Journal of Psychiatry*, 141(5), 645–50.

Kleinman, A (1995) 'Violence, culture, and the politics of trauma', in A Kleinman (ed) *Writing at the Margin*. Berkeley: CA: University of California Press, 173–89.

Laban, CJ, Gernaat, HB, Komproe, IH, Schreuders, BA, and de Jong, JT (2004) 'Impact of a long asylum procedure on the prevalence of psychiatric disorders in Iraqi asylum seekers in the Netherlands', *Journal of Nervous & Mental Disease*, 192(12), 843–51.

Laban, CJ, Gernaat, HBPE, Komproe, IH, van der Tweel, I, and De Jong, JTVM (2005) 'Postmigration living problems and common psychiatric disorders in Iraqi asylum seekers in the Netherlands', *Journal of Nervous & Mental Disease*, 193(12), 825–32.

Malloch, MS and Stanley, E (2005) 'The detention of asylum seekers in the UK—Representing risk, managing the dangerous', *Punishment & Society-International Journal of Penology*, 7(1), 53–71.

Mares, S and Jureidini, J (2004) 'Psychiatric assessment of children and families in immigration detention: clinical, administrative and ethical issues', *Australian & New Zealand Journal of Public Health*, 28(6), 520–526.

Millbank, J (2009) '"The ring of truth": A case study of credibility assessment in particular social group refugee determinations', *International Journal of Refugee Law*, 21(1), 1–33.

Miller, KE, and Rasco, LM (eds) (2004) *The mental health of refugees: ecological approaches to healing and adaptation*. New Jersey: Lawrence Erlbaum.

Miller, KE, Kulkarni, M, and Kushner, H (2006a) 'Beyond trauma-focused psychiatric epidemiology: bridging research and practice with war-affected populations', *American Journal of Orthopsychiatry*, 76(4), 409–22.

Miller, KE, Omidian, P, Quraishy, AS, Quraishy, N, Nasiry, MN, Nasiry, S, et al. (2006b) 'The Afghan symptom checklist: a culturally grounded approach to mental health assessment in a conflict zone', *American Journal of Orthopsychiatry*, 76(4), 423–33.

Miller, KE, Omidian, P, Rasmussen, A, Yaqubi, A, and Daudzai, H (2008) 'Daily stressors, war experiences, and mental health in Afghanistan', *Transcultural Psychiatry*, 45(4), 611–38.

Miller, KE, Omidian, P, Kulkarni, M, Yaqubi, A, Daudzai, H, and Rasmussen, A (2009) 'The validity and clinical utility of post-traumatic stress disorder in Afghanistan', *Transcultural Psychiatry*, 46(2), 219–37.

Modvig, J, Pagaduan-Lopez, J, Rodenburg, J, Salud, CM, Cabigon, RV, and Panelo, CI (2000) 'Torture and trauma in post-conflict East Timor', *Lancet.*, 356(9243), 1763.

Mollica, RF, Wyshak, G, and Lavelle, J (1987) 'The psychosocial impact of war trauma and torture on Southeast Asian refugees', *American Journal of Psychiatry*, 144(12), 1567–72.

Momartin, S, Steel, Z, Coello, M, Aroche, J, Silove, D, and Brooks, R (2006) 'A comparison of the mental health of refugees with temporary versus permanent protection visas', *Medical Journal of Australia*, 185(7), 357–61.

Moradi, AR, Herlihy, J, Yasseri, G, Shahraray, M, Turner, S, and Dalgleish, T (2008) 'Specificity of episodic and semantic aspects of autobiographical memory in relation to symptoms of posttraumatic stress disorder (PTSD)', *Acta Psychologica*, 127(3), 645–53.

Murphy, JM (1976) 'Psychiatric labeling in cross-cultural perspective', *Science*, 191(4231), 1019–28.

Murphy, JM (1977) 'War stress and civilian Vietnamese: A study of the psychological effects', *Acta Psychiatrica Scandinavica*, 56, 92–108.

Patel, V, Simunyu, E, and Gwanzura, F (1995) 'Kufungisisa (thinking too much): a Shona idiom for non-psychotic mental illness', *Central African Journal of Medicine*, 41(7), 209–215.

Petersen, HD (1989) 'The controlled-study of torture victims: Epidemiological considerations and some future aspects', *Scandinavian Journal of Social Medicine*, 17(1), 13–20.

Phan, T, and Silove, D (1999) 'An overview of indigenous descriptions of mental phenomena and the range of traditional healing practices amongst the Vietnamese', *Transcultural Psychiatry*, 36(1), 79–94.

Porter, M (2007) 'Global evidence for a biopsychosocial understanding of refugee adaptation', *Transcultural Psychiatry*, 44(3), 418–39.

Porter, M, and Haslam, N (2005) 'Predisplacement and postdisplacement factors associated with mental health of refugees and internally displaced persons: a meta-analysis', *JAMA*, 294(5), 602–12.

Professional Alliance for the Health of Asylum Seekers and their Children (2002) *Submission to the National Inquiry into Children in Immigration Detention*. Available at <http://www.hreoc.gov.au/human_rights/children_detention/submissions/index.html>, accessed 6 November 2011.

Pupavac, V (2006) 'Humanitarian politics and the rise of international disaster', in G Reyes and GA Jacobs (eds) *Handbook of International Disaster Psychology* Westport, CT: Praeger, Vol. 1, 15–34.

Rasmussen, OV, and Lunde, I (1980) 'Evaluation of investigation of 200 torture victims', *Danish Medical Bulletin*, 27(5), 241–43.

Robjant, K, Robbins, I, and Senior, V (2009) 'Psychological distress amongst immigration detainees: a cross-sectional questionnaire study', *British Journal of Clinical Psychology*, 48(3), 275–86.

Rousseau, C, Crépeau, F, Foxen, P, and Houle, F (2002) 'The complexity of determining refugeehood: A multidisciplinary analysis of the decision-making process of the Canadian Immigration and Refugee Board', *Journal of Refugee Studies*, 15(1), 43–70.

Ryan, DA, Benson, CA, and Dooley, BA (2008) 'Psychological distress and the asylum process: a longitudinal study of forced migrants in Ireland', *Journal of Nervous & Mental Disease*, 196(1), 37–45.

Silove, D, McIntosh, P, and Becker, R (1993) 'Risk of retraumatisation of asylum-seekers in Australia', *Australian & New Zealand Journal of Psychiatry*, 27(4), 606–612.

Silove, D, Sinnerbrink, I, Field, A, Manicavasagar, V, and Steel, Z (1997) 'Anxiety, depression and PTSD in asylum-seekers: associations with pre-migration trauma and post-migration stressors', *British Journal of Psychiatry*, 170, 351–57.

Silove, D, Steel, Z, and Watters, C (2000) 'Policies of deterrence and the mental health of asylum seekers', *JAMA*, 284(5), 604–11.

Silove, D, Steel, Z, Susljik, I, Frommer, N, Loneragan, C, Brooks, R, et al. (2006) 'Torture, mental health status and the outcomes of refugee applications among recently arrived asylum seekers in Australia', *International Journal of Migration, Health and Social Care*, 2(1), 4–14.

Silove, D, Austin, P, and Steel, Z (2007a) 'No refuge from terror: the impact of detention on the mental health of trauma-affected refugees seeking asylum in Australia', *Transcultural Psychiatry*, 44(3), 359–93.

Silove, D, Steel, Z, Susljik, I, Frommer, N, Loneragan, C, Chey, T, et al. (2007b) 'The impact of the refugee decision on the trajectory of PTSD, anxiety, and depressive symptoms among asylum seekers: A longitudinal study', *American Journal of Disaster Medicine*, 2(6), 321–29.

Silove, D, Bateman, C, Brooks, R, Zulmira, FCA, Steel, Z, Rodger, J, et al. (2008) 'Estimating clinically relevant mental disorders in a rural and urban setting in post-conflict Timor Lest', *Archives of General Psychiatry*, 65(10), 1205–12.

Sondergaard, H P, Ekblad, S, and Theorell, T (2001) 'Self-reported life event patterns and their relation to health among recently resettled Iraqi and Kurdish refugees in Sweden', *Journal of Nervous and Mental Disease*, 189(12), 838–845.

Steel, Z, and Silove, D (2000) 'The psychosocial cost of seeking and granting asylum', in A Shalev, R Yehuda, and A McFarlane (eds) *International Handbook of Human Response to Trauma*. New York: Kluwer Academic/Plenum Publishers, 421–38.

Steel, Z, and Silove, D (2001a) 'Poisoned milk—applying for asylum in Australia', in C Moser, D Nyfeler, and M Verwey (eds) *Traumatization of Refugees and Asylum Seekers: The Relevance of the Political, Social and Medical Context [Traumatiserungen von Flüchtlingen und Asyl Schenden: Einflus des politischen, sozialen und medizinischen Kontextes]* Zürich: Seismo, 31–50.

Steel, Z, and Silove, DM (2001b) 'The mental health implications of detaining asylum seekers', *Medical Journal of Australia*, 175(11–12), 596–99.

Steel, Z, Chey, T, Silove, D, Marnane, C, Bryant, RA, and van Ommeren, M (2009) 'Association of torture and other potentially traumatic events with mental health outcomes among populations exposed to mass conflict and displacement: A systematic review and meta-analysis', *JAMA*, 302(5), 537–49.

Steel, Z., Frommer, N., and Silove, D. (2004a) Part I—the mental health impacts of migration: the law and its effects failing to understand: refugee determination and the traumatized applicant. *International Journal of Law & Psychiatry*, 27(6), 511–28.

Steel, Z, Momartin, S, Bateman, C, Hafshejani, A, Silove, DM, Everson, N, et al. (2004b) 'Psychiatric status of asylum seeker families held for a protracted period in a remote detention centre in Australia', *Australian & New Zealand Journal of Public Health*, 28(6), 527–36.

Steel, Z, Silove, D, Bird, K, McGorry, P, and Mohan, P (1999) 'Pathways from war trauma to posttraumatic stress symptoms among Tamil asylum seekers, refugees, and immigrants', *Journal of Traumatic Stress*, 12(3), 421–35.

Steel, Z, Silove, D, Brooks, R, Momartin, S, Alzuhairi, B, and Susljik, I (2006) 'Impact of immigration detention and temporary protection on the mental health of refugees', *British Journal of Psychiatry*, 188, 58–64.

Sultan, A, and O'Sullivan, K (2001) 'Psychological disturbances in asylum seekers held in long term detention: a participant-observer account', *Medical Journal of Australia*, 175, 593–96.

Summerfield, D (1999) 'A critique of seven assumptions behind psychological trauma programmes in war-affected areas', *Social Science & Medicine*, 48(10), 1449–62.

Summerfield, D (2001) 'The invention of post-traumatic stress disorder and the social usefulness of a psychiatric category', *British Medical Journal*, 322(7278), 95–98.

UNHCR (1997) *The State of the Worlds Refugees: A Humanitarian Agenda*. New York: Oxford University Press.

UNHCR (2000) *State of the World's Refugees: Fifty years of Humanitarian Intervention*. Oxford, UK: Oxford University Press.

UNHCR (2006) *The State of The World's Refugees 2006: Human Displacement in the New Millennium*. Oxford, UK: Oxford University Press.

Weisaeth, L (1989) 'Torture of a Norwegian ship's crew: The torture, stress reactions and psychiatric after-effects', *Acta Psychiatrica Scandinavica, Supplementum*, 355, 63–72.

Welch, M, and Schuster, L (2005) 'Detention of asylum seekers in the UK and USA—Deciphering noisy and quiet constructions', *Punishment & Society-International Journal of Penology*, 7(4), 397–417.

Zarowsky, C (2004) 'Writing trauma: emotion, ethnography, and the politics of suffering among Somali returnees in Ethiopia', *Culture, Medicine & Psychiatry*, 28(2), 189–209.

Chapter 20

Child and Adolescent Refugees and Asylum Seekers in Australia

The Ethics of Exposing Children to Suffering to Achieve Social Outcomes

Sarah Mares and Jon Jureidini

Introduction

As the movement of people across the globe has increased, a growing number of developed nations (including Australia, the US, and the UK) have implemented harsh immigration policies. The current chapter will present a review of the conditions that faced asylum seekers including children of arriving in Australia from 2000 until late 2007, and update figures to 2011. We consider the ethical and human rights implications of these harsh policies which exposed children to abuse and neglect with negative developmental and mental health outcomes. We also consider the ethical demands on health professionals who assess and attempt to treat children and their families who are harmed by immigration policy and practice.

The Australian government maintains an offshore resettlement programme for refugees and persons in need of humanitarian assistance who receive support and assistance with resettlement on arrival in Australia. These generous programmes stand in stark contrast to the reception given to asylum seekers arriving in Australia, who were, until recently, subject to indefinite mandatory detention and restricted access to community supports and services. Many were detained for several years, in remote, privately managed detention centres. From 2001, occupants of boats intercepted at sea were held in detention on offshore islands of Australia (Christmas Island), or on other Pacific nations such as Manus Island in Papua New Guinea and the Island State of Nauru. This was known as 'The Pacific Solution'. Asylum seekers had limited access to health, legal, and other services, and were often in complete social isolation.

For those ultimately found to meet Australia's refugee protection obligations, uncertainty continued. From 1999 to 2008, Temporary Protection Visas (TPV) were offered, providing only time-limited (three to five years) refuge with no security of stay, no right of return, and no capacity for family reunification. On expiry of the TPV, refugees were required to undertake a *de novo* review of their Refugee Status in order to gain further temporary protection. The difficulties faced by already traumatized adults and children were compounded by official and media use of dehumanizing and negative language, referring to asylum seekers as unauthorized non-citizens, illegal immigrants, queue jumpers, and potential terrorists (Klocker and Dunn 2003).

The harm to children and their caregivers went beyond the failure of the state to protect children from individual acts of abuse and neglect. Rather than being unwitting, the harm was justified by politicians on the grounds that it acted as a deterrent to further attempted migration or that providing more appropriate environments would encourage asylum seekers to bring children in order to secure more favourable outcomes. The system was maintained despite increasing evidence of the negative health and mental health consequences for detainees and sustained public and professional opposition to these breaches of human rights.

Child asylum seekers and refugees

Forced migration is a major problem with increasing areas of regional armed conflict between and within nations, often complicated by environmental disaster, leading to increasing numbers of refugees, asylum seekers, and displaced persons fleeing persecution and danger. At the end of 2007, the total population under UNHCR's responsibility was 31.7 million. Information on the age breakdown is incomplete but suggests that, in refugees and refugee-like situations, 46 per cent of the refugee population are under 18, and 10 per cent are under the age of five (UNHCR 2008).

Asylum seeker and refugee children have a range of vulnerabilities related to their pre-flight experiences (Fazel and Stein 2002; Lustig et al. 2004), including exposure to violence (direct and witnessed), trauma, civil strife, family dislocation and loss and, for many families, years spent in substandard living conditions in refugee camps. Flight experiences for asylum seekers are often also traumatic. Since 1999, the journeys of those arriving in Australia frequently involve smuggling by boat from Indonesia to the northern offshore waters of Australia in overcrowded, unseaworthy vessels, many with young children on board. A number of maritime disasters and deaths have occurred as a consequence (Kevin 2004).

The experience of resettlement varies considerably depending on the welcome extended, and the way refugees are represented in the media and political debates. By definition, families found to be in need of refugee protection have not migrated voluntarily. Many live unwillingly in exile with ambivalent feelings about resettlement and the permanency of their new home. Marginalization and racism, or further traumatization during detention and the visa determination process, adversely affect the health and well-being of families and children. There is evidence that post-settlement experiences have a major impact on long term psychosocial adjustment of adult refugees and asylum seekers (Steel et al. 2006; Porter and Haslam 2005; Heptinstall et al. 2004).

The impact of immigration policies and practice on children and families—Australia as an example

Many thousands of children (0–18 years) were detained in Australia over the last decade. There are more children in immigration detention in early 2011 than ever before. In September 2001, at the height of the previous peak, there were 842 children in detention; in May 2011 there were 1,082 (Jureidini and Burnside 2011). It is assumed that, of the estimated 4089 children who arrived in Australia without valid visas between 1999 and 2003, most, if not all, were detained for some period, as until July 2005 no distinction was made in immigration law and practice between adults and children seeking asylum (Crock 2007).

Children are dependent on others to identify and meet their needs and therefore their well-being cannot be considered separately from that of their caregivers, and the wider social and cultural context (Bronfenbrenner 1979). Children who are separated from caregivers are particularly vulnerable. Two hundred and ninety unaccompanied minors, aged 8 to 17 years were detained in Australia between 1999 and 2003. For those who were detained with family, their incarcerated, traumatized, and disempowered parents and caregivers were often unable to adequately provide care and protection or fulfil parental roles and responsibilities. Separation from caregivers was offered as the only and inevitable consequence of removing children from

Box 20.1: International conventions and asylum-seekers

Australia is a signatory both to the UN Convention Relating to the Status of Refugees (UNHCR 1951) and the Convention on the Rights of the Child (CRC) (UN 1989). Under the Refugee Convention, incorporated into the Australian Migration Act, a refugee is defined as a person who 'owing to a well-founded fear of being persecuted for reasons of race, religion, nationality, membership of a particular social group, or political opinion, is outside the country of his nationality, and is unable to or, owing to such fear, is unwilling to avail himself of the protection of that country. . .' (UNHCR 1951). Asylum seekers are those who have applied for protection from persecution under the UN Refugee Convention definition but have not yet received a final decision on their application. The United Nation's CRC outlines the human rights and protections to which children are entitled. In 1990, Australia ratified the CRC and this was scheduled into the Commonwealth Human Rights and Equal Opportunity Act in 1993. However, the provisions of the CRC have not been enacted in Australian law and Australia does not have a Bill of Rights. Article 3 of the CRC states

> 1. In all actions concerning children, whether undertaken by public or private social welfare institutions, courts of law, administrative authorities or legislative bodies, the best interests of the child shall be a primary consideration.

The four core principles of the convention are non-discrimination; giving priority to the best interests of the child; the right to life, survival and development; and respect for the views of the child.

In relation to the importance of the family, the Preamble to the CRC states in part:

> Convinced that the family, as the fundamental group of society and the natural environment for the growth and well-being of all its members and particularly children, should be afforded the necessary protection and assistance so that it can fully assume its responsibilities within the community, . . .

Article 22 outlines the obligations of signatory states to refugee children:

> Parties shall take appropriate measures to ensure that a child who is seeking refugee status . . . shall, whether unaccompanied or accompanied by his or her parents or by any other person, receive appropriate protection and humanitarian assistance in the enjoyment of applicable rights set forth in the present Convention and in other international human rights or humanitarian instruments to which the said States are Parties.

In relation to detention of children, Article 37(b) states:

> Parties shall ensure that: No child shall be deprived of his or her liberty unlawfully or arbitrarily. The arrest, detention or imprisonment of a child shall be in conformity with the law and shall be used only as a measure of last resort and for the shortest appropriate period of time.

UNHCR Revised Guidelines relating to the detention of Asylum Seekers Guideline 6 (UNHCR 1999) also state that 'detention is undesirable, should not be prolonged and that children should not be detained'.

immigration detention, resulting in a choice between two negative options for children and families: continued incarceration or family break-up.

Parental mental illness increases children's vulnerability to emotional and behavioural disorders and post-traumatic symptoms and developmental disruption in children are strongly linked to their parents' well-being and level of traumatization (Sack et al. 1995; Smith et al. 2001). There is evidence of the adverse impact of parental and, in particular, maternal mental health on children's functioning both in situations of war trauma (Qouta et al. 2005; Smith et al. 2001) and while detained and seeking asylum (Mares et al. 2002; Mares and Jureidini 2004; Steel, Momartin, et al. 2004). There is also evidence that post-migration experiences have a significant impact on the mental health of refugee and asylum seeker adults and children (Porter and Haslam 2005; Steel et al. 2006).

Australia's policies have demonstrably had considerable negative mental health and developmental consequences for detained adults and children (Silove et al. 2007; Steel, Momartin, et al. 2004; Steel et al. 2006; Mares and Jureidini 2004; Momartin et al. 2006). Limited international studies support these findings (Ichikawa et al. 2006; Keller et al. 2003). Research with this population is difficult for a multitude of practical, ethical, and political reasons (Kirmayer et al. 2004; Minas 2004). Steel et al. (2004) surveyed a near complete sample of children and their caregivers in one remote detention facility. They concluded, 'All adults and children met diagnostic criteria for at least one current psychiatric disorder. Based on retrospective comparisons, adults displayed a threefold and children a tenfold increase in psychiatric disorder subsequent to detention' (p. 30). In another study (Mares and Jureidini 2004), all the children interviewed in remote detention facilities had witnessed repeated acts of self harm by their parents and other adults, including cutting, attempted hangings, self poisoning, and jumping onto razor wire. Many children had also harmed themselves. Parents felt considerable grief and guilt witnessing their children experiencing further trauma and disadvantage during prolonged periods in detention. In the detention centre setting parents were at times the source of their child's trauma as a result of their self-destructive or otherwise disturbed behaviour and mental illness.

> One young couple with an infant child lived in a donga with other unrelated detainees, from several different cultures. The tiny rooms within the donga were only separated by curtains. Many detainees became angry and complained that the infant was keeping them awake at night. The mother's response was to tape the child's mouth closed as an attempt to reduce conflict and danger. She was reported to the child protection agency but she and the child continued to be detained in the same environment.[1]

When parents or care givers are unable, for whatever reason, to provide care and protection, the state has a role 'in loco parentis' to ensure that children's needs are met. In Australia, as in many other countries, this is enshrined in child protection legislation. Australia invests considerable resources in child protection policies and programmes for its residents and citizens. Exposure to violence, physical, sexual, or emotional abuse, and neglect of children's developmental needs for love, care, and protection are all forms of maltreatment which ordinarily trigger state intervention.

> An 11 year old boy was left to care for his infant brother while his mother was in hospital with a medical condition. During that time he was sexually abused and when the state child protection agency confirmed that he had been abused, their intervention was to teach him protective behaviours so that he 'did not expose himself to the risk of further abuse'.

Detained children were knowingly exposed to violence, neglect, and abuse. Their developmental needs including education were not met and they were prevented from participation in the community and in decision-making about their lives. Australia's detention of refugee children

---

[1] These examples are adapted from the direct clinical experience of the authors and have been de-identified.

with their families and as unaccompanied minors breached children's human rights in many areas (HREOC 2004:Section 6.1, 138), and caused demonstrable harm to those detained, including children. The use of mistreatment as deterrent contravenes the 1985 United Nations High Commission for Refugees (UNHCR) Guidelines on the Detention of Asylum Seekers, which explicitly state that the use of detention to deter future asylum seekers is contrary to the principles of international protection.

The Australian government received much criticism from Australian and international bodies including the Office of the United Nations High Commissioner of Human Rights, who, in response to Australia's Migration (Further Border Protection Amendment) Bill 2002, stated detention 'for example as deterrent or as a punitive measure for illegal entry/presence is considered to be at variance with Article 31' (UNHCR 2002). These policies also resulted in sustained legal challenge (Burnside 2007) and community protest (Gosden 2006; Mares and Newman 2007).

Concerted public and professional opposition to these policies and a change of national government in November 2007 resulted in some changes to immigration policy and law including an end to detention of children (changed by regulation in 2005), indefinite detention, and Temporary Protection Visas (TPVs). The Rudd Labor government's stated key immigration values included 'mandatory detention as an essential component of strong border control', but that 'children, including juvenile foreign fishers and, where possible, their families, will not be detained in an immigration detention centre (IDC)' (Evans 2008a).

Despite this, since December 2008, the new multimillion dollar detention centre on Christmas Island (4000km from the nearest major city) has been used to detain asylum seekers. There is ongoing concern, including from members of the Parliament Standing Committee on Migration (2008) about aspects of current policy, in particular inadequate independent oversight, lack of protection against arbitrary detention, and the continuing use of off-shore detention with the associated difficulties of access to legal and medical support. Thus asylum-seeking adults and children arriving in Australia remain extremely vulnerable and detention, often in remote centres, remains standard practice. As at February 2011, there were 1027 children in immigration detention (Department of Immigration and Citizenship 2011).[2]

Deterrence as explicit policy

On 5 May 1992, the then Immigration Minister Gerry Hand made it explicit that detention legislation was intended as a deterrent.

> The Government is determined that a clear signal be sent that migration to Australia may not be achieved by simply arriving in this country and expecting to be allowed into the community. (Hand 1992)

Subsequent ministers reaffirmed this intent with specific reference to children in detention. For example, when the HREOC report was tabled in Parliament in May 2004, recommending the immediate release of all children from immigration detention (HREOC 2004), Senator Amanda Vanstone, Minister for Immigration and Multicultural Affairs and Attorney-General Philip Ruddock stated:

> The government's strong but fair border protection policies have had an impact. The number of unauthorized arrivals has dramatically reduced from 4,137 in 2000-01 to 82 in this financial year. This means

---

[2] <http://www.immi.gov.au/managing-australias-borders/detention/_pdf/immigration-detention-statistics-20110204.pdf>, accessed 3 April 2011.

that the people smuggling trade has also reduced and children have not had to undertake a hazardous journey which may have jeopardised their lives (Vanstone and Ruddock 2004).

In the face of considerable public evidence about the harmful psychological impact of detention on children and families (HREOC 2004) such statements appear to justify the damage done to children and adults in immigration detention on the grounds that there is greater benefit to others through successfully discouraging further attempts to seek asylum.

A subsequent media release confirmed this intent: 'the success of the government's strategies to deter people smugglers has seen illegal arrivals virtually cease' (Vanstone 2004), as did earlier ministerial correspondence: 'the state has the sovereign right to determine which non-citizens can enter the country, those that can remain, and the conditions under which any may be removed. . . . While deterrence is not a primary purpose of detention, it is an important incidental factor' (Ruddock, personal communication to S Mares, 28 April 2003).

Ethical implications of deterrence as policy

There are complex national and international factors that contribute to the harsh immigration policies adopted by Australia. These include perceived threat to wealth and environmental sustainability from rising numbers of displaced people. There are also valid arguments about the right of a nation state to protect and manage its borders. Likewise a complex set of interacting factors influence changes in the origin and number of asylum seekers arriving in Australia. Our focus is on the ethics of Australia's chosen response to this set of circumstances.

In addition to being contrary to Australia's treaty obligations, we examine whether detention of children as a deterrent is unethical, and ultimately also damaging to the community that it is implied to protect or advantage. Leaving aside the substantial philosophical debate[3] about the ethics of using others as a means to an end, we consider the government's argument that use of immigration detention as deterrent can be defended on the grounds that any harm done is outweighed by the good achieved. This is a consequentialist argument, whereby an act is judged morally right or wrong depending only on its consequences. According to this approach, if a cost-benefit analysis demonstrates that the benefit of mandatory detention, including the use of children as deterrence, is greater than the 'cost', the action is ethical. Recently it has been claimed that consequentialist arguments can be used to defend the use of torture in certain circumstances. It is argued that the harm caused to the person being tortured, and the person carrying out the torture (by virtue of their 'good' being diminished by engaging in demeaning behaviour) is out-weighed by the benefit. This is termed the 'ticking bomb' argument, whereby torturing a terrorist who has planted a bomb might elicit information that saves lives (Dershowitz 2006). There are a number of counterarguments, including the lack of demonstrated effectiveness of torture to elicit useful information (also see Chapter 13).

Inevitably such accounting exercises are prone to interpretation and bias, so that good evidence is needed to override the common sense conclusion that torture is inhumane or, in this case, that children should be protected. We contend that such evidence is not available to support the benefits of mandatory detention under this argument, so that even if we forego a moral

---

[3] Ethical concerns about situations in which good is secured for some people only if others suffer harm dates back to Kant: 'For all rational beings come under the law that each of them must treat itself and all others never merely as means, but in every case at the same time as ends in themselves. . . [each individual] has not merely a relative worth, i.e. value, but an intrinsic worth, that is, dignity', Kant, I (1785) *Groundwork for the Metaphysics of Morals*.

commitment to uphold and protect the well-being and the rights of asylum-seeking children and their families, we still cannot justify detention as deterrent.

Cost-benefit analysis

The first step in demonstrating favourable cost-benefit is to show that draconian measures are an effective deterrent. A causal relationship between Australia's inhumane treatment of asylum seeker adults and children, and decreasing number of boat arrivals was claimed but not demonstrated. Many other factors including political changes in origin countries and diplomatic work with Indonesia are likely to have contributed to the reduction in arrivals. The onus was on the Australian government to show that the proposed causal relationship was real, and the evidence for this is contested. Let us accept for the purposes of this argument that the possibility of a significant deterrent effect can be demonstrated.

The claimed benefits from deterring asylum seekers were:

Preventing their exploitation by people smugglers and reducing their exposure to dangerous travel in unsafe vessels

The most compelling ethical argument here is that individuals should be able to make autonomous decisions according to their own analysis of the circumstances. The fact that children are exposed to these risks by their parents without having any say in the decision raises the possibility that a third party, such as the Australian government, might have a mandate to intervene.

Fairness

Former Prime Minister Howard argued that Australia has a refugee quota that is 'quite generous' by world standards, with all asylum seekers having the right to apply to come to Australia in this way. Those who arrive by boat are then considered 'queue jumpers'. It is implied that taking too many refugees would overwhelm Australia's resources, and that the refugee assessment process must be 'fair'. This claimed benefit ignores the fact that there is no universally accessible or standardized system for refugee application. Many of the countries from which people come by boat have no 'queue' and the majority of countries do not have a refugee resettlement program but instead provide protection to asylum seekers.

Tough border protection as part of the 'War on Terror'

The argument was the need for vigilance lest one of the boat people be a terrorist. In practice, this argument found little or no empirical support, nor was it credible that terrorists would choose to enter the country through such a dangerous and circuitous route. Even if there was some merit to this concern, it was not demonstrated that detention was an effective strategy for managing this threat, with a range of community-based surveillance methods being utilized by security agencies in Australia for this purpose.

Against these claimed benefits are the costs of immigration detention. These include:

The risks and damage done to the families who do not come to Australia

There is insufficient data to quantify the potential harm caused by remaining in circumstances of persecution and danger which must be assumed to be significant.

The substantial widespread harm as a result of maltreatment of children while held in detention in Australia

These human costs are extensively documented (HREOC 2004) and include;

1. The direct effect of the harsh and depriving environment.

2. Exposure to violence and self destructive behaviour.

3. Loss of effective parenting due to the effect of the environment on parental mental health.

4. Failure of the state to adequately protect children when parents fail them or are unavailable.

Financial cost

The money spent on deterrence is unavailable for other opportunities in health, education, or overseas aid. It might be argued that deterrent policies have protected Australia from the social and economic costs of refugee processing and providing asylum. The monetary expense of running immigration detention and other deterrent policies seems likely to significantly outweigh the expense of taking asylum seekers into the community (Gauthier 2004). Former Minister Evans stated (17 November 2008):

> Neither humane nor fair, the Pacific Solution was also ineffective and wasteful. At massive cost to the Australian taxpayer—I am advised that the Department of Immigration and Citizenship expended $309.8 million between September 2001 and 29 February 2008 to run the Nauru and Manus OPCs— the Howard government sought to outsource our international protection obligations to less developed countries when we should have been shouldering them ourselves (Evans 2008b).

The cost to our national reputation, to our self-respect as citizens, and the human costs relating to harm done to those entrusted with enforcing the policy

These human costs have been considerable, resulting in the diminishment of Australia's reputation and to the national self concept as the land of the 'fair go'. Flouting of international human rights conventions can also be argued to undermine these conventions, with significant international consequences (Millbank 2004).

Taking into account the costs and benefits of justifying Australia's immigration policy, including detention of children and their families as deterrent, after some 20 years of policy implementation and development, there is evidence of both high human and material costs to individuals and to the nation, and little if any demonstrable evidence of benefit. Justification of harsh immigration policy as deterrence cannot be defended on the grounds that it can be demonstrated to achieve more good than harm.

Our final ethical point is that, if we take actions that increase a person's vulnerability, we have a greater responsibility to protect that person's welfare (Goodin 1985). Unaccompanied children, and those whose parents are incapacitated by physical or mental illness, are already vulnerable. If we wittingly add to that harm through using immigration detention as a deterrent, we render children more vulnerable by virtue of, increasing rather than diminishing our responsibility towards them. 'Someone who unwillingly suffers because of what we intend for him as a way of getting our larger goal seems to fall under our power and control in a distinctive way' (Quinn 1989:347–348). Because a person's vulnerability constitutes a reason to protect that person's welfare, responsibility for these people continues even if they are in a vulnerable position due to imprudent action, in this case, the decision to seek asylum in Australia. We argue that these vulnerable children are owed an increased duty of care by Convention Relating to the Status of Refugees and CRC signatory nations, including Australia, adding to our moral obligation to protect them.

Implications for clinicians

Clinicians who attempt to work with children and families affected by immigration policy encounter a system within which they have little power. Immigration law takes precedence over the health and child protection jurisdictions that ordinarily support the clinician's work, and this persists despite challenges in the Federal and Family Courts of Australia (Chisholm and Parkinson 2003; Freckelton 2003).

While breaches under international humanitarian law, especially of the provisions of the Convention of the Rights of the Child are unambiguous, the best response to this has not always been clear. Health professionals operate under various codes of professional conduct which are developed to inform and guide ethical professional practice. Few if any of these codes adequately anticipate the situation where a health professional is required to advocate actively against abusive government policies.

Within Australia and internationally in the political, public, and academic domains, arguments continue about the moral and ethical responsibilities of clinicians and researchers to this vulnerable population. Access to detention centres and detainees for the purposes of academic research is very limited and studies that have been undertaken were argued to be unscientific or unethical (Minas 2004). There has been little or no access to adequate clinical services for detained asylum seekers, especially those in remote centres. Medical staff employed by the private detention company have been required to sign confidentiality clauses preventing them from speaking about their observations of conditions in detention. This supports the argument made by some professional health groups that advocacy against an abusive and damaging immigration system has been preferable to employment in compromising circumstances, but this position is not universally accepted.

Despite the obstacles to detailed research information about the harmful effects of immigration policy on mental health, individual stories of harm and trauma, particularly of children, began to influence the public debate. A number of inquiries and reports (including HREOC) on the impact of immigration detention and harsh immigration policies generally were released that made the evidence increasingly difficult for politicians to dismiss. Public attention and sympathy were captured by the demonstrated harm occurring particularly to children, but it was the wrongful detention of a mentally ill Australian citizen that finally forced a government inquiry into the functioning of the immigration detention system.

Psychiatry has often been on the wrong side of the equation of human rights and mental health (Dudley and Gale 2002; Wilks 2005). In response to the human rights abuses outlined, child psychiatrists and other health professionals used knowledge of human development and the impact of trauma to demonstrate the damage done by immigration policy. They took an effective and lead role individually, as well as through professional organizations and in collaboration with community advocates, to argue for change to this policy in the political and the public domains. The emphasis was predominantly on the harmful clinical effects of detention, particularly on children rather than on the abuses of human rights, although the two were linked (Silove et al. 2007; Steel et al. 2004).

Despite the, at times considerable, personal and professional impact of these actions, we argue that health and mental health professionals are obliged to take a stand against these breaches. Health professionals have a responsibility to advocate for these already vulnerable adults and children and to remain vigilant in opposing state policies that damage one group of individuals with the stated aim of benefiting another. Not to do so is unethical and neglect of their professional duties and obligations.

Conclusion

The state, whether signatory or not to the Convention on the Rights of the Child, has a role in *loco parentis* to vulnerable children without effective parents. When state policies impact negatively on the mental health and well-being of children and adults, this constitutes a breach of human rights. This failure of the state to protect children must be distinguished from even less acceptable practice whereby state policies, such as harsh immigration policies, use the stated aim of deterrence to justify and dismiss the negative consequences for children, young people, and their caregivers. In this chapter we have examined possible defences for the government against charges that they cruelly exploited the suffering of asylum seekers, including children, for the greater good. We have shown that arguments that the cost to the children is outweighed by the benefit to others cannot be sustained because evidence that harsh detention measures are effective as deterrence is inconclusive and the human cost of the intervention is substantial. We have also argued that we have a greater duty of care to these children because our actions made them more vulnerable. Health and mental health clinicians have an obligation to document and protest against such breaches of the rights of children and their caregivers, despite the multitude of ethical, personal, and professional challenges this inevitably involves.

References

Bronfenbrenner, U (1979) *The ecology of human development: Experiments by nature and design.* Cambridge, MA: Harvard University Press.

Burnside, J (2007) *Watching Brief; Reflections on human rights, law and justice.* Melbourne: Scribe.

Chisholm, R and Parkinson, P (2003) 'The Immigration Cases', *Australian Journal of Family Law*, 219, 17.

Crock, M (2007) *Seeking Asylum Alone: a study of Australian law policy and practice regarding unaccompanied and separated children.* Sydney: Federation Press.

Department of Immigration and Citizenship (DIAC) (2008) *Managing Australia's Borders.* Available at <http://www.immi.gov.au/managing-australias-borders/> accessed 8 January 2009.

Department of Immigration and Citizenship (DIAC) (2011). *Immigration Detention Statistics Summary.* Community and Detention Services Division, DIAC. Available at <http://www.immi.gov.au/managing-australias-borders/detention/_pdf/immigration-detention-statistics-20110930.pdf>, accessed 6 November 2011.

Dershowitz, A (2006) 'Warming Up to Torture?' *LA Times*, 17 October 2006. Available at <http://www.latimes.com/news/printedition/opinion/la-oe-dershowitz17oct17,0,1026020.story>, accessed 6 November 2011.

Dudley, M and Gale, F (2002) 'Psychiatrists as a moral community? Psychiatry under the Nazis and its contemporary relevance', *Australian and New Zealand Journal of Psychiatry*, 36(5), 585–94.

Evans, C (2008a) *Government welcomes bipartisan report on immigration detention: Media Release: 01 December 2008* http://www.minister.immi.gov.au/media/media-releases/2008/ce08117.htm, accessed 6 November 2011.

Evans, C (2008b) *Refugee Policy Under The Rudd Government - The First Year. Address to the Refugee Council of Australia.* Parramatta Town Hall, Monday 17 November 2008. Available at <http://www.minister.immi.gov.au/media/speeches/2008/ce081117.htm>.

Fazel, M, and Stein, A (2002) 'The mental health of refugee children', *Archives of Disease in Childhood*, 87, 366–70.

Freckelton, I (2003) 'Migration Law, the Family Court and therapeutic jurisprudence', *Journal of Law and Medicine*, 133,11

Gauthier, K (2004) *The Cost of Detention* (Prepared for Senator A. Ridgeway). Available at <http://www.safecom.org.au/detention-cost.htm>, accessed 6 November 2011.

Goodin, R (1985) *Protecting the Vulnerable.* Chicago: University of Chicago Press.

Gosden, D (2006) 'What if no one had spoken out against this policy?: The rise of asylum seeker and refugee advocacy in Australia', *Portal*, 3, 1.

Hand, GL Migration Amendment Bill 1992: Second Reading, 05 May, 1992, Hansard pp. 2370 <http://parlinfo.aph.gov.au/parlInfo/search/display/display.w3p;query=Id%3A%22chamber%2Fhansardr%2F1992-05-05%2F0031%22>, accessed 6 November 2011.

Heptinstall, E, Sethna, V, and Taylor, E (2004) 'PTSD and Depression in refugee children: Associations with remigration and post migration stress', *European Child & Adolescent Psychiatry* 13, 373–380.

Human Rights and Equal Opportunity Commission—HREOC (2004) *A last resort? National inquiry into children in immigration detention.* Sydney: Human Rights and Equal Opportunity Commission.

Ichikawa, M, Nakahara, S, and Wakai, S (2006) 'Effects of post migration detention on mental health among Afghan asylum seekers in Japan', *Australian and New Zealand Journal of Psychiatry*, 40(4), 341–46.

Jureidini J and Burnside J (2011) 'Children in Immigration Detention: a case of Reckless Mistreatment', *Australian & New Zealand Journal of Public Health*, 35, 304–06.

Kant, I (1785 [2003]) *Groundwork for the Metaphysics of Morals.* TE Hill (ed), A Zwieg (trans). New York: Oxford University Press.

Keller, AS, Rosenfeld, B, Trinh-Shevren, C, Meserbe, C, Sachs, E, Leviss, JA et al. (2003) 'Mental health of detained asylum seekers', *The Lancet*, 362 (9397), 1721–23.

Kevin, T (2004) *A certain maritime incident: The sinking of SEIV X.* Melbourne: Scribe Publications.

Kirmayer, LJ, Rousseau, C, and Crepeau, F (2004) 'Research ethics and the plight of refugees in detention', *Monash Bioethics Review*, 23(4), 85–92.

Klocker, N, and Dunn, KM (2003) 'Who's driving the asylum debate? Newspaper and government represenations of asylum seekers', *Media International Australia incorporating Culture and Policy*, 109, 71–92.

Lustig, S, Keating, M, Grant, K W et al. (2004) 'Review of child and adolescent refugee mental health', *Journal of the American Academy of Child & Adolescent Psychiatry*, 43, 24–36.

Mares, S and Jureidini, J (2004) 'Psychiatric assessment of children and families in immigration detention: Clinical, administrative and ethical issues', *Australian and New Zealand Journal of Public Health*, 28(6), 16–22.

Mares, S and Newman, L (2007). *Acting from the heart: Australian advocates for asylum seekers tell their stories.* Sydney: Finch Publishing.

Mares, S, Newman, L, Dudley, M, and Gale, F (2002) 'Seeking refuge, losing hope: Parents and children in immigration detention', *Australasian Psychiatry*, 10, 91–96.

Millbank, A (2004) 'World's worst or world's best practice? European reactions to Australia's refugee policy', *People and Place*, 12(4), 28–37.

Minas, IH (2004) 'Detention and Deception: limits of acceptability in detention research', *Monash Bioethics Review*, 23(4), 69–77.

Momartin, S,Steel, Z, Coello, M, Aroche, J, Silove, DM, and Brooks, R (2006) 'A comparison of the mental health of refugees with temporary versus permanent protection visas', *Medical Journal of Australia*, 185, 357–61.

Parliament of the Commonwealth of Australia Joint Standing Committee on Migration (2008) *Immigration detention in Australia: A new beginning—Criteria for release from detention.* Available at <http://www.aph.gov.au/HOUSE/committee/MIG/detention/report.htm>, accessed 6 November 2011.

Porter, M and Haslam, N (2005) 'Predisplacement and Postdisplacement Factors Associated with Mental Health of Refugees and Internally Displaced Persons; A Meta analysis', *JAMA*, 294(5), 602–12.

Qouta, S, Runamäki, R-L, and Eyad, ES (2005) 'Mother-child expression of psychological distress in war trauma', *Clinical Child Psychology and Psychiatry*, 10, 135–56.

Quinn, WS (1989) 'Actions, Intentions, and Consequences: The Doctrine of Double Effect', *Philosophy and Public Affairs*, 18(4), 334–51.

Sack ,WH, Clarke, NG, and Seeley, J (1995) 'Post traumatic stress disorder across two generations of Cambodian refugees', *Journal of the American Academy of Child and Adolescent Psychiatry*, 34, 1160–66.

Silove, D, Austin, P, and Steel, Z (2007) 'No refuge from terror: The Impact of Detention on the Mental Health of Trauma-affected Refugees Seeking Asylum in Australia', *Transcultural Psychiatry*, 44(3), 359–93.

Smith, P, Perrin, S, Yule, W, and Rabe-Hesketh, S (2001) 'War exposure and maternal reactions in the psychological adjustment of children from Bosnia-Hercegovina', *Journal of Child Psychology and Psychiatry*, 4, 395–404.

Steel, Z, Mares, S, Newman, L, Blick, B, and Dudley, M (2004) 'The Politics of Asylum and Immigration Detention: Advocacy, Ethics and the Professional Role of the Therapist', in JP Wilson and B Drozdek (eds) *Broken Spirits: The treatment of traumatised asylum seekers, refugees, war and torture survivors*. New York: Brunner Routledge, 659–87.

Steel, Z, Momartin, S, Bateman, C et al. (2004) 'Psychiatric status of asylum seeker families held for a protracted period in a remote detention centre in Australia', *Australian and New Zealand Journal of Public Health*, 28, 520–26.

Steel, Z, Silove, D, Brooks, R, Momartin, S, Alzuhairi, B, and Susljik, I (2006) 'Impact of immigration detention and temporary protection on the mental health of refugees', *British Journal of Psychiatry*, 188, 58–64.

UN Convention on the Rights of the Child (1989) UN General Assembly resolution 44/25 of 20 November 1989. Available at <http://www.un.org/documents/ga/res/44/a44r025.htm>, accessed 6 November 2011.

United Nations High Commissioner for Refugees (UNHCR) (1951) *The 1951 Convention Relating to the Status of Refugees*. Geneva: United Nations.

United Nations High Commissioner for Refugees (UNHCR) (1999) *Revised Guidelines on Applicable Criteria and Standards Relating to the Detention of Asylum Seekers*. Geneva: United Nations.

United Nations High Commissioner for Refugees (UNHCR) (2008). *Global Trends: Refugees, Asylum-seekers, Returnees, Internally Displaced and Stateless Persons*. Available at <http://www.unhcr.org/statistics/STATISTICS/4852366f2.pdf>, accessed 6 November 2011.

UNHCR (2002) *Human rights envoy finds more humane approach to illegal immigration in Australia 'would be desirable': Press release hr/4619*. Available at <http://www.un.org/News/Press/docs/2002/hr4619.doc.htm> accessed 6 November 2011.

Vanstone, A and Ruddock, P (13 May 2004) *VPS 68/2004 'HREOC Inquiry into Children in Immigration Report Tabled'*. Available at <http://parlinfo.aph.gov.au/parlInfo/search/display/displayPrint.w3p;query=Id%3A%22media%2Fpressrel%2FTKC6%22>, accessed 6 November 2011.

Vanstone, A (13 May 2004) *VPS 070/2004 'No secret agenda for Brisbane detention facility'*. Available at <http://pandora.nla.gov.au/pan/67564/20070202-0000/www.minister.immi.gov.au/media/media-releases/2004/v04070.html>, accessed 6 November 2011.

Wilks, M (2005) 'A stain on medical ethics', *The Lancet*, 366(9484), 429–31.

Chapter 21

Human Rights and Women's Mental Health

Beverley Raphael, Carol Nadelson, Melanie Taylor, and Jennifer Jacobs

There are many human rights issues and their violation which may impact on the mental health and well-being of women, men, and their children. This chapter focuses on the impacts of rights violations, the failure of rights instruments, and women's mental health. It recognizes that such violations may result from many cultural, structural, and political imperatives that have arisen from the social frameworks of religion, law, work, and indeed biology. The many social and cultural constructions that exist and develop globally have for the most part meant that human rights violations affecting women's mental health are perpetrated by men. Women are also adversely affected in many instances by these structural issues, but may lack the will to move from such sanctioned roles and inequities because of the relative power differential. These factors will inform much of the discussion presented in this chapter.

In response to significant human rights violations, the United Nations adopted the Universal Declaration of Human Rights in 1948, as a common standard for all nations, followed by more detailed instruments and legislation. These are seen as fundamental rights for all people, to be applied without discrimination. They have progressively addressed specific types of discrimination and the particular vulnerability of some groups.

The International Covenant on Civil and Political Rights (United Nations 1966) emphasizes fundamental rights such as the right to life; to freedom from cruelty, inhuman or degrading treatment or punishment; to liberty, security, respect, dignity, equality, and others. Discrimination of any kind should not occur, including that related to sex or gender.

The Convention on the Elimination of all forms of Discrimination Against Women (CEDAW) (United Nations 1979) has been ratified by more than 180 countries. In Australia it is incorporated in federal law, for example, in the Sex Discrimination Act of 1984 (Commonwealth of Australia, revised version, 2006). This involves not only the prevention of discrimination, but also the active promotion of equality.

Despite such conventions and legislation, the human rights of women are persistently violated. Such discrimination against women impacts profoundly on their mental health and well-being. Women endure poverty, adversity, poor education, exposure to greater stressors, abuse and violence, a lack of access to equal work and conditions, and a lack of valuing of women's contributions. All represent violations of women's human rights which have been demonstrated to very adversely affect their mental health (Astbury 2006). For women experiencing mental illnesses, discrimination has occurred throughout the world, with social exclusion, ignorance, and rejection of those affected. Negative attitudes have extended to those providing care for people experiencing mental disorders and illnesses. This chapter will address these issues, recognizing that they are frequently interrelated.

Women and violence

Violence against women is a violation of their human rights and is widespread from childhood sexual and physical abuse to domestic violence and rape in adult life (Garcia-Moreno et al. 2005). Violence occurs in circumstances of domestic, family, and intimate partner relationships, trafficking, forced prostitution and sexual slavery, rape, and ethnic cleansing in conflict and war-affected countries. Population-based studies show that childhood and adulthood victimization leads to a three- to four-fold increase in risk of depression and other psychiatric morbidity for women.

In their review of violence against women, Watts and Zimmerman (2002) suggest 'that most forms of violence are not single incidents but chronic, repeated and continuing, often over many years'. They believe that, because of the sensitivity of issues surrounding such violence, it is under-reported across most countries and settings. Nevertheless, it is estimated that many millions of women experience such violence across the world.

In a World Health Organization (WHO) multi-centre study of women aged 15–49 from ten countries, it was estimated that domestic violence affected one in three women globally (Garcia-Moreno et al. 2005). Domestic violence impacts negatively on the mental health of women via higher rates of depression, complex and other forms of PTSD, substance abuse problems, and increased suicidal behaviours (Herman 1992; Roberts et al. 2006). Studies have shown that 29 per cent of women have experienced some form of physical violence or sexual violence before the age of 16 years, with forced intercourse, or attempted intercourse, being experienced by one in five women (Mouzos and Makki 2004). Child sexual and physical abuse is widespread, with sexual abuse being more frequently experienced by girls. Internationally, between 7–36 per cent of adult women and 3–29 per cent of adult men report such abuse (Finkelhor 1994). It is strongly correlated with childhood emotional and behavioural problems, and is well-established as a risk factor for adult mental health problems including depression, substance abuse, suicidality, and other behavioural and social vulnerabilities (Fergusson et al. 1996).

These forms of violence not only have direct consequences, increasing the risk for mental disorders and other health related problems, but are also likely to be prolonged and borne silently by women because they are fearful of further violence to themselves or their children. They develop a sense of helplessness and shame. Such violence, especially when sexualized, lowers a girl's or woman's self-esteem, and sense of personal worth; a view sometimes reinforced by societal views that it is somehow her fault.

Violence and abuse of girls and women are overt violations of women's human rights and directly contribute to poor mental health. There may be cultural and religious prescriptions which allow, or even support, such violations.

The Committee on the Elimination of Discrimination Against Women was developed with the Convention for the Elimination of Discrimination Against Women (CEDAW) (United Nations 1979) following the adoption of the Declaration of the Elimination of Violence Against Women (United Nations 1993). This group met in 2007 on the 25th Anniversary of its inception, noting the increasing acceptance of the convention in many nations. Nevertheless, at this meeting, Louise Arbour, High Commissioner of Human Rights, stated that acceptance was 'not necessarily universal' for there was a 'resurgence of notions that they should be restricted because of the imperative of culture, custom, tradition and religion', indicating that the committee had grappled with such issues since its inception. Nevertheless she concluded that there was a need to emphasize 'the universality of human rights, while respecting diversity' (United Nations 2007).

These issues are very relevant for girls and women in societies where dominant political or fundamentalist values demand that females be controlled, subservient, and subjugated. This is evidenced where women are not free to make their own choices; where female genital mutilation is culturally sanctioned; 'honour' killings are sanctioned and unpunished; and girls cannot be educated. Far more subtle forms also exist, including those societal conventions which fail to challenge the damage to women's well-being that may be associated with the range of demeaning societal prescriptions for women's identities, roles, and behaviour.

Experience of conflict and war further impacts broadly on the mental health of women. In such circumstances, women experience the loss of loved ones, destruction of home and community, torture, and other related traumatic experiences. All of these experiences profoundly impact women. Wars in recent times increasingly affect civilian populations, especially women and children. Jansen (2006) reviewed the effects of armed conflict on women's mental health. In settings of complex emergencies, such as Darfur and elsewhere, it is reported that not only is there a lack of access to basic resources for survival, but high rates of depression affect up to a third of women in such circumstances. In such instances there are multiple traumatic exposures which greatly heighten the risk of psychiatric morbidity as a likely outcome in such contexts (Joop de Jong et al. 2002).

Refugee experience in camps, detention centres, and even in new communities may be associated with ongoing trauma and grief, leading to adverse impact on mental health. Between 60–80 per cent of the world's refugees are women. In such circumstances, there is likely to have been experience of violent conflict over periods prior to refugee status, sexual assault, including in refugee camps, the experience of violence such as torture, and the traumatic deaths of husbands, children, and family members. As indicated by Joop de Jong et al. (2002) there are multiple traumatic exposures.

Human rights as they apply to children

As girls may be vulnerable with respect to the violation of their rights as female children, the United Nations General Assembly declared such rights in the Convention on the Rights of the Child (United Nations 1989). This applies to everyone under the age of 18 years; to protect them from discrimination of any kind and to ensure their rights to life, survival, and development; to protection from abuse, neglect, or exploitation; rights concerning family life and support for families; for health, education, social security, and adequate living standards; rights for care of illness and disability, including mental health problems; rights for measures to promote recovery from abuse, neglect, or violence; and to protect children in minority communities.

Despite this, the devaluation of girls, and the value placed on male babies and boy children continues in many societies. By its very nature, such a social prescription conveys to girls early in life their low relative worth. This is evidenced by sex-selective abortion and female infanticide, reflected in atypical sex ratios at birth and differential mortality (Watts and Zimmerman 2002). These authors suggest that there is a 'systematic and often fatal neglect of the health and nutritional needs of girls' (p. 1236). These discriminations result in estimates of between 60 and 100 million women and girls 'missing' in statistics across the world. Technology has increased the opportunity for early detection and selection of foetal sex, and adds to the losses. There are few data about the impact of this process on girls and women, either for those who are born despite such tendencies, or for women giving birth to girls. What does it mean for the well-being of a woman to be devalued for giving birth to a girl child, a baby 'in the image of the mother'? Clearly, for women in such circumstances it is likely that there is profound sadness, and a sense of loss—loss of self worth, but also loss of the special relationship around mother–daughter bonds.

The lack of access to education and learning impacts on girls' opportunities and may be a part of a trajectory in countries which do not support equity in these, or other, domains. Lack of education will limit the options for their futures as women. More subtle limitations may come in many societies from expectations of girls' behaviours—that they should not challenge boys, that they must always please boys. These themes, whether subtle or very overt, impact on girls' views of themselves, their identities as girls and women and, in tune with this, impact on the identities of boys and young men.

The expectation of girls as being 'quiet' or 'well behaved' may mean that their mental health problems may be unrecognized and they may similarly learn that they should not complain or protest over the way they are treated, or their 'lot' in life.

Girls, like their mothers, may be most adversely affected when subjected to sexual exploitation as may happen when taken into coerced prostitution, or other violations. Such childhood sexual abuse is a potent risk factor for adult mental health problems (Mullen et al. 1993).

Young girls may also be profoundly affected by the violence and destruction associated with conflict-affected regions. And when resources are few, girls may be provided with less than boys. They may also take over the care of others when their mothers are unable to do so. Adversities in childhood may have greater effects on the adult mental health of women than men (Pirkola et al. 2005).

Women's health, their bodies, and human rights

Girls and women may experience risk and vulnerability in terms of their mental health in relation to their female bodies, biology, physical health, and equity of access to reproductive and other health resources. The Constitution of the World Health Organization has articulated that the attainment of the highest sustainable standard of health is one of the fundamental rights of *every* human being. There should thus be no discrimination in terms of health. As noted by Astbury (2006), this may be more difficult in the implementation.

The health needs of women may be less recognized and provided for, for example with recognition of and response to heart disease. The different effects of medication for women is another. Research on broad issues of women's health has gradually improved in recent years, but still reflects many discrepancies (Greenburger et al. 2006).

Women may not have access to many preventative health practices such as cancer screening techniques for breast and gynaecological cancers, and thus present with advanced lesions, with surgical and other procedures also poorly available in low income countries or where priorities for women's health are few. The resultant health outcomes will potentially affect their mental health and well-being.

Women are affected emotionally as well as physically by cultural practices or lack of health care which deny them choices about fertility, pregnancy, contraception, and abortion. Access to health resources to support such choice may be minimal, unaffordable, or not sanctioned by dominant cultures. Similarly, reproductive health and the provision of health services, as well as opportunities for healthy birthing practices, are lacking in many low income countries or settings, reflected in higher rates of maternal and infant mortality and morbidity (UNICEF 2005).

Sexually transmitted diseases may be indicators of some women's experience of sexual assault. High rates of HIV/AIDS in many developing countries will have a profound effect on the mental health and well-being of women and their children.

Other aspects of women's sexuality may be the focus of human rights violations, which in turn affect their mental health. Women, in many cultural settings, report that that they are forced to have sexual intercourse to meet their partner's needs (Garcia-Moreno et al. 2005). Women may not believe that they can refuse to have sex within a marriage and the question of rape in these contexts remains controversial for many. Disorders of sexual function and enjoyment for women have been viewed in many instances by both the woman and her partner as her failure as a woman.

Women may suffer violence and abuse in pregnancy, with risk to themselves and their foetuses. The prevalence of post-natal depression, and the need for mental health care to screen for, and address this, is a further area of potential discrimination affecting women's mental health and well-being (Grigoriadis 2006).

The change in girls' bodies with the onset of puberty and menstruation, hormonal changes, and specific mental health problems associated for some women, such as pre-menstrual dysphoric disorder, have been poorly researched until recently and may be seen as women's problems, to be 'suffered', as part of being a woman.

Concerns over body shape and size have led to a substantial growth of cosmetic and plastic surgery for women in high income countries. Women are urged to change their bodies to meet goals that will make them more 'desirable', sexually attractive, or in competition with other women (Smolak 2006). Breast and facial procedures and liposuction predominate. Body image preoccupations for girls and women contribute also to the quest for 'thinness' and are social variables contributing to binge eating and dieting problems, as well as the emaciation of anorexia; where girls may see abnormal thinness as the ideal, a condition with a high mortality. This dissatisfaction with bodies is at odds with the emaciation and malnutrition that many women experience in countries affected by famine, or the destruction of food sources.

Menopause may be associated with changed status for women, with the need for treatment for this biological change, and with the recognition of depression or other conditions precipitated at this time in those vulnerable (Stewart and Khalid 2006).

The aging of women, and the development of disabilities such as dementia, may place them in further situations of risk. Inequity of health and social resources may mean that they are not adequately provided for in such circumstances, either in care systems or with support such as pensions. The inferior status of older women may adversely affect their mental health and well-being. Elder abuse may also occur in such contexts (Perkins 2006).

Women's roles and their mental health

As discussed, many of women's roles in society are seen as of lower status, are more poorly paid, and are often associated with significant stressors. This is exemplified by diverse challenges; additional roles as carers of children, the disabled, elderly, and the needy are prominent. Most carers are women and, although committed to such roles and rewarded by them, they are frequently stressed and distressed in terms of the 'burden' of such care. It is rarely equitably shared, nor recognized and rewarded. Women as carers for parents with dementia, handicapped children, or mentally ill family members may face particular problems if respite and support programmes are lacking. They are frequently concerned that their sons or daughters with illnesses, such as schizophrenia, will have no one to care for them when they and their husbands die. The inequities with carer roles constitute a human rights challenge.

When women do work, they are often in more lowly paid positions, lack equal access to career progression and education opportunities, and lack financial security. Social determinants, such as these, impact on health including mental health. They are associated with higher rates of depression amongst girls and women in such circumstances (Stewart 2007). Astbury (2006) highlights the profound effects of the social gradient of disadvantage on women's mental health, with depression, for instance, being 2–2.5 times higher in those experiencing the greatest social disadvantage, compared to those experiencing the least.

Racial discrimination and women's mental health

All persons have rights to freedom from such discrimination under the International Convention on the Elimination of All Forms of Racial Discrimination (ICERD) (United Nations 1965). This area of human rights is particularly relevant for women of culturally and linguistically diverse backgrounds, the more so if they are minority groups within different populations. It is in these instances that women face additional stresses which may affect their mental health. First, if they have come as immigrants, their adaptation to cultural differences added to difficulties with language for communication with the dominant populations, and difficulties understanding aspects of daily life, including television and news, can impact adversely on them. Second, many women in such circumstances remain in the home and they may not have the same opportunities for interaction as husbands and children, further hindering adaptation and acculturation in their new country.

If women have been refugees and/or escaped violence, then they may bring vulnerabilities which require special mental health expertise that may be difficult to access (Kaplan et al. 2008). In addition, the role of women in their culture of origin may be vastly different, challenging them and, as suggested above, their issues of human rights, and the new country's view of them. Practices regarding women's 'place' in society or families, independence, autonomy, reproductive rights, roles, and access to resources may challenge cultural and belief systems for their husbands, fathers, sons, and for them. Violation of their rights in these circumstances, even when they may perceive them as legitimate, for instance a husband's right to beat his wife if she disobeys (Garcia-Moreno et al. 2005) may bring repercussions for the abuser, and legal consequences in the new context. Women with mental health problems in such situations may be further disadvantaged by the lack of culturally appropriate services, and the understanding of the nature of mental illness which may be differently perceived and understood in their country of origin or cultural belief system. This may also apply to their views of the diagnosis and treatment that may be offered and the fear of stigma within their own cultural group. As with many special populations, there may be double risks of discrimination, impacting on human rights, and associated mental health effects.

Indigenous women

The human rights of Aboriginal people have been neglected in many ways, with their minority status, cultural frameworks, and socio-economic disadvantage placing many on the most adverse end of the social gradient. Many have faced significant adverse health outcomes in terms of excess morbidity and premature mortality. These effects can be exemplified by the adverse health outcomes of Australian Aboriginal people, with up to 20 years less of life, high ratios of preventable morbidity, perinatal morbidity, imprisonment, substance abuse, violence, loss of loved ones at early ages from accidents, suicide in custody, and multiple indicators of social and personal adversity (ABS/AIHW 2008). Aboriginal women are more frequently the victims of violence, and girls, of abuse. Many Aboriginal women's experience of trauma is extreme and trans-generational, with the taking away of children, the 'stolen generation', in earlier times (HREOC report 'Bringing Them Home' 1997). The ongoing disadvantages, violence, and effects of racism contribute to adverse mental health outcomes, with studies demonstrating poorer mental health than experienced by non-Aboriginal women. Addressing these inequities, preventing violence, facilitating self-determination in terms of programmes, such as those through Aboriginal Community Controlled Health Organizations, all contribute both to support human rights and mitigate the adverse mental health effects associated with their violations.

Women's experience of mental illnesses

There is much evidence of gender disparities in mental illness. Some of these may relate to the differing biology of women, others to societal, social, and psychological factors, potentially linked to human rights violations such as those identified above. Astbury (2006) notes that there has been inadequate attention in public health research and programmes to the role of human rights violations in adverse mental health outcomes, disproportionately experienced by women.

Many reports emphasize the importance of equity and social justice in improving women's mental health (WHO 2000). Nowhere is this more the case than for women with mental illnesses. Women may be differentially affected, depending on their condition, and differentially treated. The report of the Australian Human Rights and Equal Opportunities Commission (HREC 1993) on mental health and human rights highlights the specific difficulties reported by women with mental illnesses. Although recognizing the range of mental health challenges faced by women, the report focuses on four area of particular concern: diagnosis and treatment of mental illness; post natal depression; the psychological effect of violence; and the absence of adequate shelter, noting the need at that time for an urgent response to these issues.

Women with schizophrenia and other psychotic illnesses

Castle et al. (2000) provide a comprehensive overview of gender differences in schizophrenia. Women differ with respect to age of onset (for men the age is 18 to 25, for women 25 to the 30s (Goldstein and Lewine 2000)). This may be related to protective effects of oestrogen, genetic factors, and/or societal role expectations. Symptom expression may differ with more affective symptoms in women and negative symptoms in men, and women may have better social and functional outcomes, although post-menopause the courses may be more similar. Gender differences have also been reported for other psychotic illnesses, including the age of onset, frequency of psychotic symptoms, and course of these disorders.

Schizophrenia and other psychotic illnesses bring forth several health, social, and human rights issues for women. These include the effects of medication on weight, appearance, and other side effects including tardive dyskinesia. There are also greater problems in women related to gender differences in pharmaco-dynamics and pharmaco-kinetics (Burt and Hendrick 1997). Medications may bring additional stressors related to side effects, and higher risk of adverse physical health outcomes. Women who are chronically psychotic or institutionalized may experience difficulty accessing health care and prevention programmes, such as cervical cancer screening and mammography, and cardiovascular diagnosis and care.

Women may be particularly vulnerable to abandonment by their marital or other partner because of their condition. They may also be affected in their capacity to have and raise children, fearing the risk of genetic transmission, or that their children will be taken away from them (Hearle and McGrath 2000). The right to bear children and parent them is seen as a basic human right under United Nations agreements, and reproduction cannot be denied on the basis of disability alone. Women with schizophrenia or other psychotic illnesses may experience stigma, and they may be perceived as unable to parent and not entitled to pursue this aspect of life, as was frequently the case in previous times and with intellectually handicapped women who were sterilized 'for their own good'. Women with schizophrenia or other psychotic illnesses who have children may be stressed by parenting, may experience a lack of support for their parental roles, and their children may demonstrate more behavioural and emotional problems. Children, especially older girl children, may become the carers for their mentally ill mothers and their siblings (Camden-Pratt 2006).

Social disadvantage and violence may affect women with mental illnesses in additional ways, further violating human rights. Women may be more vulnerable to sexual assault in in-patient or community settings, the former if they are disinhibited, perhaps hypomanic, and make themselves more available, or if they are less aware, seeking comfort in sexual encounters. Women may become impaired functionally, unable to work or pursue a career because of the effects of their illnesses and may have fewer opportunities for work-focused rehabilitation because their roles are defined in domestic terms. They may be particularly vulnerable if they become homeless, where they may have children with them, or if they are imprisoned with a mental illness. Although men with mental illnesses experience homelessness and imprisonment at higher rates, women may be particularly vulnerable to exploitation and violence in these circumstances.

Women, PTSD, depression, and anxiety

Depression is over-represented in women, with women being twice as likely as men to suffer from major depressive episodes during their reproductive years (Robinson 2006). A wide range of factors has been implicated in the aetiology of depression in women, including genetic, hormonal, neuro-chemical, anatomical, and personality factors. Studies have indicated that social determinants, too, are relevant (Stewart 2007). These include social position in childhood and in adult life—social class, lower educational qualifications, living in government housing, parents who were divorced, and negative life events which can all contribute to mental ill health, even in mid life (Kuh et al. 2002). This, coupled with the increased likelihood that women and girls will experience early adversity, such as child abuse, further amplifies the prevalence of depression noted in women.

Women are also twice as likely to experience anxiety disorders, such as general anxiety disorder (GAD), panic disorder, phobias, social anxiety disorder, and obsessive compulsive disorder (Robinson 2006). Anxiety and depressive disorders are also likely to be co-morbid. Stressful life events, psychosocial and developmental factors have all been implicated in the aetiology of anxiety in children (Manassis 2006) and different social pressures on girls, such as body image. A greater tolerance of fearful behaviours and protectiveness towards girls may also contribute to an increased prevalence of anxiety disorders.

Women may be more adversely affected by violence and traumatic stressors, demonstrating higher rates of post-traumatic stress disorder (PTSD) than men for similar exposures, for instance with response to mass violence such as terrorism (Solomon et al. 2005). The frequency of forced sexual intercourse for women is likely to constitute a significant contribution to their mental health problems. Epidemiological studies indicate that rape and sexual assault are the most likely traumas leading to PTSD in women (Kessler et al. 2005).

Women experiencing depression, anxiety, or trauma related psychiatric symptoms may experience stigmatization associated with mental illness. They may be more likely to be abandoned by their marital or other partner, and experience economic consequences if that partner provided their primary source of income. This is particularly problematic if the woman is left to care for children while also managing her mental illness. Relationships with children can be affected, and older female children will often take over caretaking responsibilities of younger siblings. All of these factors can adversely affect women and their children's mental health.

Eating disorders

Eating disorders are another group of conditions where difficulties in terms of treatment effectiveness, the struggle for control, and the devaluing of the body may lead to treatment interactions which may impinge on the person's control of her body, or even entail involuntary treatment. This may also be the case with other mental illnesses.

Substance use

Substance abuse problems affect women also, from alcohol and tobacco to cannabis, amphetamines, cocaine, and opiates. The abuse of prescription medications occurs more frequently in women. Women's substance use problems may be more secret and silent, poorly recognized and managed. Co-morbidity is also significant, in relation to multiple mental health and substance use conditions, and physical health problems. Particular concerns include co-morbid trauma, high rates of domestic violence, and impact on parenting. Such patterns require recognition, diagnostic assessment, and management attuned to women's needs.

Diagnosis and stigma

Social exclusion and stigmatization impact on all those with mental illnesses, although campaigns to deal with these issues are improving understanding. Fear of being labelled or seen as 'mad' or inadequate may result in high levels of unmet need for prevention and treatment (Andrews et al. 2001). Women may be diagnosed and medicated without adequate assessment and understanding of the personal and social stressors and contexts which affect their well-being. This may be seen in the relative neglect of psychosocial domains in some assessment and treatment services. Women are more likely to be diagnosed, or misdiagnosed, with depression. In their recent study Magruder and Yeager (2008), noted that women were 1.6 times more likely to be incorrectly diagnosed with depression than men. This may be due to differences in the way they may present with mental health disorders, or as a possible result of gender bias in diagnosis.

Specific diagnoses may carry covert or overt stigma which will contribute to more negative perceptions for the woman, of how others will view her, or of how she will understand herself. Such diagnoses may also be viewed more negatively by mental health professions, with many women sensing such a view. Historically, hysteria was one such gender focused diagnosis. Borderline personality disorder or being a 'borderline' is a more discriminatory use of the term for what is at times a contentious diagnosis. This is an example where lack of emotional control, the self-harming and non-compliant behaviours, and chronicity may be viewed as particularly problematic and viewed negatively and pessimistically by women and by their therapists. Depression, particularly dysthymia, may be seen, like fears or anxiety disorders, as not really a 'serious mental illness', as conditions for which women could do more to 'help themselves'. Lack of hopeful and empathic understanding from those providing care may decrease its effectiveness, adding to the woman's sense that she has lost her dignity, her rights, and worth as a person.

Mental health services and care

Women may seek care in many settings: the support of friends, the family doctor working in primary care, or through referral to public or private providers. In these settings, they may be vulnerable, particularly if gender-stereotyping influences their providers' views of their problems, if they are dismissed without adequate care, if they hide their problems too well, if their health care or other professional betrays their trust through lack of knowledge or competence, or if their rights to care are exploited and abused.

Mental health carecare systems have a potential for becoming vehicles of human rights abuse. The United Nations General Assembly, in 1991, in adopting the Principles for the Protection of Persons with Mental Illness (United Nations 1991), recognized this and specified that these principles should be implemented 'without discrimination of any kind'.

With respect to equity in the resourcing of mental healthcare, the WHO Mental Health Atlas (WHO 2005); an audit of mental health policy, programmes, financing, legislative, and resource provision, demonstrates that equity is not met in a great many countries of the world, for instance, where less than 1 per cent of the health budget is provided for mental healthcare, medications, or there is less than one mental health nurse or one psychiatrist per 100,000 persons.

The specific resourcing of women's mental health care is not clearly delineated but it is likely that there is a greater focus on those with the most severe illnesses, such as schizophrenia, violence, and those associated with high levels of disability, and less for women with their greater prevalence of depression, for instance.

Particular issues for women lie in their greater risk of sexual abuse and exploitation; either by other patients or by staff; their vulnerability in terms of differential treatment effects; political or other discrimination that may apply in assessing their problems; a lack of understanding of their specific health and social needs as women with a mental illness; and specifically how their social roles and social position may adversely affect their mental health and well-being. In addition the lack of a specific research base that identifies their different needs, presentation, and management must also be addressed.

Conclusion

The fight for human rights for women, for girls, for female foetuses, and for old women, requires ongoing commitment in terms of the impact of abuses of these rights on their mental health and well-being. Not only does lesser access to education and resources create a trajectory of lesser opportunity, but the opportunities for advancement for women may be seen to be related to their capacity to meet men's needs, either in sexual behaviour, and perhaps premature sexual activity, reinforcing their lack of 'value'; or through their needing to be chosen as a partner/or gaining a husband who will secondarily confer status on them. Cycles of adversity commonly result when rights are not addressed, not protected or, indeed, are abused.

As described above, these experiences are likely to increase the women's vulnerability to mental health problems. This is particularly so if these are perceived as traumatic, shocking, degrading, humiliating, or threatening to the lives or futures of their loved ones, their children, and families (Raphael et al. 2008)

Women with existing mental health problems and mental illness may face additional significant threats to their well-being by their experience broadly, plus failures to protect their rights as people with mental illnesses, for instance in their access to and experience of treatment, the taking away of their children, and sexual assault.

Men too, have human rights and other rights violated. They also suffer as a consequence. Violent propensities and behaviours may result, contributing to further cycles of violence, abuse, assault, or other acts, including war, leading to further threats to women. The endurance, courage, and resilience of women are demonstrated in their commitment to children and loved ones including their men, to survival, and a future despite abuses or failures of rights protection. Rights instruments require systems, society, and nations to value their citizens, women, and men equally, and to institute their protection, education, support, and development as their commitment to humanity.

References

Andrews, G, Issakidis, C, and Carter, G (2001) 'Shortfall in mental health service utilisation', *The British Journal of Psychiatry*, 179, 417–25.

Astbury, J (2006) 'Women's mental health: from hysteria to human rights', in SE Romans and MV Seeman (eds) *Women's mental health: A life-cycle approach.* Lippincott Williams and Wilkins, Philadelphia, 377–392.

Australian Bureau of Statistics and Australian Institute of Health and Welfare (2008) *The health and welfare of Australia's Aboriginal and Torres Strait Islander peoples.* AIHW Catalogue No. IHW 21. Commonwealth of Australia. Available at <http://www.aihw.gov.au/publication-detail/?id=6442468085>, accessed 7 November 2011.

Burt, VK and Hendrick, VC (1997) *Concise guide to women's mental health.* Washington: American Psychiatric Press Inc.

Camden-Pratt, CE (2006) *Out of the shadows: Daughters growing up with a 'mad' mother.* Sydney: Finch Publishing.

Castle, D, McGrath, J, and Kulkarni, J (2000) *Women and Schizophrenia.* Cambridge: Cambridge University Press.

Commonwealth of Australia, Attorney-General's Department (2006) Sex Discrimination Act 1984, Updated version 27 March 2006. Available at <http://www.comlaw.gov.au/ComLaw/Legislation/ActCompilation1.nsf/0/3A1AE1C157596F93CA2571410005BFEF/$file/SexDiscrimination84_WD02.pdf>, accessed 7 November 2011.

Fergusson, DM, Horwood, LJ, and Lynskey, MT (1996) 'Childhood sexual abuse and psychiatric disorder in young adulthood: II. Psychiatric outcomes of childhood sexual abuse', *Journal of the American Academy of Child and Adolescent Psychiatry,* 34(10), 1365–74.

Finkelhor, D (1994) 'The international epidemiology of child sexual abuse', *Child Abuse and Neglect,* 18(5), 409–17.

Garcia-Moreno, C, Heise, L, Jansen, H, Ellsberg, M, and Watts, C (2005) 'Public Health: Violence against women', *Science,* 310(5752), 25 November 2005, 1282–83.

Goldstein, JM and Lewine, RRJ (2000) 'Overview of sex differences in schizophrenia: Where have we been and where do we go from here?', in D Castle, J McGrath, and J Kulkarni (eds) *Women and Schizophrenia.* Cambridge: Cambridge University Press, 111–143.

Greenburger, P, Wider, J, and Society for Women's Health Research (2006) *The savvy woman patient: How and why sex differences affect your health.* Sterling, VA: Capital Books Inc.

Grigoriadis, S (2006) 'Postpartum and its mental health problems', in SE Romans and MV Seeman (eds) *Women's mental health: A life-cycle approach.* Philadelphia: Lippincott Williams and Wilkins, 283–296.

Hearle, J and McGrath, J (2000) 'Motherhood and schizophrenia', in D Castle, J McGrath, and J Kulkarni (eds) *Women and Schizophrenia.* Cambridge: Cambridge University Press, 79–94.

Herman, JL (1992) 'Complex PTSD: A syndrome in survivors of prolonged and repeated trauma', *Journal of Traumatic Stress,* 5(3), 377–391.

Human Rights and Equal Opportunities Commission (1993) *Human Rights and Mental Illness. Report of the National Inquiry into the Human Rights of People with Mental Illness. Volume 2.* Commonwealth of Australia, ACT: Australian Government Publishing Service.

Human Rights and Equal Opportunity Commission (1997) *Bringing them home: The 'stolen children'. National inquiry into the separation of Aboriginal and Torres Strait Islander children from their families.* Commonwealth of Australia. Available at <http://www.austlii.edu.au/au/other/IndigLRes/stolen/>, accessed 7 November 2011.

Jansen, G (2006) 'Gender and War: The effects of armed conflict on women's health and mental health', *Affiliate Journal of Women and Social Work,* 21(2), 134–45.

Joop de Jong, TVM (2002) 'Public Mental Health, Traumatic Stress and Human Rights Violations in Low-Income Countries', in TMV Joop de Jong (ed) *Trauma, War and Violence: Public Mental Health in Socio-Cultural Context.* New York: Plenum Press, 1–92.

Kaplan, I, Dunsis. A, and Schwartz, R (2008) *Are there special mental health issues for refugee women?* Paper presented at the 3rd International Congress on Women's Mental Health, 17–20 March 2003, Melbourne, Australia.

Kessler, R, Wai Tat Chiu, AM, Demler, O, and Walters, E (2005) 'Prevalence, severity, and comorbidity of 12-Month *DSM-IV* disorders in the national comorbidity survey replication', *Archive of General Psychiatry,* 62, 617–27.

Kuh, D, Hardy, R, Rodgers, B, and Wadsworth, MEJ (2002) 'Lifetime risk factors for women's psychological distress in midlife', *Social Science & Medicine*, 55, 1957–73.

Magruder, KM, and Yeager, DE (2008) *Are women more likely to be incorrectly classified for depression?* Paper presented at the 3rd International Congress on Women's Mental Health, 17–20 March 2003, Melbourne, Australia.

Manassis, K (2006) 'Depression and anxiety in girls', in SE Romans and MV Seeman (eds) *Women's mental health: A life-cycle approach*. Philadelphia: Lippincott Williams and Wilkins, 53–69.

Mouzos, J and Makki, T (2004) *Women's experiences of male violence: Findings from the Australian component of the international violence against women survey (IVAWS)*. Research and public policy series, No. 56. Canberra: Australian Institute of Criminology. Available at <http://www.aic.gov.au/publications/current%20series/rpp/41-60/rpp56.aspx>, accessed 7 November 2011.

Mullen, P, Martin, J, Anderson, J, Romans, S, and Herbison, G (1993) 'Childhood sexual abuse and mental health in adult life', *The British Journal of Psychiatry*, 163, 721–732.

Perkins, C (2006) 'Aging and Cognition in Women', in SE Romans and MV Seeman (eds) *Women's mental health: A life-cycle approach*. Philadelphia: Lippincott Williams and Wilkins, 337–350.

Pirkola S, Isometsiä, E, Aro, H, et al. (2005) 'Childhood adversities as risk factors for adult mental disorders: Results from the Health 2000 study', *Social Psychiatry and Psychiatric Epidemiology*, 40, 769–77.

Raphael, B, Taylor, M, and McAndrews, V (2008) 'Women, catastrophe and mental health', *Australian and New Zealand Journal of Psychiatry*, 42, 13–23.

Roberts, G, Hegarty, K, and Feder, G (2006) *Intimate partner abuse and health professionals: New approaches to domestic violence*. Edinburgh: Elsevier.

Robinson, GE (2006) 'Gender differences in depression and anxiety disorders', in SE Romans and MV Seeman (eds) *Women's mental health: A life-cycle approach*. Philadelphia: Lippincott Williams and Wilkins, 163–178.

Smolak, L (2006) 'Part III Risks and strengths across the life span: Chapter 7. Body image', in J Worell and CD Goodheart (eds) *Handbook of girls' and women's psychological health: Gender and well-bring across the life span*. Oxford: Oxford University Press, 69–76.

Solomon, Z, Gelkopf, M, and Bleich, A (2005) 'Is terror gender-blind? Gender differences in reaction to terror events', *Social Psychiatry and Psychiatric Epidemiology*, 40, 947–54.

Stewart, DE (2007) 'Social determinants of women's mental health', *Journal of Psychosomatic Research*, 63, 223–24.

Stewart, DE and Khalid, MJ (2006) 'Menopause and mental health', in SE Romans and MV Seeman (eds) *Women's mental health: A life-cycle approach*. Philadelphia: Lippincott Williams and Wilkins, 297–309.

UNICEF (2005) *Monitoring the situation of children and women. Statistics on Child and maternal mortality*. Available at <http://www.childinfo.org/>, accessed 7 November 2011.

United Nations (1965) *The International Convention on the Elimination of All Forms of Racial Discrimination (CERD)*. Available at <http://www2.ohchr.org/english/law/cerd.htm>, accessed 7 November 2011.

United Nations (1966) *International Covenant on Civil and Political Rights*. Available at <http://www2.ohchr.org/english/law/ccpr.htm>, accessed 7 November 2011.

United Nations (1979) *The Convention on the Elimination of all forms of Discrimination Against Women (CEDAW)*. Available at <http://www.un.org/womenwatch/daw/cedaw/cedaw.htm>, accessed 7 November 2011.

United Nations (1989) *The Convention on the Rights of the Child*. Available at <http://www2.ohchr.org/english/law/pdf/crc.pdf>, accessed 7 November 2011.

United Nations (1991) *Principles for the protection of persons with mental illness and the improvement of mental health care*. Available at <http://www2.ohchr.org/english/law/principles.htm>, accessed 7 November 2011.

United Nations (1993) *Declaration of the Elimination of Violence Against Women*. Available at <http://www.un.org/documents/ga/res/48/a48r104.htm>, accessed 7 November 2011.

United Nations (2007) *Twenty-fifth anniversary of the work of the Committee on the Elimination of Discrimination against Women:* Statement by Ms. Louise Arbour, United Nations High Commissioner for Human Rights, 23 July 2007. Available at <http://www.un.org/womenwatch/daw/cedaw/cedaw25anniversary/Statement_HCHR.pdf>, accessed 7 November 2011.

Watts, C and Zimmerman, C (2002) 'Violence against women: global scope and magnitude', *The Lancet*, 359(9313), 6 April 2002, 1232–37.

World Health Organization (2000) *Women's mental health: An evidence based review.* Geneva: Department of Mental Health and Substance Dependence, WHO. Available at <http://whqlibdoc.who.int/hq/2000/WHO_MSD_MDP_00.1.pdf>, accessed 7 November 2011.

World Health Organization (2005) *Mental Health Atlas.* Geneva: Department of Mental Health and Substance Dependence, WHO. Available at <http://www.who.int/mental_health/evidence/mhatlas05/en/index.html>, accessed 7 November 2011.

Chapter 22

Trafficking, Mental Health, and Human Rights

Kathleen Maltzahn and Louella Villadiego

This chapter explores the issue of trafficking in women for prostitution, also referred to as sexual slavery, the impact of trafficking for prostitution on women's mental health, and the links with human rights in this context.

Trafficking for prostitution/sexual slavery is only one form of trafficking. Other forms of this crime and human rights violation include trafficking for labour, trafficking for marriage, trafficking children for 'adoption', and trafficking for organs. This chapter is confined to trafficking in women for prostitution, but recognizes that children and men are trafficked for prostitution, and that many people are trafficked for other purposes.

What is trafficking?—Beginning with the reality

Trafficking for prostitution is, almost by definition, an underground activity. Increasingly, however, women who have been trafficked have been able to communicate their experiences, and these provide an important starting point in understanding trafficking for prostitution/sexual slavery. Any discussion about trafficking/sexual slavery must be grounded in women's actual experiences.

While specific experiences of trafficking/sexual slavery vary from case to case, and from country to country, the following statement illustrates many of the issues in trafficking for prostitution/sexual slavery.

The statement was developed following a decision by the Australian High Court that a brothel owner, Wei Tang, was guilty of using and possessing a slave.[1] This was the first such decision in Australia. The slavery committed in this case was typical of other cases of trafficking for prostitution/sexual slavery in Australia.

Following the case, the Australian women's organization, Project Respect, ran a seminar for nine Thai and Chinese women who had been trafficked to Australia for prostitution. Using interpreters, a lawyer outlined the key findings in the High Court judgment on the *Queen v Tang*. Following this, with support from Project Respect, the women developed this shared statement.[2]

---

[1] *The Queen v Tang* [2008] HCA 39 (28 August 2008);<http://www.austlii.edu.au/au/cases/cth/HCA/2008/39.html>, accessed 12 November 2009.

[2] These statements have been developed and endorsed by the nine women mentioned above (they have endorsed the statement having read it in Cantonese or Thai, as well as English). The women have endorsed that these statements be sent to the High Court Justices, and to politicians, journalists, and the wider community, and to women in brothels who may themselves be in slavery or who may be able to help other women they meet in brothels who are.

The statement describes both many typical elements of trafficking/sexual slavery, such as long 'working' hours, threats, and violence, and the profound impact on victims' mental and physical health.

> We make this statement in response to the 28 August 2008 High Court decision on the *Queen v. Tang*. We had the same experience as the women in the Wei Tang case.
>
> What happened to us was a nightmare. We can never forget. It comes back to us in dreams. This will affect us till we die. It has changed us. We feel we are not as good as other people.
>
> We were treated very badly. We worked from 11 am to 3 or 4 am. We slept only three or four hours a night. Sometimes some of us worked for 24 hours. For four or five months, all we did was prostitution. Even when we had our period, we had to work. Even when we were sick, we couldn't stop or rest. Sometimes we worked until we couldn't walk. We had to work until we were very very sick and the customers refused to take us. Only then were we allowed to rest, for one day.
>
> Some owners were not so cruel, but even when they were friendly, they still treated us as slaves.
>
> We were made to feel like animals. Customers were violent. Some of the customers were crazy. They treated us like animals. We were sexually abused, we were dragged, we were hit. Some of us were given drugs so we could work all the time. Some of the women we know have become drug addicts and now they have to keep doing prostitution to pay for drugs.
>
> It was like we were in jail—we had no free time, we couldn't go anywhere, we never had freedom. The traffickers treated us as slaves. We didn't have anywhere to go.
>
> It felt like we survived and died at the same time. We had to keep doing what the traffickers said, for ourselves, and for the people we loved. The traffickers threatened us—we were scared they would hurt us and our families. Some of us thought we could be killed. We blamed ourselves for what happened, because we had wanted to come to Australia.
>
> This changed our lives.
>
> After we had been trafficked, if we met a good man, some of us thought we didn't deserve to be with him, that he deserved someone better. Some of us knew we deserved better, but men we loved treated us badly and told us we were dirty and couldn't expect anything better. It was hard to speak when we were treated like that.
>
> Before this High Court decision, we felt the public didn't know what happened to women like us and that they would judge us, and we felt that people like us didn't deserve anything better.
>
> But just because we have been prostitutes doesn't mean we are not good people—we had no choice. We did this to survive.
>
> Even if women chose to do prostitution, they shouldn't be treated this way.
>
> When we were told about the High Court decision, we felt glad. We felt relieved, we felt released. Now we have walked out from the darkness. We can again have a good life, like we did before we came to Australia. We can start a new life now.
>
> We feel now that people believe we are real and understand what we have been through. We feel that the High Court Justices respect and understand us. Because of what happened to us, we didn't trust people. Now it seems there are good people in the world. People outside have believed what happened to us. We feel more valuable.
>
> We agree with the Justices when they say that the situation of the women in the Tang case was slavery. Even when the traffickers were friendly to us, they still treated us as slaves. We feel good because the Justices say it doesn't matter what the women did—it was the agents' fault. What they did was slavery.
>
> What should happen now?
>
> We see that even though the government has laws, traffickers still find ways to bring women here. Because each of us has been hurt by slavery, we want to stop other women from being trafficked. We don't want other women to experience what we experienced. We want the government to find more ways to stop slavery.

> To help women who have already been hurt by slavery, we want the government to give everyone a new chance. In the past, we felt that people wouldn't give us a chance. Visas are the best thing. Secondly, we need education, so we know how to communicate, so we know how to live in Australia, so we can start a new life. We want help so we can find new jobs, otherwise we have to do the same thing, prostitution. No-one wants to stay with that many men. Of course, we can make a lot of money from prostitution, but it feel there is no respect, no love there.
>
> The High Court judgment has made us happy. We feel we have come from the darkness to the brightness.
>
> The High Court decision is important. Before, all of us were scared to talk. Now, we have hope. We can trust again. We are real. The High Court judgment feels like a blessing, something very good.
>
> Thank you from the heart to the Justices.

The day after Project Respect staff finalized the statement with the women, one of the women rang and said she had more to say for the statement. In addition to endorsing (and having contributed to) the statement, she wished to add her particular experience. This is her experience:

> It is important that people understand that the experience of being trafficked is absolutely the worst thing you can ever imagine. I want people to know that this is happening in Australia.
>
> Before I came, I had a nice life in Thailand, a nice job. I was tricked by a family member to come here, who sold me.
>
> I experienced the most extreme brutality. I was in a 24-hour brothel, where I was woken at any time to see customers. They didn't wake me up by speaking to me—they kicked me. They made me take ecstasy, so I could keep working. I had a gun pointed at my head.
>
> The people who brought us here are so bad, they damaged not just one but so many lives. It never goes away. They've made it hard for me to trust anyone again.
>
> When someone treats you like a dog for a long time, you start to believe you are a dog. You never get your voice back. You lose your confidence. You feel like you are an animal.
>
> Afterwards, sometimes I felt like I was too dirty to touch my own son. That kind of experience made me feel like I'm not human, makes me feel so dirty, even too dirty to touch my own baby.
>
> Thanks to the Judges, they help so much, they can help people to understand what we have been through.

What is trafficking?—Reflecting women's lives

'It look like I had no choice.'
Narumol, trafficking survivor[3]

Narumol, and the women who made the statement included in this chapter, are just a few of the many women—no one knows how many exactly—who have been trafficked in recent years. For many years, women's stories were largely ignored. Then, in the 1990s, women's experiences began to surface, and organizations and countries began to address trafficking/sexual slavery. It was part of a worldwide shift.

---

[3] Narumol, Santhong, Rumpueng, Daojai, and Tasanee are pseudonyms of women who have been trafficked to Australia for prostitution. The women's quotes are drawn from interviews in Australia in 2008 with Catherine Simmonds, director of the Brunswick Women's Theatre, in the course of research for the play 'Prostitute: Who is She'. The play was a partnership between the Brunswick Women's Theatre and Project Respect, which was performed in Melbourne, July 2008. For the women involved, it was a powerful way to tell their story, and help heal from the violence they experienced.

Through the 1990s, the stories of more and more women and girls like Narumol became known. While the detail varied from woman to woman, country to country, the broad pattern was the same. Women and girls were recruited, transported within or out of their country, then prostituted. Often, but not always, the movement was from poor to rich countries; almost always the victims were women or girls. Sometimes they were trafficked into street prostitution, sometimes into brothels, sometimes into other parts of the sex industry; sometimes the prostitution was legal, sometimes it was illegal. Some women were prostituted for months, then allowed to leave; others spent years in slavery. Often women were recruited from the sex industry. Inevitably, women and girls were subjected to deception, threats, battery, and rape, both rape outside prostitution and as part of being prostituted. Some were killed.

Women were not only trafficked for prostitution, and not only women were victims of trafficking. Both men and women were trafficked for labour. Others—again, predominantly women— were trafficked for marriage. Trafficking however was heavily gendered—it was overwhelmingly women being trafficked, and trafficking for sexual exploitation appeared to be the most significant form of trafficking.

While feminists had been campaigning explicitly against trafficking since at least 1987, and the first international conference on trafficking appears to have been in 1988 (Leidholdt 2003, 2004), concerted consideration of trafficking by governments and the international community began in the 1990s.

Asian feminists, amongst others, had been seeing and responding to trafficking and other violence in the sex industry for some time (Maltzahn 2008), and with the fall of the Berlin Wall and the collapse of the USSR, Europeans began to see the same phenomenon (Locher 2007:154).

As evidence of trafficking strengthened, so did the expectation that the international community would act. For an international crime such as trafficking, which can cover many jurisdictions, an international understanding of what trafficking was, and how to respond to it, was crucial. While there were existing conventions covering trafficking, they did not define what it was. This gap was filled in 2000, with the United Nations Protocol to Prevent, Suppress and Punish Trafficking in Persons, Especially Women and Children, Supplementing the United Nations Convention Against Transnational Organized Crime.

The protocol defined trafficking as:

> the recruitment, transportation, transfer, harbouring or receipt of persons, by means of the threat or use of force or other forms of coercion, of abduction, of fraud, of deception, of the abuse of power or of a position of vulnerability or of the giving or receiving of payments or benefits to achieve the consent of a person having control over another person, for the purpose of exploitation. Exploitation shall include, at a minimum, the exploitation of the prostitution of others or other forms of sexual exploitation, forced labour or services, slavery or practices similar to slavery, servitude or the removal of organs (Article 3a).

The protocol was significant in two particular ways. Firstly, and obviously, it provided a shared international understanding of what trafficking was, which increased the possibility of states working together to combat trafficking. Secondly, the definition recognised the reality of trafficking. It moved away from viewing trafficking as simply caused by force, where someone was threatened, overpowered, or deceived, and looked instead at the other ways people were made vulnerable to trafficking, including through the abuse of power. Importantly, in the protocol the consent of a victim is irrelevant where any of the means set out (such as force, abuse, or coercion) have been used. Such a definition was crucial in properly understanding the reality of women in all its complexity and truth.

While creating an international convention on trafficking may seem a necessary and obvious thing to do, in many ways it illustrated the shift that had happened within the United Nations and international law in the decade before, a shift that showed the often-ignored connections between trafficking and existing human rights instruments, and reactivated old human rights instruments.

What is trafficking?—A modern form of slavery

'I've paid f—ing $45,000; why can't they look decent.'
Trevor McIvor, convicted of sexual slavery[4]

The 1990s resurgence in international concern about trafficking in women both coincided with, and was strengthened by, growing international attention to women's human rights. The decade was characterized by a growing insistence that women's rights be fully addressed within the United Nations human rights system. Traditional approaches to human rights concentrated on the role of states in violating rights. Consequently, disturbingly often, violation of women's rights, often perpetrated by 'private' actors in domestic spheres, were seen as unrelated to the UN rights framework, and violence against women was largely ignored or trivialized. The life of women like those speaking in the statement above was invisible. It was private actors who were usually violent and exploitative in trafficking for prostitution, not a police officer, a corrupt government official, or a politician. Consequently, the violence and exploitation experienced by women such as they, was largely seen as irrelevant within the United Nations human rights system.

This changed in the mid 1990s. Feminists had been arguing that the state was not only responsible for human rights violations when its agents actively committed them; it was also culpable if it failed to stop other, non-state, perpetrators. This paved the way for a more sophisticated understanding of human rights that recognized women's experience, and in 1993, this understanding began to be reflected in United Nations statements. The first significant statement came through the Vienna Declaration and Programme of Action. 'The human rights of women and of the girl-child', it said, 'are an inalienable, integral and indivisible part of universal human rights.' More than that, it added, 'Gender-based violence and all forms of sexual harassment and exploitation, including those resulting from cultural prejudice and *international trafficking*, are incompatible with the dignity and worth of the human person, and must be eliminated (authors' italics).

Importantly, this new perspective allowed older frameworks, particularly in terms of slavery, to be better applied.

Through the 1990s, trafficking was increasingly referred to as a modern form of slavery. In doing so, one of the oldest and most powerful human rights concepts was being evoked. Slavery is both a surprisingly old, and surprisingly modern, concept. The notion of slavery often conjures up images of the slave-trade of old, of a world imagined to have long been relegated to history. However, while an age-old practice, it was not until the 1815 Declaration Relative to the Universal Abolition of the Slave Trade that there was an international instrument to condemn its practice. Recognizing this historic failure to recognize—and condemn—slavery adequately, in 2001 the World Conference against Racism, Racial Discrimination, Xenophobia and Related Intolerance stated in its final declaration that 'slavery and the slave trade are a crime against humanity and should always have been so' (Weissbrodt and Anti-Slavery International 2002:3).

While recognition of slavery seems slow, after 1815 there was significant international concern about slavery—between 1815 and 1957 there were some 300 international agreements

---

[4] 'Illegally brought here so all "could make money"', Heath Gilmore, *Sydney Morning Herald*, 6 July 2008.

implemented to suppress slavery (Weissbrodt and Anti-Slavery International 2002:3). To mention only a few, in addition to Article 4 of the Universal Declaration of Human Rights 1949 (UDHR) and Article 8 of the International Covenant on Civil and Political Rights 1966 (ICCPR), there was also the International Convention to Suppress the Slave Trade and Slavery 1926 and the Supplementary Convention on the Abolition of Slavery, the Slave Trade and Institutions and Practices Similar to Slavery 1956 prohibiting the slave trade.

It may be argued that none have been effective.

As the women's statement above shows, slavery and slavery-like practices prevail in many different forms the world over, often in contexts that at first glance are a long way from the trans-atlantic slave trade of previous centuries. The core features of slavery however—reducing a person to an object, to a thing that can be bought, sold, and disposed of by the owner at will—can be found disturbingly often. In a report on contemporary slavery for the Office of the United Nations High Commissioner for Human Rights, Weissbrodt and Anti-Slavery International (2002:3) identified the following forms of slavery in existence today: serfdom; forced labour; debt bondage; slavery of migrant workers; trafficking; enforced prostitution; forced marriage and the sale of wives; and child labour and child servitude.

The 1990s recognition of the way women's human rights should be recognized by the international human rights system allowed the enslavement of women—whether through trafficking for prostitution or marriage or in another form—to be properly identified. This in turn reinstated international law and human rights instruments as real tools that women can use.

Reflecting this, in 1998 the United Nations Working Group on Contemporary Forms of Slavery declared that 'trans-border trafficking of women and girls for sexual exploitation is a contemporary form of slavery and constitutes a serious violation of human rights' (Report of the Working Group on Contemporary Forms of Slavery 1998:para. 20).

It is particularly important that slavery has been reclaimed for women, that international law can recognize when women are enslaved. The practice of slavery has attained the status of *jus cogens* in customary international law, meaning that no derogation is permitted from its prohibition. In other words, there is an 'absolute prohibition against slavery' (Gallagher 2008) and slavery has been 'universally accepted as a crime against humanity' (Bales 2001). Understanding trafficking as slavery demonstrates how serious a human rights violation it is.

What is trafficking?—Violence against women

'I don't know why they treated me that way, as if I was not a human being'.
Trafficking survivor[5]

Alongside this, the 1990s also addressed trafficking within a human rights framework in other ways. The 1990s recognition that women's rights were human rights, and not peripheral or trivial, came with recognition of how pervasive violence against women was.

Trafficking in women for the purpose of prostitution was recognized as a form of gender-based violence, an issue which was itself identified as a critical area of concern for governments, the international community, and civil society and as a barrier to the advancement of women and the achievement of equality between men and women (Report of the Fourth World Conference on Women (Beijing, 4–15 September 1995) para. 41).

---

[5] 'Sex slave family Trevor McIvor, Kanokporn Tanuchit "psycho", victim says', Kim Arlington, *Daily Telegraph*, 14 July 2008.

Illustrative of this, one of the strategic objectives at the Beijing World Conference on Women to address violence against women was the elimination of trafficking in women and assisting victims of violence due to prostitution and trafficking (Report of the Fourth World Conference on Women 1995). The Report of the Beijing Conference called on governments to allocate resources to provide programs designed to 'heal and rehabilitate' persons who have been trafficked through legal assistance, healthcare, and to take measures to co-operate with NGOs to provide medical and psychological care of those who had been trafficked (Report of the Fourth World Conference on Women 1995).

Addressing trafficking was seen to be at the core of addressing violence against women, which was in turn central to addressing women's inequality.

This broader perspective, that links violence against women with women's inequality, means that in addition to seeing the elements of trafficking as human rights violations, trafficking can also be seen to violate other, related human rights, for example, women's able to attain the highest attainable standard of physical and mental health under Article 12 of the International Covenant on Economic, Social and Cultural Rights 1966 (ICESCR).

In addition, this approach allows us to apply a gender lens to trafficking, to see the particular impact trafficking has on women and girls.

Slavery and mental health

'If I feel sad, I never, never talk about that . . . I try not to cry . . . but if I cry, I cry by myself . . . Only myself knows that I sad.'
Daojai, trafficking survivor

There is limited research on the impact of trafficking for prostitution/sexual slavery. As the International Organization on Migration (IOM) states:

Until recently, much of the support in the fight against trafficking has focused on information exchange, police and legal cooperation, and return and reintegration assistance. In the last year, however, a number of protocols, declarations and published studies have also called attention to the serious health concerns related to trafficking. These documents highlight the need to develop minimum standards of care and provide specialized services that specifically match the needs of the victim.[6]

However, some of the impacts are clear, as the IOM again outlines:

Trafficked persons—regardless of whether trafficking is for the purpose of labour, sexual or any other form of exploitation—are exposed to a range of health-related problems. During captivity, they experience physical violence, sexual exploitation, psychological abuse, poor living conditions and exposure to numerous diseases, which may have long-lasting consequences on their physical-, in particular reproductive health, and mental health. (IOM Counter-Trafficking Handbook, in press)

However, there are important lessons from work done on other forms of violence against women. Understanding trafficking as both a form of slavery and of violence against women underlines the seriousness of this crime. Sexual slavery is a profound form of violence against women, one that, at its essence, seeks to erase the humanity of the women it enslaves. In sexual slavery, a woman becomes a thing, an object, something that can be bought and sold. Not surprisingly, slavery attacks the foundations of a person's physical and mental health.

---

[6] *The Mental Health Aspects of Trafficking in Human Beings Training Manual*, International Organization on Migration, 2004 <http://publications.iom.int>, accessed 14 November 2009.

There is a solid feminist history of showing the links between violence against women and mental health issues. The World Health Organization has found that women who have experienced violence, either as girls or in adulthood, have 'increased rates of depression and anxiety, stress related symptoms, pain syndromes, phobias, chemical dependency, substance use, suicidality, somatic and medical symptoms, negative health behaviours, poor subjective health and health service utilisation' (World Health Organization, 2000). Trafficked women's experience is consistent with this.

Importantly, trafficked women's experiences of violence often do not begin with trafficking. Many trafficked women have previously experienced domestic violence, or sexual assault as girls, or sexual harassment. Trafficking violence is on top of this violence.

Writing in 2003, Professor Liz Kelly said:

> From the work we have done, and our contacts with many activists and practitioners in central and eastern Europe we can tell horror stories: of girls dumped out of speed boats in Vlore, Albania; of women spread against walls and beaten in Macedonia; of young women kidnapped and raped in Kosovo; of weekly murders of Albanian and Nigerian women in Italy; and of women and girls literally sold in markets in Bosnia (Kelly 2003).

Importantly, however, as Kelly continued, while it is crucial that the worst cases be cited, because they were real, violence is not always life threatening:

> But just as with domestic violence and child sexual abuse most trafficking is more mundane, involving everyday, routine power and control relationships.

Both when it is life threatening and when it is not, the harmful impact of trafficking is significant.

A 2006 study of 207 women who had recently been 'released from a trafficking situation' illustrates the health impact of trafficking (Zimmerman et al. 2006). The women came from 14 countries, and were aged between 15 and 45. Ninety-five per cent reported that while they were trafficked they were subjected to physical and or sexual violence. Fifty-eight per cent reported having been injured. Significantly, 60 per cent said they had been physically and/or sexually abused before they were trafficked (Zimmerman et al. 2006).

The study tracked the women's health status over three periods, in part to ascertain the difference health and other support services made to women's health once they were outside the trafficking situation (Zimmerman et al. 2006).

The study listed the ten most common symptoms women reported: 82 per cent of women were easily tired, 81 per cent had headaches, 71 per cent had dizzy spells, the same proportion had vaginal discharge, 69 per cent had back pain, 64 per cent experienced loss of appetite, 63 per cent had difficulty remembering things, the same proportion had stomach or abdominal pain, 61 per cent had gynaecological infections, and 59 per cent had pelvic pain. Many of the women experienced several of these symptoms: the study found that 57 per cent of the women 'reported suffering between 12 and 23 concurrent physical symptoms when they entered care' (Zimmerman et al. 2006).

The study further found that 56 per cent of women 'reported symptom levels suggestive of posttraumatic stress disorder (PTSD) upon entry into care', and that the women's 'depression, anxiety and hostility levels were extremely high—with the top tenth percentile of population norms for adult females'. Thirty-eight per cent said they had had suicidal thoughts; 95 per cent said they felt depressed (Zimmerman et al. 2006).

Significantly, while many of the women's physical symptoms improved within 90 days of receiving care, the emotional impact was much harder to address. The report found that

'Women's depression, anxiety and hostility levels do not appear to decrease until after approximately 90+ days in care' and 'Depression appeared to be the most persistent symptom dimension, showing very little reduction even after 90+ days in care'(Zimmerman et al. 2006).

The study highlighted the similarities in health impacts between trafficking and other forms of violence:

> The symptom patterns detected among the women in this study are consistent with the health outcomes identified in survivors of sexual abuse, rape and intimate partner violence (Zimmerman et al. 2006).

Trafficking and links with prostitution

> 'He [the customer] say, "I pay the money for you and can do everything I want".'
> Rumpueng

In addition to the links between trafficking and violence against women such as domestic violence, there are also important questions to ask about the parallels and intersections between trafficking and prostitution, in at least two ways. (While linking prostitution causally to trafficking is highly contested, there is a vigorous discussion going on that advocates doing this, and this link has been translated into policy through the Swedish government's approach to prostitution, which identifies it as a human rights violation and a form of violence against women.[7])

Firstly, there is a historically strong link between trafficking in persons and prostitution with an estimated 80 per cent of those trafficked are trafficked for sexual exploitation (Philips 2004). At the very least, the sex industry is an important recruitment site for traffickers—prostitution makes women vulnerable to trafficking. It can be argued that both prostitution and trafficking depend on human rights violations—significant numbers of women enter the sex industry, whether through trafficking or not, because of violations of social rights such as poverty, lack of work, poor education, and homelessness, and of civil rights such as rape, battery, and sexual harassment.

Secondly, research on trafficking shows the similarities in health impacts between trafficking and prostitution. There is a growing body of work showing the links between violence against women in the sex industry and harm to women's mental health.

One important body of research, led by US researcher Melissa Farley, has found consistent and high levels of human rights violations experienced by people doing prostitution, and correspondingly significant rates of post-traumatic stress disorder.

Her latest study, of 854 people currently or recently in prostitution in nine countries, found that prostitution was multi-traumatic, and 68 per cent of the study participants met the criteria for post-traumatic stress disorder (Farley et al. 2003). This is a consequence of human rights violations that many women experience as a matter of course in prostitution. Trafficking for prostitution exposes women to this and other harm.

Interestingly, these links have been explored in previous decades. The concern at the end of the 20th century about trafficking was not the only time in recent decades trafficking has been addressed. The UN also had another long-established approach to trafficking that had been in abeyance during the second half of the 20th century.

---

[7] More information available at <http://www.sweden.se/upload/Sweden_se/english/factsheets/SI/SI_FS8_Gender%20equality/Gender_equality_300dpi.pdf>, accessed 13 November 2009.

In addition to foundational human rights agreements on slavery, the United Nations Human Rights framework includes early conventions on trafficking and prostitution.

Prior to 2000, the main international convention concerned with trafficking was the Convention for the Suppression of the Traffic in Persons and of the Exploitation of the Prostitution of Others 1949 (the Suppression of Traffic Convention) which seemed to reinforce the connection between trafficking and prostitution. Also, Article 6 of the Convention on the Elimination of All Forms of Discrimination Against Women 1979 (CEDAW) requires state parties to take all appropriate measures to suppress trafficking and forced prostitution of women. After 50 years, however, these instruments had been largely forgotten and ignored. In part, these conventions may have been ignored because of discomfort with connecting human rights violations, trafficking, and prostitution.

Conclusion

> *'I want to let people know, [you] have to be strong. Use the past to change life, to change yourself.'*
> *Tasanee, trafficking survivor*

For many years invisibilized and trivialized, trafficking for prostitution is now increasingly understood as a serious human rights violation, a profound form of violence against women, and a form of slavery.

It is important to demonstrate both the severity of this crime, and its impact on women, not to suggest that trafficked women are the sum of their negative experiences, or that they are crippled by the violence they have experienced. Rather, it is important that both professionals—police, psychologists, social workers, immigration officers—and members of the community understand what women experience so we can recognize the deep courage and resilience women have to draw on to survive, and so we can recognize honestly the destruction they have experienced. Only then can we hope both to combat trafficking, and to support trafficked women as they recover from the impact of their enslavement.

References

Acharya, AK (2006) 'International Migration and Trafficking of Mexican Women to the United States', in K Beeks and D Amir (eds), *Trafficking and the Global Sex Industry*. Oxford: Lexington Books, 21–32.

Annan, K (2001) *Message to Abuja Conference*. Available at <http://www.unis.unvienna.org/unis/pressrels/2001/sgsm7721.html>, accessed 7 November 2011.

Arlington, K (2008) 'Sex slave family Trevor McIvor, Kanokporn Tanuchit "psycho", victim says', *Herald Sun*, accessed 2 August.

Bales, K and Robbins, PT (2001) '"No One Shall Be Held in Slavery or Servitude": A Critical Analysis of International Slavery Agreements and Concepts of Slavery', *Human Rights Review*, <http://www.accessmylibrary.com/article-1G1-72116598/no-one-shall-held.html>, accessed 7 November 2011.

Bunch, C and Frost, S (2000) 'Women's Human Rights: An Introduction', in *Routledge International Encyclopedia of Women: Global Women's Issues and Knowledge*. London: Routledge.

Farley, M, Cotton, A, Lynne, J et al (2003) 'Prostitution & Trafficking in Nine Countries: an Update on Violence and Posttraumatic Stress Disorder', *Journal of Trauma Practice*, 2(3/4), 33–74.

Gallagher, A (2008) 'A Question of Bondage', The Age, 15 May 2008.

Gilmore, H (2008) 'Illegally brought here so all "could make money"', *Sydney Morning Herald*, July 6, 2008.

Global Alliance Against Traffic in Women (1999) *Human Rights Standards for the Treatment of Trafficked Persons*. Available at <http://gaatw.net/books_pdf/hrs_eng2.pdf>, accessed 7 November 2011.

Haynes, DF (2004) 'Used, Abused, Arrested and Deported: Extending Immigration Benefits to Protect the Victims of Trafficking and to Secure the Prosecution of Traffickers', *Human Rights Quarterly*, 26(2), 221–72.

Herzfeld, B (2002) 'Slavery and Gender: Women's Double Exploitation', in R Masika (ed) *Gender, Trafficking and Slavery*. Oxford: Oxfam, 50–55.

Human Rights Watch Women's Rights Project (1995) *The Human Rights Watch Global Report on Women's Human Rights*. New York: Human Rights Watch.

Jeffreys, S (2002) 'Women Trafficking and the Australian Connection', *Arena*, April–May 2002, 44.

Jordan, AD (2002) 'Human Rights or Wrongs?: The Struggle for a Rights-Based Response to Trafficking in Human Beings', in R Masika (ed), *Gender, Trafficking and Slavery*. Oxford: Oxfam, 28–37.

Kelly, L (2003) 'The Wrong Debate: Reflections on Why Force is Not the Key Issue with Respect to Trafficking in Women for Sexual Exploitation', in *Feminist Review: Exile and Asylum—Women Seeking Refuge in 'Fortress Europe'*, 73, 139–44.

Leidholdt, DA (2003) 'Prostitution and trafficking in women: A intimate relationship', in M Farley (ed) *Prostitution, trafficking and traumatic stress*. Binghamton, NY: Haworth, 167–86.

Leidholdt, DA (2004) Demand and the debate. Coalition against trafficking in women. Available at http:// action.web.ca/home/catw/readingroom.shtml?x=53793&AA_EX_Session=99887f26c70b3c9fee4456861 ebf4cfb, accessed 22/1/12.

Locher, B (2007) *Trafficking in women in the European Union: Norms, Advocacy-Networks and Police Change*. Weisbaden: VS Verlag.

Maltzahn, K (Project Respect) (2003b) *Submission to the Parliamentary Joint Committee on the Australian Crime Commission, Inquiry into Trafficking in Women for Sexual Servitude*, <http://www.aph.gov.au/ senate/committee/acc_ctte/completed_inquiries/2002-04/sexual_servitude/submissions/sub25.pdf>, accessed 7 November 2011.

Maltzahn, K (2008) *Trafficked*. Sydney, NSW: UNSW Press.

Miller, E, Decker, MR, Silverman, JG, and Raj, A (2007) 'Migration, Sexual Exploitation, and Women's Health', *Violence Against Women*, 13(5), 486–97.

Monzini, P (2005) *Sex Traffic: Prostitution, Crime and Exploitation*. London & New York: Zed Books.

Othman, Z (2006) 'Human (In)security, Human Trafficking, and Security in Malaysia', in K Beeks and D Amir (eds) *Trafficking and the Global Sex Industry*. Oxford: Lexington Books, 47–60.

Philips, J (2004) *Research Note No 20, 2004–05: People Trafficking: Australia's Response*. Parliament of Australia—Parliamentary Library. <http://www.aph.gov.au/library/pubs/rn/2004-05/05rn20.htm>, accessed 7 November 2011.

Raymond, J and Hughes, D (2001) *Sex Trafficking of Women in the United States: International and Domestic Trends*. New York: Coalition Against Trafficking In Women.

Report of the Fourth World Conference on Women (1995) (Beijing, 4–15 September 1995), A/CONF. 177/20.

Report of the Working Group on Contemporary Forms of Slavery (1998) SUBCOM Res 1998/19, UN Doc E/CN4/SUB2/RES/1998/19.

United Nations High Commissioner for Refugees (UNHCR) (2002) *Refugee Women*. Geneva: UNHCR. Available at <http://www.unhcr.org/3d4f915e4.html>, accessed 7 November 2011.

Weissbrodt, D and Anti-Slavery International (2002) *Abolishing Slavery and its Contemporary Forms*, HR/ PUB/02/4. Available at < http://www.ohchr.org/Documents/Publications/slaveryen.pdf>, accessed 7 November 2011.

Women's Empowerment Key to Achieving Millennium Summit Anti-Poverty Goals, Says General Assembly President on International Women's Day (2003) Press Release, GA/SM/308; OBV/328; WOM/1393.

World Health Organization (2000) *Women's Mental Health: An Evidence Based Review*. Geneva: WHO, 75. Available at <http://whqlibdoc.who.int/hq/2000/WHO_MSD_MDP_00.1.pdf>, accessed 7 November 2011.

Yea, S (2005) 'When Push Comes to Shove: Sites of Vulnerability, Personal Transformation, and trafficked Women's Migration Decisions', *SOJOURN: Journal of Social Issues in Southeast Asia*, 20(1), 67–95.

Zimmerman, C and Watts, C (2003) *WHO Ethical and Safety Recommendations for Interviewing Trafficked Women*. Geneva: WHO.

Zimmerman, C, Hossain, M, Yun, K, Roche, B, Morison, L, and Watts, C (2006) *Stolen smiles: The physical and psychological health consequences of women and adolescents trafficked in Europe*. Bulgaria: Animus Association Foundation, Ukraine & Moldova: International Organization for Migration, Czech Republic: La Strada, Italy: On the Road, Belgium: Pagasa, and UK: Poppy Project and London School of Hygiene & Tropical Medicine.

Chapter 23

Women's Bodies, Sexualities, and Human Rights

Şahika Yüksel, Dilek Cindoğlu, and Ufuk Sezgin

Introduction

Contrary to men, women are primarily perceived, treated, and discriminated against through their bodies. This chapter deals with the gendered nature of women's mental health issues, with special reference to women's bodies and human rights in contemporary social and political contexts. The interconnected nature of the women's bodies, sexualities, and human rights is emphasized.

Any social and cultural context that devalues the bodily and emotional well-being of women needs to be analysed thoroughly. It can be argued that some of the circumstances that women experience are primordial, stemming from their biologies, such as menstruation, birth, and menopause. Women's bodies are different than male bodies; however, most of the circumstances that women suffer are above and beyond these biological conditions. Moreover, social and cultural situations may even worsen these biological processes. The physical and emotional well-being of women suffers because of the conditions that stem from the asymmetrical gender roles in society. These gender roles prescribe women's place, roles, and positions in society as less than that of men.

Women's bodies and sexual rights

Women's bodies and boundaries

'Sexual Pleasure is a Birth Right'

Women are the symbolic representatives of the purity of their families throughout the world. Although the forms and formats are different, the girl-child's sexuality is a matter of control and concern from the most modern to the most traditional societies. In some traditional societies women's sexual conduct is thoroughly controlled via their bodies' virginity. Virginity is considered the most precious asset that the unmarried woman has to bring to the marriage. This anxiety over a woman's purity shows itself in the forms of virginity tests and virginity reconstructive surgeries (Cindoğlu 1997). In modern societies, this control is more individualistic and medicalized in the forms of forced birth control pills, fear of sexually transmitted disease (STD), illegal abortions, etc.

How a woman conducts her body, with whom she chooses to be sexually intimate, is a matter of patriarchal concern either in traditional formats, where family enforces pre-arranged marriages and punishes with honour killings when women do not abide by the rules, or modern and romantic formats when the lover does not accept the rejection or adultery of the woman and violates her body in the form of passion crimes. It is important to note that only women, not men, experience coercions and controls of their sexualities in the most life threatening ways and to this extent.

Non-mainstream sexualities and human rights

When women do not follow the expected paths of sexual intimacy via heterosexual marriages, they are either ignored, or discriminated against and harassed for their orientations. In most parts of the world, same-sex relationships are not accepted morally, socially, and politically. The claims of gays and lesbians for 'intimate citizenship' entails the rights of people to be acknowledged by the state and its institutions and being eligible for all kinds of rights to which heterosexual couples are entitled. These rights are similar to rights that come with heterosexual marriage, including tax benefits, inheritance rights, social security benefits, etc. (Plummer 2003). Women, particularly, are at the most disadvantaged end of this process. Economically, on average, women globally earn 60 per cent of what men earn and have less access to social security (<http://www.weforum.org/pdf/gendergap/report2009>) Therefore, the political acknowledgement of lesbian couples in the form of social security access through marriage and inheritance will bring more benefit to lesbians than gays.

Domestic violence

Violence against women has a negative impact on all aspects of their well-being. According to the WHO (2002), studies carried out in many countries indicate that women who have been physically and sexually assaulted and abused use health services more than those without a history of abuse. Chronic health problems such as STDs, AIDS, unplanned pregnancies, birth defects resulting from violence-related foetal injury, and premature deaths lead to a higher healthcare cost in any society (Amaro 1995).

Domestic violence and women's human rights

The Universal Declaration of Human Rights and different conventions such as Convention on the Elimination of All Forms of Discrimination against Women (CEDAW) suggest that men and women are equal and neither is in a position of control. But violence against women is a lingering problem that exists in almost all countries and societies. Women are often exposed to violence by their partners; therefore, the acknowledgement of IPV (Intimate Partner Violence) is essential in the elimination of domestic violence.

Victims of domestic violence suffer different psychological problems such as post-traumatic stress disorders (PTSD), depression, and somatic problems and are at higher risk for physical health problems. Psychological effects are more severe if the traumatic event is repeated by people close to the victim.

Women's mental health and women's human rights

Violence against women must be recognized as a human rights problem. The perception of domestic violence against women should be perceived not as a private family matter, but rather a public issue that authorities worldwide must address accordingly.

Human rights encompass civil, political, social, economic, and cultural facets of human existence. Women's civil and political rights historically have been compromised by their social and economic status. Consequently, the social and cultural limitations placed on women's activities, along with the ever-present threat of violence, often constitute an obstacle to women's participation in public and political life.

We discuss the problem within the perspective of basic human rights such as the Right to Life and Survival; the Right to Nondiscrimination; and the Right to the Highest Attainable Standards of Health (Cook 1997). Physical, psychological, sexual, and economic abuses violate women's basic human rights such as the right to live and to survive, the right to control one's body, and the right to the highest attainable standard of health. In the 1970s, the presence and prevalence of domestic violence started to be talked about within the community and medical environment; from the 1980s we were confronted with scientific proofs of its short and long-term consequences. In the 1990s the world witnessed rape publicized and discussed as a tool of violence during wars and armed conflicts.

According to several comprehensive studies, physical and sexual violence against women by family members and mostly by their intimate partners occurs in industrialized as well as in developing countries. For example, in Egypt 35 per cent of women and in New Zealand 20 per cent of women reported being beaten by their husbands at some point in their marriage (UNICEF 2000).

The stories and situations of domestic violence victims suggest unaccomplished resistances and the possibilities of opposition. Helplessness and hopelessness may decrease the motivation for change, and recent research in Turkey suggests that over the two decades, the actual level of violence did not change. However awareness of and attitudes towards domestic violence changed in a more egalitarian direction. In 2007, women do not justify male aggression in the household to the same degree as 1994. Demand for shelter also increased (Altinay and Arat 2007).

Such traumatic experiences have a negative impact on women's reproductive health and cause gynaecological disorders. Every year 500,000 women die during pregnancy or immediately after giving birth; 20 million women become handicapped due to reasons related with gender inequality; one third of all pregnancies in the world (80 million each year) are unwanted pregnancies. Sexual abuse of the child also presents a risk of gynaecological disorders and may cause infertility.

Mental health and gendered violence

Men are more exposed to violence than women in objectively defined events, such as wars or detentions (Criterion A1 for PTSD) which are potentially traumatic, with the exception of sexual violence. This is an important exception because sexual violence is associated with the highest conditional risk of PTSD in both men and women. Women appear to experience comparable events as more threatening (i.e. as involving more terror, or helplessness) (American Psychiatric Association 1994).

Women's greater risk for PTSD clearly holds in general populations and disaster-stricken communities, and is even more pronounced in the context of societies that emphasize traditional sex roles. Although gender is not the only determinant for trauma-related disorders, women show more trauma-related disorders. Other factors, such as being in poverty, being a refugee, and being uneducated are almost always gender related. The World Health Organization (2002) defines poverty as the most definite risk factor on health. Poverty leads to physiological and psychological hardship, affecting self-confidence, preventing planning, and intensifying humiliation and desperation. Poverty restricts individuals' social mobility. It is commonly accompanied by social exclusion which women suffer from the most through the ghettoization to their households as basic childcarers and elderly carers (Cockburn 1999).

Women experience traumatic stress more in the context of caregiving. Women are most of the time the only caregivers to young children, elderly, and disabled family members. Their relative lack of social and material resources to cope with trauma makes the impact of exposure more pronounced. In the United States, poor women and children tend to live together, such that 63 per cent of female-headed households are poor. Specifically, 76 per cent of women who are poor are between the ages of 18 and 44 years (Miranda and Green 1999).

In addition, there are more barriers to receiving adequate care among poor and young women. These findings are most likely pertinent for poor women throughout the world. Epidemiological studies of psychiatric disorders carried out in Africa, Asia, the Middle East, and Latin America have identified higher rates of disorders in women as opposed to men (Kimerling 2004).

The most fundamental human right is the right to live. Up to 70 per cent of the women who die due to homicide are killed by their current or former husbands or boyfriends (WHO 2002). When we consider women who are the victims of domestic violence, in different classes and different regions of the world, it is possible to see relevance between Marie Trintignant from Paris and Güldünya from Turkey, who were both killed by domestic violence (Yüksel and Sezgin 2007).

Sexual abuse

Most of the studies related to sexual abuse are conducted in Western countries and we have very limited knowledge about other parts of the world. That is why we have chosen examples from non-Western societies. The control of a woman's life has its own dynamics with its socio-political and economic sources according to the specific region in question.

Sexually assaulted women usually internalize the 'blaming-the-victim' approach at different levels. Lee et al's (2005) findings revealed that Asian and Caucasian women have different attitudes about rape. Asian students are more likely than Caucasian students to believe women should be held responsible for preventing rape, and Asians have stronger beliefs than Caucasians that victims cause the rape and most rapists are strangers.

Classical sexual abuse and rape

The classical sexual abuse or rape is the conduct of the sexual assault by a stranger (Williams 1984). Compared to intimate partner or husband rape, it is much easier for women to report and to get help in these situations.

Justified sexual abuse

'Justified' rapes range from individual rapes to more institutional rape forms. Individual sexual assaults include intimate partner rape, marital rape, and date rape which are all highly controversial crimes (Yüksel and Sezgin 2007). Institutional rapes and sexual assaults, on the other hand, involve using women's bodies in wartime and in armed conflict to intimidate the group. They happen in war zones, camps, detention centres, or occupied territories.

Marital rape The marital act has a basic understanding, which accepts sexual proximity and sexual intercourse to be 'normal' and 'legitimate'. Partner rape, sexual activity forced upon the partner without her consent, is evaluated as a private problem of the couple. When looking at general population and community studies, it is difficult to come up with a consensus definition. The social and legal recognition of marital rape is highly problematic. Russell exposed this problem, reporting that between one in ten and one in seven married women would experience rape by their husbands (Russell 1990). Indeed, most partner rape survivors have experienced multiple rapes during a relationship.

The incidence of sexual assault among battered women is five to seven times higher than that reported by ever-married women (Russell 1990). Since these samples are composed of women who sought help or who resided in women's shelters, they are not representative of all battered women. We argue, however, that many severely abused women don't seek help out of fear of their abusers, and therefore the rate of rape in the case of battered women in shelters may not be overestimated when we consider the rate of sexual violence against all battered women.

Marital rape is common in contemporary Turkey. It is reported in 21 per cent of cases by Yüksel (2010) and 51 per cent by Ilkkaracan (2000). These discrepancies may be due to sampling and measurement differences. Another striking factor is that only 1.2 per cent of women go to the police for help, rather most of them leave their houses (22 per cent) or go to their families and friends (14 per cent).

Date rape Violence against women exists in all societies, modern or traditional, in different forms and shapes. During the last decades, researchers have documented the widespread problem of date rape in American society. Two decades ago, rather than blaming the offender, it was much more common for women to blame themselves. These conflictual values and norms, reflecting internalized patriarchal guilt and shame, also discouraged legal pursuits and hindered the work of therapy (Brownmiller 1975).

Date rape, like any other sexual abuse, has hazardous effects on women's health. In social environments where the virginity of a young woman is an asset and a symbol of family honour, this phenomenon has a double binding effect. On the one hand, the woman suffers from the violation of her body; on the other hand, she suffers from humiliation and degradation of society (Cindoğlu 1997).

In Turkey, due to the value attached to virginity, lovers pay great attention to keep the hymen intact before marriage, out of respect to the woman and her reputation in the community and with prospective suitors. Our research finds that the first characteristic of date rape is that the woman has often no physical intimacy with the person and only has a platonic affair where they talk, or might have had limited sexual intimacy. In this way, a woman who has never had intercourse, experiences first intercourse as a violation of her virginity and her body. Intimate partner rape adds to this not only the violation and loss of bodily integrity, but violation by a trusted lover, and therefore an even more traumatic entry to sexuality.

The second issue in date rape is the possibility of this intercourse influencing the woman's reputation in the community and her chance of finding a suitor. If and when the family learn of her trauma, her status in the family and community are jeopardized. That is why these events usually go unreported. Furthermore, the lover who forced himself on the woman may pursue further abuse or blackmail her knowing that she is helpless and cannot seek help from the family or the police. In traditional parts of the non-Western world, young women usually do not disclose that they have boyfriends. Indeed the word for lover in Turkish is 'someone I talk'. In communities where women's contact with men is limited and closely supervised, families do not know that a woman has a man that she is 'talking to'. This may be a justification for not letting her pursue her studies or simply go out of the house without close chaperoning. In some cases, women apply for legal protection without their family knowing. Even then, the abuser may use this against her by threatening to disclose their relationship to her family (Yüksel 2010).

Honour killings Every year, thousands of women and girl-children are murdered around the world by family decision in the name of honour. Honour killings are the execution of a female family member for perceived wrongdoing vis-à-vis her body and her sexuality (Cindoğlu et al. 2008). In certain societies, it is commonly assumed that a woman's promiscuous behavior not only violates tradition, but affects and brings shame to the whole family. The family undertakes an honour killing as an attempt to wash away the shame, clear the family name, and re-establish family honour (Barakat 1999), as well as punishing women who are perceived as dishonouring their families. Pretexts include being involved in an extramarital affair, when women desire to remarry after divorce, or even when they are raped. Most of the time, the close family of the woman enforces the death sentence and the father's verdict is imposed. Once the woman marries, the spouse takes the place of the father, and also the 'powers' of trying and sentencing (Sezgin 2006).

Honour killing is therefore a form of gendered violence that takes place within the extended family, at home, and is aimed at women. While honour killing is a psychosocial problem restricted to certain geographical areas in the world, and a variety of cultural explanations have been developed as excuses for it, the geographical boundaries of this crime have expanded with increased levels of migration. Reports submitted to the UN Commission on Human Rights show that honour killings have occurred in Bangladesh, Great Britain, Brazil, Ecuador, Egypt, India, Israel, Italy, Jordan, Pakistan, Morocco, Sweden, Turkey, and Uganda.

Honour killings often remain a private family affair so official statistical data is lacking (Cindoğlu et al. 2008). According to statistics from KA-MER (a women's NGO against violence in South-East Turkey), during 2003–2006 158 women asked for help when threatened by an honour killing (Sezgin 2006). The death sentence can be issued for various reasons. The top reason was disobedience (23.4 per cent). Seventeen per cent of the women stated that a decision had been taken to kill them as a result of slander (Sezgin 2006). In 2006, several Turkish women were killed by their young male family members. Some of these women lived in Turkey, and some in European countries as migrants or refugees with citizenship. Every year, 5,000 women in developing countries are killed by their relatives in the name of honour. (<http://www.who.int/mediacentre/factsheets/fs239/en>). However, the actual number of women who face or suffer honour killings is unknown.

Even though honour crimes are well-known, mental health experts tend to disregard this subject. However, with the responsible campaigns of women's NGOs like KA-MER, these issues have become more noticeable. In recent years, murders and forced suicides in the name of virtue and honour are increasingly a focus, both in Turkey and in the world.

War Human problems increase in wartime, and as Goldstein said (2001), 'gender roles are nowhere more prominent than the war'. War disrupts social norms, releasing constraints on emotional, physical, and sexual violence. This disruption also continues to influence women's lives in their differentiated roles and status after wars. The predicament of war widows, refugee women, women affected by mass rapes, mothers, and those giving birth in situations of starvation, homelessness, devastation, and prolonged poverty, are examples. During armed conflict all civilians are at risk of violence but sexual violence is often used as a weapon of war.

Custody, torture, and women's bodies Sexual torture involves a series of enforced sexual acts, regardless of whether or not there is penetration. It is a form of violence based on the difference in power between the strong and the weak, and is a direct attack on the person's integrity. Such abuse may occur while in custody or being interrogated by state authorities or political groups, but may also occur in any situation, formal or informal, where someone is held against their will.

Testifying to sexual torture by using psychological or medical evidence is not a simple matter. People who are currently under arrest should be referred by their lawyers to a dependable trauma centre, taken regularly to their appointments, privacy should be observed during the session, and, finally, the court has to accept the medical report. During this process, specialists who have experience in evidence-based scientific clinical knowledge and who are also determined to advocate for the victim are needed.

However, the process is not merely medical. In order for the victim to be healed even partially, the medical team who has the determination to use this knowledge has to cooperate with lawyers. Despite the adverse conditions in such interviews, the psychological and social functions of victims may be improved. One of the dilemmas that it is necessary to abolish the secrecy surrounding such violence. Victims' accusations may arise in political contexts and for political reasons. But after self-disclosure, and in undergoing the processes of testimony and therapy, victims must face the individual aspects of their problems (Sezgin et al. 2000).

Forced sex and trafficking The trafficking of women happens all over the world yet remains hidden from public view. Human trafficking typically entails confinement, and often physical and psychological abuse. Research has demonstrated that violence and abuse are at the core of trafficking for prostitution. Sex trafficking occurs universally. Women are taken from their country and sold for sexual use. Prostitution dehumanizes, commodifies, and fetishizes woman. A nine-country assessment, concluded that 73 per cent of women used in prostitution were physically assaulted, 89 per cent wanted to escape, 63 per cent were raped, and 68 per cent met the criteria for PTSD (Farley et al. 2003)

Sexual health (STDs) and women

Sexual health and protection from sexually transmitted diseases is a critical issue for women. There is a growing literature on the increasing numbers of women with HIV/AIDS that discusses: (1) the woman's belief that the husband is not having any relation with others and is monogamous; (2) suffering from sexual abuse, partner rape, or incest (Melendez 2003); (3) accepting forced sex from the partner or the client because of fear of further violence (Amaro 1995); and (4) the inability to force partners to use condoms for protection. All these conditions prepare a suitable environment for infection with the HIV virus (WHO 2002). Any history of sexual abuse diminishes one's level of assertiveness for protected sex and makes one vulnerable to forced sexuality.

Conclusion

This chapter illuminated how gender is communicated through women's bodies and women's health with special reference to domestic violence, honour killings, trafficking, and STDs in contemporary social and political contexts. The interconnected nature of women's bodies, sexualities, and the violation of their human rights are mostly due to the asymmetrical gender roles stemming from the social and cultural contexts in which they live. The extensive review of the literature suggests that women's mental health, bodies, and sexualities are closely related and need to be studied together. Therefore, substantive legal and operational measures need to be taken through national and supra-national bodies in order to eliminate the hurdles for women's mental health and bodily integrity.

References

Altinay, AG and Arat, Y (2007) *Violence Against Woman In Turkey*. Istanbul: Punto Publications.

Amaro, H (1995) 'Love, Sex, and Power; considering women's realities in HIV prevention' *American Psychologist*, 50, 437–47.

American Psychiatric Association (1994) *Diagnostic and Statistic Manual of Mental Disorders. (DSM-IV)*. Washington, DC: American Psychiatric Association.

Barakat, H (1999) *Modern Arab Society: A social research*. 5th edn. Hamra, Beirut: Arab Unity Studies Center Publications.

Brownmiller, S (1975) *Against Our Will: Men, Women, and Rape*. New York: Simon and Schuster.

Cindoğlu, D (1997) 'Virginity Tests and Artificial Virginity in Modern Turkish Medicine', *Women's Studies International Forum*, 20(2), 253–61.

Cindoğlu, D, Cemrek, M, Toktas, S, and Zencirci, G (2008) 'The Family in Turkey: The Battleground of the Modern and the Traditional', in Charles B Hennon and Stephan M Wilson (eds) *Families in a Global Context*. New York: Routledge Press, 235–63.

Cockburn, C (1999). *Gender, armed conflict and political violence*. Washington, DC: The World Bank.

Cook, R (1997) *Female Empowerment and Demographic Process: Moving Beyond Cairo*. Seminar. 21–24 April. Lund, Sweden: International Union for the Scientific Study of Population.

Farley, M, Cotton, A, Lynne, J, et al. (2003) 'Prostitution and Trafficking in 9 Countries: An Update on Violence and Posttraumatic Stress Disorder', *Journal of Trauma Practice*, 2(3&4), 33–74.

Goldstein, J (2001) *War and Gender*. Cambridge: Cambridge University Press.

Ilkkaracan, P (2000). 'Exploring the Context of Women's Sexuality in Eastern Turkey', in Pinar Ilkkaracan (ed) *Women and Sexuality in Muslim Societies*. Istanbul: Women for Women's Rights Publications, 229–44.

Kimerling, R (2004) 'An investigation of sex differences in nonpsychiatric morbidity associated with posttraumatic stress disorder', *Journal American Medical Women Association*, 59(1) (Winter) 43–7.

Lee, J, Pomeroy, EL, Yoo, SK, and Rheinboldt, KT (2005) 'Attitudes Toward Rape: A Comparison Between Asian and Caucasian College Students', *Violence Against Women*, 11, 177–19.

Melendez, RM, Hoffman, S, Exner, T, Leu, CS, and Ehrhardt, AA (2003) 'Intimate Partner Violence and Safer Sex Negotiation: Effect of a Gender-Specific Intervention', *Archives of Sexual Behavior*, 32, 499–511

Miranda, J and Green, BL (1999) 'The Need for Mental Health Services Research Focusing on Poor Young Women', *The Journal of Mental Health Policy and Economics*, 2, 73–80.

Plummer, K (2003) *Intimate Citizenship: Private Decisions and Public Dialogues*. Seattle, WA: University of Washington Press.

Russell, DEH (1990) *Rape in Marriage*. Revised edn. Bloomington and Indianapolis: Indiana University Press.

Sezgin, U (2006) 'What are Honor Killings? Defining Killings Committed in the Name of Honor', in *We Can Stop This*. Turkey: Kamer Foundation Books, Berdan Publishing, 282–300.

Sezgin, U, Yüksel, Ş, and Keser, V (2000) 'Rape under detention and role of psychological reports in sexual abuse', *Treatment and rehabilitations centers reports of Turkish Human Rights Foundation*. İstanbul: TİHV publications, 25, 51–63.

UNICEF (2000) *Domestic Violence against Women and Girls*. Florence: Innocenti Research Centre, UNICEF.

Williams, LS (1984) 'Classical rape: When the victims report?', *Social Problems*, 31(4), 459–67.

World Economic Forum (2009) *World Gender Gap Report*. Geneva: WEF. Available at <http://www. weforum.org/pdf/gendergap/report2009.pdf>, accessed 7 November 2011.

World Health Organization (2002) *World Report of Violence and Health*. Geneva: WHO.

World Health Organization (2011) *Violence against Women: factsheets*. Geneva: WHO. Available at <http://www.who.int/mediacentre/factsheets/fs239/en/>, accessed 7 November 2011.

Yüksel, S (2010) 'Date rape patterns: Experiences from Turkey', in Coban Döskaya (ed) *21. Yüzyılın Eşiğinde Kadınlar: Değişim ve Güçlenme (Women in the 21th Century: Change and Empowerment)* F, Number I, İzmir, 329–334.

Yüksel, S and Sezgin, U (2007) *Discovering the truth and rebuilding trust after rape at home*, presented in 10th European Conference on Traumatic Stress, Croatia 5–9 June 2007.

Chapter 24

Human Rights, Health, and Indigenous Australians

Ernest Hunter, Helen Milroy, Ngiare Brown,
and Tom Calma

> Human rights are universal and indivisible. This means that they apply to everyone,
> everywhere, all the time and that different sorts of rights have equal importance.
> Governments should not privilege the enjoyment of one right over that of another,
> as if different rights are in competition with each other or subject to a hierarchy of
> 'more important' and 'less important' rights.
>
> *Tom Calma, 2008.*

Introduction

Australia's Aboriginal and Torres Strait Islander Social Justice Commissioner makes this statement in the foreword to his Social Justice Report for 2007 (Aboriginal and Torres Strait Islander
Social Justice Commissioner 2008). His key topics of concern are Indigenous[1] family violence and
abuse, and providing a human rights analysis of the 'Emergency Response' by the Commonwealth
government in that year in Australia's Northern Territory, ostensibly in response to allegations of
widespread child sexual abuse.[2] Calma's statement raises important issues that, at least in Australia,
are in the foreground of political and public debate. Indeed, the persistence of profound disadvantage and escalating social problems among Australia's Indigenous populations has led some to
question the wisdom or 'haste' of statutory reforms that were, supposedly, informed by social
justice concerns (Hunter 2002; Sutton 2001, 2005).

However, this is precisely the issue that Calma is challenging. The removal of racist statutes and
the repeal of discriminatory legislation without addressing directly and vigorously the barriers to
equitable participation in society that persist through denial of the means to define and realize
ideals and aspirations (education, literacy, employment, political representation...) is what Eugene

---

[1] In this chapter Indigenous (capitalized) will refer to the Aboriginal and Torres Strait Islander peoples of
Australia and indigenous (uncapitalized) will be used for indigenous peoples of all nations.

[2] The Response was announced by the conservative Liberal government in June 2007 in response to a report
by the Northern Territory Board of Inquiry into the Protection of Aboriginal Children from Sexual Abuse.
It has involved legislative change and a range of broad social and medical service interventions, some
coordinated through the military, which have been continued by the Labor government elected at the end
of 2007.

Brody referred to more than four decades ago as 'cultural exclusion' (Brody 1966). Reducing human rights to statutory reforms (as important as they were and are) trivializes the challenge and dooms the enterprise. Calma also points to the dangers inherent in privileging certain rights at the expense of others, noting that the Northern Territory intervention:

> seeks to address a breakdown in law and order in Indigenous communities. And yet it potentially involves introducing measures that undermine the rule of law and do not guarantee Indigenous citizens equal treatment to other Australians. (Aboriginal and Torres Strait Islander Social Justice Commissioner 2008:3)

The enterprise, then, is neither simple nor straightforward. It is, indeed, a global challenge and one where it should be expected that socially stable and economically privileged societies, such as Australia, should lead by example in reducing and eliminating the social, economic, and health disadvantage of indigenous citizens. Manifestly, that is not the case, and maintaining human rights progress remains as important for Aboriginal and Torres Strait Islander Australians as it does for the estimated 350 million indigenous people living in more than 70 countries worldwide, most of whom are poor by their nations' standards. Regardless of location or history they are, by and large, the most disadvantaged and vulnerable groups within the nations in which they reside.

The human rights of indigenous peoples has only recently been the focus of attention in the international human rights arena. This reflects many factors including the Eurocentric focus of this debate in the aftermath of the Second World War and, subsequently, the shifting investments in the rights of nationalities emerging with the fragmentation of the colonial order. However, it is also informed by the 'invisibility' of indigenous minorities or what, in Australia, has been characterized as 'the Great Australian Silence', a term referring to the 'disremembering' or erasure of Aboriginal Australians from the consciousness of the wider Australian society, that persisted into the latter decades of the 20th century (Stanner 1979). While that is clearly changing in Australia, as elsewhere, the 'visibility' of indigenous peoples remains obscured by their demography and diversity. Regardless, indigenous peoples share commonalities in terms of their worldviews and the nature of their relationships with the environment (Durie 2005). Most also share similar experiences of dispossession and marginalization, perhaps best described in relation to the resulting health and socio-economic consequences for the 'anglo-settler' societies of North America, Hawaii, New Zealand, and Australia (Kunitz 1994).

Health and human rights (and indigenous peoples)

> The right to health is not in Magna Carta. It is not, and never has been, a universal right. Rights have histories. They are established slowly, and usually after some great schism. (The French Revolution, in Mary Wollstonecraft's case. World War II in the case of the NHS, the Universal Declaration and the WHO). Rights are created and agreed when their existence is politically essential and technically possible. (Horton 2008:2214)

Richard Horton, editor of *The Lancet*, makes this point in considering what the right to health will mean within Britain's National Health Service in the 21st century (Horton 2008), but the point is equally relevant in terms of the slow accretion of indigenous rights. Indeed, the belated recognition of the rights of indigenous peoples must be located within the longer timeframe through which current concepts and charters of human rights developed.

Human rights are a set of universally agreed upon social, political, and cultural norms to which we are all entitled by way of our humanity. There is no hierarchy of rights, nor are the rights of one individual or population superior to another's.[3] However, while the rights of indigenous peoples are neither different nor greater, their expression and realization may assume an alternate or changing priority dependent upon cultural contexts, community priorities, and needs at any given time. The rights of indigenous peoples in relation to health cannot be considered in isolation from those contexts or from the broader rights issues of indigenous peoples.

As noted by the United Nations High Commissioner for Human Rights: 'The right to health . . . is not to be understood as the right to be healthy' (Robinson 2004:3). Rather, it refers to rights to components which assist individuals and communities to achieve the highest attainable standard of physical and mental health, including autonomy, information, education, and participation (Gruskin and Tarantola 2005).

The right to health was first identified in the World Health Organization (WHO) Constitution in 1946. The Universal Declaration of Human Rights (UDHR), ratified by the United Nations (UN) in 1948, identifies a number of aspects relevant to the right to health, Article 25 specifying that: 'Everyone has the right to a standard of living adequate for the health and well-being of himself and his family, including food, clothing, housing and medical care and necessary social services, and the right to security in the event of unemployment, sickness, disability, widowhood, old age or other lack of livelihood in circumstances beyond his control'.

Whilst not legally binding on signatories (states), the UDHR is an aspirational document with moral legitimacy. However, the right to health is most specifically and explicitly included in Article 12 of the International Covenant on Economic, Social and Cultural Rights[4] clause 1 of which states that signatories: 'recognise the right of everyone to the enjoyment of the highest attainable standard of physical and mental health'.

In 2000, the Committee on Economic, Social and Cultural Rights (one of the monitoring bodies of the UN), adopted a General Comment on the right to health.[5] General Comment 14 specifies that the right to health is dependent on a number of factors including the realization of other rights, non-discrimination, and equality. Further, it reaffirms that the right to health is understood to be: 'the right to a system of health protection which provides equality of opportunity for people to enjoy the highest attainable standard of health'. Under Article 12, Special Topics of Broad Application, it also makes specific reference to indigenous peoples, stating, *inter alia*, that: 'Indigenous peoples have the right to specific measures to improve their access to health services and care. These services should be culturally appropriate, taking into account traditional preventive care, healing practices and medicines. States should provide resources for Indigenous peoples to design, deliver and control such services so that they may enjoy the highest attainable standard of physical and mental health'.

In 1999, a number of member States of the UN proposed a resolution from the World Health Assembly (the decision making body of the WHO) to add a spiritual dimension to the WHO definition of health (Tarantola 2007); however, this was not supported due to political and

---

[3] Intersecting domains of rights may, however, result in conflicts such as has been raised in relation to female genital mutilation in the Horn of Africa (Abusharaf 1998) and subincision of adolescent males in certain desert Aboriginal communities in Australia (Hunter 2007).

[4] International Covenant on Economic, Social and Cultural Rights. Adopted and opened for signature, ratification and accession by United Nations General Assembly Resolution 2200 A (XXI) of 16 December 1966. Entered into force on 3 January 1976, in accordance with Article 27.

[5] General Comment No. 14: The Right to the Highest Attainable Standard of Health (Article 12 of the International Covenant on Economic, Social and Cultural Rights, May 2000). Adopted by the Committee on Economic, Social and Cultural Rights on 11 May 2000. UN document E/C. 12/2000/4, 11 August 2000.

religious concerns. It is interesting to note that this has since been revisited by the newly convened Human Rights Council as Resolution 2006/2,[6] which identifies the spiritual dimension of health in international rights documentation.

Indigenous rights in international context

In the 2002 Social Justice Report, the Aboriginal and Torres Strait Islander Social Justice Commissioner emphasized that, at the international level, gaining recognition for Indigenous peoples and issues has involved two processes:

> The first concerns the participation of Indigenous peoples or put differently, the struggle for recognition of our legitimate place at the negotiating table. The second is the struggle for the recognition and protection of Indigenous peoples' distinct rights in international law. (Aboriginal and Torres Strait Islander Social Justice Commissioner 2002:179)

Some five years later, three years after the International Decade of the World's Indigenous People (1995–2004) came to an end and after more than two decades of debate, the Declaration on the Rights of Indigenous Peoples was approved by the General Assembly of the United Nations.

This history, which goes back to mention of the native inhabitants in the territories of member nations of the League of Nations in its foundation Covenant in 1920 and concerns about native labour noted by the International Labour Organization (ILO) in 1921 (Havemann 1999), is reviewed in detail elsewhere.[7] Indigenous peoples themselves have been seeking recognition and representation beyond the borders of their homelands since the early 1900s. In 1923 *Haudenosaunee* (Iroquois) leader, Chief Deskaheh, traveled to Geneva to speak at the League of Nations. He planned to defend the rights of his people to live under their own laws, on their own lands, and under their own faith. The Chief was denied entry and not allowed to speak, and returned home in 1924.

Similarly, Maori religious leader TW Ratana traveled to London to petition King George in protest at the breaking of the Treaty of Waitangi in *Aotearoa*. Unable to gain access to the King, he sent part of the delegation to Geneva to the League of Nations, joining the delegation there in 1925, but was again denied the opportunity to represent his people. Indeed, it was only in 1989 that Chief Ted Moses of the Grand Council of Crees, Canada, became the first indigenous person elected to office to attend a UN meeting to discuss the effects of racial discrimination on the social and economic situation of indigenous peoples.

Indigenous rights and the United Nations

With the affirmation of the fundamental human rights of all peoples in the Charter of the United Nations in 1945 and the Universal Declaration of Human Rights in 1948, the pace of developments belatedly picked up. In the 1950s indigenous peoples were identified through consideration of labour and decolonization, and in the 1960s in the context of the International Convention on the Elimination of All Forms of Racial Discrimination (1966). In the early 1970s the

---

[6] United Nations Human Rights Council. Resolution 2006/2: Working Group of the Commission on Human Rights to Elaborate a Draft Declaration in accordance with Paragraph 5 of the General Assembly Resolution 49/214 of 23 December 1994. Geneva: Office of the High Commissioner for Human Rights, 2006.

[7] For instance see William Jonas (Aboriginal and Torres Strait Islander Social Justice Commissioner, 2002) and Tom Calma (Aboriginal and Torres Strait Islander Social Justice Commissioner, 2006).

Sub-Commission on the Prevention of Discrimination and Protection of Minorities oversighted a series of reports by Special Rapporteur José Martinez Cobo that was released from 1981 to 1984. This included a report on discrimination against indigenous peoples that in 1982 resulted in the formation of the Working Group on Indigenous Populations as a subsidiary body of the Sub-Commission on Protection and Promotion of Human Rights.[8] In 2008, the Indigenous Expert Mechanism commenced to provide guidance to the United Nations Human Rights Council (this effectively replaces the Working Group on Indigenous Populations). In 2002, the Economic and Social Council (ECOSOC) of the UN also established the Permanent Forum on Indigenous Issues which advises ECOSOC on how the UN agencies should address indigenous concerns.

What this has provided is a means for indigenous peoples to raise their issues in UN fora without being mediated through representatives of governments, and for direct dialogue with (and between) indigenous organizations. Through the 1980s indigenous ecological and resource issues were foregrounded by the UN and the World Bank, with the Working Group commencing work on the Draft Declaration of the Rights of Indigenous Peoples (the Draft Declaration) in 1985. The new Human Rights Council now also has provisions for conducting 'universal periodic reviews' of all countries' human rights records. This will ensure that the issues of indigenous peoples will be brought to international attention regardless of states' interests. The Human Rights Council is part of a United Nations institutional framework for dealing with indigenous issues that also includes the Indigenous Expert Mechanism, the Permanent Forum on Indigenous Issues, and the Special Rapporteur on the rights and fundamental freedoms of Indigenous Peoples (Davis 2006).

There are other international institutions through which the issues and rights of indigenous peoples are progressed. For instance, the ILO Convention on Indigenous and Tribal Peoples (1989)[9] provides an example of the current approach of international law frameworks to indigenous peoples' issues. ILO Convention 169 represents a shift away from the constructs of assimilation as expressed in earlier documents (Convention No. 157 1957) to a more responsive environment to Indigenous priorities. The preamble of the Convention recognizes the: 'aspirations of Indigenous peoples to exercise control over their own institutions, ways of life and economic development and to maintain and develop their identities, languages and religions, within the framework of the States in which they live'.

The position of the Australian government during the development of the draft declaration was supportive until the election of a conservative, coalition government in 1996. Canada and New Zealand were also in full support in the early years of the development of the draft declaration. However, citing the language of self-determination and concerns about territorial integrity, support for the draft declaration diminished in a number of states, specifically among what became known as the 'CANZUS alliance'—Canada, Australia, New Zealand, and the United States (these being the aforementioned 'anglo-settler' societies for all of which the implications in terms of control of land and resources are significant). Despite this, the draft declaration was presented to the Human Rights Council and adopted with minimal debate in 2006. It was then presented to the General Assembly, but as a result of intense and sustained opposition from the

---

[8] The Working Group lapsed upon the reform of the UN system in 2005 which had resulted in the abolition of the Commission on Human Rights and Sub-Commission on the Protection and Promotion of Human Rights, and the creation of the Human Rights Council.

[9] Convention No. 169 Concerning Indigenous and Tribal Peoples in Independent Countries, 27 June 1989, International Labour Conference. Entered in to force 5 September 1991.

'CANZUS alliance' adoption was deferred, the obstruction of the Australian government being noted:

> The central issue in the negotiations on the Draft Declaration is the unwillingness of States to accept that Indigenous peoples have an unqualified right to self-determination, as set out in Article 3 of the Draft Declaration.
>
> Australia has played a vital role in this process, being one of the most vocal and oppositional countries during the debates since 1997 (Aboriginal and Torres Strait Islander Social Justice Commissioner 2008:214).

Finally, on 13 September 2007, the United Nations Declaration on the Rights of Indigenous Peoples was adopted by the General Assembly of the UN, with 143 Member States voting in favour of the resolution, eleven abstaining, and four—Canada, Australia, New Zealand, and the United States—voting against it.

Indigenous rights in Australian context

Aboriginal and Torres Strait Islander Australians represent 2.3 per cent of the nation's population and are comprised of two groups.[10] Over 90 per cent are of Aboriginal origin and are the descendents of members of over 250 language groups that existed across the continent prior to colonization. While the majority now reside in urban and regional centres, Aboriginal Australians are disproportionately represented among Australians living in very remote settings. The remainder are Torres Strait Islanders from the islands between Australia's northern tip and Papua New Guinea, who themselves have two distinct languages. While the population of the Torres Strait is largely Indigenous (and includes some Aboriginal groups), the majority of Torres Strait Islanders now live in metropolitan mainland Australia.

The struggle for Indigenous rights in Australia dates back to settlement but became a public struggle only around the time of the sesqui-centenary 'celebrations' of settlement in 1938—when for the first time Indigenous Australians insisted that the language of 'invasion' be used. In the 1950s and 1960 a number of organizations, such as the Council for Aboriginal Rights and the Australian Aboriginal Fellowship, promoted equality for Aboriginal Australians using the language of rights and invoking the UDHR. The creation of the first national Aboriginal organization, the Federal Council for the Advancement of Aboriginal and Torres Strait Islanders in 1957, was for the purpose of lobbying for Indigenous social and political rights.

The rights movement in Australia gained ground during the 1960s and 1970s as Aboriginal and Torres Strait Islander peoples faced growing pressures on their lands and resources and suffered the ongoing and unresolved effects of government policy on identity, culture, and community. While a growing number of educated Indigenous Australians were aware of national and international political developments such as the Civil Rights movement in the United States, it was not for a further two decades (and multiple Commissions and Inquiries) that political acknowledgement was given to the historical violations of Indigenous rights. In December 1992, Australia's Prime Minister launched the Year for Indigenous People in the urban Aboriginal community of Redfern with a speech that: 'was and continues to be the seminal moment and expression of

---

[10] Australia also has a significant population of South Sea Islanders, descendents of indentured labourers brought to Australia over a century ago for whom there are rights issues both distinct from and overlapping with those of Indigenous Australians.

European Australian acknowledgement of grievous inhumanity to the Indigenes of this land'
(Pearson 2002). Keating said:

> And, I say, the starting point might be to recognise that the problem starts with us non-Aboriginal
> Australians. It begins, I think, with that act of recognition. Recognition that it was we who did the
> dispossessing. We took the traditional lands and smashed the traditional way of life. We brought the
> diseases. The alcohol. We committed the murders. We took the children from their mothers. We prac-
> tised discrimination and exclusion. It was our ignorance and our prejudice. And our failure to imagine
> these things being done to us. With some noble exceptions, we failed to make the most basic human
> response and enter into their hearts and minds. We failed to ask—how would I feel if this was done to
> me? As a consequence, we failed to see that what we were doing degraded all of us. (Keating
> 2005:137)

In the same year (1992), in response to the Royal Commission into Aboriginal Deaths in Custody
(1991) and the Human Rights and Equal Opportunity Commission's Report of the National
Inquiry into Racist Violence in Australia (1991), the federal government created the position of
the Aboriginal and Torres Strait Islander Social Justice Commissioner. The Commissioner's
Social Justice Reports have since placed a range of key issues within a rights framework, including
bridging the persistent gap in health status with the wider Australian population (Aboriginal and
Torres Strait Islander Social Justice Commissioner 2005), reforming the way in which governments' policy arrangements are coordinated and implemented, including Australia's responsibilities in relation to the Millennium Development Goals (Aboriginal and Torres Strait Islander
Social Justice Commissioner 2006) and, as noted in the introduction to this chapter, a rights
analysis of utilitarian, interventionist 'solutions' to Indigenous social and health 'crises'—labelled
by some commentators with view to the Northern Territory Emergency Intervention, as 'coercive
reconciliation' (Altman and Hinkson 2007).

Aboriginal and Torres Strait Islander health

By all present indicators, Indigenous Australians suffer a significant excess burden of morbidity
and mortality, and experience severe social disadvantage by comparison to the rest of the
Australian population. Indigenous children in Australia live in a landscape of risk within a nation
of wealth and opportunity. Despite substantial improvements in infant mortality during the 1970s
resulting from improved access to basic primary care services, and in contrast to the indigenous
populations of North America and New Zealand, the health differential remains entrenched, with
infant mortality rates remaining some three times higher (Fremantle et al. 2006). Many surviving
Indigenous children begin life in a state of compromise with high levels of obstetric complications, low birth weight, and exposure to substances in utero, placing them at risk for later poor
health and life outcomes (Glasson et al. 2005; Rothstein et al. 2007). Early development is often
compromised by diseases now almost non-existent in Western society (such as rheumatic fever).
Young adults experience high rates of accidents and injuries, and from early adulthood chronic
illnesses such as diabetes, renal failure, and cardiovascular disease are common, associated with
poor diet, limited exercise, and high levels of smoking, alcohol, and other substance misuse
(Trewin and Madden 2005). Mental health morbidity appears to be increasing, and attempted and
completed suicide is increasing and occurring at a much younger age (Hunter and Milroy 2006).
All of this is compounded by poor access to, and inappropriateness of, many existing services, and
beyond the clinic door Indigenous families suffer high rates of unemployment, poverty, poor
housing, overcrowding, and levels of incarceration and child removal far above that for non-
Indigenous Australians. Levels of educational attendance, retention, and achievement are low, and
the gap in education is as great as the disparity in health (Zubrick et al. 2006). The population

pyramid reveals a distorted age distribution with many children, lower numbers of adults, and very few elders. Due to the loss of human capital, the resilience-enhancing effects of extended family for Indigenous children has been significantly diminished.

However, Indigenous health is both inclusive of these realities and more, and is usually not afforded a definition separate to a whole of life understanding incorporating aspects of community and ancestry. The commonly accepted definition in Indigenous Australia draws on the World Health Organization's holistic construction (Brady et al. 1997) and was first articulated in the National Aboriginal Health Strategy in 1989 which states that: '[Health is]. . . not just the physical well-being of the individual but the social, emotional, and cultural well-being of the whole community. This is a whole-of-life view and it also includes the cyclical concept of life-death-life' (National Aboriginal Health Strategy Working Party 1989:x). This was elaborated on in the first systematic, national review of the mental health of Aboriginal and Torres Strait Islander peoples:

> The Aboriginal concept of health is holistic, encompassing mental health and physical, cultural and spiritual health. Land is central to wellbeing. This holistic concept does not merely refer to the "whole body" but in fact is steeped in the harmonised inter-relations which constitute cultural wellbeing. These inter-relating factors can be categorised largely as spiritual, environmental, ideological, political, social, economic, mental and physical. Crucially, it must be understood that when the harmony of these inter-relations is disrupted, Aboriginal ill health will persist. (Swan and Raphael 1995:13)

For Indigenous Australians, then, health, mental health, and well-being are inseparable, interconnected, and incorporate notions of balance and harmony. As is the case for indigenous peoples generally, the disruption of that balance through dispossession and trauma in its myriad forms over generations has left a legacy of profound grief and psychological distress. Consequently, the mental health needs of Indigenous Australians must be located in a human rights framework and can only be understood within an historical and social context—they cannot be reduced to the simple interplay of risk and protective factors.

'Risk' and rights

With such a burden of social adversity it should be no surprise that there has been a longstanding preoccupation with risk 'factors' that has oftentimes led to siloed, project and programme based 'solutions'. There is now an active debate regarding whether the burden of social adversity experienced by Aboriginal and Torres Strait Islander Australians is best considered in terms of risk and vulnerability, or as an issue of human rights. Indeed, it is perhaps surprising that it is only with the dawning of the new millennia that Indigenous health has clearly been placed within a human rights framework.

Regardless, the prevailing paradigms informing policy and service planning remain based on notions of risk that are, implicitly, individualistic, and presume capacities for 'choice' that are not consistent with Indigenous life experiences.[11] Developmental risk and resilience factors must also be considered in the light of social change. What was a source of resilience in traditional contexts

[11] Such paradigms often do not take account of the needs of Indigenous Australians to fulfill cultural obligations necessary for cultural survival, which may conflict with Western notions of healthy lifestyle 'choices'. Furthermore, recognition of customary law has also been contentious with William Jonas noting that the key issue is not a conflict with human rights but identifying mechanisms to ensure both can be guaranteed (Jonas 2006).

may, in contemporary settings, increase vulnerability. This has been suggested in terms of the obligations of 'demand sharing' in a subsistence-level, welfare economy (Macdonald 2000; Peterson 1993; Sutton 2001). Similarly, in terms of child development, the traditional early autonomy and self-reliance within well-buffered kinship systems that supported survival under threat (Hamilton 1981) may now predispose to negative outcomes in settings of chronic stress and compromised social support systems (Hunter 1999). Surviving in environments of racism and discrimination at times demands behaviours at variance with the norms of the wider society which, in an immediate sense, may be 'adaptive' but which ultimately embed disadvantage and eclipse potential.

Furthermore, there has been less than three decades between the first public documentation in the early 1980s of the forcible removal of Indigenous children from their families as government policy for the purposes of assimilation (Read 1981), the landmark national inquiry into those human rights violations in the mid-1990s (Human Rights and Equal Opportunity Commission 1997), and the belated but widely commended official Apology by Australia's (new) Prime Minister in 2008. Through this period Aboriginal and Torres Strait Islander children, often living in circumstances of adversity, have also had to integrate this previously suppressed history into their evolving personal and group identities, sense of safety in the world, and basic trust in humanity. For some Indigenous teenage boys outrage over this revealed history and their persistent disadvantage manifests as risk taking, aggression, and actions challenging of authority, behaviours easily pathologized as 'sociopathic' and criminalized, with entry into the youth detention and criminal justice systems often a normative rite of passage (Beresford and Omaji 1996).

Such reactions are not new and were described decades ago in terms of alcohol-associated flaunting of mainstream norms and standards as a means of asserting Aboriginal agency in a repressive society (O'Connor 1984). The marginalization and disempowerment provoking such behaviours are frequently compounded by institutional responses characterized by poor consultation, top down imposed programmes, lack of cultural understanding, unrealistic expectations, and simplistic enumeration of risk factors rather than a nuanced understanding of causal risk processes (Rutter 1994).

Indigenous mental health and rights

The rights of people suffering from mental health disorders were most dramatically raised as their systematic violation by mental health professions (specifically, psychiatrists) in the service of the racial state became known in the aftermath of the Second World War (Hunter 1993). In Australia, also, it was a series of institutional violations of patients' rights and the resulting inquiries that led to the Burdekin Inquiry into the rights of people with mental illness that ultimately informed a radical shift in Australia's mental health policies (Human Rights and Equal Opportunity Commission 1993). The Burdekin Inquiry also raised the particular vulnerability of Indigenous people suffering from mental illness who are subject to a 'triple jeopardy' (Tarantola 2007).

However, Indigenous Australians also suffer the wider mental health impacts of fundamental human rights violations. Furthermore, the damage does not necessarily end when the violations stop, such violations not only affecting those already living with mental illness but contributing to ongoing vulnerability to negative physical and psychological outcomes. This complex situation was further confused by the previous government's response to the recommendations of the 'Stolen Generations Report' (Human Rights and Equal Opportunity Commission 1997) in which attention to gross violations of human rights was diffused by a focus on one recommendation—addressing consequential mental health harms. As important as such efforts are, conflating 'treatment' with redressing the violation of human rights is to trivialize both (Nieves 2007):

> Appropriate mental health treatment is essential to reparations for indigenous peoples. But one cannot pretend to improve mental health of people who experienced grave human rights breaches through individual or clinical isolated group programs if the surrounding society refutes historical facts or fails to bring responsible persons to justice. So health care needs to be combined with state actions that acknowledge the truth about the events that happened.

Mental health ambivalence and ambiguity

As noted in the introduction, a key concern of the 2007 Social Justice Report was an assessment of human rights issues raised by the Commonwealth's Northern Territory intervention, specifically the conflict between the (stated) intentions and the methods deployed. Not surprisingly, the background to these events is complex.

Through 2007, media coverage of remote Aboriginal Australia was unprecedented, with stories of violence and community collapse in the Northern Territory followed by saturation reporting of child sexual abuse from the Kimberley, Central Australia, and Cape York. Most attention was given to the Emergency Response by the Commonwealth in the Territory (Altman and Hinkson 2007) following the release of the Anderson and Wild report (Northern Territory Board of Inquiry into the Protection of Aboriginal Children from Sexual Abuse 2007). This was certainly not new information; the widely publicized suicide of teenager Susan Taylor in a Perth fringe camp and allegations of earlier sexual abuse (Laurie and Egan 2001) having led to the Gordon Inquiry in Western Australia some five years earlier (Gordon et al. 2002). However, there are distinct similarities in the tenor of the reportage that has a much longer lineage in which the ambivalence of the wider society to Indigenous Australians is indulged and reinforced through salacious voyeurism. As an object of concern and pity, the Aboriginal victim (be it abused woman or child) is presented alongside the Aboriginal perpetrator (usually, but not always, an adult Aboriginal male). Regardless of the explicit concern for the 'victims', the subtext is invariably the ineptitude, iniquity, or both, of Aboriginal families and communities.

Ambivalence is also present within the health sector and in the attitudes of many Indigenous Australians towards health professions and professionals. While ever-present, this has changed over time with developments in the wider social and political arena (Anderson 2002; Thomas 2004) and is particularly obvious in relation to 'mental health' (Hunter 1997). However, the power base and practice of mental health service provision in Australia has been firmly lodged within mainstream, public sector institutions—near cousins to the government sectors and departments that within living memory were responsible as perpetrators or bystanders in depriving Indigenous peoples of fundamental rights (Hunter 1991). While the situation is now changing, it is thus not surprising that, historically, 'mental health' as term, concept, and practice, is contested and distrusted, and while that situation is improving, there remain different worldviews and 'ways of doing' with various degrees of discomfort and ambiguity (Hunter 2004).

Rights and ambiguities

As Tatz notes, ambiguity is a feature of policy in Indigenous affairs more broadly in Australia: '[an] unintended outcome of governmental insecurity and uncertainty about what to do or how to do it, about avoiding obvious breaches of human rights while remaining unwilling to commit Australian society to equality and to an acceptance of our native peoples' (Tatz, 2001:7). Ironically, ambiguity is most destructive and tenacious when deployed under the guise of rights. Thus, the reduction of Indigenous marginalization in Australian society to social class and economic disadvantage obscures underlying racism. Furthermore, as noted in the introduction, that various political and policy initiatives motivated by consideration of rights and social justice have had untoward (and at times frankly negative) effects, has been used to rationalize the inaction or paternalism of past times (Hunter 2002). Health professionals have contributed to the confusion and ambiguity in various ways, for instance, by supporting the medicalization of injustice and social distress, in so doing 'validating' politically expedient but, ultimately ineffective, 'solutions' to issues of enormous social complexity that are beyond the province or resources of the health sector (Hunter 2006). However, focusing solely on social change can compromise the realizable and critical role of the health sector:

> insisting only on fundamental and revolutionary social change is dooming us to programs that will take years and generations to take effect. Since it is difficult to implement such major social change, it is easy to ignore inequalities because, they say, nothing can realistically be done about them. Moral outrage about inequalities is appropriate but may be self-indulgent. If we really want to change the world we may have to begin in more modest but practical ways. (Syme 1997:9)

Autonomy and 'control'

What are the 'modest but practical ways' that health professionals can deploy in their work to support larger projects of social change? While there are clearly no approaches that, alone, will be sufficient to this task even in the fullness of time, ensuring Indigenous agency—within the health sector and more broadly—is absolutely necessary. Indeed, the provision of 'services' without supporting agency and autonomy risks increasing dependence and its vicissitudes (Trudgen 2000). Further, there is compelling evidence from Canada demonstrating that in settings where indigenous communities have greater levels of social control over their affairs and destinies, mental health-relevant, population level social indices (in this case suicide rates) are better (Chandler et al. 2003).

In the Australian context demonstrating such correlation is confounded by the illusory nature of Indigenous 'control' regardless of the overarching policy mantle (be it protection, assimilation, self-determination, self-management. . .). However, there is information from Queensland showing that where control has, historically, been most compromised as a result of discriminatory policy (including isolation, concentration, removal, and institutionalization)—that is, in discrete ex-government and mission reserve communities that have been described as 'outback ghettoes' (Brock 1993; Pearson 2007)—social and health indicators (including suicide) are worse, even by comparison to other remote areas (Office for Aboriginal and Torres Strait Islander Partnerships 2006).

How, then, do health and mental health practitioners and planners, whose practice necessarily, at times, is 'paternalistic', undertake their service roles in such settings (in the best interests of patients and consumers) at the same time as supporting Indigenous autonomy and control? Beauchamp and Childress explain that presenting beneficence and autonomy as exclusive is a false dichotomy that confuses: 'by a failure to distinguish between a principle of beneficence that competes with a principle of respect for autonomy and a principle of beneficence that incorporates the patient's autonomy' (Beauchamp and Childress 1994:272). Although this position relates to clinical practice, it has obvious implications for the wider process of social reform and, in particular, the approaches that have been adopted in northern Australia. Few would argue that the Commonwealth's intervention initiated by former Prime Minister John Howard in the Northern Territory was (and remains) paternalistic, and there would also be few who could suggest that it was undertaken in support of autonomy. The same could not so easily be said of the welfare reform interventions in Cape York in north Queensland led by Aboriginal lawyer and political spokesperson, Noel Pearson, which have both state and Commonwealth support and which have been divisive (including within the Indigenous communities of Queensland) in terms of their local implementation and wider implications (Manne 2007; Gaita 2007). While parallels have been drawn between the policy approaches in the Northern Territory and Cape York (which include suspension of elements of anti-discrimination legislation), Manne emphasizes that: 'differences between Pearson and Howard are no less important' (Manne 2007:40), a point also made by Jon Altman who observes that: 'The fundamental difference between Cape York and the Northern Territory is that in the former the state is enabling, in the latter, punitive. The language of the NT intervention is heavily "neo-paternalist" … Aboriginal people are not being invited to enter into this process; it is being forced upon them' (Altman 2007:311).

While the outcomes of these approaches in northern Australia will not be known for some time[12] three critical issues are raised. The first is how policy and practice enables meaningful decision making by Indigenous Australians in pursuit of having real control over destiny, and how the preconditions of those processes (of 'fair equality of opportunity' (Rawls 1999, Revised ed)) are ensured. That, of course, requires dialogue and contextual sensitivity, as noted by Daniels et al. (1999:246): 'In some areas of inquiry in bioethics (or ethics more generally), progress is doomed if we remain insensitive to the local texture of a problem, including the way in which a particular society's beliefs play a role in its policies'. The second issue relates to Calma's concern regarding utilitarianism noted in the introduction—the compromise of certain rights in pursuit of others.

The third issue also raised by Calma is the human rights based approach to development. The United Nations Common Understanding of Human Rights Based Approach to Development Cooperation sets out necessary elements of policy development and service delivery under a human rights based approach as follows (Office of the United Nations High Commissioner for Human Rights, 2006):

1. People are recognized as key actors in their own development, rather than passive recipients of commodities and services.

2. Participation is both a means and a goal.

3. Strategies are empowering, not disempowering.

4. Both outcomes and processes are monitored and evaluated.

5. Analysis includes all stakeholders.

6. Programmes focus on marginalized, disadvantaged, and excluded groups.

7. The development process is locally owned.

8. Programmes aim to reduce disparity.

9. Both top-down and bottom-up approaches are used in synergy.

10. Situation analysis is used to identify immediate, underlying, and basic causes of development problems.

11. Measurable goals and targets are important in programming.

---

[12] The progress report released in December 2008 focusing on the primary trigger for the intervention—the needs of children—documents screening and primary care service activity increases but little in terms of health or social outcomes, concluding that the health problems addressed: 'are the result of poor living conditions, poverty, overcrowding and lack of adequate nutrition. While these conditions can be ameliorated through health interventions, their prevention requires change to these broader determinants of health' (Australian Institute of Health and Welfare and Department of Health and Ageing 2008:xii).

12. Strategic partnerships are developed and sustained.

13. Programmes support accountability to all stakeholders.

Policy implications

While the Australian policy landscape in Indigenous affairs has changed dramatically over the course of the last half-century from being explicitly racist and discriminatory to being more inclusive and respectful of Indigenous peoples, progress has been slow and usually in response to pressure. Indigenous issues still fit uncomfortably in the national policy terrain. It is, of course, questionable whether the racism inherent in Australian society can be addressed through policy without active reflection on the racism inherent in the institutions and sectors promulgating policy—including health (Henry et al. 2004). Further, there is a substantial 'reality gap' between policy directives and implementation at the coalface. Tom Calma identifies three key policy and policy translation failures:

> First, governments of all persuasions have not activated their commitments by setting them within an achievable time frame . . . Second, they have not matched their commitments with the necessary funds and program support to realise them . . . And third, while they have accepted in health frameworks the need to address Aboriginal and Torres Strait Islander health in a holistic manner, they have not engineered their health programs consistent with this understanding nor considered the impact of their broader policy and program approaches on Aboriginal and Torres Strait Islander health. (Aboriginal and Torres Strait Islander Social Justice Commissioner 2005:11)

The Apology delivered by the Prime Minister to Indigenous Australians in 2008 may offer a new pathway to effect change in policy and programs. Although an important first step, 'a future based on mutual respect, mutual resolve and mutual responsibility' will only be possible if the power imbalance—including inequity in resources and lack of Indigenous representation—are addressed. That is, when these rights for Indigenous Australians, as well as rights in relation to health, are ALL seen as fundamental to a just society for all Australians.

References

Aboriginal and Torres Strait Islander Social Justice Commissioner (2002) *Social Justice Report 2002*. Sydney: Human Rights and Equal Opportunity Commission.

Aboriginal and Torres Strait Islander Social Justice Commissioner (2005) *Social Justice Report 2005*. Sydney: Human Rights and Equal Opportunity Commission.

Aboriginal and Torres Strait Islander Social Justice Commissioner (2006) *Social Justice Report 2006*. Sydney: Human Rights and Equal Opportunity Commission.

Aboriginal and Torres Strait Islander Social Justice Commissioner (2007) *Achieving Aboriginal and Torres Strait Islander health equality within a generation: A human rights based approach*. Sydney: Human Rights and Equal Opportunity Commission.

Aboriginal and Torres Strait Islander Social Justice Commissioner (2008) *Social Justice Report 2007*. Sydney: Human Rights and Equal Opportunity Commission.

Abusharaf, RG (1998) 'Unmasking tradition: A Sudanese anthropologist confronts female 'circumcision' and its terrible tenacity', *The Sciences*, 38(2), March/April, 22–27.

Adams, G, Fryberg, SA, Garcia, DM, and Delgado-Torres, EU (2006) 'The psychology of engagement with indigenous identities: a cultural perspective', *Cultural Diversity and Ethnic Minority Psychology*, 12(3), 493–508.

Altman, J (2007) 'In the name of the market?', in J Altman and M Hinkson (eds) *Coercive reconciliation: Stabilise, normalise, exit Aboriginal Australia*. Melbourne: Arena, 307–21.

Altman, J and Hinkson, M (eds) (2007) *Coercive reconciliation: Stabilise, normalise, exit Aboriginal Australia*. Melbourne: Arena.

Anderson, W (2002) *The cultivation of whiteness: Science, health and racial destiny in Australia*. Melbourne: Melbourne University Press.

Australian Institute of Health and Welfare and Department of Health and Ageing (2008) *Progress of the Northern Territory Emergency Response Child Health Check Initiative: Preliminary results from the Child Health Check and follow-up data collections. Cat. no IHW 25*. Canberra: Australian Institute of Health and Welfare.

Australian National Association for Mental Health (1980) *Aboriginals and mental health: Hitting our heads against a brick wall*. Paper presented at the Aborigines and mental health conference, Brisbane, July 4–6.

Beauchamp, TL and Childress, JF (1994) *Principles of biomedical ethics*. 4th edn. New York: Oxford University Press.

Beresford, Q and Omaji, P (1996) *Rites of passage: Aboriginal youth, crime and justice*. Fremantle: Fremantle Arts Centre Press.

Brady, M, Kunitz, S, and Nash, D (1997) 'WHO's definition? Aborigines, conceptualisations of health and the World Health Organization', in L Marks and M Worboys (eds) *Migrants, minorities and health. Historical and contemporary studies*. London: Routledge, 272–290.

Brock, P (1993) *Outback ghettos: A history of Aboriginal institutionalisation and survival*. Melbourne: Cambridge University Press.

Brody, EB (1966) 'Cultural exclusion, character and illness', *American Journal of Psychiatry*, 122(2), 852–58.

Chandler, MJ, Lalonde, CE, Sokol, BW, and Hallett, D (2003) 'Personal persistence, identity development, and suicide: a study of Native and Non-native North American adolescents', *Monographs of the Society for Research in Child Development*, 68(2), vii–viii, 1–130, discussion 131–138.

Daniels, N, Kennedy, BP, and Kawachi, I (1999) 'Why justice is good for our health: The social determinants of health inequalities', *Daedalus*, 128(4), 215–51.

Davis, M (2006) 'The recognition of Aboriginal customary law and international law developments', in *Indigenous Peoples: Issues in International and Australian Law*. Papers presented at a series of three seminars held between 2002 and 2004 in association with the Human Rights and Equal Opportunity Commission. Sydney, NSW: ILA.

Durie, M (2005) 'Indigenous knowledge within a global knowledge system', *Higher Education Policy*, 18, 301–12.

Fremantle, J, Read, A, de Klerk, N, McAullay, D, Anderson, I, and Stanley, F (2006) 'Patterns, trends, and increasing disparities in mortality for Aboriginal and non-Aboriginal infants born in Western Australia, 1980–2001: population database study', *The Lancet*, 367(9524), 1758–66.

Gaita, R (2007) 'Comment', *The Monthly*, August, 10–14.

Glasson, EJ, Sullivan, SG, Hussain, R, and Bittles, AH (2005) 'An assessment of intellectual disability among Aboriginal Australians', *Journal of Intellectual Disability Research*, 49(8), 626–34.

Gordon, S, Hallahan, K, and Henry, D (2002) *Putting the picture together, Inquiry into Response by Government Agencies to Complaints of Family Violence and Child Abuse in Aboriginal Communities*. Perth: Department of Premier and Cabinet, Western Australia.

Gruskin, S and Tarantola, D (2005) 'Health and human rights', in S Gruskin, M Grodin, G Annas, and S Marks (eds) *Perspectives on health and human rights*. New York: Routledge, 3–58.

Hamilton, A (1981) *Nature and nurture: Aboriginal child-rearing in north-central Arnhem Land*. Canberra: Australian Institute of Aboriginal Studies.

Havemann, P (1999) 'Chronology 2: Twentieth-century public international law and indigenous peoples', in P Havemann (ed) *Indigenous peoples' rights in Australia, Canada & New Zealand*. Oxford: Oxford University Press, 18–21.

Henry, BR, Houston, S, and Mooney, GH (2004) 'Institutional racism in Australian healthcare: a plea for decency', *Medical Journal of Australia*, 180, 517–20.

Horton, R (2008) 'What does a National Health System mean in the 21st century?', *The Lancet*, 371(9631), 2213–8.

Human Rights and Equal Opportunity Commission (1991) *Racist violence: Report of the National Inquiry into Racist Violence in Australia*. Canberra: Australian Government Publishing Service.

Human Rights and Equal Opportunity Commission (1993) *Report of the National Inquiry into the Human Rights of People with Mental Illness*. Canberra: Australian Government Publishing Service.

Human Rights and Equal Opportunity Commission (1997) *Bringing them home: Report of the National Inquiry into the Separation of Aboriginal and Torres Strait Islander Children from Their Families*. Canberra: Australian Government Publishing Service.

Hunt, L (2007) *Inventing human rights: A history*. New York: W.W. Norton.

Hunter, E (1991) 'Stains on the caring mantle. Doctors in Aboriginal Australia have a history', *Medical Journal of Australia*, 155(11–12), 779–83.

Hunter, E (1993) 'The snake on the caduceus: Dimensions of medical and psychiatric responsibility in the Third Reich', *Australian and New Zealand Journal of Psychiatry*, 27(1), 149–56.

Hunter, E (1997) 'Double talk: changing and conflicting constructions of indigenous mental health', *Australian and New Zealand Journal of Psychiatry*, 31(6), 820–27.

Hunter, E (1999) 'Considering the changing environment of Indigenous child development', *Australasian Psychiatry*, 7(3), 137–40.

Hunter, E (2002) '"Best intentions" lives on: untoward health outcomes of some contemporary initiatives in Indigenous affairs', *Australian and New Zealand Journal of Psychiatry*, 36(5), 575–84.

Hunter, E (2004) 'Commonality, difference and confusion: Changing constructions of Indigenous mental health', *Australian e-Journal for the Advancement of Mental Health*, 3(3), 1–4. Available at <http://pandora.nla.gov.au/pan/107363/20091002-1309/www.auseinet.com/journal/vol3iss3/huntereditorial.pdf>, accessed 7 November 2011.

Hunter, E (2006) *Back to Redfern: Autonomy and the 'middle E' in relation to Aboriginal health. Discussion Paper Number 18*. Canberra: Australian Institute of Aboriginal and Torres Strait Islander Studies.

Hunter, E (2007) '"Little children" and big sticks: Paternalism and autonomy in Indigenous northern Australia', in J Altman and M Hinkman (eds) *Coercive reconciliation: Stabilise, normalise, exit Aboriginal Australia*. Melbourne: Arena, 121–31.

Hunter, E (2008) 'Not quite enough: Service solutions or stagnation in Indigenous health', *Arena*, 29/30, 203–217.

Hunter, E, and Milroy, H (2006) 'Aboriginal and Torres Strait Islander suicide in context', *Archives of Suicide Research*, 10, 141–57.

Jonas, W (2006) 'The recognition of Aboriginal customary law', in *Indigenous Peoples: Issues in International and Australian Law*. Papers presented at a series of three seminars held between 2002 and 2004 in association with the Human Rights and Equal Opportunity Commission. Sydney, NSW: ILA.

Keating, P (2005) 'Speech at the launch of the Year for Indigenous People', in *Great Speeches: Words that made history*. Melbourne: Viking, 135–42.

Kunitz, S (1994) *Disease and social diversity: The European impact on the health of non-Europeans*. New York: Oxford University Press.

Laurie, V, and Egan, C (2001) 'Susan's story', *The Weekend Australian Magazine*, 15–16 December, 38–43.

Macdonald, G (2000) *An economy out of kilter: Demand sharing among the Wiradjuri. Department of Archaeology and Anthropology seminar, October Seminar*. Canberra: Australian National University.

Manne, R (2007) 'Pearson's gamble, Stanner's dream: The past and future of remote Australia', *The Monthly*, August, 30–40.

National Aboriginal Health Strategy Working Party (1989) *A national Aboriginal health strategy*. Canberra: Department of Aboriginal Affairs.

Nieves, G (2007) 'Healing hidden wounds', *Cultural Survival Quarterly*, 31(3).

Northern Territory Board of Inquiry into the Protection of Aboriginal Children from Sexual Abuse (2007) *Ampe Akelyernemane Meke Mekarle—'Little Children are Sacred': Report of the Northern Territory Board of Inquiry into the Protection of Aboriginal Children from Sexual Abuse.* Darwin: Northern Territory Government.

O'Connor, R (1984) Alcohol and contingent drunkenness in Central Australia. *Australian Journal of Social Issues,* 19(3), 173–83.

Office for Aboriginal and Torres Strait Islander Partnerships (2006) *Partnerships Queensland: Future directions framework for Aboriginal and Torres Strait Islander Policy in Queensland 2005-2010—Baseline report.* Brisbane: Department of Communities, Queensland Government.

Office of the United Nations High Commissioner for Human Rights (2006) *Frequently asked questions on a human rights-based approach to development cooperation.* Geneva: United Nations. Available at <http://www.ohchr.org/Documents/Publications/FAQen.pdf>, accessed 7 November 2011.

Pearson, N (2002) 'The need for intolerance', In P Craven (ed) *The best Australian essays 2002.* Melbourne: Black Inc, 21–30.

Pearson, N (2007) 'Vale hope in outback hellhole', *The Australian: Inquirer,* February 17.

Peterson, N (1993) 'Demand sharing: Reciprocity and the pressure for generosity among foragers', *American Anthropologist,* 94(5), 860–74.

Rawls, J (1999) *A theory of justice.* Revised edn. Cambridge, MA: Belknap Press, Harvard University Press.

Read, P (1981) *The stolen generations: The removal of Aboriginal children in New South Wales 1883-1969. Occasional paper No 1.* Sydney: Ministry of Aboriginal Affairs.

Robinson, M (2004) 'Health, human rights and development', on *OECD Forum, May 12, 2004: Health of Nations.* Paris: Organisation for Economic Cooperation and Development.

Rothstein, J, Heazlewood, R, and Fraser, M (2007) 'Health of Aboriginal and Torres Strait Islander children in remote Far North Queensland: findings of the Paediatric Outreach Service', *Medical Journal of Australia,* 186(10), 519–21.

Royal Commission into Aboriginal Deaths in Custody (1991) *Final report.* Canberra: Australian Government Publishing Service.

Rutter, M (1994) 'Stress research: Accomplishments and tasks ahead', in R Haggerty, L Sherrod, M Garmezy, and M Rutter (eds) *Stress, risk and resilience in children and adolescents: Processes, mechanisms and interventions.* Cambridge: Cambridge University Press, 354–85.

Stanner, WEH (1979) *White man got no dreaming: Essays 1938-1973.* Canberra: Australian National University Press.

Sutton, P (2001) 'The politics of suffering: Indigenous policy in Australia since the 1970s', *Anthropological Forum,* 11(2), 125–71.

Sutton, P (2005) *The politicisation of disease and the disease of politicisation: causal theories and the Indigenous health differential.* Paper presented at the 8th Rural Health Conference, Alice Springs, 11 March. Available at <http://nrha.ruralhealth.org.au/conferences/docs/8thNRHC/Papers/KN_sutton,%20peter.pdf>, accessed 7 November 2011.

Swan, P, and Raphael, B (1995) *'Ways forward': national consultancy report on Aboriginal and Torres Strait Islander mental health* (No. 0644357592 (pbk. set)). Canberra: Australian Government Publishing Service.

Syme, SL (1997) 'Individual vs. community interventions in public health practice: Some thoughts about a new approach', *Health Promotion Matters,* 2(July), 2–9.

Tarantola, D (2007) 'The interface of mental health and human rights in Indigenous peoples: Triple jeopardy and triple opportunity', *Australasian Psychiatry,* 15(Supplement), S10–S17.

Tatz, C (2001) *Aboriginal suicide is different: a portrait of life and self-destruction* (No. 0855753714). Canberra: Aboriginal Studies Press.

Thomas, DP (2004) *Reading doctors' writing: Race, politics and power in Indigenous health research 1870-1969.* Canberra: Aboriginal Studies Press.

Trewin, D, and Madden, R (2005) *The health and welfare of Australia's Aboriginal and Torres Strait Islander peoples, 2005*. Canberra: Australian Bureau of Statistics and the Australian Institute of Health and Welfare.

Trudgen, R (2000) *Why warriors lie down and die: Towards an understanding of why Aboriginal people of Arnhem Land face the greatest crisis in health and education since European contact*. Darwin: Aboriginal Resource and Development Services.

Zubrick, SR, Silburn, SR, De Maio, JA, Shepherd, C, Griffin, JA, Dalby, RB, et al. (2006) *The Western Australian Aboriginal Child Health Survey: Improving the educational experiences of Aboriginal children and young people*. Perth: Curtin University of Technology and Telethon Institute for Child Health Research.

Chapter 25

Human Rights for People with Intellectual Disabilities

Ian Hall and Evan Yacoub

Introduction

People with intellectual disabilities are perhaps some of the most vulnerable in our society, and as such may have more difficulty than most in protecting themselves from human rights abuses. In this chapter we give a brief historical account of human rights violations that people with intellectual disabilities have experienced. Having considered recent policy developments, which would tend to protect against such violations, we then assess to what extent people with intellectual disabilities continue to experience them. Finally we consider potential solutions to further protect the human rights of people with intellectual disabilities. Because our experience is mostly in the United Kingdom, we have adopted a UK focus, but used international examples where appropriate.

Historical perspective

In pre-industrial times, infant mortality rates were much higher than now, and fluctuated depending on economic conditions (Wrigley 1972). Those people with intellectual disabilities who survived tended to live with their families in small communities. With industrialization came population expansion, rural–urban drift, and the development of more institutional models of care for people with intellectual disabilities. Such models did bring some benefits for people with intellectual disabilities, such as a degree of protection from exploitation, improved nutrition, and ready access to a peer group. In the latter part of the 19th century, these institutional models began to be informed by eugenic theories that held that for the improvement of society, people with intellectual disabilities should be separated from the rest of society and prevented from procreation (Jackson 1996). This deprivation of a family life was officially sanctioned at the highest level, for example by the British 'Royal Commission on the Care and Control of the Feeble Minded' in 1908 (Jackson 2000) and by state organized sterilization programs, for example in Sweden and Canada (Kevles 1999). The right to liberty was removed for many with intellectual disabilities who were admitted to institutional settings. In England for example, the concept of 'voluntary' admission to 'mental handicap' hospitals was only introduced by the 1959 Mental Health Act.

State sponsored abuse of the human rights of people with intellectual disabilities reached its peak in the late 1930s and early 1940s. The Nazi regime in Germany developed eugenic theory into a 'euthanasia' program. The pilot gas chambers were in institutions for people with intellectual disabilities, with some of the first systematic murders being of children with 'incurable' conditions. The programme was carried out with the cooperation of medical staff, and in secret from the inmate's families (Weale 2001).

Post war, institutional models of care continued for people with intellectual disabilities, and with them some well described human rights abuses. There are many examples from all over the world, including Willowbrook in New York State, a centre which was closed in the 1970s after the poor conditions of people with intellectual disabilities living there came to light. However, perhaps the best documented of these concerns a deinstitutionalization project in the early 1990s at the PIKPA asylum on the Greek island of Leros (Tsiantis et al. 2000).

There were 165 residents aged 8–46, out of which 32 were children and adolescents. Living conditions and sanitation were found to be 'unacceptable and completely degrading', nutrition was poor, residents were packed into 40-bed wards which were insufficiently heated, there were no elevators or mobility aids, and the majority of patients remained bed-ridden, without mobility support. There was also a lack of trained personnel, a lack of medical, nursing, and physiotherapeutic care, a total absence of special equipment or educational material, and an extensive use of violence and physical restraint by staff. In general, it was found that the residents of this asylum on Leros had, since their childhood, suffered appalling forms of institutionalization, extreme deprivation, neglect, and ill-treatment, with tragic consequences to their physical and social development.

Policy

Since the Second World War there have been major shifts in public policy concerning people with intellectual disabilities away from the eugenic segregation, sterilization, and euthanasia programmes. The post-war human rights agenda and increasing affluence were important factors in enabling the development of the normalization movement and related concepts such as social role valorization (Wolfensberger 1972). People with intellectual disabilities were increasingly recognized as individuals and respected and valued members of society. Proponents of normalization were highly critical of the conditions which had developed in large institutions, even though many of these institutions had been set up with good intentions. They called for making available to people with intellectual disabilities the kinds of experiences and environments considered normal in society.

These concepts are now often embedded in public policy in many parts of the world. For example, in the Republic of Ireland, 'A Vision for Change' (Department of Health 2006) promotes the principles of citizenship, inclusion, access, and community-based services for people with intellectual disabilities. Similarly, the English policy document 'Valuing people' (Department of Health 2001) includes the principles of rights, independence, choice, and inclusion into mainstream society. They have also been developed with more focus on equality principles. For example, in the UK the Disability Equality Duty (Office for Disability Issues 2006) places a legal duty on all public sector organizations to promote equality of opportunity for disabled people, including those with intellectual disabilities. It covers the full range of what public sector organizations do, including policy making and services that are delivered to the public.

One might predict that one effect of integrating people back into the mainstream of society would tend to protect people from human rights abuses. However, as the examples discussed below illustrate, it is debatable how much of a reality these policy principles are in the everyday lives of people with intellectual disabilities. Community environments can sometimes replicate the problems of institutional care, and be hidden from public view.

Human rights issues for people with intellectual disabilities

The UK Parliament's Joint Committee on Human Rights (2008) identified the following reasons as to why people with intellectual disability especially might be especially vulnerable to infringements of their human rights:

- People with intellectual disabilities may not be aware of their human rights due to the lack of accessible information.

- Expectations have traditionally been low for people with intellectual disabilities.

- The existence of negative attitudes, e.g. people with intellectual disabilities are somehow worth less than other people.

- People with intellectual disabilities are often marginalized and isolated.

- People with intellectual disabilities are often dependent on carers.

- Difficulties in understanding and communicating with people with intellectual disabilities.

In the light of this, we review below specifically the rights to life, liberty, a fair hearing, family life, freedom from inhuman and degrading treatment, and the prohibition on discrimination, and consider where people's rights have been infringed. We have used the European Court of Human Rights Articles as a framework for our analysis, grouping them into three broad (and somewhat overlapping) themes: the protective role of human rights legislation, promoting autonomy, and promoting economic and social rights.

The protective role of human rights legislation

Article 2, European Convention for the Protection of Human Rights and Fundamental Freedoms: The right to life

People with an intellectual disability have a reduced life expectancy compared to the general population (McGuigan et al. 1995). There are several potential explanations for this, including increased incidence of physical illness in people with intellectual disability. However there are two other factors that may particularly interfere with a person with intellectual disability's right to life:

1. The concept of '*diagnostic overshadowing*' (Reiss and Szyszko 1983), which will be familiar to many practitioners working with people with intellectual disability. This is where symptoms of mental or physical disorder are mistakenly attributed to the learning disability per se, so that the causative mental or physical disorder is not treated (which may have life threatening consequences).

   Example: a man with a severe intellectual disability starts to hit the side of his face. Although this is unusual for him, he does have a history of self injurious behaviour, so maybe it is just part of his learning disability. It is decided not to investigate further. A few days later, he is very sweaty and won't get out of bed. He has developed a life threatening septicaemia that started with a dental abscess. It was the toothache that was causing him to hit the side of his face. If he had been treated earlier he might not have developed the septicaemia.

2. Problems accessing healthcare. This can arise because health care organizations fail to make reasonable adjustments to meet the needs of people with learning disability. This has been described by MENCAP as 'institutional discrimination' in their report 'Death by Indifference' (MENCAP 2007) where they highlight the stories of six people with learning disability who have died through neglect in physical health care settings:

   …institutional discrimination results when organizations fail to make changes in the way they deliver services to take into account people's differing needs. Nor does the organization deal with ignorance and prejudice within the workforce and culture of the organization. We believe that there is a fundamental lack of understanding and respect towards people with a learning disability and their families and carers. This lack of understanding and respect leads to—and is demonstrated by—the poor design of systems, policies and procedures to meet the particular and differing needs of patients with a learning disability.

   Such institutions could not be said to be fulfilling their Disability Equality Duty.

   Notwithstanding these problems with diagnostic overshadowing and access to health care, it is important to remember that, in the general population, living conditions are important determinants of health, often more so than access to health care. This may also be true in people with intellectual disabilities, although interestingly, in one study Cooper et al. (2007) found that factors such as living in deprived areas and being unemployed were not associated with the mental health of people with intellectual disability.

Article 3, European Convention for the Protection of Human Rights and Fundamental Freedoms: Prohibition of torture or inhuman or degrading treatment

Despite improvement in standards of care, there are still frequent examples of people being subject to inhuman and degrading treatment in many countries including 'developed' ones. This is in a wide variety of settings including residential care, family homes, specialist inpatient units, and in general hospitals.

Amnesty International (2003) was particularly alarmed that in Russia, children with intellectual disabilities—including those with Down Syndrome and autism—are denied their human rights purely because of their disability. Such children are kept in close confinement with little or no sensory stimulation, with low staff numbers and effectively no attempt to provide education or other developmental care.

Recent inquiries in the UK have identified institutional abuses of people in the intellectual disabilities in Cornwall and Sutton and Merton (Healthcare Commission 2007; Healthcare Commission & Commission for Social Care Inspection 2006). The Cornwall report identified systematic abuses, assaults, lack of care, and lack of clinical responsibilities including the inappropriate use of psychotropic medication to control behaviour. The Sutton and Merton report revealed a lack of external scrutiny and physical and sexual abuses of people with intellectual disabilities.

The Mental Disability Advocacy Centre investigated the use of cage beds in four Eastern European countries shortly before they joined the European Union. They report the routine use of cage beds 'to restrain people with severe intellectual disabilities who exhibit "challenging" or "difficult" behaviour, sometimes for years'. Lack of adequate resources, staff, and training were cited as explanations. Their report describes the experience as invariably 'degrading, frightening, disempowering and damaging' (Mental Disability Advocacy Centre 2003). There have been recent press reports about their continued use in children.

It is certainly true that there are much more humane methods of successfully managing challenging behaviour, including improving communication, functional behavioural analysis, addressing mental and physical health needs, and the judicious use of medication as a second line in conjunction with other approaches. There are established guidelines describing this in detail (Royal College of Psychiatrists, British Psychological Society and Royal College of Speech and Language Therapists 2007). In a humane society there is no place for the use of excessive restraint, punishment regimes, or physical abuse in the management of challenging behaviour.

Promoting autonomy (self-governance) through human rights legislation

Article 5, European Convention for the Protection of Human Rights and Fundamental Freedoms: The right to liberty

Article 5 concerns the right to liberty and security of the person, and states that 'No one shall be deprived of his liberty save. . .in accordance with a procedure prescribed by law'. There is specific reference to the 'lawful detention of. . . persons of unsound mind', whereby:

1. The detention must be effected in accordance with a procedure prescribed by law.
2. Except in emergency cases, the individual concerned must be clearly shown to be of unsound mind.

3. The mental disorder must be of a kind or degree warranting compulsory confinement.

4. The validity of continued confinement depends upon the persistence of such a disorder.

It is controversial whether intellectual disability per se constitutes a mental disorder and different countries have taken differing legal views. In the recent reform of mental health law in the UK, it was argued by many stakeholders that people with intellectual disabilities should not be subject to mental health legislation (and at risk therefore of deprivation of liberty) unless they have a mental disorder in addition to their intellectual disabilities. Nevertheless, people with intellectual disabilities are sometimes detained in hospitals because of their learning disability, rather than any (other) mental disorder. This has sometimes been without using mental health legislation.

The 'Bournewood' case (*HL v United Kingdom* 2004) illustrates the issue of depriving someone with an intellectual disability of their liberty without a formal legal process. A man with an intellectual disability and autism was admitted to psychiatric hospital informally (not under a 'procedure prescribed by law'). He did not have the mental capacity to decide for himself whether to be admitted to hospital or not. He was 'compliant' in that he did not obviously object to being in hospital. However it was decided that he should not leave, and his paid carers were not allowed to visit. This was subsequently judged to amount to a deprivation of his liberty.

In the UK the final European Court of Human Rights judgment has led to the government bringing in new legal procedures to authorize deprivation of liberty for people lacking capacity where it is judged to be in their best interests and where they will not be subject to mental health legislation (Ministry of Justice 2008).

Notwithstanding this, in the UK there have been several recent examples of adults with intellectual disabilities being effectively locked up in a way that is clearly detrimental to their human rights and without recourse to the legal safeguards that exist (e.g. in England the Mental Health Act 1983), for example:

1. The Commission for Health Improvement (CHI) (2003) was disturbed to find in its investigation of Bedfordshire and Luton Community NHS Trust that:

    All bedrooms are kept locked so that clients cannot use them in the day. Staff hold the keys. Patio doors and windows are chained. The purpose is to contain one person with particularly complex needs who was assessed by the JCS two years ago. . .

    CHI found examples in other homes where clients have complex needs and where bedrooms are locked…There did not appear to be clear criteria for when a client's bedroom should be locked or when clients should hold their own keys if their room is locked during the day. This needs to be resolved so that the human rights of people with learning disabilities are not infringed.

2. The Healthcare Commission (2007) investigation team into Sutton and Merton Primary Care Trust found that:

    When people are restrained on a regular basis in a hospital setting they should be assessed to see if their rights and treatment needs could best be met through the use of the Mental Health Act 1983. None of the people who lived in these houses had participated in such as assessment and no one was actually detained under the Act.

Promoting economic and social rights through human rights legislation

Article 6, European Convention for the Protection of Human Rights and Fundamental Freedoms: The right to a fair trial

The Bournewood case and other examples above illustrate that people are being deprived of the liberty without access to a fair hearing to authorize this detention. People detained under mental health legislation will usually have access to hearings, but people with intellectual disabilities are sometimes subject to mental health legislation when others might be subject to criminal proceedings (e.g. an act of violence against another person is treated as 'challenging behaviour' in need of treatment as opposed to an offence such as assault or grievous bodily harm). Criminal proceedings usually have a higher standard of proof, and if found guilty a defined punishment ensues, rather than the more open-ended detention for treatment under mental health legislation. So it can be argued that in circumstances such as these, people with intellectual disabilities do not have access to the same fair hearings as others.

If people with intellectual disabilities are sent to prison, they may be excluded from the offending behaviour programmes. Participation in such programmes can form a crucial part of the evidence considered by hearings that decide parole and resettlement from prison, so to deny people with intellectual disabilities access to such programmes effectively denies them a fair hearing.

Adults with intellectual disabilities have a higher risk of being victims of crime and abuse, face greater hurdles to achieving justice, yet are less likely to report the crime and abuse they have suffered (Respond, Voice UK & Ann Craft Trust 2007). The Joint Committee on Human Rights (2008) analysed why people with intellectual disabilities may have low confidence in dealing with the criminal justice system. Firstly, they may not know what is being done to them is a crime. If they do know this, they may not know how to report a crime, or may have difficulty doing so because of communication problems. People with intellectual disabilities are often in dependent relationships with their carers, so if the complaint is about a carer, the person may fear losing their care and support. Alternatively, they may rely on carers to help them report crimes, and this support may not be forthcoming. When it comes to criminal investigations, police officers may not have sufficient training in identifying or interviewing people with intellectual disabilities. Prosecutors may consider that people with intellectual disabilities may not make reliable witnesses, and may be unaware of strategies to enhance reliability, and so may decide there is insufficient evidence to prosecute perpetrators. So it is both as victims of crime, and when accused of criminal acts or otherwise said to merit detention against one's will, that people with intellectual disabilities may be denied access to a fair hearing.

Article 8, European Convention for the Protection of Human Rights and Fundamental Freedoms: The right to respect for private and family life

Encompassed in the right to respect for private life (Article 8 ECHR) is the right to respect for an individual's physical and psychological integrity, and the right to form relationships with others. It also requires respect for an individual's family life and home. Article 8 has been interpreted by the European Court of Human Rights as including a right to participate in the life of one's local community. The Court has also recognised that States are under a positive obligation to facilitate such participation.

Perhaps the most fundamental aspect of family life is being brought up by one's own parents. Many countries ran institutions for children with intellectual disabilities where contact from parents was discouraged, although these institutions were often the first to close in reprovision programmes. However, there have been recent reports of parents being discouraged from bringing up their children: in Russia, Amnesty International (2003) have reported that for many children with intellectual disabilities, shortly after birth parents would be told by hospital staff that their baby is suffering from an intellectual disability. Parents would then be advised to renounce their legal rights, and the child becomes a 'social orphan', condemned to live out his or her life in a grossly understaffed children's home. This sometimes happens without parents even seeing their new-born babies.

Old institutional models often prevented a proper family life for adults with intellectual disabilities too. Unfortunately there is lots of evidence that adults with high levels of need, particularly challenging behaviour, are still often placed a long way from home with no meaningful contact with their family. A survey of independent learning disability units in the UK (Healthcare Commission and Valuing People Support Team 2004) identified the average distance from home for clients to be 74 miles. The furthest placement was 385 miles from home.

Family life includes parenthood, and with the right support many people with intellectual disabilities can become successful parents, particularly if they live in cultures that are accepting of this. Parents with intellectual disabilities may face many barriers however. Legislation that concerns the protection of children quite rightly puts the needs of the child paramount, but too often this can be misused to ignore the needs of parents, and to remove children rather than provide the necessary support to parents. The Joint Committee on Human Rights (2008) reported that children of people with intellectual disabilities are more likely to be removed from the care of their parents which, unless justified and proportionate to a risk to the child, may lead to a serious risk of a breach of the rights of the child.

Organized mass sterilization programmes such as those in Sweden and Canada (Kevles 1999) arose out of the eugenics movement. These were a clear intrusion on the right of people with intellectual disabilities to have a family life, especially as decisions about sterilization were made because someone had a particular label of intellectual disabilities, as opposed to a decision being made in the person's best interests taking into account their individual circumstances and wishes. The Center for Reproductive Rights (2002) argues that laws and policies affecting women's reproductive rights and services, when not blatantly discriminatory, are often silent where women with disabilities are concerned.

Sexual offences legislation can deprive people with learning disability from a sexual life. In the UK, the legislation has moved from a diagnosis based approach (it used to be unlawful to have sex with a 'female mental defective') to one that is based around an individual's capacity to consent to sexual relations. Many have argued that this is the best approach, although others are concerned that it may deny a sexual life to those who lack capacity, even though they have sexual wants and desires.

Article 14, European Convention for the Protection of Human Rights and Fundamental Freedoms: Prohibition on discrimination

Most of the human rights infringements experienced by people with intellectual disabilities described in this chapter are also examples of discrimination against people with intellectual disabilities and therefore infringe their rights in this way too. People with intellectual disabilities are denied access to health care, perhaps because those controlling access place less value on their lives; victims of hate crime are denied access to justice because the criminal justice system fails to make reasonable adjustments to their needs; mothers with intellectual disabilities are denied a proper chance at looking after their own children because authorities deny them the assessment and support offered to other parents in need.

Potential solutions

Many of these issues have come to light through case law as well as institutional scandals and inquiries. These have sometime had the effect of increasing public awareness and changing public policy. However we want to end this chapter by considering other potential ways to improve the human rights of people with intellectual disabilities.

Enshrining human rights principles and obligations into national law can be a helpful start. In the UK this was achieved by incorporating the European Convention on Human Rights through the Human Rights Act 1998. This has not been without its problems, and one in particular for people with intellectual disabilities has been the fact that the Act is limited in its remit to the action of public bodies. Case law determined that privately run care homes are not included in the remit, even if the care they provide is funded by a public authority (Halstead 2001). The UK government are taking steps to close this loophole.

More recently, in 2008, The United Nations Convention on the Rights of Persons with Disabilities (United Nations 2006) came into force. This convention is intended 'to promote, protect and ensure the full and equal enjoyment of all human rights and fundamental freedoms by all persons with disabilities, and to promote respect for their inherent dignity'. It builds on existing texts in order to promote human rights of people with disabilities. The Articles of the convention include the right to live independently, to personal mobility, rehabilitation, and to participation in political and public life, and cultural life, recreation and sport. Clearly, incorporating these rights in national law would be very beneficial to people with intellectual disabilities.

Having a clear legislative framework for decision-making when people lack the mental capacity to make decisions for themselves can also guard against some human rights abuses. If decisions really are made in the 'best interests' of the person with intellectual disabilities who lacks capacity to decide for him or herself, then hopefully their right to life, to a family life and freedom from inhuman or degrading treatment can be upheld.

Decision-making can be improved by a balanced approach taking into account all relevant information, and with independent advocacy. For example, the Code of Practice for the Mental Capacity Act for England and Wales (Department of Constitutional Affairs, Department of Health & Welsh Assembly Government 2007) offers a 'best interests checklist' requiring the decision-maker to consider matters such as whether the person is likely to regain capacity in the future and the need to include the person as far as possible in decision-making. Account must be taken of the past and present wishes of the person concerned and the views of other people concerned with the person who lacks capacity. For serious decisions where there is no family or friend to advise, then an independent advocate must become involved by law. A balanced approach is important: in making decisions on behalf of people, there is a danger that, in the management of risk, services' preoccupation with possible negative outcomes are not properly balanced with the opportunity to be maximize independence (e.g. to travel independently, or meet friends unsupervised). This 'risk conundrum' is further explored by Manthorpe et al. (1997).

Some of the worst human rights abuses have occurred in institutions that are relatively closed to the outside world and which have little external scrutiny. Promoting the closure of such institutions, or at least their regular inspection, might have an important role in prevention. However it is important not to focus exclusively on such institutions, and we make some suggestions below as a systematic way to improve the human rights of people with learning disabilities living in care settings.

Developing explicit standards for the full range of social and health care settings that support people with intellectual disability is crucial. These will vary in details country by country, depending on the general living standards available, but we would suggest the following as particularly important to consider:

- Equality of access to health care and to justice.

- Freedom to make choices where people have the mental capacity, and to contribute to decision making when they don't.

- The avoidance of punishment as a means of controlling or changing challenging behaviour.

- Restraint and deprivation of liberty can only be carried out under a proper legal process and as a last resort.

- Recognizing that an overwhelmingly risk-averse approach may lead to depriving people of the opportunity to be more independent, and it is important to strike an appropriate balance between empowerment and autonomy, and providing support.

For such standards to be effective there need to be appropriate checks that they are being implemented. In England, we have had different standards and until very recently different inspectorates depending on the type of support being offered—in the health care or social care sector, and whether privately managed health care institutions or state run ones. The two recent scandals in state run health care institutions (Healthcare Commission 2006, 2007) are perhaps a reflection of the 'lighter touch' inspection they experienced.

Social inclusion and citizenship for people with intellectual disabilities, so that they are seen as full members of society, has been advocated for the past 40 years. Much progress has been made in many countries, and we would see this as a crucial element in their protection against human rights abuses. It is much more difficult to sanction people's abuse if they are your neighbours, your friends, people you encounter in your daily life.

The individualization of support packages for people with intellectual disabilities can also be protective. Two recent developments may be particularly helpful. Aiming to meet a person's individual needs is important (rather than just trying to fit people into existing services). However 'Person Centred Planning' (Department of Health 2001) takes this a step further. It aims to put the person with intellectual disabilities at the centre of the planning process, in particular their views about their own needs, and their wishes about how such needs might be met. Another liberating development is 'direct payments' where people with intellectual disabilities (with appropriate support) are given individualized budgets with which to purchase the care and support they need.

Of course users and carers sometimes have difficulty speaking up for themselves, and the promotion of user and carer advocacy in recent years as done much to guard against and expose human rights abuses. The charitable sector has an important role in this regard, for example MENCAP has campaigned on exposing poor standards of care in state run institutions for people with intellectual disabilities (Healthcare Commission 2006) and poor access to physical health care (MENCAP 2007).

Much of the human rights abuse described in this chapter has occurred with the collusion of professionals. This is an uncomfortable truth for people who have made their career choices wanting to help and support people with intellectual disabilities. We know that professional isolation and closed institutions can make such collusion more likely. Much has been done in recent years about making professional standards more explicit, and particularly the development of appraisal and continuing professional development may help guard against this. Many employers have also developed 'whistle blowing' policies.

This brings us to our last point, the implementation of policy. The potential solutions we have discussed are not new, and have been part of public policy in many countries for a number of years. It is one thing to persuade a government to issue a policy, and another to ensure that it is comprehensively implemented so that every person with intellectual disabilities benefits. Introducing a positive duty on public authorities to promote respect for human rights might help ensure this (Joint Committee of Human Rights 2008). It is sometimes those with the best advocates, or those who are good at speaking for themselves that are first to benefit from more enlightened policy. We need to remember those with more challenging needs, without people to speak up for them, and ensure they benefit too.

References

Amnesty International (2003) *Russian Federation: Far From Justice in the Russian Federation.* EUR 46/056/2003. London: Amnesty International.

The Center for Reproductive Rights (2002) *Reproductive Rights and Women with Disabilities: A Human Rights Framework.* Briefing paper. New York: Centre for Reproductive Rights.

Commission for Health Improvement (2003) *Investigation: Learning Disability Services—Bedfordshire and Luton Community NHS Trust.* London: The Stationery Office.

Cooper, SA, Smiley, E, Morrison, J, Williamson, A, and Allan, L (2007) 'Mental ill-health in adults with intellectual disabilities: prevalence and associated factors', *The British Journal of Psychiatry* 2007, 190, 27–35.

Department of Constitutional Affairs, Department of Health & Welsh Assembly Government (2007) *Mental Capacity Act 2005 Code of Practice*. London: The Stationery Office.

Department of Health (2001) *Valuing People. A new strategy for Learning Disability in the 21st century*. (CM 5086).

Department of Health (2006) *A vision for Change: Report of the Expert Group on Mental Health Policy*. London: The Stationery Office.

Halstead, S (2001) 'The Human Rights Act 1998: The Lion That Snored', *Learning Disabilities Psychiatry*, 3(1), 2–3, 5.

Healthcare Commission (2007) *Investigation into the service for people with learning disabilities provided by Sutton and Merton Primary Care Trust*. London: Commission for Healthcare Audit and Inspection.

Healthcare Commission and Commission for Social Care Inspection (2006) *Joint investigation into the provision of services for people with learning disabilities at Cornwall Partnership NHS Trust*. London: Commission for Healthcare Audit and Inspection.

Healthcare Commission and Valuing People Support Team (2004) *The Private and Voluntary Healthcare Survey of Independent Mental Health Hospitals For People With Learning Disabilities*. London: Healthcare Commission.

HL v United Kingdom (2004) European Court of Human Rights, Application no 45508/99, decision of 5 October 2004.

Jackson, M (1996) 'Institutional provision for the feeble-minded in Edwardian England: Sandlebridge and the scientific morality of permanent care', in D Wright and A Digby (eds) *From Idiocy to Mental Deficiency—Historical perspectives on people with learning disabilities*. London: Routledge, 161–183.

Jackson, M (2000) *The Borderland of Imbecility* Medicine, Society and the Fabrication of the Feeble Mind in Late Victorian and Edwardian England. Manchester: Manchester University Press.

Joint Committee on Human Rights, Seventh Report (2008) *A life like any other? Human Rights of adults with Learning Disabilities*. HL Paper 40–IHC 73-I by authority of the House of Commons. London: The Stationery Office.

Kevles, DJ (1999) 'Eugenics and human rights', *British Medical Journal*, 319, 435–38.

Manthorpe, J, Walsh, M, Alaszewski, A, and Harrison, L (1997) 'Issues of risk practice and welfare in learning disability services', *Disability and Society*, 12(1), 69–82.

McGuigan, SM, Hollins, S, and Attard, M (1995) 'Age-specific standardised mortality rates in people with learning disability', *Journal of Intellectual Disability Research*, 39, 527–31.

MENCAP (2007) *Death By Indifference*. London: MENCAP Campaigns.

Mental Disability Advocacy Centre (2003) *Cage Beds: inhuman or degrading treatment or punishment in four EU Accession countries*. Budapest: MDAC.

Ministry of Justice (2008) *Mental Capacity Act 2005 Deprivation of Liberty safeguards Code of Practice to supplement the main Mental Capacity Act 2005 Code of Practice*. Norwich: The Stationery Office.

Office for Disability Issues: HM Government (2006) *Disability equality: a priority for all*. London: Office for Disability Issues.

Respond, Voice UK, and Ann Craft Trust (2007) *Submission to the Joint Committee on Human Rights Inquiry into the Human Rights of Adults with Learning Disabilities: Crime and Abuse against Adults with Learning Disabilities*. Available at <http://www.publications.parliament.uk/pa/jt200708/jtselect/jtrights/40/40we78.htm>, accessed 7 November 2011.

Reiss, S and Szyszko, J (1983) 'Diagnostic overshadowing and professional experience with mentally retarded persons', *American Journal of Mental Deficiency*, 87, 396–402.

Royal College of Psychiatrists, British Psychological Society, and Royal College of Speech and Language Therapists (2007) *Clinical and service guidelines for supporting people with learning disabilities who are at risk of receiving abusive or restrictive practices*. College Report CR144. London: Royal College of Psychiatrists.

Tsiantis, J, Diaremme, SP, and Kolaitis, G (2000) 'The Leros PIKPA Asylum Deinstitutionalization and Rehabilitation Project: A follow-up study on care staff fears and attitudes', *Journal of Intellectual Disabilities*, 4(4), 281–92.

United Nations (2006) *Convention on the Rights of Persons with Disabilities*. New York: United Nations.

Weale, A (2001) *Science and the Swastika*. London: Channel 4 Books.

Wolfensberger, W (1972) *Normalization: the principles of normalization in human services*. National Institute on Mental Retardation: Toronto.

Wrigley, EA (1972) 'Mortality in pre-industrial England: the example of Colyton, Devon, over three centuries', in: DV Glass and R Revelle (eds) *Population and social change*. New York: Crane, Russak, 243–73.

Chapter 26

Missing Voices

Speaking up for the Rights of Children and Adolescents with Disabilities

Myron L. Belfer and Diana Samarasan

Introduction

At the base of classic Western theories of justice is an assumption that the rules and boundaries which create justice are contracted by people with roughly equal powers who do so for mutual advantage. This conception of justice manufactures outliers—people who, because they do not have and have never had equal powers to negotiate the rules on which society is based, are—as noted law professor and philosopher, Martha Nussbaum has said—at the 'frontiers of justice.' One such group is people with disabilities,[1] in particular people with severe disabilities as well as children with disabilities, who have long had their voices neglected.

The numbers of children who survive disabling medical conditions as a result of technological advances and children who are recognized and identified as having disabilities are increasing. (Goldson 1997) Some 200 million children—ten per cent of the world's young people—are born with an impairment or acquire an impairment before age 19. Ten per cent of these children have a serious impairment leading to significant disability. Eighty per cent of children with disabilities live in the developing world, and there, make up some of the poorest of the poor. As noted in the UNICEF Innocenti publication, *Promoting the Rights of Children with Disabilities*, 'statistics such as these demonstrate that to be born with or acquire an impairment is far from unusual or abnormal.' (UNICEF 2007, <http://www.unicef-irc.org/publications/pdf/digest13-disability.pdf>).

The historical understanding of children and childhood must be appreciated to realize how children, in particular, can suffer drastic consequences as a result of being considered disabled (Hibbard and Desch 2007). In the modern history of civilization children were seen as property (Slee 2002). The role of children was to increase the productivity of the family and propagate to continue the family line (Slee 2002). There was until the past century no concept of a developing child with potentials that could be enhanced or thwarted by environmental or attitudinal factors. There was little understanding that there was a developmental trajectory for children and that they were not simply little adults. Lastly, in many cultures it was felt that 'children should be seen and not heard.' Both because of a better scientific understanding of child development and the

---

[1] The term, 'disability', as used in this paper refers not to individual impairment but to the disenfranchisement which occurs as a result of the interaction between a person with an (physical, sensory, psychosocial, or intellectual) impairment and attitudinal and environmental barriers. Often described as the social (rather than the medical) model of disability, this understanding forms the basis for the recent UN Convention on the Rights of Persons with Disabilities.

evolution of social thinking, children are now viewed differently by many, but certainly not by all, segments of society. However, the potential of children with disabilities, for the most part, continues to be ignored. '. . .widespread underestimation of the abilities and potential of children with disabilities creates a vicious cycle of underexpectation, under-achievement and low priority in the allocation of resources.' (<http://www.unicef-irc.org>).

Children, with or without disability, are at a particular disadvantage both historically and in contemporary society for being heard and being accorded their rights for inclusion. As noted by Levine (2005), when it is a child who is disabled, it is usually a parent, probably a mother, who must push for acceptance by society, or doors remain closed. This chapter attempts to focus a light on the barriers which children with disabilities continue to face in being considered active members of society, who are involved in decisions about their lives.

Concepts crucial to understanding the impact of disability

There is a conflict between the value of including all people in society's benefits, with whatever accommodations and expenditures are necessary to make that possible, and the devaluing of those with impairments and more visible dependence needs. In simplistic terms, it is a conflict between acceptance and avoidance, with a lot of ambiguity in between. It is a perhaps a sign of progress that such conflicts have become part of public debate. In earlier generations, it was not remarkable that people with disabilities either did not live very long or were kept out of sight at home or in institutions. If their appearance was unusual enough, they were given sensational names like 'Elephant Man' and displayed in circuses and medical schools. Non-Western societies are sometimes described as more tolerant of those with disabilities, but this is a partial and highly romantic view. A few studies, for example in Northern Mexico and Botswana, have shown that children with disabilities may be particularly valued as gifts of God, but these instances are rare (Whyte and Ingstad 1995).

Cultures that maintain a strong belief that 'bad' outcomes reflect bad behavior somewhere in the past, whether by the person with a disability or by the person's family, are far less sympathetic to people whose disabilities have been present since birth (Room et al. 2001) than those that do not endorse an historical causality. In cultures where shame is a prominent value, children with disabilities are considered retribution for the family's sins. In cultures that believe in reincarnation, the child herself may be held at fault for transgressions in a previous life (Groce 1999; Whyte and Ingstad 1995). This same scenario can be divined in unconscious attitudes in the most 'advanced' of societies.

Consequences of disability

In many countries, children with disabilities are placed in institutions at birth or as toddlers and remain there until death. All available data show that children in institutions do far worse socially, educationally, medically, and psychologically than children raised in supportive community settings (Groce and Paeglow 2005; UNICEF-IRC 2007). Human Rights Watch found that the death rate among institutionalized children with disabilities was almost twice that of the general population and of children kept at home. In some institutions in some countries the mortality rate exceeds 75 per cent (Human Rights Watch 2001).

According to the United Nations and UNICEF, girls with disabilities are twice or three times more likely to experience sexual and physical abuse than their non-disabled peers. Where the ability to contribute economically to family survival is critical, children with disabilities have little value, other than as objects displayed for pity or money. The most common employment around the world for disabled people is begging (Groce 1999). Isolation both self-imposed and socially created is common, particularly for those who look different.

Emotional and behavioral problems affect between 10 per cent and 20 per cent of children worldwide (Belfer 2008). Recognizing childhood emotional and behavioral problems in the context of disability rights remains a challenge and, to date, has not had the prominence warranted (Stewart-Brown 2003). The data on the cost to society of mental disability in children is yet to be fully calculated, but those studies that are available show dramatic costs comparable to those with other disabilities and with equal issues related to participation in society (Hsia and Belfer 2008).

The special nature of the relationship of children to society and the family establishes patterns of approach to access, care, and participation that differ from adults, but perhaps apply to others with disabilities. There is a 'propensity for exploitation' (Levine 2005); when society defaults the family is left to try to fulfill unmet needs, no matter the cost. This global pattern has allowed society to abdicate its responsibility to this group.

Children who have impairments suffer a spectrum of abuse from the most obvious physical and sexual abuse, bullying, and mortal assaults, to more subtle but equally devastating isolation and non-participation. The lost potential and costs to society are only now being recognized through advocacy and the uncovering of rights processes.

Concept of participation

Approaches to clinical care for people with disabilities are too often conceived from a deficit model focusing on individual impairment. This has consequences for how the person is viewed and unreasonably limits expectations. The Convention on the Rights of the Child (Article 12) redefines the role of children in society as participants and, through their participation, as critical contributors to their own health and that of the community in which they live. If the clinician and policy maker move from a deficit model to the concept of maximizing participation and focus on the barriers faced by people with disabilities in seeking full participation, then many opportunities for creative programming are opened. It requires a considerable shift in the mindset of the clinician and policy maker but, once adopted, can be seen as freeing up opportunities or identifying barriers that can readily be overcome.

The World Health Organization has attempted through the International Classification of Impairments, Disabilities and Handicaps (ICIDH-2) to disseminate a model for professionals to use to approach care for people who have impairments from this concept of participation. The ICIDH-2 covers three dimensions of disability: impairment in bodily functions and structures; limitation in activity; and restriction in participation. This classification recognizes that someone with an impairment may or may not have a limitation in activity or even a disability, depending on the environment and society (Clark and MacArthur 2008).

The human rights approach to disability shifts the focus from the limitations of individuals to the barriers within society that prevent the full participation of people with impairments on an equal basis with others.

UN Convention on the Rights of the Child

The UN Convention on the Rights of the Child clearly advocates for the inclusion of all children in the life of the community with strong recommendations for access to education and services. Furthermore, it argues against discrimination of any kind. However, experience with the Convention has shown that it has lacked meaningful implementation (WHO 2005). In particular, children and adolescents with disabilities including psychosocial disabilities have not seen meaningful inclusion.

UN Convention on the Rights of Persons with Disabilities

Going one step further, the Convention on the Rights of Persons with Disabilities, drafted with the strong activism and unprecedented participation of persons with disabilities, mandates the involvement of people with disabilities (including children with disabilities) and their representative organizations in implementation and monitoring of programmes concerning them.

The CRPD attempts to address a gap in justice which has occurred, not because people with disabilities were explicitly excluded from other more general human rights legislation (in fact, in the CRC, children with disabilities were specifically included), but because the moral platform which we use to interpret such documents has been skewed to leave out certain populations. The social model of disability, from which the convention is derived, places the obligation for inclusion squarely back on the shoulders of society. In this model, disability is not inherent in the person but rather, occurring with the interaction between a person with impairment and societal, attitudinal, and environmental barriers.

In a way, the existence of the CRPD points to the fact that it is (again) the larger philosophical construct of the omnipotent 'we' which is the problem. Since the Enlightenment, as previously marginalized segments of society have demanded and realized their voice, the conception of who 'we' are has gradually expanded. Sixty years after the adoption of the Universal Declaration on Human Rights, thanks largely to the persistence of the disability rights movement (whose slogan is 'nothing about us without us'), there is recognition that disability is part of the human experience.

As Law Professor Amita Dhanda (2008, <http://www.surjournal.org/eng/conteudos/getArtigo8. php?artigo=8,artigo_dhanda.htm>) writes, 'It is my view that the CRPD has done the following for persons with disabilities: it has signaled the change from welfare to rights; introduced the equality idiom to grant both the same and different to persons with disabilities; recognized autonomy with support for persons with disabilities and most importantly made disability a part of the human experience.' Whether the CRPD and the growing disability rights movement will give a voice to children remains to be seen.

Rights-based approaches to children with disabilities

It is an indictment of society that children and adolescents have not seen meaningful inclusion and participation when they have been born with impairments or suffered disability. Remedies have been proposed, and in some cases demonstrated to be effective, but their implementation is patchy and often not sustained. Two prominent examples of initiatives to address the lack of voice for the rights of children with disabilities are the Guardianship Councils in Brazil and the Social Charter of the European Union. These are very different approaches but both draw heavily on legal remedies and due process with respect for the plaintiff.

Guardianship Councils

The 1988 Federal Brazilian Constitution emphasized popular participation in governance. Municipal Participatory Administrative Councils were formed. The child rights perspective embedded in the authorizing legislation and implementation has transformed a disadvantaged population of children into a population of citizens whose current and future rights should be respected (Duarte et al. 2007; Rizzini et al. 2002). The authorizing legislation covers all children under the age of 21, and notably does not single out one 'at risk' group. The legislation is broad but focuses on the entitlement to rights. The legislation determined that children's rights will be guaranteed through the activities of municipal Administrative Councils. The Brazilian Child and

Adolescent Rights Act (ECA) mandates that every one of approximately 5,700 Brazilian municipalities should have two Municipal Child Councils: a Child Rights Council and a Child Guardianship Council. In addition each state should have one state Child Rights Council. The Child Rights Council has the responsibility for addressing child and adolescent rights at the macro level. The Guardianship Councils ensure that children in need or at risk receive the best possible assistance. Their task is to make referrals and guarantee the delivery of service, but not act as a provider. Access to the Guardianship Councils can be by children themselves, parents or a wide range to other interested parties.

European Social Charter

The European Social Charter (Council of Europe) is a rights-based document that can and has been applied in the case of apparent discrimination of people with disabilities. A notable example is the successful appeal by Autism Europe to the European Committee of Social Rights complaining that in France '. . . children and adults with autism do not and are not likely to effectively exercise, in sufficient numbers and to an adequate standard, their right to education in mainstream schooling or through adequately supported placements in specialized institutions that offer education and related services.' In essence, the complaint alleged that France is not taking enough action as required under the revised European Social Charter to secure children and adults with autism a right to education as effective as that of all the other children. While this is a specific example that has led to remediation, the Articles themselves serve as a model. The Code of Social Action states that, '. . .whenever the aptitudes of the person with a disability and the capabilities of the family so allow, ensure access to the minor or adult with disability to those institutions open to the whole population.' 'Social and medico-social action shall . . . promote the autonomy and protection of individuals . . . prevent exclusion and correct its effects. It shall be based on continuous evaluation and needs and of expectations . . . in particular of those people with disabilities . . . action shall respect the equal dignity of all human beings. . .'

It will be interesting to see if and how models such as these gain uptake in implementation of the new Convention on the Rights of Persons with Disabilities.

Paradigm shifts for clinicians

'Integrating the principles of children's rights, equity and social justice into practice will require a fundamental shift in the education of child health professionals at all levels of training.' (Waterston and Goldhagen 2008). If a high priority is to be given to providing rights-based services to children with disabilities, it will be increasingly necessary to engage, train, and prepare non-government organizations, professionals, parents of children with disabilities, and children with disabilities themselves to work together to effect change. Professional training programmes today still focus on medicalization of disability. The focus on specialization for working with differing populations of children with disabilities thwarts the desire to lessen discrimination in services and the participation of children in the mainstream of society.

Future concerns

In an era with the increasing use of genetic testing and intrauterine intervention for congenital abnormalities there has arisen a line of reasoning that suffering associated with disability might be eliminated (Edwards 2001). In fact, as stated by Edwards (2001) a common justification for the human genome project is that it will reduce the incidence of suffering. Professor John Harris states that if one intentionally brings a child with a disability into the world the wrong done is that of '…deliberately choosing to increase the suffering in the world when [one] could have avoided so doing' (Harris 2000). The implications of Harris's thesis are chilling! Adopted as policy, this misuse of genetic testing could lead to unwarranted and unwanted abortion, which amounts to further discrimination against people with disabilities, and to euthanasia. Fortunately, previous proposals for such sweeping screening have been turned aside by even the most conservative governments, but the danger of using screening in the name of science requires continued societal vigilance.

Conclusions

It is quite remarkable that in the modern era the rights of children with disabilities remain such a challenge. The maltreatment of children with disabilities must be considered a critical public health issue (Hibbard et al. 2007). Contrast the available resources for children with a host of medical illnesses, to those available to children with disabilities. International agreements are in place to end the era of isolation, abuse, and neglect. The challenge is to increase awareness of the current situation and to educate a broad range of individuals to exercise their rights. Incrementally increasing participation of people with disabilities will lead to a lowering of the barriers that now prevent full participation in society.

'The inclusion of children with disabilities is a matter of social justice and an essential investment in the future of society. It is not based on charity or goodwill but is an integral element of the expression and realization of universal human rights.' (<http://www.unicef-irc.org>).[2]

References

Belfer, ML (2008) 'Child and adolescent mental disorders: the magnitude of the problem across the globe', *Journal of Child Psychology and Psychiatry*, 49(3), 226–36.

Clark, P and MacArthur, J (2008) 'Children with physical disability: Gaps in service provision, problems joining in', *Journal of Pediatrics and Child Health*, 44, 455–58.

Convention on the Rights of the Child. Available at <http://unicef.org/crc/>, accessed 7 November 2011.

Council of Europe, European Social Charter, Available at <http://www.coe.int/T/DGHL/Monitoring/SocialCharter/>, accessed 7 November 2011.

Dhanda, A (2008) 'Constructing a new Human Rights lexicon: Convention on the Rights of Persons with Disabilities', *Sur International Journal on Human Rights*, 5(8), 42–59. Available at <http://www.surjournal.org/eng/conteudos/getArtigo8.php?artigo=8,artigo_dhanda.htm>, accessed 7 November 2011.

Duarte, CS, Rizzini, I, Hoven, CW, Carlson, M, and Earls, F (2007) 'The evolution of child rights councils in Brazil', *International Journal of Child Rights*, 15, 269–82.

Edwards, SD (2001) 'Prevention of disability on grounds of suffering', *Journal Medical Ethics*, 27, 380–82.

Groce, NE (1999) 'Disability in cross-cultural perspective: rethinking disability', *The Lancet*, 354, 756–57.

Groce, NE and Paeglow, C (2005) *Violence against Disabled Children. UN Secretary Generals Report on Violence against Children. Thematic Group on Violence against Disabled Children.* New York: UNICEF.

Goldson, EJ (1997) 'Commentary: gender, disability and abuse', *Child Abuse Neglect*, 21, 703–705.

Harris, J (2000) 'Is there a coherent social conception of disability', *Journal Medical Ethics*, 26, 95–100.

Hibbard, RA, Desch, LW, and the Committee on Child Abuse, Neglect and the Council on Children with Disabilities (2007) 'Maltreatment of children with disabilities', *Pediatrics*, 119(5), 1018–25.

---

[2] <http://www.unicef-irc.org/publications/pdf/digest13-disability.pdf>, p. v.

Hsia, RY and Belfer, ML (2008) 'A framework for the analysis of child and adolescent mental disorders', *International Review of Psychiatry*, 20(3), 251–59.

Human Rights Watch (2001) *Easy Targets: Violence Against Children Worldwide*. New York: Human Rights Watch.

Levine, C (2005) 'Acceptance, avoidance, and ambiguity: Conflicting social values about childhood disability', *Kennedy Institute of Ethics Journal*, 15(4), 371–83.

Rehabilitation International. Available at <http://rehab-international.org/>, accessed 7 November 2011.

Rizzini, I, Barker, G, and Cassaniga, N (2002) *From Street Children to All Children: Improving the Opportunities of Low-Income Urban Children and Youth in Brazil*. Cambridge: Cambridge University Press.

Room, R, Rehm, J, Trotter II, RT, Paglia, A, and Ustun, TB (2001) 'Cross-cultural views on Stigma, Valuation, Parity, and Societal Values Towards Disability', in TB Ustun, S Chatterji, JE Bickenbach, et al. (eds) *Disability and Culture: Universalism and Diversity*. Geneva: Hogrefe & Huber Publishers, Seattle and World Health Organization, 247–291.

Slee, PT (2002) *Child, Adolescent and Family Development*. Cambridge: Cambridge University Press

Stewart-Brown, S (2003) 'Research in relation to equity: Extending the agenda', *Pediatrics*, 112(3), 763–65.

UNICEF-IRC. (2007) *Promoting the Rights of Children with Disabilities*. Innocenti Digest No. 13. Florence: UNICEF-IRC. Available at <http://www.unicef-irc.org/publications/pdf/digest13-disability.pdf>, accessed 7 November 2011.

Waterston, T and Goldhagen, J (2008) 'Why children's rights are central to international child health', *Archives Diseases of Children*, 92, 176–80.

Whyte, SR and Ingstad, B (Eds) (1995) *Disability and culture*. Los Angeles: University of California Press.

World Health Organization (2005) *Child and adolescent Atlas: Resources for child and adolescent mental health*. Geneva: World Health Organization.

Chapter 27

The Mental Health and Rights of Mentally Ill Older People

Carmelle Peisah, Henry Brodaty, and Nick O'Neill

What is it to be an older person and what constitutes a life worth living as an ageing member of our society? Human rights law maps out the terrain of the struggle for human well-being and dignity (Reid 2004). A number of frameworks exist that enshrine human right issues for older persons, perhaps the most well known of which is that developed by the United Nations (see Table 27.1) (<http://home.vicnet.net.au/~ac99vic/principles.html>). The realization of these rights is a challenge in any ageing society, particularly so for disabled, marginalized, and/or mentally ill older people who are especially vulnerable to abuse. From this general framework of human rights, the following are particularly salient for the disabled mentally ill elderly:

1. Independence/Autonomy—Older people have the right to make their own decisions on matters affecting their lives and their death.

2. Safety and dignity—Older people have the right to live safely, free of violence, abuse, exploitation, and neglect.

3. Care—Older persons should benefit from family and community care and protection. They should have access to healthcare to help them to maintain or regain the optimum level of physical, mental, and emotional well-being and to prevent or delay the onset of illness.

There is a degree of overlap between rights such that the failure to exercise one right—such as the right to care—is also failure to exercise another right, the right to safety and dignity. The failure to exercise either of these rights is often brought about by inaction which constitutes a type of abuse. In a similar way, the failure to permit older people to exercise autonomy in decisions regarding sexual relationships can constitute a failure to allow the right to live safely and with dignity, again a type of abuse.

Rights have different sources and statuses. Some have emerged from the common law and are part of Australian domestic law as a result of judicial decisions; some are based on the international covenants; while others still emerge from statements of principles which are taken into account when awarding funding, but are not enforceable in their own right. A 'right' which can be enforced by an action in damages in a court is different from a 'right' that is stated in an international covenant which has moral but not legal strength, and different again from a 'right' which is set out in a policy document which has no legal standing as a 'right' but may be effective in justifying the removal of governmental financial support from a service-provider who breaches such a 'right'.

In this chapter we will discuss the sources and status of these human rights and illustrate how certain conditions which confer disability and vulnerability on older persons might compromise the exercise of their human rights. By way of illustration, we will use hypothetical but commonly encountered clinical vignettes as a focus for discussion of these issues.

Table 27.1 The United Nations Principles for Older Persons

Independence	
1.	Older persons should have access to adequate food, water, shelter, clothing and healthcare through the provision of income, family and community support and self-help.
2.	Older persons should have the opportunity work or to have access to other income-generating opportunities.
3.	Older persons should be able to participate in determining when and at what pace withdrawal from the labour force takes place.
4.	Older persons should have access to appropriate education and training programmes.
5.	Older persons should be able to live in environments that are safe and adaptable to personal preferences and changing capacities.
6.	Older persons should be able to reside at home for as long as possible.
Participation	
7.	Older persons should remain integrated in society, participate actively in the formulation and implementation of policies that directly affect their well being and share their knowledge and skills with younger generations.
8.	Older persons should be able to seek and develop opportunities for service to the community and to serve as volunteers in positions appropriate to their interests and capabilities.
9.	Older persons should be able to form movements or associations of older persons.
Care	
10.	Older persons should benefit from family and community care and protection in accordance with each society's system of cultural values.
11.	Older persons should have access to healthcare to help them to maintain or regain the optimum level of physical, mental and emotional well being and to prevent or delay the onset of illness.
12.	Older persons should have access to social and legal services to enhance their autonomy, protection and care.
13.	Older persons should be able to utilise appropriate levels of institutional care providing protection, rehabilitation and social and mental stimulation in a humane and secure environment.
14.	Older persons should be able to enjoy human rights and fundamental freedoms when residing in any shelter, care or treatment facility, including full respect for their dignity, beliefs, needs and privacy and for the right to make decisions about their care and the quality of their lives.
Self-fulfilment	
15.	Older persons should be able to pursue opportunities for the full development of their potential.
16.	Older persons should have access to the educational, cultural, spiritual and recreational resources of society.
Dignity	
17.	Older persons should be able to live in dignity and security and be free of exploitation and physical or mental abuse.
18.	Older persons should be treated fairly regardless of age, gender, racial or ethnic background, disability or other status, and be valued independently of their economic contribution.

Why are older people vulnerable to human rights abuses?

External factors: ageism and discrimination

Systemic and societal attitudes towards ageing per se provide fertile ground for human rights abuses. Discrimination against people on the grounds of older age is common. Older people are commonly seen by care staff as an homogenous group characterized stereotypically as warm but incompetent, dependent, and diseased (Peisah 1991). Such attitudes are often driven by fear—of disease, infirmity, dependence, or death (Montepare and Zebrowitz 2002).

Ageing persons may be vulnerable to discrimination or 'Ageism' manifesting as negative perceptions and attitudes which devalue and disempower older people and influence health resource allocation. This may be exacerbated by the adverse effects of discrimination and stigmatization conferred by having a mental illness, the 'double jeopardy' of psychiatric stigma and stigma against old age (Lindesay 2005:124). Discrimination may reduce or nullify the equal enjoyment of human rights of mentally ill people through acts of avoidance, withholding help, coercion, or segregation (Corrigan and Watson 2002).

Ageist perceptions can be found amongst community members and healthcare professionals alike (Lookinland and Anson 1995; Kearney et al. 2000; Gunderson et al. 2005), all the more towards ageing people with mental illness. These forms of discrimination may be compounded by:

◆ gender discrimination;

◆ discrimination on basis of social class, wealth, education—those with the least resources are the most vulnerable;

◆ minority ethnicity, race, religion, and language barriers to access to culturally appropriate services;

◆ lack of a support infrastructure within some community groups particularly among indigenous groups and rural and remote communities which present another set of challenges associated with distance, availability, and access to services.

Disability and dependency

As well as the extremely variable biopsychosocially determined ageing processes, older age can be associated with a number of conditions which cause disability and dependency on others. With increasing dependency, the carer becomes central to maintaining the life of the older person. The carer may or may not be living with the impaired person, but close and frequent contact between the carer and the impaired person leads to a special relationship and puts the carer in a unique position of influence. Where there is an imbalance of power in relationships there is a risk of abuse by the dominant person or persons.

Mental disorder

Mental disorders afflicting older people such as dementia, mood disorder, and various psychoses such as schizophrenia may confer vulnerability in several ways, through discrimination, disability, and dependency and by virtue of altered perceptions and impaired cognition, particularly judgement and reasoning. With regards to the latter, many mentally ill older people are either unaware of their rights or unable to recognize the kind of healthcare or environment which would maximize their physical, mental, and emotional well-being.

Salient human rights issues for mentally ill elderly

Participation and autonomy

Autonomy is defined as a person's ability and opportunity to make decisions relating to his or her own wishes (Rosin and van Dijk 2005). Older people with disability have the right to make their own decisions on personal, financial, domestic, and health-related matters as far as they are competent to do so and their freedom of decision and action restricted as little as possible. They should be encouraged as far as possible to be as self-reliant in matters relating to their personal domestic and financial affairs and to live a normal life in the community. This should also include access to spiritual and pastoral care, of particular importance to many older adults at the end of their lives (Wallace and O'Shea 2007).

Autonomy in healthcare

Older people of sound mind have the right to determine what is or is not done to their body and this must be respected and accepted, irrespective of what others, including doctors, may think is in the best interests of that person. Accordingly, older people have the right to refuse treatment and doctors have an obligation to obtain consent to treat, this right being ratified in judicial law. Thus, informed consent for treatment, including the use of medications, and for involvement in drug trials or other research must be obtained from the person or, if he or she is incompetent, from the person's proxy. Failure to do so constitutes trespass if the treatment is carried out without consent, except in the case of an emergency in which the principle of necessity upholds the actions of treating 'agents' who are unable to get instructions from the person, to act in a way that is in the best interests of the person. Despite these regulations, treatment of older people without their consent or that of their proxy is common. In one study in nursing homes of psychotropic use for older people who were mentally incompetent, proxy consent was provided in writing for only 6.5 per cent of residents and orally for another 6.5 per cent (Rendina et al. 2009).

When older people become incompetent to make decisions regarding their healthcare, personal care, and accommodation they have the right to have these decisions made in their best interests, ideally by people that they themselves have previously appointed autonomously, and, in accordance with their previously expressed wishes, if such are known. This can be effected by means of enduring guardianship, enduring power of attorney, and advance directives or through guardianship or financial management orders.

Personal relationships and sexuality

Case 1

Mrs S is an 85-year-old widow who suffers from Parkinson's disease and early dementia and is living in a nursing home. She has little insight into her need for care and desperately wants to return home. A man in his early 50s, who is a male friend of a fellow resident, has befriended her and offered to take her home permanently and care for her in return for a car and a trip overseas. The family are concerned that the younger man is exploiting Mrs S and are particularly concerned because there have been reports from staff that the two have been intimate with each other.

The right to form relationships is a fundamental human right into which neither the courts nor family nor doctors have a right to interfere unless the exercise of that right involves abuse or exploitation. While it is sometimes difficult to ascertain whether or not a sexual relationship involving an older disabled person involves abuse or exploitation, most commonly sexual abuse of older disabled people is often ignored or underestimated. Importantly, the risk of emotional harm as a result of sexual abuse is sometimes underestimated with regards to older cognitively impaired people such as those with Alzheimer's disease (AD) who cannot recall recent events and experiences (Sabat 2005). In particular, it has been argued that the burgeoning literature regarding implicit memory shows that people with AD can still be affected in a lasting manner by experiences that they may not be consciously able to recall having had (Sabat 2005).

Therefore, when the appropriateness of a sexual relationship involving at least one cognitively impaired individual is called in to question, two issues need to be considered: (i) do the individuals have capacity? and (ii) is there harm or abuse? There are no specific tests or criteria designed to cover consent to sexual relations, although some of the factors that might be relevant to an assessment of such capacity include an understanding of what is involved in sexual intercourse and an awareness of the identity of the partner, and perhaps, the nature of the relationship (although this is clearly difficult to assess). In the absence of harm or abuse, a lack of capacity to consent formally to sexual relations does not necessarily mean that the relationship should be prevented or discouraged (BMA 2004:100).

More importantly, careful consideration should be given to the existence of any the following indicators of harm, abuse, or exploitation:

◆ What kind of relationship do they have? Is there a power imbalance or element of coercion?

◆ Is the relationship associated with other exploitation, e.g. financial?

◆ Is there a significant discrepancy between the two people's cognitive capacity?

◆ What pleasure (or otherwise) do they experience in the relationship? Are they willing or content for it to continue?

Should there be interference in the relationship between Mrs S and her 'friend' where there is a significant discrepancy both in cognitive capacity and age? This issue commonly arises in community and residential care settings, but it is in residential care where the subject of sexual behaviour is particularly fraught with complex systemic, legal, and ethical issues. It is the need to consider two human rights issues simultaneously that makes this issue so complex. Older people have the right to personal liberty and autonomy was well as the right to be protected from abuse or exploitation. Accordingly, residential care facilities have a dual responsibility to provide residents with the freedom to associate with others—both intimately and sexually—while protecting them from abuse, injury, and neglect (Kamel and Hajjar 2004).

End of life

Case 2

Mr G is a 92-year-old man living at home with his son, daughter-in law, and grandchildren. Over the last 12 months he has suffered repeated episodes of delirium usually related to urinary tract infections although he is known to have also a history of ischaemic heart disease and chronic obstructive pulmonary disease. All but one of these episodes was treated at home, the one inpatient episode resulting in marked worsening of confusion, hallucinations, and distress. Subsequently his cognitive recovery has not been full and he may be developing dementia. After presenting with a recurrence of confusion associated with paranoid delusions and visual hallucinations, initially responsive at home to an antipsychotic drug and antibiotics, he develops a cough and deteriorates. He is no longer competent to make decisions about his treatment and there is debate and uncertainty between his family and treating doctors about whether to hospitalize him or leave him at home. His son recalls the disastrous impact of his last inpatient treatment and his previously expressed verbal wishes (made some three years earlier) not to be treated needlessly: 'I don't want to go on forever and lie in some hospital like a vegetable if I haven't got my marbles.'

Older people have the right to die in dignity and comfort and to decide the manner in which they will die. They have the right to expect treating teams to act in good faith in relation to advance directives, and to adapt or change treatments to meet their verbal or written wishes, except where doing so would cause suffering which the person did not anticipate when making the advance directive (Treloar 1999; Biegler et al. 2000). In the absence of previously expressed wishes it is lawful in Australia to withhold or withdraw treatment where the commencement or continuation of it would be futile and not in the incapable person's best interests.

In addition to the right to autonomy in end of life decisions, there is a right to die a 'good death', i.e. free of pain and suffering where possible. Brennan discusses the human right to palliative care in terms of the right to freedom from unnecessary suffering and the provision of all possible measures to enable that relief to be met, including adequate housing, nutrition, water, and sanitation. Yet, there are major disparities in the provision of palliative care around the world, and this has led to statements of advocacy, objectives, and obligations directed at individual governments to ensure that this fundamental human right to a dignified death is respected (Brennan 2007).

Conversely in many developed countries, the pursuit of a 'good death' has also led to increasing interest and debate about physician assisted suicide (PAS), the active and intentional termination of a patient's life at the explicit request of a patient. That mental disorders in old age such as depression and dementia are often at the heart of such debate highlights the importance of mental health assessments and the role of mental health professionals in the determination of competence to choose euthanasia (Ganzini et al. 2000; Hertogh 2005). The clinical, ethical, and legal dilemmas associated with PAS and older people with mental health disorders are discussed elsewhere at length (Draper et al. 2010; Post 1997).

Safety and dignity

Older persons with disability should be protected from abuse, exploitation, and neglect.

Elder abuse

The definition of elder abuse endorsed by all Australian states and territories through the Healthy Ageing Taskforce (HATF) (a joint federal, state, and territory body) on 8 December 2000 is:

> Any act occurring within a relationship where there is an implication of trust, which results in harm to an older person. Abuse can include physical, sexual, financial, psychological and social abuse and/or neglect.

There are several types of abuse identified. Abuse or mistreatment of older people can occur in the following domains (<http://www.eapu.com.au>):

◆ Financial abuse: The illegal or improper use of an older person's money or possessions;

◆ Psychological abuse: Causing fear or shame, intimidation, humiliation, or making threats;

◆ Physical abuse: Inflicting pain or injury, e.g. hitting or slapping, restraining, over medicating, or refusing medicine;

◆ Sexual abuse: Sexually abusive or exploitative behaviour, including rape, indecent assault, sexual harassment, and indecent behaviour;

◆ Social abuse: Preventing a person from having social contact with family or friends;

◆ Neglect: The intentional or unintentional failure to provide necessities of life and care;

◆ Access: Kidnapping by families, denying elderly people access to those they wish to see by not allowing those others to see them; the overbearing of the will of the elderly so that they cut off contact with others not approved by those (often family members) supporting them;

◆ Autonomy in asset disposition: Older people may be coerced or influenced to change their wills or make gifts during life with the result that the legitimate beneficiaries under their wills receive very little or nothing because the person's estate has little in it when they die.

Despite increased awareness of elder abuse, it continues to be a major problem in many societies. A disproportionate number of older women are victims of abuse compared to men, although older men are more likely to be victims of abandonment (<http://www.elderabusecenter.org>). Women also represented nearly half (47.5 per cent) of the perpetrators of abuse while adult sons and daughters combined to form the single biggest category of abusers. Children perpetrate many of the above categories of abuse, commonly financial abuse which may be increasing:

> the variety, complexity, and creativeness of ways to take financial advantage of older people are also increasing. Today, there are scores of scams, misdeeds, and rip-offs designed to take advantage of vulnerable older people (Kemp et al. 2005)

Abuse within the residential care setting is a subject of increasing debate and public awareness. Nursing home residents are particularly vulnerable to abuse, with one-fifth to one-third of these institutions in the United States cited for abusive activities that result in actual harm (Liang 2006). Both overt abuse by staff and neglect (an issue addressed below in regards to the human right to care) and more commonly, resident-to-resident abuse have been identified in nursing homes (Lachs et al. 2007).

A particular focus of concern has been the misuse of physical and chemical restraints for dealing with disabled or mentally ill (often dementing) elderly people within aged care facilities (Turnham 2003). In Australia, a number of policies have been developed to deal with this issue. For example, some years ago the Australian Society for Geriatric Medicine put out a Position Statement on physical restraint use in the elderly (<http://www.anzsgm.org/documents/POSITIONSTATEMENTNO2.PhysicialRestraint-Revision.pdf>). In 2004 the Australian government Department of Health and Ageing released a Decision-Making Tool responding to issues of chemical, physical, and environmental restraint and the use of aversive treatment or practices in aged care (<http://www.health.gov.au/internet/wcms/publishing.nsf/Content/ageing-decision-restraint.htm>). Similarly, the Guardianship Tribunal of New South Wales (<http://www.gt.nsw.gov.au>) supports the provision of care with minimal restraint in the least restrictive environment for people with dementia who require management of their challenging behaviour. This may involve empowering an appointed guardian to consent to behavioural intervention and support that includes restrictive practices (eg. physical restraint or exclusionary 'time out') that are used to contain and reduce challenging behaviours when it is clearly in the best interests of the person to do so. The tribunal may also be approached to consent to medication that is used to control challenging behaviour, or to authorize an appointed guardian to be able to consent to medication as a means of behavioural intervention and support.

Care

The right to health

There has been a general consensus between academia, governments, non-governmental organizations, and international bodies, including agencies of the United Nations, regarding the link between the promotion and protection of human rights and health (Brennan 2007) An extensive body of literature has focused on the right to health, especially in the context of the significant inequalities in access to healthcare throughout the world (Brennan 2007). Viewing the provision of healthcare in terms of equality and social justice, Farmer and Gastineau (2002) called for programmes to rectify the inequalities of access to services that can help all humans lead free and healthy lives and to ensure that everyone has a share in scientific advancements and developments.

Advanced age is one of a number of factors, in addition to employment, education, income, and race, that determine a person's ability to acquire healthcare (Papadimos 2007). Older people have the right to equal access to the treatment and care they want or need to maintain or regain an optimum level of physical, mental, and emotional well being and to prevent or delay the onset of illness. This means reasonable access to new and expensive treatments from which older persons could derive genuine benefit, when barring them from that treatment because of their age has no ethical basis.

The connections between health and human rights have been directed to advocacy, the provision of services, research, and defining health policy (Brennan 2007), particularly needed for disabled, marginalized, and/or mentally ill older people. For example, expenditures per recipient are substantially higher for younger individuals with disabilities, largely as a result of more effective advocacy (Kane et al. 2007). Private psychiatric service provision to older people is inequitable when compared with younger adults (Draper and Koschera 2001). The proportion of Medicare private psychiatry expenditure on older adults has declined since 1985–1986 and older people are only one third as likely to see a psychiatrist compared with the younger adult population and then for briefer consultations (Draper and Koschera 2001).

Indeed, it has been suggested that human rights law has been better at protecting older people from unwanted or unnecessary treatment and care than it has been at securing necessary treatment and care for them. This is particularly so with regards to mental health (Hale 2007). In relation to mental health, international human rights law affirms that everyone has a right to the enjoyment of the highest attainable standard of mental health. It contains both freedoms and entitlements including the right to control one's own health and the right to be free from non-consensual treatment and experimentation (Reid 2004).

Other theorists have been critical of the concept of an individual 'right to health,' describing it as a privilege not a right, illusory, meaningless, or, in the context of a world with limited resources and escalating health expenses, unattainable (O'Neill 2001; Goodman 2005; Papadimos 2007). In the face of this increased competition for finite resources, greater efficiency and equity between expenditure on younger and older disabled individuals might be achieved by finding commonalities in care needs, care models, and programmes for young and old and consolidating formerly separate care agencies, while acknowledging that approaches across groups may not be identical (Kane et al. 2007).

Community care

The basic human right to care includes the right of older persons to access appropriate levels of community and institutional care that provide protection, rehabilitation, and social and mental stimulation in a humane and secure environment. Community care means effective community support services, advocacy services, self help or support organizations (e.g. Alzheimer's Association), and educational programmes such as the Living with Memory Loss Program for people with early dementia and their family carers.

In Australia, the provision of these services helps many people to continue to live in their own homes for much longer than they would otherwise be able. This gives effect to the right to reside at home for as long as possible, which is part of the right to independence.

Case 3

Mr X is a 90-year-old man with mixed Alzheimer's disease and vascular dementia complicated by behavioural problems such as negativity, irritability, resistiveness, and verbal aggression, usually directed at his wife, his primary carer. Although his behavioural disturbances are pronounced, his overall cognitive function is only mildly impaired as is his functioning in everyday activities of daily living for which he merely needs prompting in order to carry them out independently. His wife has found it increasingly difficult to deal with his behaviours which have been resistant to treatment with behavioural therapy and pharmacological agents. She feels she cannot cope with him at home any more, but he refuses to accept residential care.

Just as exercising the right to healthcare is constrained by finite health resources, the right to reside at home is constrained by finite carer and community resources. The case of Mr X illustrates the competing needs of Mr and Mrs X. Whose human rights take priority: the right of Mr X to live at home as long as possible or the right of Mrs X to be free of abuse? Rosin and van Dijk (2005) discuss the question of how far a family is obliged to respond to the demand of a parent (or spouse) for care and attention and the limits of the responsibility of a child to a parent to provide care. In this context the clinician has to deal with the complex environment of the older person and exercise a 'moral and medicosocial' judgment:

> If he thereby became convinced that the damage inflicted on the family outweighs significantly any benefit that the old person derives from their immediate care, and that an alternative solution need not objectively affect him adversely, it would be justified to give priority to the family's needs (Rosin and van Dijk 2005:357).

A vital part of any process that deals with these complicated situations is the assessment of the person's decision-making capacity (Strang et al. 1998). Can the person make decisions regarding care, and specifically, is any apparent indifference to the needs and interests of others a manifestation of premorbid personality or impaired judgment? If the former, the solution lies in the resolution of conflict and enhanced communication within the family, while if the latter, a determination of incompetence will often make it easier for family members to accept a decision that is both in their best interests and that of the older person, albeit against the person's wishes. Sometimes the limits to autonomy must be accepted, especially where others' interests are threatened (Strang et al. 1998).

Residential care

The achievement of basic human rights within the residential care environment form the basis of standards policy developed by the Australian government Department of Health and Ageing which specifies that:

(1) Residents retain their personal, civic, legal, and consumer rights and are assisted to achieve active control of their own lives within the residential care service and in the community

(2) Residents' physical and mental health will be promoted and achieved at the optimum level in partnership between each resident (or his or her representative) and the healthcare team.

(3) Residents live in a safe and comfortable environment that ensures the quality of life and welfare of residents, staff, and visitors. (<http://www.health.gov.au/internet/main/publishing.nsf/Content/ageing-rescare-index.htm>)

To this end, the User Rights Principles 1997 under the Aged Care Act 1997 includes a Charter of Residents' Rights and Responsibilities (<http://www.health.gov.au>), in which each resident of a residential care service has the right:

◆ to full and effective use of his or her personal, civil, legal, and consumer rights;

◆ to quality care which is appropriate to his or her needs;

◆ to full information about his or her own state of health and about available treatments;

◆ to be treated with dignity and respect, and to live without exploitation, abuse, or neglect;

◆ to live without discrimination or victimization, and without being obliged to feel grateful to those providing his or her care and accommodation;

◆ to personal privacy;

◆ to live in a safe, secure, and homelike environment, and to move freely both within and outside the residential care service without undue restriction;

◆ to be treated and accepted as an individual, and to have his or her individual preferences taken into account and treated with respect;

◆ to continue his or her cultural and religious practices and to retain the language of his or her choice, without discrimination;

◆ to select and maintain social and personal relationships with any other person without fear, criticism or restriction;

◆ to freedom of speech;

◆ to maintain his or her personal independence, which includes a recognition of personal responsibility for his or her own actions and choices, even though some actions may involve an element of risk which the resident has the right to accept, and that should then not be used to prevent or restrict those actions;

◆ to maintain control over, and to continue making decisions about, the personal aspects of his or her daily life, financial affairs, and possessions;

◆ to be involved in the activities, associations, and friendships of his or her choice, both within and outside the residential care service;

◆ to have access to services and activities which are available generally in the community;

◆ to be consulted on, and to choose to have input into, decisions about the living arrangements of the residential care service;

◆ to have access to information about his or her rights, care, accommodation, and any other information which relates to him or her personally;

◆ to complain and to take action to resolve disputes;

◆ to have access to advocates and other avenues of redress; and

◆ to be free from reprisal, or a well-founded fear of reprisal, in any form for taking action to enforce his or her rights.

To what extent do residential care homes uphold these rights? Institutional elder abuse still occurs and quality care is not always available. A report form the United Kingdom showed that nearly 50 per cent of care homes for the elderly failed to meet national minimum standards for the provision of medication. Older people in these homes are routinely given the wrong doses of drugs or no drugs at all (Editorial 2006).

Involuntary treatment and care: the rights of involuntary patients

The European Court of Human Rights protects the human rights of persons subjected to involuntary psychiatric commitment by creating 'supranational' laws in the following areas: definition of 'unsoundness of mind'; conditions of lawfulness of detention; right to a review of detention by a court; right to information; right to respect for private and family life; and conditions of confinement which address inhuman and degrading treatment (Niveau and Materi 2007).

In Australia, mental health legislation and guardianship laws protect the rights of elderly people who require involuntary care. Involuntary detention is otherwise considered false imprisonment if the person wishes to leave. However, the border between care and involuntary detention is often fuzzy in settings outside mental health. 'Duty of care' is the frequent reason for the detention of older people with impaired cognition in hospitals and nursing homes despite their objections. Mostly the older person's lack of will, means or attempts to leave is held to justify this practice. Even if the older person attempts to escape, a legal framework is seldom applied.

Summary

The rights of older people have been considered as regards independence/autonomy, safety, and dignity and care. In each of these domains, rights may be encroached upon for benign or malignant reasons. The former may result from lack of thought, insensitive systems of care, or mistaken beliefs. The latter, which may take the form of physical, sexual, psychological, or financial abuse, may result from material or psychological motives by others.

Older people, despite having contributed taxes, employment, child rearing, and voluntary work over a lifetime, are vulnerable to being treated as inferior citizens or being denied opportunities available to younger members of the community. The independence, autonomy, and rights of older people may be abrogated because they lack occupational or financial status or because of mental illness or declining cognitive abilities. While most families, carers, and healthcare professionals respect and provide loving care to older people, the vulnerability of those with mental illness or mental impairment makes them targets for abuse by a minority.

The maintenance of human rights of older people with mental illness requires effort. Societies constantly strive to find the right balance between beneficence and autonomy, between paternalism and independence. Legislation provides only partial protection and needs to be bolstered by positive community attitudes such as those articulated in the United Nations Principles (Table 27.1). On 30 March 2007 the Convention on the Rights of Persons with Disabilities (CRPD) opened for signature at the United Nations Headquarters in New York. It clearly applies to older persons who have long-term physical, mental, intellectual, or sensory impairments which hinder their full and effective participation in society on an equal basis with others. Article 1 of the CRPD declares its purpose to 'promote, protect and ensure the full and equal enjoyment of all human rights and fundamental freedoms by all persons with disabilities, and to promote respect for their inherent dignity'.

The convention came into force generally on 3 May 2008 and for Australia on 17 July 2008. It has not yet been incorporated into Australian domestic law. Nevertheless, Australia has ratified the Optional Protocol to the convention with effect from 20 September 2009. Consequently, individuals may complain to the Committee on the Rights of Persons with Disabilities about rights guaranteed under the convention; but only after they have exhausted their domestic remedies and only in relation to events occurring after 20 September 2009. The impact the convention will have on community attitudes to the rights of those with disabilities and on government programmes to protect and enhance those rights has yet to be seen.

References

Australian Government Department of Health and Ageing. *Decision making tool: Responding to issues of restraint in Aged Care*. Available at <http://www.health.gov.au/internet/main/publishing.nsf/Content/ageing-decision-restraint.htm>, accessed 8 November 2011.

Australian Government Department of Health and Ageing. *Publications, Statistics & Resources*. Available at <http://www.health.gov.au/internet/main/publishing.nsf/Content/Publications+Statistics+&+Resources-1>, accessed 8 November 2011.

Australian Government Department of Health and Ageing. *Standards of care in aged care homes*. Available at <http://www.agedcareaustralia.gov.au/internet/agedcare/publishing.nsf/Content/Standards+of+care-2>, accessed 8 November 2011.

Australian Society for Geriatric Medicine. *Position Statement No.2: Physical Restraint Use in Older People*. <http://www.anzsgm.org/documents/POSITIONSTATEMENTNO2.PhysicialRestraint-Revision.pdf>, accessed 8 November 2011.

Biegler, P, Stewart, C, Savulescu, J, and Skene, L (2000) 'Determining the validity of advance directives', *Medical Journal of Australia*, 172, 545–48.

BMA (British Medical Association) and The Law Society (2004) *Assessment of Mental Capacity—Guidance for doctors and lawyers*. 2nd edn. London: BMJ Books.

Brennan, F (2007) 'Palliative care as an international human right', *Journal of Pain Symptom Management*, 33, 494–9.

Corrigan, PW and Watson, AC (2002) 'Understanding the impact of stigma on people with mental illness', *World Psychiatry*, 1, 16–19.

Draper, BM and Koschera, A (2001) 'Do older people receive equitable private psychiatric service provision under Medicare?', *Australian and New Zealand Journal of Psychiatry*, 35, 626–30.

Draper, BM, Peisah, C, Snowdon, J, and Brodaty, H (2010) 'Early dementia diagnosis and the risk of suicide and euthanasia', *Alzheimer's & Dementia*, 6(1), 75–82.

Editorial (2006) 'Institutional elder abuse', *The Lancet*, 367, 624.

Elder Abuse Prevention Unit. <http://www.eapu.com.au/>, accessed 8 November 2011.

Farmer, P and Gastineau, N (2002) 'Rethinking health and human rights: time for a paradigm shift', *Journal of Law, Medicine & Ethics*, 30(4), 655–66.

Ganzini, L, Leong, GB, Fenn, DS, Silva, JA, and Weinstock, R (2000) 'Evaluation of competence to consent to assisted suicide', *American Journal of Psychiatry*, 157, 595–600.

Goodman, T (2005) 'Is there a right to health?', *Journal of Medicine & Philosophy*, 30, 643–62.

Gray, N and Bailie, R (2006) 'Can human rights discourse improve the health of Indigenous Australians?', *Australian and New Zealand Journal of Public Health*, 30, 448–52.

Guardianship Tribunal. <http://www.gt.nsw.gov.au/>, accessed 8 November 2011.

Gunderson, A, Tomkowiak, J, Menachemi, N, and Brooks, R (2005) 'Rural physicians' attitudes toward the elderly: evidence of ageism', *Quality Management in Health Care*, 14, 167–76.

Hale, B (2007) 'Justice and equality in mental health law: The European experience', *International Journal of Law and Psychiatry*, 30, 18–28.

Healthy Aging Taskforce (2000). Cited in <http://www.eapu.com.au/>.

Hertogh, CMPM (2005) 'End-of-life care and medical decision making in patients with dementia', in A Burns (ed) *Standards in dementia care—European Dementia Consensus Network (EDCON)*. London/New York: Taylor & Francis, 339–54.

Kamel, HK and Hajjar RR (2004) 'Sexuality in the nursing home, Part 2: managing abnormal behavior—legal and ethical issues', *Journal of American Medical Director's Association*, 5(S2), S48–52.

Kane, RL, Priester, R, and Neumann, D (2007) 'Does disparity in the way disabled older adults are treated imply ageism?', *Gerontologist*, 47, 271–9.

Kearney, N, Miller, M, Paul, J, and Smith, K (2000) 'Oncology healthcare professionals' attitudes toward elderly people', *Annals of Oncology*, 11, 599–601.

Kemp, Bryan J and Mosqueda, Laura A (2005) 'Elder Financial Abuse: An Evaluation Framework and Supporting Evidence', *Journal of the American Geriatrics Society*, (53), 1123–27.

Lachs, M, Bachman, R, Williams, CS, and O'Leary, JR (2007) 'Resident-to-resident elder mistreatment and police contact in nursing homes: findings from a population-based cohort', *Journal of the American Geriatrics Society*, 55(6), 840–5.

Liang, BA (2006) 'Elder abuse detection in nursing facilities: using paid clinical competence to address the nation's shame', *Journal of Health Law*, 39(4), 527–50.

Lindesay, J (2005) 'Destigmatization of elderly people with early or late-onset schizophrenia', in A Hassett, D Ames, and E Chiu (eds) *Psychosis in the elderly*. Abingdon: Taylor & Francis, 94–100.

Lookinland, S and Anson, K (1995) 'Perpetuation of ageist attitudes among present and future health care personnel: implications for elder care', *Journal of Advanced Nursing*, 21, 47–56.

Montepare, JM and Zebrowitz, LA (2002) 'A socio-developmental view of ageism', in TD Nelson (ed) *Stereotyping and Prejudice Against Older Persons*. Cambridge, MA: MIT Press, 77–128.

Niveau, G and Materi, J (2007) 'Psychiatric commitment: Over 50 years of case law from the European Court of Human Rights', *European Psychiatry*, 22, 59–67.

O'Neill, O (2001) *Autonomy and trust in bioethics*. Cambridge: Cambridge University Press, 78–79.

Papadimos, TJ (2007) 'Healthcare access as a right, not a privilege: a construct of Western thought', *Philosophy, Ethics, and Humanities in Medicine*, 2, 2.

Peisah, C (1991) 'Caring for the institutionalised elderly: how easy is it?', *Australian Journal of Public Health*, 15, 37–42.

Post, SG (1997) 'Physician-assisted suicide in Alzheimer's disease', *Journal American Geriatric Society*, 45, 647–51.

Reid, EA (2004) 'Health, human rights and Australia's foreign policy', *Medical Journal of Australia*, 180, 163–65.

Rendina, N, Brodaty, H, Draper, B, Peisah, C, and Brugue, E (2009) 'Substitute consent for nursing home residents prescribed psychotropic medication', *International Journal of Geriatric Psychiatry*, 24(3), 226–31.

Rosin, AJ and van Dijk, Y (2005) 'Subtle ethical dilemmas in geriatric management and clinical research', *Journal of Medical Ethics*, 31, 355–59.

Sabat, SR (2005) 'Capacity for decision-making in Alzheimer's disease: selfhood, positioning and semiotic people', *Australian and New Zealand Journal of Psychiatry*, 39, 1030–5.

Strang, DG, Molloy, DW, and Harrison, C (1998) 'Capacity to choose place of residence: autonomy vs beneficence?', *Journal of Palliative Care*, 14(1), 25–29.

Treloar, A (1999) 'Advance directives: Limitations upon their applicability in elderly care', *International Journal of Geriatric Psychiatry*, 14, 1039–43.

Turnham, R (2003) *Quality care or human rights abuse? Physical restraint of people with dementia in residential aged care*. Paper Presented at AASW Annual Conference, Canberra, September 2003.

Wallace, M and O'Shea, E (2007) 'Perceptions of spirituality and spiritual care among older nursing home residents at the end of life', *Holistic Nursing Practice*, 21, 285–9. Available at <http://home.vicnet.net.au/~ac99vic/principles.html>, accessed 8 November 2011.

Chapter 28

Sex and Gender
Biology, Culture, and the Expression of Gender
Louise Newman

Introduction—sex, gender

Concepts of gender, sex-role behaviour, sexual difference, and sexuality have been central to psychiatric discourse and concepts of mental disorder. Non-conformity to particular models of gender roles and sexual preference has been linked to mental disorder since the emergence of psychiatric classification systems (Seil 1996). Concepts of healthy psychological functioning or 'normality' have been linked to models of gender behaviour and sexuality assuming that gender conformity is intrinsic to mental health. Psychiatry as a discipline has been implicated in the explicit and implicit use of its theory to pathologize and stigmatize individuals with gender and sexual variance, and continues to be involved in mediating access to certain medical interventions such as 'sex-reassignment procedures' for transsexual individuals. Historically, for example, concepts of mental disorder such as hysteria were attributed to excesses of female sexuality, and homosexuality has been seen as intrinsically disordered and indicating a variety of possible mental disorders ranging from psychopathy to personality disorder and neurosis to psychosis. Psychiatry has been involved in the design and implementation of 'treatments' for homosexuality aimed at elimination of homosexual desire and a heterosexual outcome. Psychiatry then has been seen as reinforcing a particular view of the categories of sex, sexuality, and gender which reflects a heteronormative model and which sees gender as an essential and fixed category of human subjectivity. This chapter will focus on the role of psychiatry in the regulation of gender categories and the creation of a category of gender identity disorder.

In current use, sex is defined as the biological status of a person as either male or female, based on anatomical characteristics, and gender as its socialized aspect. Gender identity refers to the individual subjective sense of maleness or femaleness and a self-definition and perception of the self as gendered. Gender role refers to the socially ascribed characteristics and expectations—attitudes, behaviours, beliefs, and values—associated with being male or female. Whilst there is social and cultural variation in the behaviours and attributes defined as masculine or feminine these are incorporated in the individual sense of self—I am a male or female with these core characteristics. In other words, biology is seen as determinant of psychology.

Gender identity is seen as linked to anatomical sex. In normative development, biological males develop male anatomy and a corresponding sense of self as male and this is reflected in the development of attitudes, behaviours, and personality attributes that are socially identified as masculine. In this account, anatomical sex is linked to subjective sense of gender and reflected in corresponding social and cultural categories. This model essentially marginalizes the role of culture and meaning in shaping gender identity.

The tension between essentialist and constructivist views is central to the ongoing debate around gender identity disorder (GID), the condition defined by a desire to be the other sex. Essentialism refers to the view that the category of gender is irreducible and is a universal biologically-determined category. Constructivists, on the other hand, argue that gender and sexual differences are the result of complex social processes and are social constructs (Kessler and McKenna 1978; Garber 1992) which shape the perception of biology. Psychiatry and medical discourse have taken an essentialist account of sex and gender which sees a natural connection between the biological and the social—biology determines psychology and social gender roles. This account also assumes that the phenomenology of gender dysphoria is historical and independent of culture.

'Throughout the ages there have been men who wished to be women and women who wished to be men. Individuals with cross-gender wishes and cross-gender behaviour have existed in every major culture in the world, knowing no boundaries of race, creed or color. Thus historical study reveals that transsexualism and related disorders of gender identity are not conditions peculiar to modern times' (Steiner 1985; Usher 1997, 2006).

Anthropological and historical approaches have pointed to the significant variation in definitions of sex differences across time and culture and the related variations in how particular cultures understand and theorize gender diversity. In this sense, current medical accounts of GID and related conditions very much reflect a particular theory of gender identity and its pathology.

The existence of individuals with experiences of gender non-conformity and non-heterosexual orientation has troubled psychological theory and continues to raise fundamental issues about our conceptualization of the development of the sense of gender identity and its relationship, if any, to sexual identity and behaviour. Individuals experiencing gender non-conformity present with a variety of questions around their sense of maleness and femaleness and the relationship to the body. Some will describe an essential split or lack of fit between the body or anatomical sex, and gender as a sense of subjective identification; others present with questions around a sense of identity that may not appear fixed or easy to define as male or female regardless of their experience of the body. Cultural and social responses to individuals with gender variant experience vary widely from reverence to stigmatization and discrimination in terms of civil liberties and legal status. Gender variant experiences raise issues as to the complexity of early development, the interactions of the biological and sociocultural domains, and the rights of the individual to free expression of varyingly gendered behaviours and sexual orientations.

Gender identity disorder

Following considerable debate and lobbying, homosexuality was removed from the American Psychiatric Association's Diagnostic and Statistical Manual of Mental Disorders (DSM) classification system of mental disorders in 1973. In 1980, the DSM-III introduced the new category of gender identity disorder, a broad category including transsexual and non-transsexual types. Cross dressing behaviour was concurrently classified as transvestic fetishism, as one of a group of paraphilias. DSM describes transsexualism as a 'persistent discomfort and sense of inappropriateness about one's assigned sex' and persistent preoccupation for at least two years with getting rid of one's primary and secondary sex characteristics and acquiring the sex characteristics of the other sex. GID is defined as a broader designation inclusive of transsexualism, gender identity disorder of childhood, and non-transsexual type gender identity disorder. In essence, this represents a shift from the pathologization of a type of sexual behaviour to a disorder of identity. Gender identity disorder by definition implies that there is a normative form of gender identity linked to biological categories of anatomical sex. Immediately this raises the debate concerning genetic and biological contributing factors, as opposed to social and environmental influences on gender identity and sexual difference. The 'disorder' of cross-gender identification (GID) still embodies a model of strict gender conformity and a binary gender model. Recent surgical and medical developments provide the option of gender change, but only between male and female categories. The term 'transsexualism' then is defined by the desire for medical and surgical interventions and was introduced concurrently with the development of hormonal and surgical interventions in the 1950s. Publicity surrounding the case of Christine Jorgensen (Benjamin 1954) who underwent genital surgery and oestrogen treatment raised awareness of the newly available synthetic hormones and a corresponding in increase in the requests for treatments occurred, although many were from homosexual and/or effeminate men and transvestites. Transsexualism was largely seen as an extreme form of transvestism and this subsequently became linked to the emerging accounts of the development of gender identity. Increasingly, transsexual individuals themselves described early experiences of a dissonance or split between their subjective sense of gender and their anatomical sex—the notion of being trapped in the wrong body and the corresponding demand for medical and surgical interventions to allow 'sex change'. The arguments that circulate around the body of the transsexual are the very same arguments that reveal the tensions in the sex-gender model: how much is biology, how much is culture, what is sexed subjectivity, and what are the ethical issues surrounding the individual's ownership of and right to change their own body? (Lewis 1995). In the majority of countries where sex reassignment surgical interventions are available, the mental health and competency of the person requesting sex change is a major focus of assessment and the psychiatrist or mental health professional acts as a gatekeeper for access to treatment. However, there is clear cultural variation in the understanding of gender diversity and the notion of sex change itself which further problematize the dominant model of gender identity in the West.

The study of non-Western cultures shows significant variation in models of sex roles and gender identity. In some cases, anatomical sex is not necessarily seen as a fixed biological given and is open to cultural interpretations, and there are several examples of cultural groups having more than two genders (Herdt 1994). In Western psychology, gender identity is generated primarily by sex assignment as male or female at birth. Mixed gender roles, ambivalent gender identity, or a gender identity that fluctuates over the life span are seen as problematic and usually as pathological. There is a need for unambiguous identity and considerable cultural anxiety around those who do not neatly fit into a binary gender model. Intersex infants, for example, with ambiguous genitalia have traditionally been treated as a medical emergency largely because of the social need to assign gender and the fear of poor developmental outcome if a child is not raised as one sex or the other from birth. Recent interest in 'brain sex' and the possible prenatal hormonal and neurodevelopmental basis of gender identity has again highlighted the nature/nurture debate, with some arguing that the assignment of sex to these children should be delayed until these biological contributions become apparent in sex typed behaviours and characteristics.

Acceptance and tolerance of sex change and gender role fluidity also varies considerably across cultures. The well know 'penis at 12' syndrome of the Dominican Republic, and found in some parts of Papua New Guinea and the South Pacific, is a culturally accepted phenomenon where children with ambiguous genitalia and a 5-alpha-reductase deficiency virilize at puberty, essentially changing from girls to boys. Even those raised clearly as girls appear to adapt to their new male role in an unproblematic way. The Hijras of India also pose a challenge to the Western model of gender and sex. This diverse group of hermaphrodites, ceremonially castrated men, and effeminate men constitute a recognized religious subculture and perform on ceremonial occasions. They exist within a Hindu tradition where deities are frequently sexually ambiguous or change sex. In the Tantric sect, for example, the supreme being is a hermaphrodite and male transvestism is used in religious devotions. Hinduism appears to allow for many sexual contradictions and ambiguities (Newman 2002).

In Western culture, the situation is somewhat different. Sexual ambiguity is less well tolerated and this has contributed to the development of an adversarial system in which the psychiatrist has become the gatekeeper and is seen by the transsexual as a barrier to surgical treatment. Some may not want to discuss psychological issues and may define their problem 'as medical, surgical, or hormonal', and see the mental health professional as unwanted intruder (Brown and Rounsley 1996). The current system where the psychiatrist provides opinions as to the suitability of individuals for medical and surgical intervention is essentially one which works to dissuade transsexuals from discussing concerns or psychological issues and in which they fear rejection. The surgical approval system also encourages gender conformity along traditional lines and encourages conformity of the new 'opposite' gender role.

Homosexuality and mental disorder

Similar essentialist *vs.* constructivist debates have surrounded the category of homosexuality and the debates in the history of psychiatry as to its status as a mental disorder. While same-sex sexual activity (homosexual behaviour) has been described since antiquity in many cultures, the notion of homosexual identity is a relatively recent phenomenon and reflects the attempts of psychoanalytic theory to account for the development variations in sexual identification. Early biological accounts around sexual orientation have historically confounded sex and gender with the implication that sexual object choice logically follows from normal development of gender role. Homosexuality was originally seen in medical accounts as a 'third sex' (Hirschfeld 1938) or a form of hermaphroditism leading to the trial of hormonal treatments—on males, the treatment involved unilateral castration followed by transplant of testicular tissue from a heterosexual male (Schmidt 1984).

Freud himself is widely known for his 'liberal' views and is quoted in a letter to the mother of a homosexual man as saying that he did not see homosexuality as a mental disorder per se (Freud 1951). The medicalization of the category of homosexuality occurred in the 19th century when the word homosexuality itself was first used to describe same-sex attraction and when this was seen as a sign of medical disorder as opposed to a moral failure. The early debates focused on the issue of whether homosexuality was inborn or acquired, but by the mid 20th century a plethora of medical approaches for the 'treatment' of homosexuality began to emerge, all with very little success. Behavioural psychology influenced the development of aversive techniques designed to reduce homosexual arousal to erotic stimuli, such as electrical aversive therapy (Feldman 1977), or the use of the drug apomorphine to induce nausea (McConaghy et al. 1972). These approaches not only make the assumption that homosexuality is a disease, but also that human sexual orientation is malleable even in adult life. More recently, psychological approaches have focused on the need to undo or 'repair' homosexual interest (Nicolosi 1991:615), and use psychotherapeutic techniques to reinforce traditional gender roles and to build an identification with a male role model. The underlying assumptions of the pathological nature of homosexuality and the confounding of sexual orientation with gender identity and gender role are clear, but less overt are the links between psychological theory and particular religious and moral approaches to sexual orientation conversion.

Psychoanalysis as a body of theory has been used to support reparative approaches and includes writers clearly seeing homosexuality as a personality disorder and those looking at the emergence of sexual orientation in terms of early relationships in the family and the way in which the child negotiates separation from the mother and development of identity.

During the 1950s, many psychoanalytic and psychological accounts of homosexuality expressed a clear view of inherent pathology: Albert Ellis (1965), for example, stated that—'Although I once believed that exclusive homosexuals are seriously neurotic...considerable experience...has convinced me that I was wrong: most fixed homosexuals, I am convinced, are borderline psychotic or outrightly psychotic' (Ellis 1965).

Ironically, Freud's original accounts of the development of gender identity and sexual identity were based on a view that sexuality was 'polymorphously perverse' or objectless (in infancy), and that sexual orientation was the outcome of a complex developmental process. Freud described the constitutional bisexuality of humans and the existence of homosexual desire as a normal part of psychosexual development. Much of the radical constructivist account of early Freud was questioned by later analysts with an investment in maintaining the diagnostic category of homosexuality and seeing the aim of psychoanalytic therapy as exclusively heterosexual orientation (Socarides 1978).

Research conducted on clinical samples of homosexual men was used to support the link between homosexuality and pathology, and this research bias was not challenged until Hooker (1957) compared non-clinical homosexual and heterosexual men and found no differences in psychological adjustment. The rise of the more critical approaches to the conceptualization of mental disorder such as the anti-psychiatry movement (Szasz 1961) was also significant in a move towards the removal of homosexuality as a mental disorder from the DSM system. The first edition of DSM had included homosexuality within a category of sexual deviation as a subset of sociopathic personality disturbance. Homosexuality was mentioned as an example of sexual deviation along with transvestism, fetishism, sadism, and paedophilia. The second edition of DSM in 1968 listed homosexuality separately as a sexual deviation under the category of personality disorders.

In 1973, the American Psychiatric Association (APA) adopted the well-known statement opposing discrimination against homosexuals and support of civil liberties:

> whereas homosexuality per se implies no impairment in judgment, stability reliability or general social or vocational capabilities, therefore, be it resolved the APA deplores all public and private discrimination against homosexuals in such areas as employment, housing, public accommodation, and licensing and declares that no burden of proof of such judgment, capacity or reliability shall be placed upon homosexuals greater than that imposed upon any other persons. Further the APA supports and urges the enactment of civil rights legislation at the local, state and federal level that would offer homosexual citizens the same protection now guaranteed to others on the base of race, creed, color etc. Further the APA supports and urges the repeal of all discriminatory legislation singling out homosexual acts by consenting adults in private (APA 1974).

Leading up to the acceptance of this resolution was a debate cutting near to the heart of psychiatry around the definition of mental disorder itself. Stoller (1973) argued that homosexuality did not itself constitute a disorder and that psychiatry's attitude towards homosexuals put the discipline in the role of an agent of social control (Stoller 1973). Spitzer (1973) stated that the definition of a mental disorder should include subjective distress and that the majority of homosexuals did not meet this criterion as they are happy with their sexual orientation. As a compromise to opposing views, a category of 'sexual orientation disturbance' was created to apply to homosexual individuals who were distressed by or wished to change their sexual orientation. In 1980, with the publication of DSM-III, the category of sexual orientation disturbance was renamed ego-dystonic homosexuality. This again proved controversial, with arguments put that it was inappropriate to include culturally-induced homophobia as a mental disorder—in other words, that the pathology lies in the negative and discriminatory attitudes towards homosexuals rather than with the individual. Others argued that it was clinically useful to describe the significant conflict over sexual orientation and subsequent distress that an individual could experience and which needed to be a focus of treatment and support. In the 1987 revision of DSM-III this category was removed, with the notion of 'persistent and marked distress about one's sexual orientation' remaining as an example of a sexual disorder not otherwise specified.

The rise of biological models and research into the aetiology of mental disorder also impacted on models of sexual orientation. Paradoxically, a purported biological basis for homosexuality has been used to argue for a tolerance and acceptance of biological diversity on the one hand, and for the need for medical interventions for abnormal biological condition, on the other.

Biological accounts of homosexual orientation have been used to advocate preventive 'treatment' including surgical and hormonal interventions. Durner et al. (1987), for example, hypothesize that the cause of homosexuality is an abnormal level of sex hormones during prenatal brain differentiation, and advocated altering foetal hormones as a preventive measure (Durner et al. 1987). The impact of the medicalization and pathologization of homosexuality has been profound with the inappropriate 'treatment' of thousands of individuals. For a review, see Cabaj and Stein (1996).

Gender dysphoria and the right to treatment

Regardless of the philosophical debates, individuals presenting with gender dysphoria experience considerable distress with potentially major impact on psychosocial function and mental health. The subjective experience of being 'in the wrong body' or of not having a coherent sense of self may be associated with depression, self harming behaviours, substance abuse, relationship difficulties, and social isolation. Discrimination and a sense of marginalization compound any individual difficulties. Some individuals experience genital aversion and an intense desire to change their anatomy. Reports of self surgery are not uncommon. Children with gender dysphoria may experience difficulties with peer relationships, academic performance and behaviour, and the experience of bullying and teasing. Many parents of a child with GID feel isolated and there are limited services and supports available for parents and families. There are also clear difficulties in access to support and mental health services and a view that mainstream services do not understand the experiences of gender-variant individuals.

The development of hormonal interventions, and advances in surgical techniques have created treatment possibilities, on the one hand, and a complex system of regulating access to treatment, on the other. International guidelines such as those of the Harry Benjamin International Gender Dysphoria Association (known as the Standards of Care) have emerged as guides to clinical practice including the assessment, diagnosis, and psychological support of individuals requesting intervention. The individual presenting with a request for medical intervention is required to live as the gender of their choice (the 'real life test') for a period of at least 12 months and their adaptation to the new role is monitored. Treatment then is monitored and staged and progresses from hormonal to surgical approaches. Critics point out that 'success' in this situation amounts to conformity to an opposite and narrowly defined gender stereotype and that this serves only to reinforce a notion of stable and fixed gender identity. In practice, individuals seeking interventions may be discouraged from discussing emotional issues and any difficulties in exploring a new identity through fear of 'not passing' the 'test' and being refused support. There are significant ethical dilemmas for clinicians when treatment is declined and the individual continues to see this as the solution to their predicament. Mental health services may not see the long-term support of individuals experiencing gender dysphoria as central to their role and may only provide crisis responses. In some ways, this can be seen as reinforcing behaviours such as self-harm and their emergency presentations as the individual has very limited options for support. Worldwide, the number of specialist gender identity clinics has declined and remaining services do not often provide comprehensive psychosocial and psychological interventions and supports for those not accepted onto surgical and other treatment programmes. The gender 'non-conformists' and those whose gender dysphoria is complicated by other mental health issues tend to be the marginalized of mental health approaches to GID, and are essentially denied intervention or a validation of their subjective experience.

The question of access to treatment and processes surrounding decision-making remains problematic. The individual requesting gender-change presents with a self-diagnosis intrinsic to their narrative account. In other words, there is an account of early-onset cross-gender identification and identity that is the normative account of 'primary transsexualism' that allows entry to treatment. Stories of identity confusion or ongoing questioning about gender wishes are not usually the ones told to the clinician where the clinical encounter is seen as a barrier to service access. This in effect invalidates the potential psychotherapeutic nature of an assessment of the individual's gender dysphoria, and creates an encounter based on an adversarial model and fundamental mistrust and dissimulation. There is a fundamental conflict where the clinician is at once the gatekeeper and the confidant or psychotherapist that may only be resolved by separation of those functions. The creation of a separate process of the regulation of access to treatment and separation of this from psychological support function might allow for a more meaningful discussion of the gender issues.

Policing gender and sex—the mental health professional

To what extent does contemporary psychiatric and mental health practice continue to reinforce particular ideologies of gender and sexuality? Certainly, debates around 'reparative therapies' for homosexuality are ongoing with a (usually religious) minority arguing on the basis of moral belief that the mental health disciplines should be involved in these approaches. Similarly, the view of gender non-conformity as related to mental disorder (at least in some cases) is discussed particularly in the literature relating to childhood trauma and abuse, where there is seen to be an association between early abuse and disruption and development of gender identity.

The debate around treatment of childhood GID also raises some of these issues. Childhood gender non-conformity is frequently anxiety-provoking for families and schools. The young child is often puzzled by the social response to their interests and not in a position to understand the 'rules' around gender behaviour and questions the seemingly arbitrary nature of the gender system. The clinician essentially faces a dilemma—to 'treat' to reduce the gender aberrant behaviour, or to explore and support development regardless of gender identity outcome? The sociocultural context and related belief system may influence the decision—a gender 'rigid' social system may find the gender 'disordered' child intolerable and demand conformity (Newman 2000), whilst in other situations ideas and practices around gender may allow for more flexibility. Conservative psychology advocates for behavioural approaches to the eradication of gender non-conforming behaviours in the face of evidence that behaviour modification has little impact on the child's sense of self and may, in fact, result in depression and low self-esteem. These practices are based on a view that there is a moral imperative to prevent the development of transsexuality and homosexuality if possible, and do not consider the broader context of social and cultural determinants of gendered behaviour. This then returns to the debate concerning the nature of gender identity itself and whether social reform and increasing tolerance of gender diversity will 'depathologize' the aberrant gender behaviour. The persistence of a diagnostic category of GID, in the absence of developmental and social context, reinforces psychiatry's role as a key regulatory body in a system of gender and sexuality and producer of specifically gendered and sexed subject (Butler 1990).

Spade comments that the diagnostic criteria for GID

> produces a fiction of natural gender in which normal, non-transsexual people grow up with minimal or no gender trouble or exploration . . . This story isn't believable but because medicine produces it not through a description of the norm, but through a generalized account of the transgression,

it establishes a surveillance and regulation effective for keeping both non–transsexuals and transsexuals in adherence to their roles. In order to get authorization for body alteration, this childhood must be produced, and the GID diagnosis accepted, maintaining an idea of two discrete gender categories that normally contain everybody but occasionally are wrongly assigned requiring correction to reestablish the norm (Spade 2006).

Supporting diversity and human rights

The right to self-determination of gender expression and sexuality are fundamental and reinforced in international conventions such as the International Covenant on Civil and Political Rights (1966) (Articles 2, 26). Despite this, persecution on the grounds of homosexuality or gender variant expression remains widespread and is recognized as a valid ground for seeking political asylum under the 1951 United Nations Convention Relating to the Status of Refugees and related 1967 Protocol. Denial of civil, political, social, and economic rights of homosexual and transgender people are common, with criminal sanctions, imprisonment, and death penalties operating in several countries. The right to health and mental health is at conflict with discriminatory policies and practices and the pathologization of these experiences. Within health systems this may be reflected in anxiety and negative attitudes amongst clinicians and health workers, lack of basic knowledge within health services, and a culture which assumes heterosexuality and gender normativity.

The real mental health needs of transgender people are simultaneously raised as a concern in psychiatric discourse and research and poorly responded to within medical services. Concerns about rates of depression and suicide, for example, are not met with specific services or training for mental health staff but are subsumed within an already burdened health system. Gaining 'cultural competency' in the needs of transgendered individuals is complex but underlies any moves toward an inclusive approach: 'Acknowledging the cognitive-conceptual limit for providers that creates barriers to health care for people with non-normative bodies does not excuse those providers from their ethical responsibility to grapple with their limits' (Singer 2006).

A shift toward an inclusive medical model involves a shift from a binary and polarized gender system to one that conceptualizes gender along a continuum of experiences and acknowledges individual autonomy and capacity to find, with support if needed, a place along that continuum to accommodate their subjective experience of gender. The concept of informed consent for gender-change procedures is perhaps more useful than the current approach of the meeting of standard criteria and allows for assessment of the individual's understanding and insight into their own gender position and supports self-determination. Moving toward a framework that accepts gender complexity in a non-pathologizing context is a challenge for current psychological and psychiatric theory, but one that is necessary for the protection of basic rights to gender and sexual expression.

References

American Psychiatric Association (1974) 'Position statement on homosexuality and civil rights', *American Journal of Psychiatry*, 131, 497.

American Psychiatric Association (1980) *Diagnostic and Statistical Manual of Mental Disorders*. 3rd edn. (*DSM-III*). Washington, DC: American Psychiatric Association.

Benjamin, H (1954) 'Transsexualism and transvsetism as psychosomatic and somato-psychic syndromes', *American Journal of Psychotherapy*, 8, 219–30.

Brown, ML and Rounsley, CA (1996) *True Selves: Understanding Transsexualism—For Families, Friends, Co-workers, and Helping Professionals*. San Francisco: Jossey-Bass.

Butler, J (1990) *Gender Trouble. Feminism and the Subversion of Identity*. New York: Routledge.

Cabaj, R and Stein,T (eds) (1996) *Textbook of Homosexuality and Mental Health*. Washington: American Psychiatric Press.

Dixen, JM, Maddever, H, Van Maasden, J et al. (1984) 'Psychosocial characteristics of applicants evaluated for surgical gender reassignment', *Archives of Sexual Behaviour*, 13, 269–77.

Durner, G, Gotz, F, Rohde, W et al. (1987) 'Sexual differentiation of gonadotrophin secretion, sexual orientation and gender role behaviour', *Journal of Steroid Biochemistry*, 27, 1081–87.

Ellis, A (1965) *Homosexuality: its causes and cure*. New York: Lyle Stuart.

Feldman, P (1977) 'Helping homosexuals with problems: a commentary and a personal view', *Journal of Homosexuality*, 2, 241–50.

Freud, S (1951) 'Historical notes: a letter from Freud (1935)', *American Journal of Psychiatry*, 107, 786–87.

Garber, M (1992) *Vested Interests*. New York: Routledge, Chapman and Hall.

Herdt, G (ed) (1994) *Third Sex. Third Gender: Beyond Sexual Dimorphism in Culture and History*. New York: Zone Books.

Hirschfeld, M (1938) *Sexual Anomalies and Perversion*. London: Encyclopaedic Press.

Hooker, EA (1957) 'The adjustment of the overt male homosexual', *Journal of Projective techniques*, 21, 17–31.

Kessler, S and McKenna, W (1978) *Gender: An Ethnomethodological Approach*. New York: John Wiley.

Lewis, F (1995) *Transsexualism in Society*. Melbourne: MacMillan.

McConaghy, N, Procter, D, and Barr, R (1972) 'Subjective and penile plethysmography responses to aversion therapy for homosexuality: a partial replication', *Archives of Sexual Behaviour*, 2, 65–78.

Newman, LK (2000) 'Transgender issues', in J Ussher (ed) *Women's health. Contemporary international perspectives*. London: British Psychological Society Books, 394–405.

Newman, LK (2002) 'Sex, gender and culture: issues in the definition, assessment and treatment of gender identity disorder', *Clinical Child Psychology and Psychiatry*, 7, 352–59.

Nicolosi, J (1991) *Reparative therapy of male homosexuality: a new clinical approach*. Northvale NJ: Jason Aronson.

Schmidt, G (1984) 'Allies and persecutors: science and medicine in the homosexuality issue', *Journal of Homosexuality*, 10(3–4), Winter, 127–40.

Seil, D (1996) 'Transsexuals. The boundaries of sexual identity and gender', in R Cabaj and T Stein (eds) *Textbook of Homosexuality and Mental Health*.Washington: American Psychiatric Press, 743–63.

Singer, TB (2006) 'From the medical gaze to Sublime Mutations. The Ethics of (Re)Viewing Non-normative Body Images', in S Stryker and S Whittle (eds) *The Transgender Studies Reader*, 616.

Socarides, C (1978) *Homosexuality*. New York: Jason Aronson.

Spade, D (2006) 'Mutilating Genders', in S Stryker and S Whittle (eds) *The Transgender Studies Reader*. New York: Routledge, 315–33.

Spitzer, RL (1973) 'A proposal about homosexuality and the American Psychiatric Association nomenclature: homosexuality as an irregular form of sexual behaviour and sexual orientation disturbance as a psychiatric disorder', *American Journal of Psychiatry*, 130, 1214–1216.

Steiner, BW (1985) 'Transsexuals, transvestites and their partners', in BW Steiner (ed) *Gender Dysphoria: Development, Research, Management*. New York: Plenum, 351–64.

Stoller, RJ (1973) 'Criteria for psychiatric diagnosis', *American Journal of Psychiatry*, 130, 1207–1209.

Szasz, TS (1961) *The Myth of Mental Illness*. New York: Harper and Row.

Usher, JM (1997) *Body Talk. The maternal and discursive regulation of sexuality, madness and reproduction*. London: Routledge.

Usher, JM (2006) *Managing the Monstrous Feminine*. London: Routledge.

Walker, PA, Berger, JC, Green, R et al. (1990) *Standards of Care: the hormonal and sex-reassignment of gender dysphoric persons*. Palo Alto, CA: Harry Benjamin International Gender Dysphoria Association.

Chapter 29

The Rights of Individuals Treated for Drug, Alcohol, and Tobacco Addiction

Adrian Carter and Wayne Hall

Introduction

Individuals with a drug addiction are a uniquely vulnerable and stigmatized group among persons with mental disorders. Unlike other mental disorders, the status of addiction, dependence, or substance use disorder[1] as a mental illness is hotly contested—by the public, politicians, and policy makers. The behaviours that define some types of addictions are criminal offences, such as the possession and distribution of proscribed substances (e.g. heroin, cocaine), and persons with a history of criminal convictions are more likely to become dependent on alcohol and illicit drugs. Addiction also has an enormous negative impact upon the health and welfare of the rest of society. Consequently, those dependent on drugs are often discriminated against as a result of their status as 'addicts' and/or criminals.

Policies towards those with an addiction are often motivated by a combination of strong moral disapproval of drug use and a need to protect society from the harmful behaviour of the minority who abuse drugs. The goal of treating a debilitating and chronic condition often receives a much lower priority. This can lead to discrimination and inappropriate restrictions on, or violation of, the rights of those with an addiction. It can also affect the type and quality of treatment offered to individuals with a substance use disorder and the manner in which it is provided.

Addiction, drug policy, and human rights

Drug addiction is the habitual or repeated use of an addictive substance, such as heroin, cocaine, amphetamines, cannabis, benzodiazepines, alcohol, and tobacco. Addiction usually begins as occasional or infrequent use of addictive drugs that becomes habitual in a small population of users. Individuals with a substance use disorder find their use of drugs difficult to control and continue to use drugs despite often wishing and attempting to stop, and despite the enormous harm that it causes to themselves, their friends and family, and the broader public.[2]

The chronic abuse of addictive drugs can cause serious physical harm, such as: fatal overdose or brain damage (e.g. with opiates, alcohol, and benzodiazepines); cancer (e.g. with nicotine and alcohol); infectious diseases from sharing injecting equipment (e.g. contraction of human immunodeficiency virus (HIV) and hepatitis C virus (HCV)); and accidents arising from

---

[1] Different terms to describe addiction have been used in the literature for a number of reasons. We will use these terms interchangeably.

[2] These features are codified in the diagnostic criteria for addiction, drug dependence, or substance use disorders, such as the Diagnostic and Statistical Manual for Mental Disorders, 4th ed. (DSM-IV) and the International Classification of Diseases, 10th ed. (ICD-10).

drug-intoxication (e.g. driving or operating heavy machinery while intoxicated) (Gerstein and Harwood 1990). Chronic drug use can also precipitate psychiatric symptoms such as psychosis, depression, and anxiety (e.g. with amphetamines, alcohol, and cannabis abuse) and produce significant cognitive deficits.

Addiction and drug abuse are also associated with a number of social harms that include: increased crime and violence (often to fund expensive drug habits); increased suicide and demand for mental health care; loss of employment and increased social welfare; family breakdown; and child abuse and neglect (Gerstein and Harwood 1990). All these harms lead to significant increases in disability, morbidity, and mortality that impose a substantial economic, as well as emotional, burden upon society (SAMSHA 2006).

Addictive disorders are often co-morbid with one or more other psychiatric conditions, such as depression, anxiety, personality disorders, and psychoses. Addictive drugs may be used to alleviate symptoms of these co-morbid disorders (e.g. self-medication), and psychiatric symptoms or disorders may result from the chronic use of addictive drugs (e.g. amphetamine- and cannabis-related psychoses).[3] Addiction is also a developmental disorder that gradually emerges over time as drug use worsens. This can make it difficult to distinguish between addictive drug use and the harmful abuse of drugs without addiction (e.g. harms arising from acute intoxication).[4] In reality, addictive disorders occur along a spectrum of problems that is correlated with a continuum from drug abuse to addictive drug use, and complicated by co-morbid psychiatric disorders.

In response to the harms caused by drug abuse and addiction, most nation states have criminalized some forms of drug use in order to deter non-users from using drugs and becoming addicted, to protect society from drug-related harm, and to punish those whose drug use harms others. These punitive policies include the prohibition of the possession, manufacture, and distribution of many addictive substances on pain of imprisonment (derogation of the right to liberty and freedom), forced addiction treatment with or without detention (derogation of the right to bodily integrity and consent), compulsory drug testing (derogation of the right to privacy), and child protection orders (derogation of the right to family).

Addiction is increasingly being recognized as a mental health disorder that requires treatment (Dackis and O'Brien 2005). Most developed and developing countries employ a range of medical or therapeutic approaches to minimize the harm that addiction and drug abuse cause to those who abuse them. Social policies towards drug use and addiction are therefore ambivalently motivated by competing aims: a punitive or judicial approach that aims to protect society and punish 'addicts'; and a therapeutic, often medical, approach that aims to treat and prevent addiction. Confusion about the aims and motivation of policies to deal with addictive behaviour—to treat a valid medical condition, or to punish criminal behaviour—can lead to inappropriate or unjustified violation of the human rights of those who are addicted.

Basic human rights for addicted individuals

Under human rights law, people with an addiction should be afforded the same rights as all other members of society: they should be treated equally and with dignity, irrespective of their age,

---

[3] Understanding whether drug use is a consequence or cause of other psychiatric conditions is a very active area of research. At present, research would suggest that the aetiology of addiction and a co-morbid mental illness can occur in both directions.

[4] Difficulty in making this distinction is part of the reason why the term addiction was dropped in favour of substance use disorder in the DSM-IV.

gender, ethnicity, or other status (Gilmore 1995; Gostin 2001).[5] Individuals suffering from an addiction cannot have their rights denied simply by virtue of being addicted. People with an addiction who are also involved in criminal activities should not be discriminated against by virtue of their status as criminals or as a result of their incarceration, other than the legal restrictions entailed in their punishment (United Nations General Assembly 1988). All prisoners are entitled to 'equivalence' in treatment, and to have access to the same medical health care that is available to the broader public.

Any restrictions on the rights of those addicted must be in accordance with the harm that their behaviour causes to others, and in line with restrictions imposed on someone else convicted of the same crime. Addicted individuals may have some rights derogated, such as: the right to freedom and liberty (e.g. when imprisoned after being convicted of a criminal offence); and some social and economic rights (e.g. removal of children into protective custody because of child abuse, or quarantining social welfare payments to ensure that the money is spent on children's education rather than the purchase of drugs). These derogations must also be protected by due process. Importantly, individuals with an addiction maintain a right to health that cannot be derogated under any circumstances, including imprisonment for a serious crime (Gostin 2001). To do so violates the most basic of human rights, and is an extreme form of extrajudicial punishment that is cruel and inhumane. A number of countries and multilateral agencies have produced charters and codes of ethics that explicitly outline what these human rights principles require of governments and their agencies (ANCD 2007; UNODC and WHO 2008; WHO 1995).

The validity of the restrictions and derogations of the rights of addicted individuals often depends upon balancing: (1) the rights of the individual to liberty and freedom; (2) the obligation of the drug dependent individual not to harm society; and (3) the state's obligation to protect other individuals' health, liberty, and freedom from harm caused by addictive drug use. Whether we think that particular drug policies inappropriately violate an individual's human rights will depend on whether we see addiction as a wilful and immoral act for which individuals with a substance use disorder should be made responsible, or as a mental illness requiring medical treatment. If we accept the latter, what is an effective and appropriate form of treatment for a condition where control over behaviour is impaired? How should this treatment be provided? We discuss these issues next.

The right to access to effective treatment of addiction

Many politicians, policy makers, and members of the public see addiction as a self-serving excuse for the abuse of recreational drugs (Szasz 1975; Davies 1997). Those who hold such views are often sceptical about whether addiction is a 'real' mental disorder. On this view, addiction and the choice to abuse drugs is a moral weakness: users choose to continue to use drugs despite the negative impact that consumption has on them or the rest of society. Addiction sceptics see punitive responses as the most appropriate way of deterring people from using illicit drugs and punishing those that break laws against using some drugs.

---

[5] This is formally recognized in the Universal Declaration of Human Rights, and codified in legally binding instruments such as the International Covenant of Civil and Political Rights (ICCPR) and the International Covenant of Economic, Social and Cultural Rights (ICESCR).With the Universal Nations Charter, these four documents comprise the International Bill of Rights, and are the primary source of all human rights law. Human rights are also protected by regional declarations in Europe, the Americas, Africa, Asia, and in Arab countries. See the General Introduction to this volume and references to particular standards and treaties in the Index.

Such sceptical views about addiction are inconsistent with a number of observable facts: (1) addiction is more likely to occur in people from socially disadvantaged groups or with a family history of drug problems; (2) addiction risk varies in ways that depend on which drugs are used and how they are administered (i.e. more common for short-acting drugs that are injected); (3) it is responsive to pharmacological treatment; and (4) has a significant genetic basis (Ball 2008). Punitive approaches to dealing with addiction have also been largely unsuccessful in reducing its incidence or the harm that it causes to drug dependent persons and others (Gerstein and Harwood 1990).

The case for medical treatment of addiction

In recent years, scepticism about addiction has been partially replaced by the view that addiction is, to some extent, a mental disorder that can be treated medically. This shift has largely occurred because of scientific evidence that many addictive phenomena arise from the effects of chronic drug use on the brain (Volkow and Li 2004).

Neuroimaging has identified changes in the brains of those addicted that neuroscientists argue explain drug craving and their *apparent* inability to refrain from drug use (Volkow and Li 2004). Chronic abuse of addictive drugs disrupts the central dopaminergic reward pathway that is thought to explain why individuals with a drug dependence focus their attention on drug use at the expense of all other activities. There is also significant dysfunction in the frontal cortical areas of the brains of addicted individuals—regions of the brain that are responsible for the regulation and control of behaviour (Volkow and Li 2004). These changes appear to underlie the intense cravings that are such a potent motivator of drug use and trigger of relapse in addiction, and that makes impulses to use drugs more difficult to resist.

Twin and adoption studies indicate that there is a substantial genetic contribution to vulnerability to addiction to alcohol, nicotine, and other drugs (Ball 2008). Neuroscience research suggests that genetic vulnerability to addiction may reflect variations in the way that drugs of dependence are metabolized or in the effects that drugs have on neurotransmitters in key brain regions involved in reward, motivation, and decision-making (Ball 2008).

Neuroscience research thus supports the idea that chronic use of addictive drugs produces changes in the brains of addicted persons that reduces their ability to control their drug use. It has led to the view that addiction is a 'chronic, relapsing brain disease' (Volkow and Li 2004). While the brain disease model of addiction is not without concerns, which we will discuss below, the confluence of scientific evidence and clinical observation suggests that the right to health obliges nation states to provide access to the most effective and safest forms of addiction treatment that they can afford.

Effective treatment of addiction

The stigma attached to addiction has meant that sufferers in many developing and some developed countries have been denied access to effective treatment. People who hold moral or sceptical views of addiction often believe that abstinence from all drugs is the only appropriate goal of treatment and that this can be achieved by coercing drug users to become abstinent. Research suggests that this expectation is unrealistic because most people addicted to drugs will relapse to drug use without pharmacological and psychosocial support (Gerstein and Harwood 1990).

Addiction sceptics often oppose addiction treatments that involve replacing a drug of dependence with less harmful drugs that produce similar (although not identical) effects to the drug of dependence in controlled, supervised doses of known strength and purity (e.g. agonist or partial agonist treatment using methadone or buprenorphine). These treatments are known as drug substitution, replacement, or maintenance treatments of addiction. Their aim is to stabilize the behaviour of addicted individuals and reduce the harm that their drug use causes while encouraging them to use psychological counselling and social support. These treatments also yield significant reductions in the social harm and public health costs associated with addiction (e.g. reduced crime and violence), a fact which is often used to garner public support for them.

The most well known form of maintenance therapy is methadone maintenance therapy (MMT) (Ward et al. 1998). Despite good evidence of the effectiveness of MMT, some countries have denied addicted individuals access to this form of treatment by banning its use (e.g. Russia and Malaysia). Drug dependent individuals in many of these countries have minimal access to a limited range of less effective treatments, exposing them to greater harm from their continued use of illicit drugs. In the case of opiate addiction, those who relapse to opiate use following a period of abstinence (whether voluntary or enforced) are at significant risk of overdose if they use their usual doses of the drug (Darke and Hall 2003). Failure to provide addicted individuals with more effective forms of medical treatment is arguably a denial of their right to health, and indeed life in the case of fatal overdose.

When agonist substitution treatments are allowed, a punitive attitude by treatment staff can still mean that these treatments are operated in ways that impair addicted individuals' right to health. Treatment centres in countries such as China, Viet Nam, and Lao PDR often resemble work camps, where patients are treated under compulsory orders and made to work in order to pay for their 'treatment'.

The size of the dose of methadone provided to individuals in MMT is another example (Ward et al. 1998). The dose needs to be high enough to reduce the symptoms of withdrawal and cravings, but not so high that it harms the individual, or can be diverted to the black market. An inadequate dose will often cause many individuals to return to illicit drug use to alleviate the symptoms of withdrawal and craving. The dose may also be reduced in order to punish sufferers for non-compliance with programme rules. This is often counterproductive in that it leads to expulsion from the programme and a return to illicit drug use, increasing risk to the individual and society. Continued illicit drug use during MMT is better seen as a signal that the dose is not high enough and needs to be increased.

The right to access harm reduction measures

An addicted individual's right to health also includes access to measures that enable them to reduce harms caused by their drug use (Elliott et al. 2005). For example, needle exchange programmes offer clean needles to injecting drug users to reduce sharing of contaminated equipment and hence infection with blood borne viruses, such as HIV and HCV.

Opponents of needle exchange programmes argue that these programmes implicitly condone the injection of illicit drugs. However, epidemiological studies of these programmes have shown that they have no effect on levels of injecting drug use (Elliott et al. 2005). These arguments also ignore the fact that people with an addiction find it difficult to abstain from drug use. Given that continued drug use is expected, failure to provide relatively cheap harm reduction programmes such as needle exchange denies addicted drug users their right to health, and in the case of HIV, life. These programmes have recently been supported by the United Nations and the World Health Organization (UNODC 2006; UNODC and WHO 2008). Access to these programmes has gradually expanded, even in countries with more punitive policies towards drug addiction (e.g. South-East Asia) although, all too often, only as small scale 'pilot' programmes.

The right to effective medical treatment for other medical conditions

The rights of addicted individuals to equal access to effective medical treatment is most often advocated for the treatment of HIV/AIDS: the right to equal access to antiretroviral drugs (ARVs).

In many countries, such as in Asia and the former Soviet Union, injecting drug users (IDUs), who make up the majority of HIV positive cases, are much less likely to receive ARVs (Wolfe 2007). While access to ARVs for HIV-positive IDUs is increasing via the Global Fund (<http://www. theglobalfund.org/en/>) and similar initiatives (e.g. in Viet Nam and China), access for HIV infected drug users is still limited in many high need areas.

A common reason used to justify the failure to treat HIV in IDUs is that they will not adhere to ARV treatments, allowing the virus to develop viral resistance (WHO 2006). However, research has consistently found no difference between IDU and non-IDU populations in compliance with ARV treatment, particularly when it is provided in conjunction with substitution treatment (Wolfe 2007).

HIV treatment programmes often discourage IDUs from seeking or remaining in treatment by policies that require them to pay for their medication or hospitalization, have their name recorded in government registries which may be subsequently used to discriminate against them (e.g. denial of employment), or submit to drug tests with the threat of criminal prosecution for a positive test. Inequity in access may also result from structural inadequacies within the health system: many AIDS clinics will refuse to treat current IDUs, and few substance abuse clinics provide HIV treatment. This is a denial of the right to health and poor public health policy that increases HIV infection rates among the general population (WHO 2006).

The use of unevaluated, invasive, and risky treatments of addiction

Neuroscience research on addiction has yielded a number of novel medical technologies that could be used to treat and, purportedly, cure addiction. Some of these are invasive, costly, and can cause significant harm to the patient.

Ultra-rapid detoxification (UROD) was a radical treatment promoted to opioid dependent individuals as a 'cure' for opioid addiction. UROD was based on the belief that opioid addiction was the result of the state of the addicted individual's opioid receptors. It involved the use of an opioid antagonist (naltrexone) to flush out all exogenous opioids from the brain, while under general anaesthesia for 24–48 hours. It was expensive and required intubation of the patient in an intensive care unit. Several deaths were recorded during treatment, and when clinical trials were conducted, most patients relapsed to heroin use with an increased risk of fatal overdose when they did so. More recently, clinicians in China and Russia have used neurosurgery to 'treat' addiction (Hall 2006). These invasive and risky treatments were performed without proper evaluation of their safety or efficacy, or any systematic effort to identify any adverse side-effects of the treatment.

The premature use of these technologies is often justified by appealing to neurobiological models of addiction. Proponents employ simplistic, yet plausible misrepresentations of the neurobiology of addiction to suggest that it is simply the result of a 'diseased organ' (in the case of neurosurgery) or a 'neurochemical imbalance' (for UROD) that the treatment will correct. This gives patients and families a dangerously unrealistic expectation of the effectiveness of the treatment and their ability to remain abstinent, with potentially fatal consequences.

Individuals with an addiction and their families are extremely vulnerable: they are often marginalized within society and desperate for a cure. The use and promotion of potentially dangerous and highly invasive neurological treatments without evidence of their safety and efficacy obtained from properly conducted clinical trials denies sufferers of addiction the right to safe and effective healthcare. Individuals with a substance use disorder have the right to treatments that have been assessed for their safety and efficacy as would be expected for any other disorder.

Respecting human rights when treating under legal coercion

A persistent problem in the treatment of addiction is attracting sufferers into and retaining them in treatment. One response has been to use the coercive power of the state to force individuals with an addiction into treatment (e.g. by threatening them with imprisonment if they do not comply). Coerced treatment of addiction is most often justified on the grounds of protecting the public by reducing the harms caused by drug use. However, the chronic, relapsing brain disease model of addiction may increase the use of treatment under coercion to prevent individuals from harming themselves. Forced treatment of addiction to prevent individuals from harming themselves would need to demonstrate that the individual in question is unable to choose not to use drugs, or in some other way cognitively impaired, so as to undermine their autonomy, either as a result of chronic drug use, or a co-morbid psychiatric disorder.

Some bioethicists have used neuroscience research to argue that drug dependent individuals lack the autonomous decision-making capacity to refrain from using drugs; they are driven to use drugs by the state of their neurotransmitters and so their choices are not their own (Caplan 2006). They argue that, as dependent persons are unable to refrain from using drugs, the state should, and is in fact obligated to, treat them 'for their own good'.

Proponents of this paternalistic policy understate the capacity that many with an addiction have to refrain from using drugs. Many drug dependent individuals manage to quit drug use without assistance, while others quit for periods to deal with life changes (e.g. birth of a child), to take a break from the rigours of the drug lifestyle or to reduce physical or psychological harm, or to lower tolerance so as to get a 'bigger hit' (Gerstein and Harwood 1990).

Neuroscientific research has shown how the chronic abuse of drugs can produce long-lasting neuroadaptations in the brain that can affect the ability to choose not to use drugs. This provides a stronger argument that addiction is, to some degree, a neuropsychiatric condition in need of treatment. This research does not, however, show that addicted individuals lack *any* ability to refrain from using drugs. Both neuroscience and social science show that *most* addicted individuals retain *some* autonomous decision-making capacity in regards to drug use (see Carter and Hall (2008) for a review).

Coerced treatment involves a derogation of a number of human rights, including the right to liberty and freedom and to bodily integrity (Gilmore 1995). Given that addiction, as a rule, does not override autonomy, the state is not justified in detaining and forcing individuals into treatment simply by virtue of the fact that they are addicted (often referred to as *compulsory treatment*). Coerced treatment may be justified if offered in response to harm caused by the addicted individual to others (e.g. theft, child neglect), or when it is offered as an alternative to imprisonment or removal of child into custody, if the addicted person refuses or fails to comply with the treatment (referred to as *legally coerced treatment*). In the latter case, the addicted individual is able to refuse treatment, but would have to suffer the same punishment as anyone adjudged to be responsible for the offence for which they have been convicted. It is important that, where coerced treatment is used, individuals are offered the choice of treatment from a range of effective treatments (Porter, Arif, and Curran 1986).

Human rights in the treatment of addiction in prisons

The treatment of addiction and injecting drug use within prisons is an area in which the respect for the rights of addicted individuals has been inadequate (Jurgens and Betteridge 2005). Few prisons in developed or developing nations provide effective treatment for addiction. When addicted individuals enter prison, they more often than not receive little or no treatment for their condition. Consequently, many are forced to undergo unsupervised detoxification, or 'cold turkey'. This can produce severe withdrawal symptoms, including nausea and diarrhoea, convulsions, anxiety, and dysphoria. It may also have serious medical consequences, particularly for pregnant women and their foetuses, immuno-compromised individuals (common amongst intravenous drug users), and those with co-morbid medical disorders (e.g. depression), potentially increasing the risk of suicide (Fiscella et al. 2005).

Very few prisons operate drug substitution programmes. Consequently, many individuals stabilized on methadone or buprenorphine maintenance treatment prior to entering prison are also forced to go through detoxification and withdrawal. This amounts to a violation of the right not to be subjected to cruel and inhumane punishment. Forced detoxification would be unacceptable in the wider community, and should not be accepted as part of prisoners' punishment. Given that the freedom and liberty of prisoners are restricted by the state, they are unable to take action themselves to prevent symptoms of withdrawal. This increases the burden upon the state to ensure that these symptoms are properly treated.

The lack of adequate addiction treatment can lead to the use of drugs within prison, increasing the risks of drug overdose, and HIV and HCV infection. The human rights claims for this failure would be significant for someone on a legitimate and widely accepted treatment programme prior to incarceration, such as methadone maintenance, who contracted HIV after injecting drugs in prison. '[B]y entering prisons, prisoners are condemned to imprisonment for their crimes; they should not be condemned to HIV and AIDS.' (United Nations Commission on Human Rights (UNCHR) 1996). Forced detoxification can also lead to overdose if individuals with no opioid tolerance relapse to opioid use in prison or upon release, as many often do (Kariminia et al. 2007).

Few prisons provide access to sterile injecting equipment for IDUs. This is despite high rates of HIV (10–20 per cent) and HCV (30–40 per cent) infection occurring in prisons (Jurgens and Betteridge 2005). Approximately a third of prisoners report injecting drugs while incarcerated and a high proportion share injecting equipment. These individuals are at a very high risk of contracting HIV or HCV. Failure to provide prisoners with the means to avoid these diseases arguably denies them access to health measures available to the rest of society, violating the 'principle of equivalence' and the right to health (UNAIDS 2006).

Human rights in the treatment of pregnant women

Substance abuse during pregnancy is a significant problem. In the US, almost 5 per cent of pregnant women under the age of 44 have abused illicit drugs in the last month, 10 per cent have abused alcohol, and up to 18 per cent of pregnant women are smokers (SAMSHA 2006). Substance abuse during pregnancy can have adverse effects on both the mother and the developing foetus, and may increase the risk of medical complications during birth (Campbell and Fleischman 1992). Individuals born to substance-using mothers often suffer from significant structural brain abnormalities (e.g. significant neuronal loss and smaller brains) and lifelong cognitive and behavioural deficits for the abuse of drugs such as alcohol (e.g. foetal alcohol syndrome), cocaine, and methamphetamine (Campbell and Fleischman 1992).

The treatment of substance abuse or addiction during pregnancy raises the challenging ethical issue of balancing the interests of the foetus and the freedom of the mother. Society often imposes limits on the autonomy of individuals when their behaviour impacts on the rights of others, such as overriding a competent patient's refusal of treatment to prevent the spread of an infectious disease. However, the case of overriding the autonomy of drug abusing pregnant mothers to protect the foetus from harm is complicated by the uniquely interdependent relationship between the mother and foetus, and the uncertain legal status of the foetus.

There are two arguments against state-sanctioned coercive treatment and detention of pregnant mothers: (1) the stress and anxiety associated with forced detention or medical intervention, or the experience of intense withdrawal symptoms, can have serious adverse effects on the mother and foetus; and (2) the threat of compulsory treatment programmes may deter women from presenting themselves early for prenatal care and pre-term health checks in order to avoid compulsory detention or intervention (Ridgely et al. 2004). Both of these outcomes would adversely affect the health and welfare of the child and mother in ways that may offset any benefits of coerced treatment.

Increasing access to addiction treatment for consenting addicted mothers is a preferable option. Given the potential harms from enforced addiction treatment for pregnant women, treatment programmes should rely on less restrictive and coercive forms of treatment that do not override the mother's autonomy. This may involve improving engagement with clinicians and education, reinforcing abstinence using vouchers, offers of free prophylactic support to prevent relapse, less punitive responses to positive drug tests, and offers of effective and safe substitution treatments (Ward et al. 1998).

Future challenges for human rights practitioners

A contentious issue in drug policy is whether a respect for human rights entails the decriminalization of currently illicit drugs for adult use. Some have produced cogent arguments for doing so (Husak 1992). The major problem is that international covenants on human rights are overridden by international drug control treaties that most states have also signed. These prohibit the legalization of the production, sale, and use of proscribed drugs such as amphetamines, cannabis, cocaine, and heroin. These treaties have strong support from the international community and from public opinion in most developed countries. Any country that decided to establish legal markets for these drugs would need to renounce or ignore these international treaties and bear the strong international disapproval that would follow either action.

There are significant social factors that contribute to addiction. These include: coming from a lower socio-economic background; early exposure to drug use in the family and among peers; a family history of drug abuse; and lack of access to quality education. Social policies that address these issues can have a significant impact on the incidence and burden of drug use and addiction (Spooner et al. 2001). The role of co-morbid psychiatric disorders, such as personality disorders, in the development of addiction is another area that requires grater attention (Chambers 2008). Better diagnosis, treatment, and early intervention is urgently required. Imprisonment of individuals for illicit drug use to deal with an inadequately treated psychiatric disorder could be argued to be an inappropriate derogation of the right to freedom and a denial of the right to health. There is significant debate in the human rights literature, however, as to how, if at all, human rights law can contribute to social policies that address social and structural disadvantage. This is a large topic that is beyond the scope of the present chapter (see Spooner et al. (2001) for further discussion).

Conclusions

Rights in the treatment of addiction, particularly within criminal populations, have been largely ignored by most nation states, despite clear UN and WHO guidelines. Given that those with a substance use disorder are marginalized within society and suffering from a condition which impinges on their ability to access proper treatment, there is arguably a greater burden on society to ensure that those addicted are able to access effective medical treatment.

The right to health requires that addicted individuals have access to the most effective forms of addiction treatment available, where treatment is motivated by an intention to treat a neuropsychiatric disorder, rather than a form of extrajudicial punishment. When the behaviour of addicted individuals causes harm to society, they should be treated the same as other individuals who commit such acts. Those incarcerated should be given access to effective addiction treatments, such as MMT, as well as other harm reduction measures (e.g. needle exchange programmes). Where coercion is used, it must be done in a way that does not unduly deny the right to liberty and freedom. The right to effective health care should not be denied simply by virtue of their status as a criminal or an 'addict'. Human rights law would suggest that the treatment of addiction be recognized as a health issue, and not simply a criminal justice one.

References

ANCD (2007) *The Australian alcohol and other drugs charter*. Canberra: Australian National Council on Drugs.

Ball, D (2008) 'Addiction science and its genetics', *Addiction,* 103, 360–7.

Campbell, DE and Fleischman, AR (1992) 'Ethical challenges in medical care for the pregnant substance abuser', *Clinical Obstetrics and Gynaecology*, 35, 803–12.

Caplan, A (2006) 'Ethical issues surrounding forced, mandated, or coerced treatment', *Journal of Substance Abuse Treatment*, 31, 117–29.

Carter, A and Hall, W (2008) 'Informed consent to opioid agonist maintenance treatment: Recommended ethical guidelines', *International Journal of Drug Policy*, 19, 79–89.

Chambers, RA (2008) 'Impulsivity, dual diagnosis, and the structure of motivated behavior in addiction', *Behavioral and Brain Sciences*, 31, 443–44.

Dackis, C and O'Brien, C (2005) 'Neurobiology of addiction: Treatment and public policy ramifications', *Nature Neuroscience*, 8, 1431–36.

Darke, S and Hall, W (2003) 'Heroin overdose: Research and evidence-based intervention', *Journal of Urban Health*, 80, 189–200.

Davies, JB (1997) *The myth of addiction*. Amsterdam: Harwood Academic Publishers.

Elliott, R, Csete, J, Wood, E, and Kerr, T (2005) 'Harm reduction, HIV/AIDS, and the human rights challenge to global drug control policy', *Health and Human Rights*, 8, 104–38.

Fiscella, K, Moore, A, Engerman, J, and Meldrum, S (2005) 'Management of opiate detoxification in jails', *Journal of Addictive Diseases*, 24, 61–71.

Gerstein, DR and Harwood, HJ (1990) *Treating drug problems (vol 1). A study of effectiveness and financing of public and private drug treatment systems*. Washington DC: Institute of Medicine, National Academy Press.

Gilmore, N (1995) 'Drug use and human rights: Privacy, vulnerability, disability and human rights infringements', *Journal of Contemporary Health Law and Policy*, 12, 355–447.

Gostin, LO (2001) 'Beyond moral claims: A human rights approach in mental health', *Cambridge Quarterly of Healthcare Ethics*, 10, 264–74.

Hall, W (2000) 'UROD: An antipodean therapeutic enthusiasm', *Addiction*, 95, 1765–6.

Hall, W and Carter, L (2004) 'Ethical issues in using a cocaine vaccine to treat and prevent cocaine abuse and dependence', *Journal of Medical Ethics*, 30, 337–40.

Hall, W (2006) 'Stereotactic neurosurgical treatment of addiction: Minimizing the chances of another "great and desperate cure"', *Addiction*, 101, 1–3.

Husak, DN (1992) *Drugs and rights*. Cambridge, England: Cambridge University Press.

Jurgens, R and Betteridge, G (2005) 'Prisoners who inject drugs: Public health and human rights imperatives', *Health and Human Rights*, 8, 46–74.

Kariminia, A, Law, MG, Butler, TG, et al. (2007) 'Suicide risk among recently released prisoners in New South Wales, Australia', *Medical Journal of Australia*, 187, 387–90.

Porter, L, Arif, A, and Curran, WJ (1986) *The law and the treatment of drug- and alcohol-dependent persons: A comparative study of existing legislation*. Geneva: WHO.

Ridgely, M, Iguchi, M, and Chiesa, J 2004) 'The use of immunotherapies and sustained-release formulations in the treatment of drug addiction: Will current law support coercion?', in HJ Harwood and TG Myers (eds) *New treatments for addiction: Behavioral, ethical, legal, and social questions*. Washington, DC: National Academies Press, 173–87.

SAMSHA (2006) *Results from the 2005 National Survey on Drugs Use and Health: National findings*. Rockville, MD: Substance Abuse and Mental Health Services Administration.

Spooner, C, Lynskey, M, and Hall, W (2001) *Structural determinants of youth drug use*. Canberra: Australian National Council on Drugs.

Szasz, TS (1975) *Ceremonial chemistry: The ritual persecution of drugs, addicts, and pushers*. London: Routledge.

UNAIDS (2006) *International guidelines on HIV/AIDS and human rights (consolidated version)*. Geneva: Office of the United Nations High Commissioner for Human Rights and the Joint United Nations Program on HIV/AIDS.

UNCHR (1996) *Fifty-second Session, Item 8 of the agenda. HIV/AIDS in prisons, statement by the joint United Nations programme on HIV/AIDS*. Strasbourg: UNAIDS.

UNODC (2006) *HIV/AIDS and custodial settings in South East Asia: An exploratory review into the issue of HIV/AIDS and custodial settings in Cambodia, China, Lao PDR, Myanmar, Thailand and Viet Nam*. Thailand: United Nations Office on Drugs and Crime.

UNODC and WHO (2008) *Principles of drug dependence treatment*. Vienna: United Nations Office on Drugs and Crime.

United Nations General Assembly (1988) *Body of principles for the protection of all persons under any form of detention or imprisonment, adopted by general assembly resolution 43/173 of December, 9, 1988*. Geneva: United Nations High Commissioner for Human Rights.

Volkow, ND and Li, TK (2004) 'Drug addiction: The neurobiology of behaviour gone awry', *Nature Reviews Neuroscience*, 5, 963–70.

Ward, J, Mattick, RP, and Hall, W (1998) *Methadone maintenance treatment and other opioid replacement therapies*. Sydney: Harwood Academic Press.

WHO (1995) *European charter on alcohol*. Copenhagen: WHO Regional Office for Europe.

WHO (2006) *HIV/AIDS treatment and care for injecting drug users: Clinical protocol for the WHO European region*. Copenhagen: WHO Regional Office for Europe.

Wolfe, D (2007) 'Paradoxes in antiretroviral treatment for injecting drug users: Access, adherence and structural barriers in Asia and the former Soviet Union', *International Journal of Drug Policy*, 18, 246–54.

Commentary 6

The Veil of Silence

Human Rights and Suicide

Lakshmi Viijayakumar and Lillian Craig Harris

Three young Indian girls hanged themselves after writing the following note to their parents:

'Dear Mom and Dad,

Please forgive us for doing this. We curse the fate which gave you only daughters and no son. Why is the world so unfair? We do not want to burden you. We are not earning and we do not have money to be married. We feel bad to see you both worried, anxious and know that you are desperate to get us married. You have treated us with love and we have given you only misery. We have been good children as you have taught us, but the world wants money and not goodness. We will repay all your love and care in our next lives. We hope at least one of us will be a son for you.
Mallika, Devi and Swarna'

The size of the problem

It is evident that one need not be mentally ill to be suicidal. Although mental illness is a factor in many suicides, there are many other conducive situations—as illustrated by the above sad statement by three young women—in which cultural, economic, religious, and other factors play a role. The World Health Organization estimates that between 850,000 and one million people die by suicide every year and more people are lost annually by suicide than because of war (WHO 2001). In persons between the ages of 15–34 suicide is officially regarded as the third leading cause of death. However, this is certainly a gross underestimate, as for roughly half the countries (47 per cent) and more than one quarter of the world population (27 per cent), there are no data on suicide (Vijayakumar et al. 2005). There remain large geographical areas, particularly in Asia and Africa, where the toll of annual death by suicide remains completely unknown. Developing countries are said to contribute 73 per cent of suicides and even that is an underestimate due to a variety of factors such as unreliable population count, inefficient civil registration systems, and non-reporting of deaths, including the non-reporting of suicides due to legal and social consequences (Joseph et al. 2003).

In some countries, attempted suicide is a punishable offence. If the purpose of the law was to prevent suicide by legal methods it is counter productive. Emergency care to those who have attempted suicide is denied as many hospitals and practitioners hesitate to provide the needed treatment since they are fearful of the legal repercussions. The actual data on attempted suicide becomes difficult to ascertain as many attempts are assigned as accidental to avoid entanglement with police and courts (Leenaars 2003).

Each one of these deaths is of a suffering individual who felt her or his life no longer worth living—and many of them were pushed by seemingly hopeless circumstances including having mental or physical illness. Despite the enormity of the problem, there is a lack of awareness about the various psychological, social, and cultural factors associated with suicide and of the urgent need for intervention. Moreover, the insidious chain of human rights violations which are likely to occur along the path to suicide is often ignored.

There are many reasons for rising national and international suicide rates. These include, apart from the various risk and protective factors, the lack of public awareness of the signs of suicidal intention, lack of mental health services for those at risk, and cultural preconditioning or acceptance of suicide as a 'natural' phenomenon. There is also concern that even the thought that suicide is an individual right in which others ought not to interfere has diverted attention from the multitude of people who suffer social ostracism, cultural pressures, and health, including mental health, circumstances which eventually lead them to take their own lives.

For these reasons, although discussion of euthanasia—or assisted suicide with consent of the one to die as it is sometimes called—is an important topic, we shall not discuss it here other than to say that the phenomenon seems to us more a religious violation for some people and more a legal issue for others. To deny an individual the right to end his or her life of terminal and painful illness which will impoverish his family seems itself to border on a human rights violation. There is much to discuss in this area of concern but our focus is on a much more widespread phenomenon: the suffering of millions of individuals who may or may not be terminally ill but all of whom face stigmatization and violation of their rights which can eventually result in death by their own hands.

We are not so naïve as to hope that all suffering can or even should be abolished. Indeed pain and suffering can be signals of need for individual growth and change of direction. Rather, we hope to focus on those millions of people in every culture and on every continent whose humanity has been discounted in a variety of ways so that eventually they take refuge in death by suicide.

Human ambivalence towards suicide

Both national and individual beliefs and attitudes towards suicide are complicated. Because suicide can be regarded as either noble or abominable depending on the circumstances, ambivalence towards suicide is in our international and national heritages. All depends on the circumstances and suicide can be depicted as craven cowardice and utterly sinful or as entirely praiseworthy and in accordance with 'God's will'. Adulation of suicide was seen in the official Japanese use of Kamikaze pilots during World War Two and in the response by the British public to the suicidal charge of the Light Brigade at Balaclava during the Crimean War. Modern recurrence of hero worship for those who kill themselves for a cause is evident in homage paid to Muslim terrorists who destroy themselves to draw attention to their historical and political grievances. But in all cultures 'noble suicides'—as occur as self sacrifice in battle or in saving a drowning child—are acceptable and even to be lauded for they are seen as patriotic and/or public service.

On the contrary, suicides for reasons of despair, illness, financial ruin, or other personal causes are generally labelled shameful and morally wrong. For millions of people this second, seemingly self centred rather than society centred, suicide is stigmatized as cowardly, sinful, and repugnant. Not only are suicidal people labelled, they are also treated as outlaws and even as though they were psychologically contagious. Attempters may be given delayed or inadequate care in hospitals or denounced as time wasters. In some situations family members of the person who has committed or attempted suicide may also be stigmatized, avoided, and criticized. Historically, unhappy Chinese women killed themselves by jumping into a well, their deaths serving not only to pollute the water supply but to shame and stigmatize the family into which they had been unhappily married. Moreover, maintenance of one's 'good name' has always been important in all societies and in historical China, according to American sinologist John Fairbank, 'People whose reputations had been blackened could redeem themselves by suicide.' (Fairbank 1994).

Around the world modern families are not infrequently branded by the phenomenon of suicide and their members shunned or even prevented from receiving the social support which other bereaved families expect and receive. Such treatment naturally enhances the possibility of additional suicidal risk. Moreover, people with both mental illness and suicide in their families face double jeopardy. Few parents wish for their children to marry into such seemingly dangerous and wounded families. In public opinion, therefore, suicide becomes an apparently contagious act.

The stigma of suicide

To be stigmatized is to be treated disdainfully and differently from the way in which 'normal' people are treated. According to the Mental Health Services Director of the US Substance Abuse and Mental Health Services Administration, disrespect is at the core of stigmatization and therefore 'Stigma deters individuals from seeking the care they need and deters the public from wanting to pay for that care.' (Kankiewiez 2007). Sadly it is possible that social alienation of those who suffer from suicidal inclinations due to their psychological or physical conditions or circumstances may be stimulated to attempt suicide.

Those working with the despairing and suicidal often encounter individuals whose fear, self loathing, and/or anger are intense due to their perception that they have been labelled as 'hopeless nut cases', 'time wasters', and 'chronic complainers'. Can there be any greater disrespect than to have one's humanity discounted?

To understand the dangers connected to stigmatization it is necessary to look at the broad range of those who are stigmatized and thus potentially put at greater suicidal risk. Among them are the poor, the mentally ill, the handicapped, the imprisoned, the sexually abused and sex workers, the addicted, refugees, migrants, and minority religious groups. We also tend to stigmatize people who are trapped in unpleasant situations and therefore stigma often attaches to those who are or have been imprisoned, those who are being bullied, women in forced marriages or who are the victims of domestic violence, and the members of oppressive religious movements whose members not infrequently turn to suicide. Moreover, many people carry more than one stigma, just as one violation of a person's human rights often leads to another. There is as well the crippling shame and guilt which attaches to those who have lost someone to suicide and, in turn, increases the risk of suicide.

The results of stigmatization can be appalling violation of human rights. Authorities, for example, often treat refugees as guilty until they are proven worthy. Not infrequently people who have attempted suicide are stigmatized for life. Inadequate support or help may be given to depressed and/or violent persons. Because suicide is, tragically, sometimes an attempt to regain self control, it is a tribute to the human spirit that more people do not attempt.

Areas of particular vulnerability and concern

Worldwide, there are 10 million refugees and asylum seekers. The majority of them live in developing countries. Genocide, war, imprisonment, violence, and crime are often the reasons why millions become refugees or internally displaced. These are also the circumstances where gross violations of human rights occur. Post-relocation difficulties like discrimination, detention, destitution, delayed decision on refugee status and denial of work, and health are also grave human rights issues. Hence it is not surprising that the prevalence of suicidal behaviour is high (3.4 to 34 per cent) among refugees (Vijayakumar and Jotheeswaran 2010). There are many other areas where suicide and human rights are intertwined but we focus here on a few of particular concern.

Suicide in prisons

Suicide is the leading cause of death in prisons in most Western countries (Paton and Jenkins 2005). Unfortunately there is a scarcity of data from other countries. Studies also reveal high levels of mental disorders and drug abuse in prison suicides and show that suicides occur disproportionately in the early stages of custody (Shaw et al. 2003). Suicides due to prison-specific factors such as loss of autonomy, inactivity, and fears for physical safety are of human rights concern and suicidal thoughts are higher in prisoners who report unfairness and feel unsafe (Liebling et al. 2003). When a prisoner is suicidal he may be isolated in a 'suicide proof' room which is bare and undignified, a situation invariably seen as victimization and an assault on human dignity. Hancock and Snow (2001) reported that in some US prisons 'Prisoners wore leg irons and were chained to beds that precluded the use of hands to aid self harm.'

The search for humane alternatives continues. The European Convention on Human Rights has, for example, raised the potential for legal challenge to some constraints on the ground that they constitute inhumane or degrading treatment (Council of Europe 2001). In response to these concerns, some countries have developed 'crisis suites' which, by providing a supportive atmosphere, seek to make suicide as difficult as possible. In Tanzania and Kenya, the use of shared accommodation may be an explanation for a very low rate of prison suicides (Aardema et al. 1998). The importance given to prison suicides has resulted in better listening to human rights and quality of life for prisoners in a few countries (Paton and Jenkins 2005). It is hoped that this practice will be copied elsewhere.

Marriage, human rights, and suicide

In many Asian, Middle Eastern, and African countries 'arranged marriages' remain prevalent. When a young person attains marriageable age according to his or her culture, families decide on a partner. Often young women and sometimes men are forced into marriage against their wishes. In cultures in which divorce is unacceptable, many young people feel trapped and some consider suicide an option.

Another aspect of this problem, sometimes known as 'love failure', occurs when young people who desire to marry one another are refused permission by their families for social, economic, religious, caste, or other reasons. Such disappointed lovers may then die by suicide either alone or together. During 2006 at least 2500 people killed themselves in India for these reasons (Accidental Deaths & Suicides in India 2006). Although these parental actions are human rights violations which lead to suicide, they are so embedded in culture and tradition that the enormity of the problem remains submerged.

Suicide pacts

Another distressing occurrence in developing countries, including China, India, and Sri Lanka, is the frequency of suicide pacts and family suicides, mutual arrangements between two or more people to die together, usually in the same place (Vijayakumar and Thilothammal 1993) Often there is a dominant partner who instigates the idea, and family suicides may include several people in suicidal/homicidal agreement in which adults first murder their children and then kill themselves.

In India 148 suicidal pacts involving 324 persons were studied. Contrary to the prevalent statistics in individual suicides, in suicide pacts women (55.7 per cent) outnumber men (44.3 per cent). In individual suicide, psychopathology is an important risk factor, whereas in pacts social situations and stressors play an important role. Thus, pacts can be viewed as a form of protest against archaic social norms and expectations (Vijayakumar and Thilothammal 1993).

In India in 2006, 105 children were involved in family suicides. In effect they were murdered, and yet this violation against the rights of children has not received the major attention from human rights activists and suicidologists which it deserved.

Domestic violence

Violence against women has been acknowledged as a significant health problem worldwide (Dubnova and Joss 1997; Heise et al. 1994). Abused women are five times more likely to attempt and complete suicide than non-battered women (Heise et al. 1994). Women who have experienced violence are more likely than women who have not experienced violence to report physical symptoms (Leserman et al. 1998) and poor mental health outcomes such as panic, depression, anxiety, and alcohol and substance abuse (Heise et al. 1994), all of which can lead to suicide.

Wife abuse is one of the most significant precipitants of female suicide as shown by studies conducted in Papua New Guinea where domestic violence was found to be a normal part of marital relationships and the major trigger to suicide was identified as physically violent domestic argument. Abused, shamed, and powerless wives take their own lives to shift the burden of humiliation from themselves to their tormentors. In Fiji, and South American societies, suicide associated with marital violence is also common. Data from a number of societies indicate that wife abuse remains one of the most important precipitants of female suicide and suicide attempts (Counts 1987). Domestic violence is a fairly common occurrence in most Asian societies and in the rural areas of many developing countries and its practice is to a large extent socially and culturally condoned (Heise et al. 1994).

A highly significant relationship between domestic violence and suicidal ideations has been found in population samples of women from many developing countries. In Brazil (48 per cent), Egypt (61 per cent), India (64 per cent), Indonesia (11 per cent), and the Philippines (28 per cent) of women had significant correlation between domestic violence and suicidal ideation (Leskauskas 2002). In a study conducted in a General Hospital in Durban, significantly more married women than men cited marital violence, spousal alcohol abuse, and extramarital affairs as precipitants of their self-destructive behaviours (Pillay et al. 2001). Physical and emotional abuse experienced in the family were statistically more frequent among suicide attempters than among their non-suicidal peers according to a research finding in Lithuania on adolescent girls (World Health Organization 2001).

Child sexual abuse and suicide

The child, when sexually abused, does not even realize that his or her rights have been violated. Many studies have shown that child sexual abuse is related to suicidal behaviour and that the odds of attempting suicide are three to four times greater when the abuse occurred prior to the age of 16. A meta-analysis of the effects of child sexual abuse reveals that the average weighted and unweighted score was 0.64 and 0.44 (Paolucci et al. 2001).

Time may not heal the wounds caused by child sexual abuse and thus such abuse at an early age is associated with an increased lifetime risk of attempted suicide. A recent study found that suicidal ideation and suicide attempts among depressed women of middle age and older correlated with having been abused sexually as a child. Multiple attempts were also commonly found (Talbot et al. 2004).

The way forward

While writing this chapter, we were asked to visit a young foreigner in a Tunisian prison who had been on hunger strike for over 40 days. A beating administered by prison guards hoping to make him give up the strike had only increased his anger over his lack of rights and his resolve to continue fasting even if this led to his death. I (Lakshmi) was able to listen to his grievances and, because I know his language, to support him to pull back from death. He ended his hunger strike while we were with him and I (Lillian) had the access and privilege to follow up.

When hope vanishes death beckons. An old hymn speaks of 'hope which sends a shining ray far down the future's broadening way'. It is the duty and privilege of all who retain hope in their lives, and especially those with access and resources, to reach out to people who have been marginalized, discounted, and stigmatized. To listen compassionately to the pain of another human being is to recognize his humanity. Medical, economic, and legal work as well as awareness raising are, of course, also necessary. But although many organizations both local and international are engaged in such efforts, abundant opportunity remains for individual participation. To be listened to, no matter what the circumstances, is a human right.

It is also among our human rights to be educated, to have adequate medical and psychological services, not to be marginalized, stigmatized, or forced into marriage against our will and to live in dignity and equality. Fortunately, stigmatized suicide survivors and the families of some of those who have died have now begun to rise up to ask government and mental health professionals to examine the laws and to raise public awareness of the dangers.

References

Aardema, A, Blaauw, E, Gatherer, A, Kerkhof, A, and Themeli, O (1998) *Mental health in European prisons*. Amsterdam: Department of Clinical Psychology, Vrije Universiteit.

Accidental Deaths & Suicides in India (2006) Government of India: National Crime Records Bureau, Ministry of Home Affairs.

Council of Europe (2001) 11th General report on the CPT's activities covering 1 January to 31 December 2000. Available at <http://cpt.coe.int/en/annual/rep-11.html>.

Counts, DA (1987) 'Female suicide and wife abuse—a cross-cultural perspective', *Suicide and Life Threatening Behavior*, Fall, 17(3), 194–204.

Dubnova, I and Joss, DM (1997) 'Women and domestic violence: Global dimensions, health consequences and intervention strategies', *Work*, 9, 79–85.

Fairbank, JK (1994) *China: A new history*. Cambridge, MA: Harvard University Press, 232.

Hancock, N and Snow, L (2001) 'Suicide prevention in North America: fewer deaths but at what cost?', *Prison Service Journal*, 138, 24–6.

Heise, LL, Raikes, A, Watts, CH, and Zwi, AB (1994) 'Violence against women—a neglected health issue in less developed countries', *Social Science Medicine*, 39, 1165–1171.

Joseph, A, Abraham, S, Muliyil, JP, George, K, Prasad, J, Minz, S, Abraham, VJ, and Jacob, KS (2003) 'Evaluation of suicide rates in rural India using verbal autopsies, 1994–9', *British Medical Journal*, 326, 1121–122.

Kankiewicz, K (2007) *Combating Harmful Misperceptions. The Stigma of Mental Illness*. Available at <http://kim-kankiewicz.suite101.com/the-stigma-of-mental-illness-a12505>, accessed 9 November 2011.

Leenaars, A (2003) 'Ethical and Legal issues', in L Vijayakumar (ed) *Suicide Prevention—Meeting the challenge together*. Chennai: Orient Longman, 85–110.

Leserman, J, Li, Z, Drossman, DA, and Hu, YJ (1998) 'Selected symptoms associated with sexual and physical abuse history among female patients with gastrointestinal disorders: The impact of subsequent health care visits', *Psychological Medicine*, 28, 417–25.

Leskauskas, D (2002) 'Relationship between the suicidal attempts of adolescent girls and risk factors in the family', *Medicina (Kaunas)* [Article in Lithuanian]. 38(4), 387–392.

Liebling, A, Durie, L, van Den Bueckel, A, and Tait, S (2003) *Legitimacy prison suicide and the moral performance of prisons*. Paper presented to the American Society of Criminology conference Roundtable, Denver, 13 November, 2003.

Paolucci, EO, Genius, ML, and Ucolato, C (2001) 'A meta-analysis of the published research on the effects of child sexual abuse', *Journal of Psychology*, 135(1) 17–36.

Paton, J and Jenkins, R (2005) 'Suicide and suicide attempts in prisons', in K Hawton (ed) *Prevention and treatment of suicidal behaviour—From science to practice*. Oxford: Oxford University Press, 307–334.

Pillay, AL, van der Veen, MB, and Wassenaar, DR (2001) 'Non-fatal suicidal behaviour in women—the role of spousal substance abuse and marital violence', *South African Medical Journal*, 91(5), 429–432.

Shaw, J, Appleby, L, and Baker, D (2003) *Safer prisons; a national study of prison suicides 1999–2000 by the National Confidential Inquiry into Suicides and Homicides by People with Mental Illness*. London: Department of Health.

Talbot, N, Duberstein, R, Cox, C, Denning, D, and Conwell, Y (2004) 'Preliminary report on childhood sexual abuse, suicide ideation and suicide attempts among middle aged and older depressed women', *American Journal of Geriatric Psychiatry*, 12, 536–539.

Vijayakumar, L and Jotheeswaran, AT (2010) 'Suicide in refugees and asylum seekers', in D Bhugra, T Craig, and K Bhui (eds) *Mental Health of Refugees and Asylum-seekers*. Oxford: Oxford University Press, Chapter 14, 195–211.

Vijayakumar, L and Thilothammal, N (1993) 'Suicide Pacts in India', *Crisis*, 14(1), 43–47.

Vijayakumar, L, Nagaraj, K, Pirkis, J, and Whiteford, H (2005) 'Suicide in developing countries: Frequency, distribution and association with socio-economic indicators', *Crisis*, 26(3), 104–111.

World Health Organization (2001) *World Health Report: Mental Health–New understanding–New Hope*. Geneva: WHO.

Part 4

Protection of Mental Health: Current Provisions and How They may be Strengthened

This theme moves to the area of intervention, in surveying a range of response to the challenges outlined in the book.

Crick Lund, Tom Sutcliffe, Alan Flisher, and Dan J. Stein overview key international human rights instruments and note their relevance for people suffering from mental disorders in poor settings. This includes for example providing support to stopping rights violations, making legislation and policy compatible with the latest conventions (e.g. the CRPD), monitoring progress towards achieving a rights-based approach to mental health service provision, and lending weight to providing and scaling up appropriate, accessible, and affordable mental health care. After briefly analysing human rights aspects of legislation, oversight, and mental health systems in four African countries, the authors examine recent South African legislative reforms in detail, and the role of review boards, which has significantly helped protect rights in an affordable way. The final section makes recommendations for strengthening key areas of human rights protection.

François Crépeau and Anne-Claire Gayet argue that improving the effectiveness of human rights standards relevant to mental health depends firstly on being aware of the existing framework. This they do by considering the specific responsible institutions — international and regional treaty bodies which receive periodic reports, produce 'soft law', hear individual and collective complaints, and undertake on-site visits; the procedures of independent experts and UN Special Rapporteurs; the work of international courts and tribunals, national judicial tribunals and human rights institutions, and other inquiries and investigations, both at international and national levels. They provide examples about the work of these bodies. They also explore how human rights standards can be actively promoted and protected, through cross-sectoral cooperation, inter-institutional consultation, and mobilizing civil society and human rights education for all. These arguments particularly draw on the Canadian context.

Non-governmental mental health organizations and the 'consumer' movement as human rights advocates provide the focus for the chapter by John Copeland, Eugene Brody, Tony Fowke, Preston Garrison, and Janet Meagher. They outline how the World Federation of Mental Health since 1948 advocated for rights, opposed abuses, and gradually included self-help groups and consumer organizations, and also discuss the World Psychiatric Association's programme to reduce stigma. They chart the history of the mental health consumer advocacy movement, its spectrum of views and messages, and its increasing profile. Unfinished business includes the disempowerment and rights violations of people with mental illnesses in many countries, frequent absence or obsolescence of mental health legislation, and UN signatory nations not fulfilling their obligations. Emphasizing the voice of lived experience in national and international associations, the authors make the case for consumer involvement and representation in mental health care, in all levels of organizations, services, policy formulation, evaluation, promotion, and prevention. They signal the crucial role of families and carers. They flag the WFMH's Global Consensus programme, and attempt to demonstrate agreement on key messages to governments and regarding what fundamental issues should guide the policy of the United Nations and its Agencies.

In a challenging perspective, David Oaks discusses oppressive aspects of psychiatry, the sanism that ostracizes citizens whom society calls mad, and the Mad Pride movement's response. He observes how users and survivors, formerly marginalized, now influence international developments through (for example) participation in the drafting of the CRPD, and how language usage of mental health professionals accommodates terms like empowerment, peer support, advocacy, trauma, alternatives, recovery, and self-determination. Questioning the widening ambit of psychiatry through avenues such as community treatment orders, and school screening and referral, he argues that users and their families should be presented with a range of mental health service choices, not just the conventional mental health system or the medical model. He warns against the rising tide of mental health export packages to developing countries, comprising drugs and electroshock (including without anaesthetic) but little by way of information, advocacy, alternatives, and activism. He asks about the long-term brain effects of neuroleptics. Probing normality to reveal its reductionism and silent complicity with the (potentially suicidal) status quo, he argues for creative maladjustment: while being fully aware that 'not all strange thoughts are necessarily good', pleads that madness as dissent may represent imagination and ingenuity.

The Right to Health is central to this book. In their commentary, Gunilla Backman and Judith Mesquita consider its history, its grounds in both civil–political and socioeconomic/cultural rights thinking and practice, and the legal sources and norms for this. They contemplate the desiderata for (mental) health care, and further examine those norms that are highly relevant to mental health care, such as non-discrimination and equality, development of costed national health plans, progressive realization, participation, accountability, and international assistance and cooperation. They describe the implementation of the right to health in policy, in terms of both protecting and promoting rights, and in seeking more resources, and monitoring and accountability. Examples of Special Rapporteur and treaty monitoring processes are both given. The authors emphazise how the right to health has been increasingly used by the health sector, civil society, and national human rights institutions as a framework for structuring analysis and to demand action to improve mental healthcare.

In a chapter that reminds the reader of the importance of broad participation in the flourishing of democracies, Oliver Lewis and Nell Munro argue that the participation of people with mental disabilities in legal and policy reforms relating to their lives is critical in realizing a full range of rights. Participation improves the relevance, credibility and outcome of reforms, empowers people with mental disabilities, and communicates an inclusive message about equity to wider society. The practice of societies excluding mental health (or health) service users when designing laws and policies affecting their lives has changed in recent decades: the authors explore the reasons. This entitlement, embedded in General Comment No. 14 of the Convention on Economic, Social and Cultural Rights, is confirmed by the CRPD's shift from welfare to rights. In addition, user involvement may ensure broader human rights compliance, assist securing equality and the dignity of one's identity (so easily violated by coercion, stigma, and social exclusion), and it strengthens democracy. They consider means of enhancing participation, who should be consulted, the costs of participating or not, and questions surrounding user status (this may be future as well as past or present). Governments and mental health professionals have special responsibilities to ensure participation of service users.

The challenges in undertaking research that attends to both mental health and human rights are explored by Susan Rees and Derrick Silove. They consider the possible translations of such research into practice, and offer a provisional typology of human rights and mental health research methods. These range from documentary research undertaken by international NGOs, through primary mental disorder and/or trauma research that implicitly considers human rights, empiricist rights-focused research in mental health, and social science research in disaster and conflict, to participatory action research in human rights. The problems of emancipatory research allegedly colliding with natural science models of research 'objectivity', and also the implicit assumption that research translation should respect the status quo, are discussed. Research case examples with asylum-seekers and the East Timorese community consider and address these tensions.

With particular reference to a mother–infant intervention in South Africa, Mark Tomlinson, Peter Cooper, Leslie Swartz, and Mireille Landman report frank, human rights-based reflections on international research collaborations between rich countries and low- and middle-income countries. They notice the bias in research publication between rich countries and LAMICs. They consider the ethics and power in research and researcher relationships, notably between researchers in rich and LAMI countries, within the LAMI country (a new observation), and also with research participants. The authors actively reflect on inter-group differentials of privilege, the question of insiders and outsiders and who speaks on behalf of the research or community. Challenges with researching motherhood in South Africa arose from race and gender relations in the context of institutionalized racial discrimination and cultural imperialism, and related problems with defining who was expert in infant care, creating a space for reflection about infants' needs, and negotiating the traumas associated with childhood. Partnership models that address power and sharing the fruits of research are vital.

Returning to the needs of those with severe and persistent mental illness, Peter Walker and colleagues review the use of cognitive-behavioural therapy (CBT) as a human rights-promoting intervention for psychosis. Recent emphasis on continuity between normal and psychotic experiences and study of cognitive processes in the context of psychotic symptoms, has revised understandings of 'madness' and has had the effect of socially including sufferers through making their experiences understandable. The authors review the self-help movement that supports those who hear voices. CBT in this context has been seen as promoting consumer empowerment and advancing their rights. This assists to change their experience of mental health systems from a coercive to cooperative model, counteracts internalized stigma, and promotes freedom of expression, self-determination, and narratives of recovery. Such collaborative therapeutic alliances, where the therapist acts as witness often over a sustained period, where formulations of the problem are shared, and where users are active participants in designing their own recovery, are new to many users, breaking through a dominantly coercive pattern of care. The practitioner acts as a human rights advocate pursuing issues of social justice. Similarities to testimony therapy documenting the person's story in other contexts are remarked.

Following up their earlier chapter, and with particular reference to the inheritance of the Nazis and the Nuremberg trials, Fran Gale and Michael Dudley ponder challenges in promoting social goodness and preventing human rights violations. They interrogate professional ethics about the social responsibilities of helping professionals, the place of social justice within mental health, and ask ethical questions about medical technology with particular reference to the 'new eugenics'. For nations and communities undertaking post-genocide interventions, the struggle for remembrance and justice, the attractions and elusiveness of forgiveness, and the mixed results attending reconciliation are surveyed with reference to individual and community mental health — such as the benefits of testifying at a TRC, or how to support witnesses. What of the needs of children in conflict zones, the rearing of children to prevent or halt violence? Warning systems that prevent genocide and the question of development programmes that promote social goodness are also discussed. The necessity to renew democracy should not be underestimated. Lastly they contemplate the role of socially engaged helping professionals, the mandate in international standards for such engagement, and their contribution to strengthening of civil society.

Chapter 30

Protecting the Rights of the Mentally Ill in Poorly Resourced Settings

Experiences from Four African Countries*

Crick Lund, Tom Sutcliffe, Alan J. Flisher, and Dan J. Stein

Introduction

In poorly resourced countries, the mentally ill are particularly vulnerable to a range of human rights abuses. Establishing mechanisms to protect the mentally ill from these abuses is therefore vital. This chapter will provide a broad overview of key international human rights instruments that are relevant for these settings. A brief analysis of the human rights aspects of mental health systems in four African countries will then be presented, to illustrate the interaction between international instruments and country realities. This will be followed by a more detailed examination of recent legislation reforms in South Africa, and the role of review boards in human rights protection. The final section of the chapter makes recommendations for a way forward, highlighting key areas of human rights protection that need to be strengthened in poorly resourced countries.

Throughout this chapter we will be emphasizing the relatively low levels of service provision in low- and middle-income countries (LMICs). This is not to equate increased service resources with increased protection of human rights. Clearly the relationship between service resources, economic development, and human rights protection is complex. There are dangers in a form of cultural imperialism which assumes that 'Western' models of human rights should be imported uncritically to low resource settings, and that increased economic development and resources for mental health care will necessarily translate into improved human rights protection in these settings. These assumptions should be critically examined, and the assumptions of Western human rights frameworks interrogated in terms of the culture and values of the countries in which they are to be applied. During the course of this chapter we will attempt to demonstrate that both increased mental health service resources (designed and delivered on the basis of human rights and evidence-based care) and strengthened legislative provisions are required to protect the human rights of the mentally ill in low resource settings.

In addition it is important to note that a lack of resources for research is also relevant. The results of mental health service and epidemiological research can inform service planning, improve legal systems, and protect human rights, and the absence of such research can thus have the reverse effect.

* Tragically, Professor Alan Flisher died of leukemia during the writing of this book. Please see the Acknowledgements section at the end of this chapter.

Key international human rights instruments

There are a number of international human rights instruments that are relevant for mental health. A primary instrument is the 'International Bill of Rights', which comprises the Universal Declaration of Human Rights (1948), the International Covenant on Civil and Political Rights (ICCPR), and the International Covenant on Economic, Social and Cultural Rights (ICESCR, 1966). Among the issues that are relevant to mental health that are enshrined in the International Bill of Rights are protection against discrimination; the rights to health (including the right to access rehabilitation services, dignity, community integration, reasonable accommodation, liberty, security of person); the need for affirmative action to protect the rights of people with disabilities (which includes those with mental disorders); and the right to protection against torture, cruel, inhuman, and degrading treatment (including in medical institutions such as those providing psychiatric care).

Another instrument is the UN Convention on the Rights of the Child, which includes the right to life, survival, and development; respect for the views of the child; protection from all forms of physical and mental abuse; and non-discrimination. Also, the UN Convention Against Torture and Other Cruel, Inhuman Treatment or Punishment (1984) obliges signatory states to prevent acts of cruel, inhuman, or degrading treatment or punishment. Finally, the UN Convention on the Rights of Persons with Disabilities (2007) is based on the following principles: respect for inherent dignity, individual autonomy including the freedom to make one's own choices, and independence of persons; non-discrimination; full and effective participation and inclusion in society; respect for difference and acceptance of persons with disabilities as part of human diversity and humanity; equality of opportunity; accessibility; equality between men and women; and respect for the evolving capacities of children with disabilities and respect for the rights of children with disabilities to preserve their identities. In addition to these instruments that are applicable globally, there are a number of instruments that are applicable to certain regions; for example, in the African region, the African Charter on Human and Peoples' Rights (1981), and the African Court on Human and People's Rights.

What are the practical benefits for the inhabitants of a poorly resourced country that is a signatory to these instruments? First, throughout the world, there are a number of examples of human rights violations experienced by recipients of psychiatric care. So far as inhuman or degrading treatment is concerned, for example, one may encounter a lack of a safe environment, inadequate health care facilities, and unnecessary limitations on movement. All such circumstances are more likely to be applicable in poorly resourced countries, and are explicitly proscribed by the instruments mentioned above. In this context, the instruments can serve to galvanize public sentiment about the human rights violations, and thus inspire civil society actions and movements that aim to ensure that such violations are terminated. Furthermore, if service users or their advocates challenge the health care system in a court of law, the fact that the country is a signatory to an instrument in which these practices are proscribed will increase the chances of a successful legal challenge.

Second, according to the commitments that are embraced by the signing of an instrument or treaty, a country commits itself, *inter alia*, to give expression to the contents of the instrument in legislation and policy (WHO 2005b). Thus, the instruments should—indeed, must—inform the development of legislation and policy at all levels, from the initial drafting by a team of experts, to the passage through statutory processes, to implementation. Poorly resourced countries are less likely to have modern legislation and policies than well resourced countries. So far as legislation is concerned, for example, 30.0 per cent and 16.7 per cent of countries in Africa and South-East Asia respectively had initiation of the latest mental health law after 1990, compared to

58.4 per cent and 76.6 per cent in the Americas and Europe respectively (WHO 2005a). There is an opportunity for poorly resourced countries that are in the process of developing new legislation to do so in a way that it is compatible with the latest conventions such as the Convention on the Rights of Persons with Disabilities. This does not apply just to legislation and policy in the health sector. Many other sectors are also obliged to address mental issues that are included in the instruments. For example, as mentioned above, the Convention on the Rights of Persons with Disabilities is based on the principles of full and effective participation and inclusion in society and respect for the evolving capacities of children with disabilities; these principles need to inform the development of legislation and policy in the labour and education sectors respectively.

Thirdly, the instruments can be used as a basis for monitoring progress towards achieving a rights-based approach to mental health service provision. This requires three steps: a clear specification of the rights applicable to people with mental health problems; provision for delivery of these rights (which can include legislation and policies); and the documentation of the outputs and outcomes in relation to standards and interventions (Bentley 2003; Bray and Dawes 2007). Such monitoring is particularly important in low resource settings where the barriers to establishing and maintaining a rights-based approach to mental health care provision are greater. As will become evident below, substantial challenges remain in this regard.

Finally, the instruments can lend weight to the provision and scaling up of appropriate, accessible, and affordable mental health care. A major challenge in low resource settings is human rights violations of people with mental disorders who are not accessing mental health treatment (WHO 2005b). These include chaining of people in huts in remote rural villages, subjection to public humiliation, ostracism, and abusive 'traditional' healing practices of faith healers and alternative practitioners, such as exorcisms and floggings. There are dangers in assuming that 'traditional' practices in low-income countries are necessarily effective or humane. Expansion of the coverage of humane, evidence-based treatment for mental disorders may, therefore, be a crucial means of protecting human rights and implementing the range of international instruments that have been developed to protect these rights.

Human rights scenarios in four African countries: Ghana, South Africa, Uganda, and Zambia

As shown in the previous section, there are a number of international instruments that have bearing on human rights protection for the mentally ill in low resource settings. But what is the situation on the ground in low resource settings in Africa? Are these instruments used in practice and what protection do they offer? We provide a brief review of the situation in four African countries, which represent a variety of scenarios in low- and middle-income countries: Ghana, South Africa, Uganda, and Zambia.

Legislation

The four countries currently have various forms of legislation in place (see Table 30.1). In Ghana, the 1972 Mental Health Decree (which replaced the Asylum Ordinance of 1888) is in force. Many stakeholders in Ghana have agreed that the 1972 legislation is inadequate for protecting human rights, and in partnership with the WHO, a new Mental Health Bill has been drafted (Doku et al. 2008). The Bill has been lauded by WHO as best practice in the protection of human rights for the mentally ill. It provides several mechanisms and incentives for the provision of community-based mental health services, which are intended to reduce stigma and improve access to care. However, there have been a number of delays since the Bill was first presented to Cabinet in 2006.

Table 30.1 Legislation, review boards, and mental health service resources in four African countries

Country	Mental health legislation	Review boards present	Psychiatrists per 100,000 population	Beds per 100,000 population in mental hospitals	Mental hospitals	% of beds located in mental hospitals	Psychiatric inpatient units in general hospitals
Ghana	Mental Health Decree of 1972	No	0.05	5.4	4	87	10
South Africa	Mental Health Care Act (No. 17 of 2002)	Yes	0.28	18.0	23	56	41
Uganda	Mental Health Treatment Act of 1964	No	0.08	1.8	1	48	27
Zambia	Mental Disorders Act of 1951	No	0.01	1.8	1	100%	0

Several attempts to lobby the Minister of Health and other key stakeholders have proved fruitless. At the time of going to press the Bill had been reviewed by Cabinet and was due to be presented to Parliament.

In South Africa, the current legislation is the Mental Health Care Act (No. 17 of 2002) which replaced the previous Mental Health Act (No. 18 of 1973). The intention of the new Mental Health Care Act (MHCA) is to safeguard the rights of the mentally ill persons through a number of legal requirements that dictate the procedural flow and clinical management of service users (Lund et al. 2010). The MHCA is a significant departure from the previous legislation, which was developed during the apartheid era, and offered only limited protection of human rights. The development and adoption of the MHCA was conducted through a thorough consultation process that included a wide range of mental health stakeholders in the country. During the debate of the Bill in Parliament and its eventual adoption, the MHCA enjoyed widespread support from a variety of political parties.

In Uganda, current legislation is the Mental Health Treatment Act of 1964. As with Ghana, many stakeholders state that the Act is outdated and does not provide adequate protection of human rights for the mentally ill (Cooper et al. 2010). For example, the Act does not distinguish between voluntary and involuntary care, it uses derogatory language that leads to further stigmatization of the mentally ill, and it makes no provision for review bodies to inspect facilities and review admissions. There are plans under way to reform the legislation, and a new draft Bill has been developed. One magistrate in Uganda expressed his concerns regarding the protection of people with mental illness as follows:

> . . . even in society . . . the way society looks at them, it is like they don't mind about them. And even when assaulted, you may not see anyone reporting to police that a mad man has been assaulted there. And if this mad man committed an offence, even court may not take the case serious (Magistrate, Uganda) (Kigozi et al. 2008:84).

In Zambia, legislation from the colonial era, the Mental Disorders Act of 1951, remains on the statute books. Like the Ugandan law, Zambian legislation makes no distinctions between voluntary and involuntary care, uses language currently construed as stigmatizing (such as 'idiot' and 'imbecile'), and makes no provision for review bodies or other mechanisms to protect human rights of people with mental disorders (Banda et al. 2008). One Zambian service user describes the effect of this legislation:

> Who am I? The identity that I am given by the law … [is] to call me an imbecile, an idiot. This is very critical to me because immediately you just label me as an idiot, that in itself has got a lot of repercussions, . . . because everyone will be looking at me as an idiot then I attract the very negative attitude that we receive from the community. Because the community is meant to believe that S is an idiot. An idiot is one person who is not worth actually staying with and maybe the better place is being out there at the edge of society. That I think is where I really find my law inadequate and very cruel to people with mental health problems.
>
> (Mental health service user, Zambia) (Banda et al. 2008:54)

A Mental Health Service Bill of 2006 to repeal the 1951 Act is awaiting a consensus meeting and is expected to be submitted to the Attorney General in Zambia shortly.

Review/oversight mechanisms

Of the four countries, only South Africa has review bodies that oversee human rights issues, such as inspecting mental health facilities, reviewing involuntary admissions, and investigating complaints. *Inter alia*, the MHCA requires that the Member of the Executive Committee for Health (MEC) in each of the nine Provinces in South Africa must establish a Review Board (or Boards). These Boards must be set up to function as appropriately skilled and resourced bodies that are able to act independently and autonomously in ensuring the proper implementation of the MHCA and its regulations.

Service resources

Service resources have a major role to play, not only in supporting the right of access to mental health care, but also, through services, providing information and treatment options that equip service users to protect their own rights within communities.

When reviewing resources across the four countries, it becomes immediately apparent that there are wide discrepancies (see Table 30.1). Psychiatrists per 100,000 population range from 0.01 to 0.28 in public sector services (Banda et al. 2008; Doku et al. 2008; Kigozi et al. 2008; Lund et al. 2010). The differences in decentralization of services are also stark, e.g. while Zambia has all inpatient resources concentrated in the single mental hospital, Uganda has a relatively well developed decentralized inpatient service, through the establishment of psychiatric inpatient units in general hospitals throughout the country. Making use of a grant from the African Development Bank to supplement Ministry of Health budgets and build infrastructure for mental health care, such units improve access to care and, through their setting in general hospitals, reduce stigma associated with admission. Thus, in spite of the limitations in the legislative environment in Uganda, some important steps have been taken to improving access to care and reducing stigma.

Nevertheless, compared to high income countries, these service resources paint a stark picture of mental health care, and the threadbare system of human rights protection that accompanies it. While international human rights instruments such those mentioned above offer protection, the lessons from these African countries seem to indicate that, unless this is translated into national level legislation, and service resources are made available, there is little protection of people with mental illness. A key mechanism by which such international measures can become translated into country realities appears to be via the use of international tools and agencies (such as the WHO) in providing support for the reform of national legislations, as has occurred in South Africa, and is continuing to occur in Ghana, Uganda, and Zambia.

It is also important to understand these legislative provisions, review mechanisms and service resources in the context of the wider human rights and social situations in these countries. While all four countries have democratically elected governments, and (except for the north of Uganda) are free of major civil conflict, all face ongoing human rights challenges. For example, in South Africa there are high levels of interpersonal violence, including some of the highest incidences of rape and violence against women in the world. South Africa has unemployment rates exceeding 40 per cent in places and one of the highest rates of economic inequality in the world, with the Gini coefficient rising from 0.64 to 0.72 between 1995 and 2005 (Bhorat et al. 2009). There are also ongoing public debates around the HIV epidemic and the right to health (Hassim et al. 2007; United Nations High Commissioner for Human Rights 2003). This context adds a new dimension to the prospect of discharging people with mental illness from mental health facilities into communities with high levels of crime and violence, distressed families, and limited opportunities for employment, rehabilitation, and participation in social and economic development (Lund et al. 2008).

Case exemplar: mental health legislation reform and review boards in South Africa

In the context of varying scenarios across Africa, we now present some recent legislation reforms and associated human rights protection mechanisms in South Africa, as a case exemplar.

The Mental Health Care Act (2002)

The MHCA specifies a number of rights that are consistent with those upheld in the international instruments described above. In addition, the MHCA specifies that Review Boards must be established in each province. Each Review Board must comprise at least three but no more than five members, one of whom must be a mental health care practitioner, one a representative of the community, and one a person with legal training. The main role of Review Boards is to consider the appropriate admission, transfer, and discharge of involuntary and assisted mental health care users. Also, the Board must satisfy itself that users have been informed of their rights, including the right to appeal against their classification and their right to receive legal representation. The new Act provides fixed timeframes for the submission of admission forms. This ensures that a user's circumstances are reviewed by the Board and, in the case of involuntary care users, by the High Court without lengthy delays.

The Review Board in the Western Cape Province

The Review Board was appointed by the MEC for Health in the Western Cape on 1 April 2005. It comprises five members and serves the entire province (population: 3,496,499). According to the MHCA, the Review Board must consist of at least a mental health practitioner; a magistrate, an attorney, or an advocate admitted in terms of the law of the country; and a member of the community. The early and successful establishment of the Board was largely due to the determination of the MEC for Health and senior members of the Health Department.

At the outset the Review Board was fully briefed on the new Act and its regulations. Following a month studying the new Act and assessing the nature of the workload, the Board drew up a methodology for 'best practice' in a document titled, 'The Governance and Operational Charter of the Western Cape Review Board'. This guides the Review Board's functions and is updated regularly. Protocols and procedures for holding formal hearings were developed by members of the Board with legal experience. These were ratified by the State Legal Advisor. The Board has taken the view that it should be financially accountable at all times.

At the outset, some members of the Board had limited experience with mental illness. A series of lectures was arranged on a wide range of relevant mental health topics and training is ongoing. The Board draws up a regular annual roster of visits to psychiatric hospitals and other health facilities, including primary care clinics and facilities in rural areas. The intention of these visits is to make the role and function of the Review Board better known and to receive input from health care professionals regarding the implementation of the MHCA. They also provide an opportunity for members of the Board to assess conditions in hospitals and clinics, but this is not the primary reason for the visits. Except on one occasion where an extremely serious incident had been reported, no visit is made unannounced.

The Review Board had a pocket-sized User's Rights card made which briefly describes to users what their rights are and how to contact the Board. Cards are printed in all three official languages of the Province and the Board's instruction is that they be issued to each and every user, no matter at what level they enter the mental health services. Similarly, pamphlets describing mental health care users' rights and how to contact the Review Board have been provided to all health care establishments and posters containing similar information have been put up in wards. In addition, the Review Board has set up tables at many non-governmental organizations' (NGOs) mental health functions and has prepared a series of PowerPoint presentations that are tailored to suit a variety of audiences including mental health care nurses in training, the general public, judges of the Cape High Court, and the National Prosecuting Authority (NPA).

The Review Board holds a planning workshop each year to address key requirements and to formulate strategies to improve operational performance and promote awareness of the Board. The Review Board has met with, or made presentations to, a range of key stakeholders. These included the NPA, relevant non-profit organizations (NPOs), private sector mental health care providers, Correctional Services, military health services, and Health Facility Boards. As a result of concerns expressed by some judges of the Cape High Court around issues of interpretation of the Act and its Regulations, the Review Board made a presentation to, and held an informative discussion with, the full bench of the Cape High Court under the Chairpersonship of the Judge President of the Cape High Court.

The national Department of Health has held national workshops and produced a set of guidelines to assist in the establishment and management of Review Boards and in interpreting the Act. Apart from ongoing administrative support and assistance, the Review Board is included in provincial departmental meetings attended by relevant public sector mental health care providers. The Western Cape Board has met with other Review Boards with a view to exchanging information and operational experiences.

The Review Board has made a number of presentations to mental health care professionals and allied workers. The Review Board has met with representatives of press and media in order to secure articles that promote a better understanding of the Review Board. Members of the Board have also taken part in radio programmes with the same intention. The Review Board conducts ward or home visits to users when there is any indication of possible neglect or abuse or when a user lodges an appeal against his or her status. Reports are drafted following each visit. The report and its recommendations are presented to the full Board for ratification and a copy referred to the relevant hospital head.

The Board provides the MEC with regular quarterly and annual reports. These reports give relevant statistical data for the period in question, observations the Review Board has made on relevant aspects of mental health services, and actual case studies without sacrificing user confidentiality.

In LMICs an important question to ask is how attainable is the establishment of Review Boards given funding constraints and the growing demand for resources, both financial and human? The reality is that hard choices need to be made in most LMICs to fund a wide range of competing needs. This is also the case in the Provincial Department of Health in the Western Cape. However, if the annual budget of the Review Board is compared to the overall budget for mental health services in this province, the Review Board consumes an extremely small percentage of that budget.

In considering what effect the Review Board has had on mental health care services and user rights in the Western Cape Province it is important to first interrogate the scale of work undertaken by the Board. To illustrate the caseload of the Board: in fulfilling its principal role of reviewing involuntary and assisted admissions, the Board has to date reviewed 9713 admissions of mentally ill users since its inception. Of these, 2480 were applications for assisted care and 7233 were for involuntary care. In the same period, the Board reviewed 1094 periodic reports.

Flowing from this workload, the Board considered and responded to 259 appeals from users, family members of users, concerned members of the public, or other parties. The breakdown of these appeals is set out in Table 30.2. Of particular interest is that the number of appeals received by the Board is growing each quarter, presumably as awareness of the Board and its role increases.

In terms of human rights, the Mental Health Care Act has clearly provided an important avenue for mentally ill users, and indeed any other concerned party, to be heard. What has the effect of this been?

In appeals against involuntary status, the recommendations of the Review Board are likely not to have been perceived by users as helpful in that, in all cases seen by the Board thus far, the user's appeal could not be supported. However, all appeals against involuntary status are addressed by visiting the applicant, or by holding a hearing, or consulting with attending health care practitioners, or a combination of all three. The Board's findings are communicated to the applicant in a carefully worded letter. Notwithstanding the outcome, the mere fact that an appeal against involuntary status has received consideration from an independent body is, in the main, perceived positively by users.

In appeals against degrading treatment, neglect, or abuse, the positive effect of the Board's role can be stated with greater surety. Each appeal is carefully investigated and the Board compiles a report on its findings with recommendations that seek to address the problem and to prevent a recurrence.

Table 30.2 Appeals to the Western Cape Review Board from users, family members of users, concerned members of the public, or other parties, July 2005–February 2008

Reason for appeal	Number of appeals
Appeal against involuntary admission	86
Accusations of sexual abuse	12
Reports of alleged physical abuse	37
Concerns about physical or environmental conditions in hospitals or primary care facilities	23
Appeals about poor access to services	20
Appeals against state patient status	14
Perceived poor quality of clinical management	26
Allegations of degrading or neglectful treatment	18
Miscellaneous appeals	23
Total	**259**

Apart from receiving formal appeals, the Board follows up on informal written or verbal complaints as well as on press articles reporting abuse of mentally ill persons. In addition, users whose medical records report evidence of physical injury are visited by the Board in order to determine whether the user had been physically abused or not.

In cases of alleged abuse, neglect, or degrading treatment, the user and, if necessary, any other concerned parties, are visited. In the main, these visits take place at a ward level, but there have been many instances where members of the Board have visited users in their homes or in institutions.

The impact visits have on improving service delivery, or in addressing infringements of human rights, is difficult to determine, but they do appear to be beneficial. Benefits stem from the mere presence of members of the Review Board in a ward, a home, or an institution which, given the powers of Review Boards, clearly must act as a form of deterrent or disincentive to further violations or sub-optimal service delivery.

Secondly, reports written by the Board on its investigations, interviews, and visits always contain a set of recommendations. These recommendations identify actions the Board believes will help to prevent further abuse, comment on the need for redress, or recommend correction of any deficiencies in service delivery. Finally, in each Quarterly Report submitted to the MEC for Health, the Review Board draws the Minister's attention to matters it believes are serious enough to invite his consideration and possible intervention. The quarterly and annual reports are also circulated to senior public sector mental health care managers, to the National Department of Health, and to a senior judge of the Cape High Court. However, there are no clear indications that the Reports of the Review Board have led to significant increases in service resources for mental health in the province.

A number of challenges face the Review Board. First, there is a challenge in communicating to the public the role and function the Board can fulfill in the interest of mental health care users, their families, and care givers. This is an issue of improving awareness to the widest community of the province. The findings thus far are that awareness and understanding of the Mental Health Review Board remains low in the communities served, and in some instances, even among professional mental health care practitioners. However, there is discernable improvement in the metropolitan area of Cape Town in the three years the Board has been operational. This is measured by the increasing number of members of the public drawing the Board's attention to exploitation, neglect, or abuse outside of the psychiatric hospital setting, in other words concerning people living in the community. Of significance recently has been the growing numbers of reports to the Board of financial exploitation in community settings.

It is likely that communities living in more rural areas still remain significantly uninformed about the Review Board. Issues of language, the geographic separation of more isolated communities, and the relative lack or absence of mental health care services in these areas compounds this problem. Second, the Mental Health Care Act itself, and its accompanying regulatory forms, are ambiguous in places and many of the forms are not user-friendly. The Western Cape Board has re-drafted the most important forms with a view to streamlining them and to improving clarity. This process was done in consultation with all relevant role-players including clinical staff. The Review Board has submitted the draft revised forms to the National Department of Health to consider for inclusion in future amendments to the Act. Third, the exact extent of the executive authority that resides in a Review Board is still not clear. For example, to what extent can a Review Board determine that additional funds are allocated to services, where it perceives services are under-resourced? The new Act certainly does not confer such powers. The view of the Board is that Review Boards are empowered only to submit written recommendations to the MEC recommending matters such as budget revision or resource allocation where the Board has identified deficiencies in user care. However, in the event of a mental health care provider acting in a negligent manner, or abusing users, the Board would be free to recommend that the matter be referred to the Health Professions Council of South Africa (HPCSA). The Board is also free to recommend that an internal disciplinary investigation be undertaken and that it receive a copy of the findings. In the case of serious offences, the Board has in the past recommended that particular cases be referred to the police for investigation, or to the NPA. However, at all times the MEC is free to overrule the Board on any of its considerations. While recommendations of the Review Board clearly carry a lot of weight, the Board is not another arm of management.

To summarize, the introduction of the new Mental Health Care Act, and in particular the provision within the Act for the establishment of Review Boards, has facilitated improved care of people with mental illness (including management at district hospital level) and has significantly helped to protect their rights. In addition, Review Boards would appear to be efficient and affordable in LMICs. While this conclusion is drawn by comparing the current annual budget for mental illness in the Western Cape Province to the annual cost of running its Review Board, it is our view that, even in significantly under-resourced countries, the establishment of independent, oversight bodies such as a Review Board is essential and, if properly run, would represent an efficient use of available resources.

The way forward: strengthening human rights protection in poorly resourced countries

Strengthening human rights protection in low resource settings ideally requires multiple interventions at different levels. These include policy, legislation, service planning, education, research, consumer awareness, and advocacy. The challenge remains that in many of these settings the resources and political will do not exist to mobilize these resources, at least not in the short term. In this light it is necessary to highlight certain fundamental 'non-negotiable' mechanisms that should be in place. From our assessment, the following provisions need to be in place to offer basic human rights protection for the mentally ill:

1. Legislation needs to be enacted that is consistent with international human rights standards.

2. Mechanisms for implementation of the legislation need to be put in place. An example is Review Boards, which are relatively efficient, with powers to sanction and enforce the legislation.

3. Legislative mechanisms need to be linked to service provision and resource allocation. Ideally policy/planning and legislative processes should be linked, but in situations where they are not (as is the case in most low resource settings), legislative mechanisms should have a right to compel services to increase resource allocation to mental health care, in order to protect the right to care for people with mental illness and at least ensure parity with other health service provision.

Of interest in the four African countries examined in this chapter, is that none have all three of these mechanisms in place. While Ghana, Uganda, and Zambia are in the process of reforming their legislation (provision 1), and South Africa has legislation and Review Boards in place (provisions 1 and 2), South Africa still faces major challenges regarding adequate service provision, in particular the lack of access to mental health care among poor and marginalized communities.

Ongoing documentation and further research into existing practice is essential, both to allow for monitoring of human rights protection in these settings, and to generate lessons that can further promote the human rights of the mentally ill in low resource settings.

Acknowledgements

Professor Alan J. Flisher died of leukemia in April 2010, after a relatively short period of illness. As his co-authors on this chapter, we would like to acknowledge his contribution to this work, including his thoughtful comments on the structure of the chapter, his writing of the section on key international human rights instruments, and his comments on successive drafts. His contributions to this chapter were characteristic of many facets of his life and work, and exhibited his generosity, robust intellect, attention to detail, and unflinching integrity. He was committed to protecting and promoting the rights of people who suffered from mental illnesses, particularly children and adolescents, and we would like to dedicate the chapter to his memory.

References

Banda, M, Mwanza, J, Sikwese, A, and Mayeya, J (2008) *A situation analysis of mental health policy development and implementation in Zambia. Phase 1 Country Report.* Lusaka: Mental Health and Poverty Project, University of Zambia.

Bentley, K (2003) *A child-rights approach to monitoring and indicator development.* Presentation given at the HSRC's Child, Youth and Family Development Indicators Project Planning Seminar, HSRC, Cape Town, 17–18 July.

Bhorat, H, Van der Westhuizen, C, and Jacobs, T (2009) *Income and Non-Income Inequality in Post-Apartheid South Africa: What are the Drivers and Possible Policy Interventions?* Development Policy Research Unit, University of Cape Town, DPRU Working Paper 09/138 ISBN: 978-1-920055-74-5. Cape Town.

Bray, R and Dawes, A (2007) 'Monitoring the well-being of children: historical and conceptual foundations', in A Dawes, R Bray, and A Van der Merwe (eds) *Monitoring Child Well Being: A South African Rights-based Perspective.* Johannesburg: Human Sciences Research Council Press, 5–28.

Cooper, S, Ssebunnya, J, Kigozi, F, Lund, C, Flisher, AJ, and MHaPP Research Programme Consortium (2010) 'Viewing Uganda's Mental Health System through a Human Rights Lens', *International Review of Psychiatry*, 22(6), 578–588.

Doku, V, Ofori-Atta, A, Akpalu, B, et al. (2008) *A situation analysis of mental health policy development and implementation in Ghana. Phase 1 Country Report.* Accra: Mental Health and Poverty Project.

Hassim, A, Heywood, M, and Berger, J (2007) *Health and democracy: a guide to human rights, health law and policy in post apartheid South Africa.* Johannesburg: Siber Ink.

Kigozi, F, Ssebunnya, S, Kizza, D, et al. (2008) *A situation analysis of the mental health system in Uganda. Phase 1 Country Report.* Kampala: Mental Health and Poverty Project, Makarere University.

Lund, C, Kleintjes, S, Campbell-Hall, V, et al. (2008) *Mental health policy development and implementation in South Africa. Phase 1 Country Report.* Cape Town: Mental Health and Poverty Project, University of Cape Town.

Lund, C, Kleintjes, S, Kakuma, R, Flisher, A, and the MHaPP Research Programme Consortium (2010) 'Public sector mental health systems in South Africa: inter-provincial comparisons and policy implications', *Social Psychiatry and Psychiatric Epidemiology*, 45, 393–404.

United Nations High Commissioner for Human Rights (2003) *The right to health. Factsheet no 31.* Geneva: United Nations High Commissioner for Human Rights.

WHO (2005a) *Atlas: mental health resources in the world.* Geneva: WHO.

WHO (2005b) *WHO Resource book on mental health, human rights and legislation.* Geneva: WHO.

Chapter 31

Human Rights Standards Relevant to Mental Health and How They can be Made More Effective

François Crépeau and Anne-Claire Gayet

Mental health is an inherent component of human dignity to which every human being is entitled as enshrined in the Universal Declaration of Human Rights. Human rights standards relative to mental health embody the right to health for everyone and should therefore be considered to be as fundamental as standards pertaining to all other civil, political, social, economic, and cultural rights. Social rights are indeed also subject to legal action (Aliprantris 2006). However, mental health tends to be neglected as a human rights issue: some criticize insufficient, inadequate, and inequitably distributed resources (Horton 2007). Such standards are important, as to protect mental health is key to elevating the quality of health in the entire society. It is therefore essential to find ways to make such a social right more effective.

The argument will be twofold. As mental health standards are enshrined in international law and sometimes domestic law, the first element of the solution is to make better use of the existing international and national mechanisms entrusted with respecting, fulfilling, protecting, and promoting human rights. The first step is to be aware of the existing human rights framework regarding mental health. To do so, the specific institutions in charge of implementing human rights standards—including treaty bodies, national institutions, as well as tribunals, both at international and national levels—will be presented, with an evaluation of what they can do to enhance the effectiveness of human rights standards relative to mental health. Secondly, the maximal use of these institutions can only happen if all actors, including civil society, take an active role. This will result from cross-sectional cooperation and inter-institutional consultation, as well as human rights education for all. These arguments will be based primarily, though not exclusively, on the Canadian context.

Using existing international and national institutions to their full potential

Previous chapters advocate in favour of a broadening and deepening of human rights standards relative to mental health. To complement this, a more efficient implementation of those already in place is needed, by using the existing human rights institutions, both international and national, to their full potential. Composed of various international treaties, international law has set up a complex machinery in order to establish standards, monitor implementation, promote compliance, and investigate violations of human rights: be it treaty bodies, judicial tribunals, or other mechanisms, these institutions aim at enhancing the implementation of human rights standards. At national level, some institutions are specifically mandated for ensuring the respect, fulfilment, protection, and promotion of human rights. When the latter institutions do not exist, their creation should be a top political priority.

Treaty bodies

Many international human rights conventions create treaty bodies whose task is to monitor the implementation of their provisions by state parties. Let's consider the treaty bodies that are important for our topic. Those belonging to the United Nations (UN) are the Human Rights Committee (HRC) which monitors the implementation of the 1966 International Covenant on Civil and Political Rights (ICCPR), the Committee on Economic, Social and Cultural Rights (CESCR) which monitors the implementation of the 1966 International Covenant on Economic, Social and Cultural Rights (ICESCR), the Committee against Torture (CAT) which monitors the implementation of the 1984 Convention against Torture and Other Cruel, Inhuman or Degrading Treatment or Punishment (Torture Convention), and the Committee on the Rights of Persons with Disabilities (CRDP) which, since 2009, monitors the 2006 Convention of the Rights of Persons with Disabilities. The regional treaty bodies are the European Committee of Social Rights (ECSR) established by the Council of Europe's European Social Charter (adopted in 1961 and revised in 1996); the European Committee for the Prevention of Torture (CPT) established by the 1987 European Convention for the Prevention of Torture and Inhuman or Degrading Treatment or Punishment (European Torture Convention); and the Inter-American Commission on Human Rights (IACHR), whose mandate is found in the 1948 Charter of the Organization of American States and the 1969 American Convention on Human Rights (American Convention).

Periodic reporting

States parties to human rights conventions must submit reports to the treaty body on how the rights are being implemented. Such reports are submitted periodically (the period varies from two to five years, depending on the convention). Each committee examines the report, as well as the information submitted by the state or coming from other sources. In particular, it has become a regular practice that non-governmental organizations (NGOs) from the state in question submit 'shadow' reports containing additional information or alternative explanations. The committee then addresses its praise, concerns, and recommendations to the state party in the form of 'concluding observations', which may declare that rights violations have taken place, urge the State party to desist from any further violations, or call on the authorities to adopt measures to improve the situation.

For example, the 2006 concluding observations of CESCR regarding Canada's implementation of the ICESCR report both positive and negative aspects regarding mental health (CESCR 2006). 'The Committee notes with satisfaction the numerous health programmes conducted by the State party, such as the 10-Year Plan to Strengthen Health Care and the launch of the Public Health Agency' (§8). 'However, the Committee is concerned by the significant disparities still remaining between Aboriginal peoples and the rest of the population in access to health' (§15). 'The Committee also recommends that the State party give special attention to homeless girls, who are more vulnerable to health risks and social and economic deprivation, and that it takes all necessary measures to provide them with adequate housing and social and health services' (§57).

The ICCPR does not contain any specific provision relating to health. Nevertheless, since the covenant's provisions apply fully to all members of society, persons with disabilities (including mental illness) are clearly entitled to the full range of rights recognized in the ICCPR, including the right to liberty and security of the person, the right to vote, the right to associate, the right to property, the right to freedom from torture, the right to family life, to name only a few. The most recent HRC's Concluding Observations on Canada (HRC 2006) include specific considerations toward persons with mental disabilities, substantiated thanks to reports from Canadian NGOs. The Committee is concerned that, in some provinces and territories, people with mental disabilities or illness remain in detention because of insufficient provision of community-based supportive housing (§17): it recommends that the state party, including all governments at provincial and territorial level, 'should increase (their) efforts to ensure that sufficient and adequate community-based housing is provided to people with mental disabilities, and ensure that the latter are not under continued detention when there is no longer a legally based medical reason for such detention'. Canada is thus expected to make appropriate changes and report on its efforts to conform to such observations.

In its 2005 Concluding Observations on the Fourth and Fifth Periodic Reports of Canada (submitted in 2002 and 2004), CAT expresses its satisfaction regarding 'the general inclusion in the 2002 *Immigration and Refugee Protection Act* (IRPA) of torture within the meaning of article 1 of the [Torture] Convention as an independent ground qualifying a person as in need of protection …and as a basis for non-refoulement …, where there are substantial grounds for believing that the threat of torture exists'. However, CAT is concerned by 'the failure of the Supreme Court of Canada, in *Suresh v. Minister of Citizenship and Immigration*, to recognize in domestic law the absolute nature of the protection of article 3 of the Convention', which states that 'no State Party shall expel, return or extradite a person to another State where there are substantial grounds for believing that he would be in danger of being subjected to torture'. Therefore, CAT recommends that 'the State party unconditionally undertake to respect the absolute nature of article 3 in all circumstances and fully to incorporate the provision of article 3 into the State party's domestic law' and 'remove the exclusions in the IRPA … thereby extending to currently excluded persons entitlement to the status of protected person, and protection against refoulement on account of a risk of torture' (CAT 2005). The relationship between immigration detention and mental health is documented and the CAT clearly indicates that the dignity of the person should prevail in immigration implementation mechanisms.

The ECSR has to decide on the conformity of the law and practice of Council of Europe (CoE) member states with the European Social Charter (or the Revised European Social Charter, if ratified by the state). The provisions relative to mental health can be found in the 'right to safe and healthy working conditions' (Article 3) and the 'right of persons with disabilities to independence, social integration and participation in the life of the community' (Article 15). In its General Introduction to its 2007 Conclusions, the Committee recalls that 'the underlying vision of Article 15 is one of equal citizenship for persons with disabilities' (ECSR 2007). In its 2007 Conclusions on France, regarding the respect of Article 15, the ECSR notes with satisfaction that specific results regarding children with mental disabilities had been achieved: 'recommendations on the early diagnosis of autism have been elaborated and are currently spread among medical and non-medical staff; the Departmental Centres for Autism have been established; 801 places for children and 678 for adults were financed in 2005'. However, the Committee also observes that 'at the end of 2005, only 38% (301) of the 801 places for autistic persons financed in 2005 has been actually established' and concludes 'that the situation in France is not in conformity with Article 15§1 on the ground that equal access to education (mainstreaming and special education) of persons with autism is not yet guaranteed in an effective manner' (ECSR 2007). The monitoring done by the ECSR therefore ensures that States are precisely and publicly informed of their shortcomings in implementing the rights guaranteed in the European Social Charter. This has a pedagogical effect which in itself constitutes an element of promotion of such rights and helps the rights-holders and the NGO community to exercise pressure in favour of a higher degree of respect, fulfilment, and protection on the part of the state.

Production of soft law

The treaty bodies may also have an important influence in the production of 'soft law', as soft law can be used to guide interpretation of treaties. The Principles for the Protection of Persons with Mental Illness and for the Improvement of Mental Health Care, adopted by the General Assembly of the United Nations (UNGA) in 1991 (UNGA 1991) and the Standard Rules on the Equalization of Opportunities for Persons with Disabilities (UNGA 1993)—the purpose of which is to ensure that all persons with disabilities 'may exercise the same rights and obligations as others'—constitute particularly valuable reference guides in identifying more precisely the relevant obligations of states parties under the ICESCR.

Article 12.1 of the ICESCR refers explicitly to the right to 'the highest attainable standard of physical and mental health'. Commenting this article in its General Comment No. 14, the CESCR notes that this 'reference…is not confined to the right to health care. On the contrary, [it] acknowledge(s) that the right to health embraces a wide range of socio-economic factors that promote conditions in which people can lead a healthy life, and extends to the underlying determinants of health, such as food and nutrition, housing, access to safe and potable water and adequate sanitation, safe and healthy working conditions, and a healthy environment' (CESCR 2000). This comprehensive understanding of the right to health is not easily enforceable because of its broadness, but it provides a strong statement of the necessity to preserve health in most dimensions of our daily lives. In its General Comment No. 5, Persons with disabilities, the CESCR notes that, in its experience, states parties devote very little attention to this issue in their reports. It underlines that it is consistent with the Secretary-General's conclusion that 'most Governments still lack decisive concerted measures that would effectively improve the situation' of persons with disabilities (CESCR 1994).

Such soft law is important as it reflects an emerging consensus, mainstreams certain concepts, and is often the precursor of 'harder' standards. It is regularly used by treaty bodies or tribunals to support their interpretation of the law. Thus, the IACHR expressly quoted the 1991 Principles in its decision in the case of *Victor Rosario Congo v Ecuador*, thus lending them some force of law as precedent within the inter-American human rights system (IACHR 1997). In order to enhance the implementation of the rights of persons with disabilities, it is therefore appropriate to review and disseminate the observations and other forms of 'soft law' made by the treaty bodies that concern persons with disabilities.

Individual complaints mechanisms

Individual complaints against violations of human rights can be brought to the attention of certain treaty bodies. They may be submitted by an individual, a group, or a state under a number of procedures. The ability of individuals to complain about the violation of their rights in an international arena brings real meaning to the rights contained in the human rights treaties. Although inter-state complaints are provided for, none has ever been filed at universal level under any of the human rights conventions regimes: the individual complaints procedure is the only mechanism that has ever worked regarding individual cases.

Several human rights treaty bodies may, under certain circumstances, consider individual complaints. CAT may consider individual communications relating to states parties who have made the necessary declaration under Article 22 of the Torture Convention. HRC may consider individual communications relating to states parties to the First Optional Protocol to the ICCPR. The Committee on the Elimination of Racial Discrimination may consider individual communications relating to States parties who have made the necessary declaration under Article 14 of the Convention on the Elimination of All Forms of Racial Discrimination (ICERD). The Committee on the Elimination of All Forms of Discrimination against Women (CEDAW) may consider individual communications relating to state parties to the Optional Protocol to the Convention on the Elimination of All Forms of Discrimination against Women. For example, CEDAW adopted views on the Communication No. 2/2003, *Ms A v Hungary*: the victim, a Hungarian national, said 'that her physical integrity, physical and mental health and life [had] been at serious risk and that she [lived] in constant fear'. The Committee concluded that the state party had failed to fulfil its obligations and had thereby violated the rights of the claimant. The Committee recommended Hungary to 'take immediate and effective measures to guarantee the physical and mental integrity of A. T. and her family' and 'ensure that A. T. is given a safe home in which to live with her children, receives appropriate child support and legal assistance as well as reparation proportionate to the physical and mental harm undergone and to the gravity of the violations of her rights' (CEDAW 2005). Other committees in charge of receiving and considering individual communications on rights violations have been recently established. The treaty body of the Convention on the Rights of Persons with Disabilities has held its second meeting in November 2009. The Optional Protocol to the ICESCR, that establishes an individual complaints mechanism, was adopted on 10 December 2008 by the General Assembly and has now to be acceded to by States (UNGA 2008). The treaty body of the International Convention on the Protection of the Rights of All Migrant Workers and Members of Their Families was established in 2004, and will entertain individual complaints when ten countries have accepted the procedure: At present, only Mexico and Guatemala have done so.

IACHR is expressly authorized to examine complaints or petitions regarding specific cases of human rights violations. In the case *Victor Rosario Congo v Ecuador,* the Commission reported that although 'the victim was diagnosed as mentally ill, he was kept in isolation and his basic physical needs were disregarded in the knowledge that he was in no condition to care for himself.' The Commission concluded that 'the fact that the State [had] no special facilities for the admission of prisoners with mental illness [did] not exempt it from the obligation to provide medical care to the persons in its custody.' IACHR reiterated its recommendations to Ecuador that it should 'provide medical and psychiatric care for persons suffering from mental illness and confined in penitentiary facilities' and 'assign to the health services of the penitentiary system specialists able to identify psychiatric disorders that can affect the lives and the physical, mental and moral integrity of those confined in it' (IACHR 1998).

Such individual complaints mechanisms are therefore available for denouncing human rights violations, including those related to mental health issues. A more widespread use of such mechanisms, for example with the help of NGOs, would go a long way towards adding pressure on governments. The reticence of many states to accept that treaty bodies be empowered to hear individual complaints is an indirect recognition of the power of such a mechanism to exert pressure on state authorities to change their laws and practices so as to ensure a better implementation of the concerned rights.

Collective complaints mechanisms

Collective complaints mechanisms allow specific organizations to complain about situations of human rights violations. For example, the ECSR can receive collective complaints from trade unions, business associations, and international NGOs enjoying participatory status with the Council of Europe, but only 12 countries have acceded to the 1995 protocol that provides for this possibility.

The ECSR declared admissible several complaints relative to the protection of health. For example, on Complaint No. 13/2002 of the *International Association Autism—Europe (IAAE) v France*, alleging insufficient educational provision for autistic children, ECSR concluded that there was a violation of Articles 15 (the right of persons with disabilities), 17, and E (non-discrimination) of the Social Charter (ECSR 2003). Following ECSR's deliberation, the Committee of Ministers adopted Resolution ResChS(2004)1 to 'take note of the statement made by the respondent Government indicating that the French Government undertakes to bring the situation into conformity with the Revised Charter and that measures are being taken in this respect' (CoE Committee of Ministers 2004). On Complaint No. 41/2007 of the *Mental Disability Advocacy Centre (MDAC) v Bulgaria,* the Committee concluded in 2008 that there was a violation of the Revised Charter as children with moderate, severe, or profound intellectual disabilities residing in homes for mentally disabled children in Bulgaria did not have an effective right to education and were subject to disability-based discrimination, as a result of the low number of such children receiving any type of education when compared to other children (ECSR 2007).

Although not widespread, such a collective complaint mechanism can provide for a meaningful debate around pressing human rights issues.

On-site visits

The Optional Protocol to the United Nations Convention against Torture (UNGA 2002, entered into force 2006) allows in-country inspections of places of detention—e.g. prisons, police stations, immigration detention centres, and psychiatric hospitals—by the Subcommittee on Prevention of Torture (SPT) in collaboration with national institutions. The SPT favours a preventive approach, which aims at protecting people deprived of their liberty rather than condemning states. It therefore communicates its recommendations and observations confidentially to the state party. Since 2007, the SPT has conducted six on-site visits, in Mauritius, Sweden, and Mexico among others.

The European Committee for the Prevention of Torture (CPT) has also the mandate to examine the treatment of persons deprived of their liberty, and, contrary to the SPT, has an *unlimited access* to all places of detention. It must notify the state concerned but does not need to specify the period between notification and the actual visit: the CPT often notifies a government only a few hours before the actual visit. Governments' objections to the time or place of a visit (to an institution or to a person) can only be justified on very specific grounds (national defence, public safety, serious disorder, medical condition, or an inquiry in progress) and the state must take steps to enable the Committee to visit as soon as possible. The CPT makes confidential reports on its visits and addresses recommendations to national governments. If a country fails to cooperate, the CPT may decide to make a public statement.

The CPT gives specific considerations to the conditions of detention of mentally disabled persons. In its Response to the report of the [CPT] on its visit to Albania from 28 to 31 March 2006, the Albanian government addressed the Committee's concern regarding 'the issue of those chronic patients who were held in the psychiatric hospitals "because of a lack of services and the lack of the appropriate alternatives in the actual health system" as well as of mentally disabled persons who were held in psychiatric hospitals "because of a lack of appropriate structures for their stabilization". It said that the issue was on the agenda of the Department of Health and the Department of Labour, Social Affairs and Equal Opportunities, that 'no concrete results [had] been achieved', but that they would 'immediately inform the CPT' as soon as both parties would find a 'concrete solution' (CPT 2007).

The IACHR also carries out on-site visits to countries to engage in in-depth analysis of the general situation and/or to investigate a specific situation. In its 2003 Report on the Situation of Human Rights in Venezuela, the Commission observed that 'the worsening of the institutional conflict in Venezuela has spilled over into acts of violence that have led to violations both of the right to life … and of the right to humane treatment' and recommended Venezuela to 'ensure that acts of torture are categorized and punished as such by the courts; conduct meaningful, thorough and impartial investigations into acts of torture and other cruel, inhuman or degrading treatment; initiate, through the Office of the Prosecutor General of the Republic, a thorough investigation of all complaints of abuses of physical integrity, in particular concerning persons deprived of liberty' (§364) (IACHR 2003).

Treaty bodies, whether at international or regional level, are therefore essential tools to increase the respect, the protection, the fulfilment, and the promotion of human rights standards relative to mental health.

Special procedures

The independent experts appointed by the United Nations to investigate and report on the human rights situations in specific countries or on thematic issues often address concerns pertaining to the rights of persons with mental health issues or confronted with violations of the right to mental health. Their conclusions and recommendations are published and debated, bringing the issues to international attention and serving as guidance for the governments.

The 'Special Rapporteur of the Commission on Human Rights on the Right of Everyone to the Enjoyment of the Highest Attainable Standard of Physical and Mental Health' was established by the Commission on Human Rights Resolution 2002/31 with the mandate to collect and share information from all relevant sources on the realization of this right, to foster dialogue and cooperation with all relevant actors, to report on 'good practices most beneficial to its enjoyment and obstacles encountered domestically and internationally to its implementation', and to make recommendations on measures to promote and protect the realization of this right in order to support 'States' efforts to enhance public health' (OHCHR 2002:5.c and d).

In his report from a mission to Sweden, the Special Rapporteur was concerned by the deterioration of mental health in Sweden: 'Sleeping disorders, depression, anxiety and other types of nervous problems are increasing, and sales of anti-depressant drugs increased fivefold between 1992 and 2003'; 'unless the situation is urgent, waiting times for mental health care are lengthy'; although 'up to a quarter of refugees and asylum-seekers are affected by post-traumatic stress disorder, … refugees, asylum-seekers and homeless persons all reportedly have difficulty accessing mental health care'. As a consequence, the Rapporteur 'urges the Government to ensure that it takes measures to address causes of psychosocial disabilities among vulnerable and marginalized groups, including children, adolescents, homeless persons, women, asylum-seekers, and lesbian, gay, bisexual and transgender persons. He urges the Government to ensure that mental health care, including psychiatric care and other therapies, is made more accessible for marginalized groups' (UN Special Rapporteur 2007).

Such special procedures can have an important fact-finding role and can bring issues to the international scene.

International courts and tribunals

International human rights tribunals are independent judicial bodies aiming at sanctioning violations of specific human rights conventions. The European Court of Human Rights (ECHR) has been created to implement the 1950 European Convention on Human Rights (European Convention): it is the oldest, most productive, and most effective regional human rights tribunal. The Inter-American Court of Human Rights (IACourtHR) was established by the American Convention. The African Court of Human and Peoples' Rights, established in 2004 to implement the 1981 African Charter on Human and Peoples' Rights, has yet to start its judicial work.

In *Kucheruk v Ukraine*, the ECHR held that there had been a violation of Article 3 of the European Convention ('no one shall be subjected to torture or to inhuman or degrading treatment or punishment'): the solitary confinement and handcuffing for seven days of a person who suffered from schizophrenia, without psychiatric justification or medical treatment, had to be regarded as constituting inhuman and degrading treatment. The domestic authorities had not provided appropriate medical treatment and assistance to the applicant (ECHR 2007).

In *Ximenes-Lopes v Brazil*, the IACourtHR reaffirmed several fundamental rights for mentally ill persons. The victim was mentally ill and died while under treatment in a mental health institution. The Court reaffirmed that states must give special attention to 'persons with mental disabilities for they are particularly vulnerable', especially since 'such vulnerability is greater when they are admitted to mental health institutions.' Furthermore, 'any health treatment administered to persons with mental illness should aim at achieving the patient´s welfare and the respect for his or her dignity as a human person, which is translated into the duty to adopt the respect for the intimacy and autonomy of persons as guiding principles for administering psychiatric treatment.' The Court conceded that the principle of autonomy 'is not absolute, since the patients' needs themselves may sometimes require the adoption of measures without their consent.' However, 'mental illnesses should not be understood as a disability for determination and the assumption that persons with mental illness are capable of expressing their will, which should be respected by both the medical staff and the authorities, should prevail.' The Court also stressed that 'States have the duty to ensure the creation of the conditions required to prevent the violations of (the) inalienable right (to life and to humane treatment), and particularly, the duty to prevent their agents from infringing it.' Therefore, the Court declared that Brazil violated the rights to life and humane treatment enshrined in the American Convention and ruled, among other things, that 'the State must keep developing an education and training programme for staff in health care, psychiatry, psychology, nursing, and for any person involved in mental health services, in particular, covering the principles that govern treatment to patients with mental illness, according to international standards and the provisions of the instant Judgment' (IACourtHR 2006).

National judicial tribunals

National tribunals are naturally important for making human rights standards relative to mental health more effective. Civil and criminal courts, as well as judicial and quasi-judicial administrative bodies—such as the Canadian Immigration and Refugee Board (IRB)—have a clear role to play in the implementation of human rights standards applicable to mentally ill persons: very specific practices do emerge.

As a social right, the right to mental health care should be justiciable in domestic courts, although states have rarely provided for that possibility (Aliprantis 2006). One such example is provided by the Indian Supreme Court. In the case of *Rakesh Chandra Narain etc v State of Bihar*, acting on the complaints of citizens regarding the living conditions of patients in three mental hospitals (more precisely, 'the abysmal living conditions, the inadequate diet, the budgetary limits on medicine and the absence of staff'), the Supreme Court requested the Indian National Human Rights Commission to supervise the functioning of the psychiatric hospitals at Ranchi, Agra, and Gwalior and improvements were noticed in the working of these institutions (Dhanda 2005; Supreme Court of India 1995).

National human rights institutions

Beyond national courts, the effective enjoyment of human rights calls for the establishment of a national infrastructure of human rights bodies. While their tasks may differ from country to country, they share a common purpose: the respect, fulfilment, protection, and promotion of human rights and for this reason are collectively referred to as National Human Rights Institutions

(NHRIs). The majority of existing national institutions can be grouped in two broad categories: human rights commissions and ombudspersons (OHCHR 1993).

A NHRI is a quasi-governmental agency occupying a unique place between the judicial, representative, and executive functions of the state. The UN General Assembly adopted the 1993 Principles relating to the Status of National Institutions (Paris Principles) to assess the effectiveness of existing NHRIs and to ensure that new ones are set up with the requisite ingredients for effective and independent functioning. They are not an alternative to an independent, impartial, properly resourced, and accessible judiciary whose rulings are enforced. They can however constitute an effective complement to the judiciary and other institutions within the state in promoting and protecting human rights standards.

The Paris Principles suggest that national institutions can advise authorities on situations, promote harmonization of national legislation and practices with international human rights instruments, encourage ratification of such instruments, contribute to the reports which states are required to submit to treaty bodies, contribute to human rights education, research, and public awareness programmes, and engage in international cooperation with like minded institutions. Their mandate should include the protection and promotion of the rights of those in society who are particularly at risk of human rights violations, especially women and children, people with disabilities, persons belonging to aboriginal peoples or minorities, human rights defenders, refugees, asylum-seekers, and migrant workers.

The ombudsperson's primary function is to ensure fairness and legality in public administration and, more specifically, to protect the rights of individuals who suffer injustice at the hands of civil servants. Human rights commissions are more specifically concerned with discrimination and will often address the actions of private actors, as well as of the government (OHCHR 1993). For example, besides the prevention and communication aspects, the Discrimination Prevention Branch of the Canadian Human Rights Commission is responsible for ensuring that federally regulated employers meet the requirement of the Employment Equity Act (1995) that aims at achieving 'equality in the workplace so that no person shall be denied employment opportunities or benefits for reasons unrelated to ability and, in the fulfillment of that goal, to correct the conditions of disadvantage in employment experienced by women, Aboriginal peoples, persons with disabilities and members of visible minorities'. It recognizes that these persons (including mentally ill persons) have to be treated in the same way but that they also require special measures and accommodation for their difference (Canada, Employment Equity Act 1995, s. 2).

Although NHRIs have essentially an advisory capacity, governments are under growing pressure to respond publicly, within a reasonable time, to case-specific as well as to more general findings, conclusions, and recommendations. When the government fails to respond or refuses to implement recommendations, Amnesty International (AI) recommends that the NHRI continue to press the government, for example, through pressure by the media or Parliament, as well as by bringing the case to the attention of international human rights bodies, such as treaty bodies or special mechanisms (AI 2001). The French Haute Autorité de Lutte contre les Discriminations et pour l'Egalité (HALDE) made public its Decision No. 2006–128 of June 2006 referring to a State Prosecutor's objection to the marriage of an asylum seeker of Algerian nationality and a person suffering from cerebral palsy to a degree of 80 per cent: 'although this disease is characterized by motor dysfunction that does not worsen over time and has no effect on the sufferer's mental faculties, a series of extrapolations led to the assumption that the claimant's physical disability and resulting appearance amounted to mental disability and legal incapacity'. The HALDE considered that the claimant had been victim of discrimination on the grounds of disability (HALDE 2006).

Other national institutions

At national level, other institutions can have a positive impact on human rights standards relative to mental health. Two examples will be useful.

In Australia, the Palmer Inquiry came about after an Australian resident of German origin (Cornelia Rau) was detained in view of her deportation for 11 months. Due to mental illness, she called herself by a different name ('Anna'), maintained that she was a German tourist and spoke German. The inquiry report showed that the mental health assessment of the victim had been inadequate and that the mandatory detention policy for unauthorized foreigners had structural shortcomings and was poorly managed. The six-month detention of Ms Rau in a criminal detention facility was especially inappropriate since 'she was not a prisoner, had done nothing wrong and was put there simply for administrative convenience' (Palmer 2005). Following the Palmer report, the Australian government asked the Commonwealth Ombudsman to investigate some 201 immigration detention matters that had been referred to Mr Palmer. As of June 2008, the Ombudsman had tabled in Parliament 413 individual reports on immigration detainees. The reports show that many have mental health issues and that mental health care is often inadequate (Commonwealth Ombudsman 2008, 2009).

In Canada, the Office of the Correctional Investigator (OCI) investigates and attempts to resolve complaints from individual offenders under federal jurisdiction. It also has a responsibility to review and make recommendations on the policies and procedures of Correctional Services Canada (CSC) that relate to individual complaints. In its 2007 report, the OCI expressed concern over the services available to inmates with mental health issues and to those with a history of self-injury. The competence of clinical personnel and the quality of assessments as to the mental state of an inmate were sometimes put into question. Some institutions lacked a multidisciplinary mental health team. In several cases, suicide watch was observed as being *de facto* segregation and that it did little to respond to the inmate's mental health needs (Correctional Investigator Canada 2007). In its recent Mental Health Strategy, the CSC conceded that its intake assessment of offenders' mental health upon admission was inadequate, consisting only in a few questions on such matters as previous psychiatric hospitalizations and prescriptions for psychotropic medications. Only culprits with evident, serious mental health issues are referred for a more comprehensive psychological assessment. The report also suggests that a sound and comprehensive mental health intake assessment is required for CSC to implement a more effective suicide and self-injury prevention strategy. It also calls for significant investments in the care, treatment and support of inmates with mental health issues (Canada 2002).

This first section showed the importance of all democratic institutions in safeguarding the legal and political foundations upon which human rights are based. National human rights institutions cannot be expected to solve all by themselves those problems which governments and the international community have been unable to effectively address. Neither are they set up to replace the human rights organs of the United Nations or the NGOs working in the same area. The roles of all these actors are clearly complementary to one another, and the strengthening of one such institution can only enhance the effectiveness of the others, thus reinforcing both national and international systems for the protection and promotion of human rights. Human rights standards relative to mental health can only benefit from the strengthening of such institutions (OHCHR 1993).

Practices that enhance the effectiveness of human rights standards

Enforcing human rights requires institutions having the mandate and resources to respect, fulfil, protect, and promote such rights. Many of them already exist, but will remain powerless unless sustained by cooperation practices and an effective mobilization of the population behind them. This implies a multi-level cooperation between institutions, a mobilization of civil society and the availability of human rights education for all.

Cross-sectional cooperation and inter-institutional consultation

In order to make human rights standards relative to mental health more effective, consultation and cooperation between actors are essential.

One can illustrate the cross-sectional cooperation hypothesis with the case of an asylum seeker in Canada at the end of 2007. This example shows that cooperation among actors may enhance the respect, fulfilment, and protection of the human rights of persons with mental illness. *A contrario*, a lack of cooperation—be it refusing to assume one's responsibility ('passing the buck') or misunderstanding each actor's role—can deeply endanger human rights protection.

The example is one of good practice. It is the case of an asylum seeker whose symptoms are akin to those of schizophrenia and who benefited from the implementation of existing standards protecting her rights (both national and international) and from the cooperation among the actors in her social network. This person claimed asylum upon her arrival in Montreal. However, her identity was not established and the officer believed that she represented a high flight risk, meaning it was likely that she would not come to the hearing during which the Immigration and Refugee Board (IRB) would determine her refugee claim. Therefore, detention was ordered by the Canadian Border and Services Agency (CBSA), in application of the Immigration and Protection Refugee Act (IRPA) and its Regulations (Canada 2001).

According to the United Nations High Commissioner for Refugees' Detention Guidelines, detention of asylum seekers is 'inherently undesirable'. This is even more so in the case of vulnerable groups, such as those with special medical or psychological needs. 'Freedom from arbitrary detention is a fundamental human right and the use of detention is, in many instances, contrary to the norms and principles of international law.' Besides, detainees' mental health is likely to deteriorate over the course of their detention. Detention of mentally ill asylum seekers not only contradicts human rights standards but also endangers their already weakened health. Best practices would proscribe detention for mentally ill persons, and encourage finding appropriate solutions, such as transfer to a mental health facility. However, the issue is more frequently the *availability* of alternatives, such as shelters or appropriate lodging offering some kind of 'control' over and protection of the person (UNHCR 1999).

Shortly after she was detained, CBSA's agents complained that the individual was violent and needed specific care for a mental health disorder. Therefore, she was assigned a 'designated representative' from a provincial programme to help new immigrants and asylum seekers. The designated representative is responsible for defending the interests of a person subject to refugee determination proceedings and who, because of age or health issues, is unable to understand the nature of the proceeding (Roy 2003). Their mandate includes the preparation of the individual for the hearings, collaboration with the professional network that surrounds the individual (doctor, social worker, psychologist, etc.) in order to report to the IRB on the individual's difficulties.

The law provides for regular reviews of detention and sets forth the conditions under which a person may be released. Efforts were made to adapt the hearing to this person's needs, in accordance with Guideline 8 on Procedures with Respect to Vulnerable Persons Appearing before the IRB. The IRB acknowledges that appearing before an immigration officer is a difficult process for several reasons: the painful challenge of telling one's traumatic story, the stress of appearing in front of government officials, the utmost importance of the outcome of the hearing for those involved. Therefore, all persons appearing before the IRB have to be treated with sensitivity and respect. Persons who are particularly vulnerable, such as mentally ill persons, need to have their case processed taking into account their specific vulnerability. 'Vulnerability' is defined as the impairment of one's ability to present one's case due to a psychological or physical frailty. The intention of Guideline 8 is therefore to 'provide procedural accommodation(s) for individuals who are identified as vulnerable persons by the IRB'; it articulates the 'IRB's commitment to making procedural accommodations for such persons so that they are not disadvantaged in presenting their cases', whether it be for admissibility, detention, removal, refugee protection, permanent resident status, or family reunification—all of these being matters that affect the lives of individuals directly and profoundly (IRB 2006).

At the third monthly detention review, the CBSA officer argued that the asylum seeker, if released, would not have the financial means to pay for her medication, without which she would become aggressive, and requested prolonging the detention. However, the designated representative and the counsel suggested an alternative to detention. The lawyer obtained the assurance that a social service would cover the costs of the medication upon release. An NGO proposed to accommodate the person until she would find an apartment. She was willing to respect the conditions of her release: to check in once a week at the immigration office in Montreal and to take her medication daily. The IRB member welcomed these efforts to find an appropriate arrangement and the individual was released subject to the agreed upon conditions.

Several conclusions can be drawn from this example. Canadian law contains several provisions that aim at ensuring a fair hearing for mentally ill persons. In addition to appointing a designated representative and to adopting particularly comprehensive practices towards such asylum seekers, the institutions and individuals at work (IRB, CBSA, designated representative, and counsel) had to cooperate to find the appropriate solutions in the case, that is, solutions that would better protect the right to dignity of a person with mental health issues.

The mobilization of civil society

Civil society intervenes at different levels. Non-governmental organizations are key actors in the respect, fulfilment, protection, and promotion of human rights. Being in the field, they may have an easier access to victims, and gain their trust more readily than government officials. They can be involved in mediation. They may sensitize international and national public opinion by providing timely information to governmental and intergovernmental bodies on factual situations or on governments' policies and practices. They can work with international organizations, such as the UN (Human Rights Council, treaty bodies, special procedures, etc.), and contribute to the development of human rights standards and the monitoring of government and private actors' implementation of such standards. In particular, NGOs can submit alternative reports to human rights treaty bodies and play an important role during the examination of state party reports by bringing to light information about serious human rights situations. They can also contribute to the implementation of the decisions and recommendations of the treaty bodies and special procedures. The Canadian Institute for Health Information published in 2007 a report on Improving the Health of Canadians: Mental Health and Homelessness: such reports are important for underlining the specific needs of these vulnerable populations. NGOs are particularly well placed to provide such information, especially when their action is supported rather than opposed by governmental authorities. NGOs can also provide the necessary support to victims when access to courts or NHRIs proves difficult. They can also initiate 'test cases' (Federal Court of Canada 2007).

Academics should also participate more in the process of assessing the needs for human rights respect, fulfilment, protection, and promotion and identify current gaps in law and practice. For example, numerous studies have shown the negative effect of family separation (and the positive effect of family unity) on the psychosocial adjustment of individuals, and more specifically on their mental and physical health, especially in a context of forced migration (*inter alia* Ayotte

2001; Montgomery et al. 2001; Rousseau et al. 2001). This academic input strengthens pronounce-ments by international organizations that emphasise the right to family reunification as enshrined in some international conventions such as the European Social Charter, the 1977 European Convention on the Legal Status of Migrant Workers, and the 1990 International Convention on the Protection of the Rights of All Migrant Workers and Members of Their Families (see, notably, 'Toward a Migration Management Strategy' 2000).

Human rights education

Individuals who benefit from human rights education will be in a better position to claim their rights and to respect, fulfil, protect, and promote the rights of others, in particular in the field of mental health. Furthermore, a population who is knowledgeable about human rights and can in turn carry out human rights education is an asset to international and national human rights bod-ies. Educating the population about human rights is a task that governments, NHRIs, NGOs, academics, and other members of civil society working even under the most repressive govern-ments are able to attempt. It is important that it be done effectively. Specific audiences must be targeted, such as those working in mental health institutions, detention centres, schools, tribunals, as well as with communities and NGOs. The 2006 brochure 'The Right to Adequate Housing: How to Fight for Your Rights' done by the Centre for Equality Rights in Accommodation, is a good example of a document designed to inform and to educate people about their right to ade-quate housing: it explains Canada's obligation under international and domestic laws and shows possible remedies for victims of discrimination (CERA 2006).

The review of existing institutions and mechanisms that have an impact on the protection of human rights, at international, regional, and national levels, reveals all the tools that are already at our disposal to make human rights standards relative to mental health more effective. In order to maximize their potential, every actor is important: international organizations, governments, national institutions, NGOs, and individuals all have a role to play and cooperation between them is essential. They all contribute to consciousness-raising and policy and practice modifica-tions in favour of sustainable societal changes that make mental health a fundamental right for the individual as well as a global concern.

Abbreviations

Institutions:

Amnesty International (AI)
Canadian Border and Services Agency (CBSA)
Canadian Immigration and Refugee Board (IRB)
Committee against Torture (CAT)
Committee on the Elimination of All Forms of Discrimination against Women (CEDAW)
Committee on Economic, Social and Cultural Rights (CESCR)
Committee on the Rights of Persons with Disabilities (CRDP)
Correctional Services Canada (CSC)
Council of Europe (CoE)
European Committee of Social Rights (ECSR)
European Committee for the Prevention of Torture (CPT)
European Court of Human Rights (ECHR)
General Assembly of the United Nations (UNGA)
Haute Autorité de Lutte contre les Discriminations et pour l'Égalité (HALDE)

Human Rights Committee (HRC)
Immigration and Refugee Board (IRB)
Inter-American Commission on Human Rights (IACHR)
Inter-American Court of Human Rights (IACourtHR)
Non-Governmental Organizations (NGOs)
Office of the Correctional Investigator (OCI)
Subcommittee on Prevention of Torture (SPT)
United Nations (UN)
United Nations High Commissioner for Refugees (UNHCR)
National Human Rights Institutions (NHRIs)

Instruments:

American Convention on Human Rights (American Convention).
Convention against Torture and Other Cruel, Inhuman or Degrading Treatment or Punishment (Torture Convention)
Convention on the Elimination of All Forms of Racial Discrimination (ICERD)
Convention on the Elimination of All Forms of Discrimination against Women (CEDAW)
European Convention on Human Rights (European Convention)
Immigration and Protection Refugee Act (IRPA)
International Covenant on Civil and Political Rights (ICCPR)
International Covenant on Economic, Social and Cultural Rights (ICESCR)
European Convention for the Prevention of Torture and Inhuman or Degrading Treatment or Punishment (European Torture Convention)
Principles relating to the Status of National Institutions (Paris Principles)

References

Doctrine

Aliprantris, N (2006) 'Les droits sociaux sont justiciables', *Droit Social*, 2, 158–64.

Ayotte, W (2001) *Separated Children Seeking Asylum in Canada*. Ottawa: UNHCR Canada.

Dhanda, A (2005) 'The Right to Treatment of Persons with Psychosocial Disabilities and the Role of the Courts', *International Journal of Law and Psychiatry*, 28(2005), 155–70.

Horton, R (ed) (2007) 'Launching a New Movement for Mental Health', *The Lancet Series on Global Mental Health*. The Lancet Global Health Network. Available at <http://multimedia.thelancet.com/pdf/mental_health_comments.pdf>, accessed 8 November 2011.

Roy, G (2003) *Pratique sociale interculturelle au SARIMM (Service d'aide aux réfugiés et aux immigrants du Montréal métropolitain)*. (Intercultural Social Practise at SARIMM, service that provides help to refugees and new immigrants in Montreal, now known as PRAIDA). Montreal: CLSC Côte-des-Neiges.

Montgomery, C, Rousseau, C, and Shermarke, M (2001) 'Alone in a strange land: Unaccompanied minors and issues of protection', *Canadian Ethnic Studies*, 33(1), 102–119.

Rousseau, C, Bertot, J, Mekki-Berrada, A et al. (2001) *Étude longitudinale du processus de réunification familiale chez les réfugiés*. Montreal: Conseil québécois de la recherche sociale.

International publications

Amnesty International (2001) *National Human Rights Institutions: Amnesty International's Recommendations for Effective Protection and Promotion of Human Rights*.

European Committee on Migration (2002) *Toward a Migration Management Strategy*. Strasbourg: Council of Europe.

European Committee of Social Rights (2007) *General Introduction—Conclusions 2007*. Strasbourg: Council of Europe.

Office of the High Commissioner for Human Rights (OHCHR) (1993) *Fact Sheet No. 19, National Institutions for the Promotion and Protection of Human Rights*. Geneva: OHCHR.

United Nations High Commissioner for Refugees (UNHCR) (2009) *Revised Guidelines on Applicable Criteria and Standards relating to the Detention of Asylum Seekers*. Geneva: UNHCR.

World Health Organization, WHO (1999) *Mental Health of Refugees, Internally Displaced Persons and Other Populations Affected by Conflict*. Geneva: WHO.

WHO (2001) *Mental Health: Strengthening Mental Health Promotion*. Geneva: WHO.

National publications

Canadian Institute for Health Information (2007) *Improving the Health of Canadians: Mental Health and Homelessness*. Available at <http://secure.cihi.ca/cihiweb/en/downloads/mental_health_summary_aug22_2007_e.pdf>, accessed 8 November 2011.

Centre for Equality Rights in Accommodation (2006) *The Right to Adequate Housing: How to Fight for Your Rights*. Available at <http://www.equalityrights.org/cera/wp-content/uploads/2010/04/Adequate-Housing-2-page-E.pdf>, accessed 20 October 2011.

Commonwealth Ombudsman (2008) *Immigration reports tabled in Parliament*, 25 November 2008. Available at <http://www.ombudsman.gov.au/reports/immigration-detention-review/tabled-in-parliament/2008-11-25>, accessed 8 November 2011.

Commonwealth Ombudsman (2009) *Immigration detention review reports tabled in Parliament*, 17 June 2009.

Correctional Service of Canada (2002) *The 2002 Mental Health Strategy For Women Offenders*. Ottawa: The Correctional Investigator of Canada.

Correctional Investigator Canada (2007) *Deaths in Custody. Final Report submitted by Thomas Gabor*. Ottawa: The Correctional Investigator of Canada.

Immigration and Refugee Board Canada (2006) *Guideline 8. Guideline on Procedures with Respect to Vulnerable Persons Appearing Before the IRB*. Ottawa: Immigration and Refugee Board Canada.

Independent High Commission for Equality and Against Discrimination (Haute Autorité de Lutte contre les *Discriminations et pour l'Egalité*) (2007) *Annual Report 2006*. Available at <http://www.halde.fr/rapport-annuel/2006/>, accessed 8 November 2011.

Palmer, Mick (2005) *Inquiry into the Circumstances of the Immigration Detention of Cornelia Rau*, July 2005 (Palmer Report). Available at <http://www.immi.gov.au/media/publications/pdf/palmer-report.pdf>, accessed 8 November 2011.

International and national decisions, judgments, views, concluding observations, reports, and national legislation

Canada, *Employment Equity Act*, S.C. 1995, c. 44.

CESCR (1994) *General Comment 5. Persons with Disabilities*.

CESCR (2000) *General Comment No. 14 (2000). Substantive Issues Arising in the Implementation of the ICESCR*. E/C.12/2000/4.

CESCR (2006) *Concluding Observations on Canada*. E/C.12/CAN/CO/4 and E/C.12/CAN/CO/5.

CEDAW (2005) *Communication No:2/2003, Ms. A. T. v. Hungary*.

CEDAW (2005) *Views of the Committee under article 7, paragraph 3, of the Optional Protocol of CEDAW*.

Committee against Torture (2005) *Conclusions and Recommendations: Canada*. CAT/C/CR/34/CAN.

Committee of Ministers, CoE (2004) *Resolution ResChS(2004)1 on the Collective complaint No. 13/2002, Autisme-Europe against France*.

ECSR (2003) Complaint No. 13/2002. *International Association Autism—Europe (IAAE) v. France*.

ECSR (2004) Complaint No. 14/2003. *International Federation of Human Rights Leagues (FIDH) v. France.*

ECSR (2007) Complaint No. 41/2007. *Mental Disability Advocacy Centre (MDAC) v. Bulgaria.*

ECSR (2007a) *Conclusions 2007 (France).*

European Committee for the Prevention of Torture (2007) *Response of the Albanian Government to the report of the CPT on its visit to Albania from 28 to 31 March 2006.*

European Court of Human Rights (2007) *Kucheruk v. Ukraine. No. 2570/04 (Sect. 5).*

Federal Court of Canada (2007) *Canadian Council for Refugees* et al. v. Canada. [2007] FC 1262.

General Assembly of the United Nations (2002) *Optional Protocol to the Convention against Torture and other Cruel, Inhuman or Degrading Treatment or Punishment.* A/RES/57/199.

General Assembly of the United Nations (2008) *Optional Protocol to the International Covenant on Economic, Social and Cultural Rights.* A/RES/63/117.

General Assembly of the United Nations (1991) *The protection of persons with mental illness and the improvement of mental health care.* A/RES/46/119.

Haute Autorité de Lutte contre les Discriminations et pour l'Egalité (HALDE) (2006) *Délibération relative à l'opposition au mariage prise par le Procureur de la République à l'encontre de l'union d'un demandeur d'asile et d'une personne handicapée. n° 2006-128 du 05/06/2006.*

Inter-American Commission on Human Rights (1997) *Victor Rosario Congo v. Ecuador, Case 11.427, Report n°12/97 on Admissibility.*

Inter-American Commission on Human Rights, IACHR (1998) *Victor Rosario Congo v. Ecuador, Case 11.427, Report 51/98,* as cited in *IACHR (1999) Victor Rosario Congo v. Ecuador, Case 11.427, Report 63/99.*

Inter-American Commission on Human Rights, IACHR (2003) *Report on the Situation of Human Rights in Venezuela.* Chapter 5: 'The Right to Humane Treatment'.

Inter-American Court of Human Rights, IACourtHR (2006) *Ximenes-Lopes v. Brazil. (Merits, Reparations and Costs).*

Office of the High Commissioner for Human Rights (2002) *The right of everyone to the enjoyment of the highest attainable standard of physical and mental health.* Commission on Human Rights resolution 2002/31.

Supreme Court of India (1995) *Rakesh Chandra Narayan vs State of Bihar.* [AIR 1995 SC 208].

United Nations Human Rights Committee, HRC (2006) *Concluding Observations on Canada.* CCPR/C/CAN/CO/5.

UN Special Rapporteur on the Right of Everyone to the Enjoyment of the Highest Attainable Standard of Physical and Mental Health (2007) *Report of the Special Rapporteur on the right of everyone to the enjoyment of the highest attainable standard of physical and mental health, Paul Hunt. Mission to Sweden.* Human Rights Council. A/HRC/4/28/Add.2.

Chapter 32

The Role of World Associations and the United Nations

John Copeland, Eugene Brody, Tony Fowke,
Preston Garrison, and Janet Meagher

Introduction: four important human rights to establish internationally

Amongst the many human rights that intersect with mental health, four are surely outstanding: the rights of a person who experiences a mental health problem or disorder to expect to be dealt with respectfully; the right to receive appropriate interventions directed towards recovery; the right not to be abused socially, emotionally, physically, or financially, and the right to be appropriately protected by law and against discrimination. Sadly, the world has some distance to go to achieve all four. In spite of repeated calls to scale up mental health services most governments have failed to comply. It has been pointed out (Jacob et al. 2007) that important strides have been made in a small number of low- and middle-income countries, demonstrating that poverty is not in itself an excuse. But the consumer voice is strengthening and there is a sense that at last the mental health world is stirring and moving forward to grasp the important issues. It can only succeed by identifying the common ground, uniting around that, and insisting that human rights and mental health be central to governmental policy.

Where are we coming from: the background to the international movement?

Non-governmental mental health organizations as advocates for human rights (Brody 1998)

In 1942, prior to the end of World War II, United States president, Franklin D. Roosevelt declared: 'Today we are faced with the pre-eminent fact that if civilization is to survive we must cultivate the science of human relationships, the ability of peoples of all kinds to live together.' He suggested the formation of a new intergovernmental organization to be called the 'United Nations' (UN). The UN's founding on 25 June 1945 was soon followed by the emergence of organizations acting as consultants and advocates to its specialized agencies. Free of governmental constraints they were known as NGOs, non-governmental organizations. One of the first, founded in 1948, was the World Federation for Mental Health (WFMH). The first International Congress of Mental Health was convened in London in 1948 by the British National Association for Mental Hygiene (Bertolote 1993). At the end of the congress the International Committee was superseded by the formation of WFMH. The International Committee on Mental Hygiene had its origins in the mental hygiene movement started by Clifford Beers, himself a consumer in the US, after the publication of his book 'A Mind that Found Itself' in 1908 (Beers 1908, 1937). WFMH for many years remained the only international mental health NGO. It quickly gained formal consultative status with the United Nations and its Agencies including the World Health Organization. Although it replaced a mental hospital reform movement its mental health concerns were not primarily expressed through a focus on psychiatric disorders, but on world peace and human rights. Its founding document, Mental Health and World Citizenship, referred to 'an informed, reflective, responsible allegiance to mankind as a whole . . . Common humanity' living together 'in a world community built on free consent and respect for individual and cultural differences'. Its view of human rights antedated by four months the 10 December 1948 UN Universal Declaration of Human Rights. The freedoms and entitlements which the declaration defined as rights were regarded by WFMH as essential to optimal development and function. They also allowed a focus on issues relevant to patient care such as a right to refuse treatment.

In 1971 WFMH was the first NGO to condemn the practice of incarcerating political dissidents in mental hospitals followed by the World Psychiatric Association in 1977 expelling the powerful Soviet Union Psychiatry Association from its ranks. It was not until 1982, though, that it began to include leaders of self-help groups and consumer (patient) organizations in its annual meetings. In 1985 several NGOs worked together to formulate and have passed by the UN General Assembly a Declaration of Basic Principles of Justice for Victims of Crime and Abuse of Power. In the middle and late 1980s WFMH, the International Commission of Jurists, the International Council of Psychologists, and the International Commission of Health Professionals for Health and Human Rights collaborated with WHO in regard to its protection of patients' rights.

In 1989 WFMH adopted its own Declaration of Human Rights and Mental Health. It 'recognizes the Federation's concern not only with people defined as mentally ill, but also with those vulnerable to or at risk of mental and emotional illness or distress . . . human rights transcend political, social, cultural and economic boundaries and apply to the human family as a whole.' It also collaborated with other NGOs in an effort to influence UN deliberations on issues relevant to mental health. A major effort with the International Social Science Council culminated in a volume on human rights concerns raised by advancing biomedical technology (Brody 1993) which led to a Division of Bioethics in UNESCO, the UN's Educational, Scientific and Cultural Organization. In the 1990s a mental health group of NGOs was initiated in UN New York consulting to the agencies associated with ECOSOC, the Economic and Social Council.

In the late years of the 20th century the WFMH focus on human rights was gradually replaced by a concern with essentially psychiatric issues, similar to that of the many professional and voluntary associations which by then had attained NGO status. But as WFMH became less concerned with patient rights and related issues, and lost some of its claim to uniqueness, the theme was picked up by others such as the World Psychiatric Association's programme aimed at reducing the stigma attached to mental illness. It does, however, retain its special status as an ecumenical organization not limited to members of any profession and free of governmental constraints.

In some ways the World Federation for Mental Health has come full circle and is once again, in the 21st century, showing its concern for the continuing abuses that are constantly being revealed in every country, whether it be in out-dated mental hospitals whose staff are deprived of adequate training and resources, or in modern states where community care has rarely been adequately funded, or nursing home care for older people with mental health problems adequately monitored and their staff adequately trained, or in the practices of some native healers.

The evolutionary role of non-governmental organizations in mental health advocacy

Advocacy to improve awareness of mental illness and the right to receive appropriate treatment directed towards recovery has emerged as an important part of the NGO remit.

During the past 30 years, there have been major changes in the way in which the general public's voice has been heard on issues relating to mental health and mental illnesses. Until the late 1970s and early 1980s, advocacy and public awareness efforts on behalf of these issues came primarily from a very few 'umbrella' citizen advocacy organizations—primarily represented by national mental health associations (National MHA-US, the Canadian Mental Health Association, the Finnish Association for Mental Health, Mind-UK, Mental Health Ireland, Philippine Mental Health Association, Zimbabwe National Association for Mental Health, etc.).

The Mental Health Associations were often characterized as 'speaking for the mentally ill', and were made up of a variety of constituencies including mental health professionals, citizen volunteers, and, to a lesser extent, family members of those with a mental illness. In most instances, people with mental illnesses and their family members constituted a minority—and usually a silent one—of MHA memberships.

During the late 1970s and early 1980s, the 'megatrend' that affected all of the traditional 'umbrella' voluntary health agencies in North America began to bring about significant changes and fracturing of the citizens' mental health movement. During this time, parents of adult children with severe and persistent mental illnesses became more vocal about their frustration with the public policies of 'deinstitutionalization' and 'community-based care,' and they voiced concerns about the burden of care placed on families, and the fear for their adult children's future when parents died or were unable to provide care. This active involvement of parents of people with mental illness was solidified in the United States with the founding of the National Alliance on Mental Illness (NAMI); the development of national family member/carer movements spread more slowly to other countries in succeeding years and continues to expand today through organizations like EUFAMI and the World Fellowship for Schizophrenia and Related Disorders (WFSAD).

At around the same time in the United States other organizations began to evolve, some driven by people with mental illnesses who were no longer institutionalized and supported by funding from the National Institute of Mental Health (such as the National Consumer Self Help Clearinghouse), and others representing families and people with a specific disorder (the National Depressive and Manic-Depressive Association—now DBSA—and the Anxiety Disorders Association of America, etc.). It is interesting to note that the leading forces behind the development of 'diagnosis-specific' advocacy groups were typically leading researchers and clinicians working on those disorders. Many of these new 'patient/support' organizations received early funding from the pharmaceutical companies. As with the family support organizations, diagnosis specific and patient/service user organizations have spread to countries around the world, including into low-income countries (e.g. the Zambia Mental Health Service Users Network).

A third group of 'service user/survivor/ex-patient' organizations also developed in the 1970s and 1980s (e.g. the World Federation of Psychiatric Users (WFPU) and the World Network of Users and Survivors of Psychiatry (WNUSP)) bringing a decidedly negative view of psychiatry and its effects, including hospitalization and medication use, and also of the 'mainstream' mental health advocacy movement. These activist groups remain active and maintain their distance, for the most part, from the major professional, family member, patient, and citizen advocacy organizations. In some instances, 'anti-psychiatry/anti-medication' groups are forming interesting alliances with other organizations opposed to, or wishing to heavily regulate, mental health treatment methods and practices, including medication and any kind of involuntary treatment.

Similar fracturing of the citizens' mental health movement has occurred in the other developed countries of the world. Among the results of this evolution of 'diagnosis-specific' and patient–family support and advocacy organizations have been sometimes significant 'disconnects' in the key advocacy messages directed to policy makers, professional associations, the general public, and the funding community. As more organizations have developed, the degree of competition for funding, strategic position, and miscommunication has also increased.

The more recent active engagement of the pharmaceutical industry, the national and global psychiatric associations, the World Health Organization (WHO) Department of Mental Health and Substance Abuse, and the European Union with the mental health advocacy community has also enhanced the competition for status and support among the consumer, family, and citizen advocacy organizations (and at all levels—local, state/provincial, national, and international).

During this period of development and emergence of new international organizations and networks of consumer/patient and family member/caregiver organizations, there has been limited connection, communication, and cooperation between these newer organizations—or between them and the longer-existing national mental health associations and international organizations such as WFMH.

One of the historical roles and strengths of the World Federation for Mental Health has been that of a convener and as a forum for the sharing of mutual interests among diverse elements of the global mental health movement. WFMH, as the 'oldest' of the international mental health 'movement' organizations, has sometimes been able to provide a non-threatening meeting ground where ideas can be explored, mutual interests identified, and collaborative strategies can be agreed to and promoted that benefit the entire sector—and most importantly—the people directly affected by mental illnesses, their treatment, and the public policy decisions impacting them.

Where are we now? Unfinished business

Disempowerment, universal human rights, rights to self-determination, and protection of human rights

It is well documented that many people living with mental illness are disadvantaged. Poverty, social exclusion, educational disadvantage, and illiteracy are still risk factors for some disorders. Mental illnesses tend to be chronic, or remitting and relapsing, and are associated with considerable social disability.

Those affected may not fulfill their educational potential, find it difficult to establish or maintain a livelihood, may be socially isolated, and are less likely to marry and have children. The discrimination and stigma still experienced by many with mental disorders, and their families, greatly exacerbates these disadvantages and undermines the potential for networking, lobbying, and advocacy among users and consumers of mental health services. The disempowerment of people living with mental illnesses leaves them especially vulnerable to human rights abuses. Human rights violations both result from, and enhance inequities.

Universal human rights—to food, shelter, clothing, sufficient income, and general health care—are not assured in many countries to this day, particularly for those living in institutionalized settings. Civil and political rights—to marry, to raise children, to own and dispose of property, and to vote—are likewise often circumscribed. Many of the worse violations of human rights are at the hands of the very services that have been established to care for those with mental illness. Some of this is attributable to neglect. The under-funding and under-resourcing of mental health services means that up to 90 per cent of those with the most severe forms of mental illness receive no mental health care whatsoever, particularly in the least developed countries, and for those living in rural and remote areas.

Rights to self-determination are also routinely violated—treatments are sometimes provided without informed consent, and there is well documented unnecessary and unmonitored coercion, detention, and physical restraint. Some mental illnesses can cause temporary or longer-lasting impairment of decision-making capacity. Most states therefore make some provision for compulsory admission and treatment. However, the principles that mental health care for the incapacitated client should be provided in the least restrictive possible setting, and with the minimum degree of coercion, and only in the best interests of the patient, are not always applied. Procedures for determining the application of compulsory treatment or detention orders are often inadequate.

The World Health Organization's project ATLAS (WHO 2005a: 540) has recently established that one quarter of all countries lack a Mental Health Act. There is little available information on the suitability of provisions in those countries that do have Mental Health Acts, many of which were enacted long ago and lack necessary safeguards such as the right to independent appeal, inspection, and monitoring. In many countries the physical facilities and quality of psychiatric and nursing care in the hospitals in which patients are detained are grossly deficient. In others, the mentally ill can be detained, entirely inappropriately, in prison.

Enhancements in the protection of human rights of people with mental illness will come about through the actions of policy makers and legislators in the countries concerned, assisted by technical experts, particularly in the mental health and legal professions. Most of these governments will be signatories to relevant intergovernmental charters, conventions and agreements, including the United Nations' Universal Declaration of Human Rights (1948); the United Nations General Assembly, Declaration on Rights of Mentally Retarded Persons, GA Resolution 2856 (XXVI), UN Doc. A/8429 (1971) the first UN document to pay attention to a mental health issue; The United Nations General Assembly, Principles for the Protection of Persons with Mental Illness and for the Improvement of Mental Health Care, A/RES/46/119 (1991); and the Convention on the Rights of Persons with Disabilities (2006). Such governments need to be reminded of their obligations.

There are a number of national and international organizations whose primary mission is to address concerns and abuses of human rights of people living with mental disorders. Among those organizations are the Mental Disability Advocacy Center (MDAC) (<http://mdac.info/>), Disability Rights International (DRI) (<http://www.disabilityrightsintl.org/>), and the Global Initiative on Psychiatry (<http://www.gip-global.org/>).

The World Health Organization's Department of Mental Health and Substance Abuse plays a central role in attempting to improve the policies and practices of countries in regard to ensuring and protecting the human rights of people living with mental illnesses. The WHO 'Resource Book on Mental Health, Human Rights and Legislation' (WHO 2005b) (<http://www.who.int/en/>) provides an essential guideline for addressing these issues.

As outlined in 'Mental Health, Human Rights and Legislation: WHO's Framework' (<http://www.who.int/mental_health/policy/legislation/en/index.html>), there are a number of common human rights violations of people living with mental disorders as we have detailed above—often associated with stigma about mental disorders. Impetus for change will come about when civil society and people in general have understood the nature and extent of the problem for themselves. The more people who have a common understanding, the more they are empowered to effect change. This can come about through the testimonies and activism of those most affected; users of mental health services, and their families; bolstered by advocacy training, and amplified by accurate and informative reporting by print and broadcast media.

An informed national debate in a spirit of partnership and solidarity with those most affected is most likely to bring about reform and ensure sustained implementation of measures to protect their human rights.

The important voice of consumer/user/survivor participation in world associations

The role of consumers in advocacy is of crucial importance. Mental health and human rights have long been so closely aligned that they are inextricably linked by both circumstance and need. Indeed, the interrelationship is so solid that in either the mental health sector, or in the human rights arena, when one or the other is compromised then the other becomes susceptible or impacted upon. Looking at human history there are multiple examples of this co-dependence and its human impact on mental health balance and rights infringement. Where warfare, cruelty, intimidation, economic deprivation, exploitation, or disaster occurs there is collateral increase of emotional disturbance, breakdown and trauma amongst populations involved. Correspondingly, in such environments, persons and organizations (governmental and private) rise up and exert considerable power over those who are vulnerable or disempowered. At this juncture, the human rights of those caught up are at extreme risk. Wherever there is disengagement or disempowerment there is the likelihood of abuse or exploitation.

Persons who have experienced a mental health problem or disorder can be considered as belonging to this 'at risk' group. Historically they have, as an identified cohort of vulnerable individuals, been involved in every possible dimension of human rights abuse.

Reports, enquiries, revelations, articles, anecdotes, and court cases proliferate, attempting to raise awareness, seek redress, change practice, and engage political or public outrage. Sometimes these set out to protect, enact prevention activity, or engage public empathy over human rights violations of people who are identified as having a mental health problem or disorder. These types of awareness raising actions have proliferated in first and second world countries over the last 100 years. Looking at Australia as an example, the fact that during the last 20 years there have been over five national inquiries and countless state and territory formal reports cataloguing an inventory of abuse, inappropriate or unacceptable treatment regimes, and neglect and personal trauma in formal mental health or psychiatric care environments serves to illustrate that the correlation between mental health issues and human rights violations is pronounced. Australia is not unique. A parallel experience of such reporting of human rights infringements can be found in one form or another in a variety of European countries, North America, and parts of Asia and Africa, from institutional failures of care to abuse justified by some native healers. States have put into place legislative and regulatory devices and there are multiple rights protection resources locally, nationally, and internationally, from local one-on-one interactions through to the United Nations: all are framed to protect rights. Despite all of this, matters are still regularly reported. Regardless of any number of historic determinations to avoid and prevent their re-occurrence, it goes on unabated, merely changing slightly from time to time. After all the above, there would be a temptation to begin to view rights protection in the psychiatric sector, locally and worldwide, with a degree of cynicism. To maintain enthusiasm for the moral imperative society as a whole needs to assess and reassess the rights protection mechanisms that are traditionally in place and view these from a new perspective.

The history of the consumer movement for mental health and the case for their involvement in mental health care

Some earliest beginnings of the move toward an international voice for consumers/users/survivors can be found in the 'Search for Mental Health, a History and Memoir of WFMH' (Brody 1998) in which Brody states . . . 'the 1983 (WFMH) (Washington, D.C.) Congress did feature a symposium of self-help and ex-patient contributors for the first time . . . This was the beginning of independent and vital participation by these groups . . . in all succeeding World Congresses'. And further on he states 'In 1989 during the World Congress for Mental Health in Auckland (New Zealand) . . . a proposal to form a new WFMH-affiliated organization, the World Federation of Mental Health Consumers, was supported.' The 1991 World Congress in Mexico included a sub-congress of consumers. Consumers/users/survivors meeting during the congress formally founded the World Federation of Psychiatric Users (WFPU) 'to facilitate the development of user groups worldwide and to expose and stop violations of user rights and self-determination.' It had met again in Japan at the Tokyo Congress in 1993.

In 1993 there were over 400 members from 16 countries in the WFPU. Its next meeting was at the Dublin Congress (Ireland) in 1995. The WFPU was growing and had developed by-laws, had an irregular newsletter and position paper by this time.

The initial pre-eminence of the World Federation of Psychiatric Users faded. The change of leadership of the WFPU did not take the network forward. Attempts to revitalize the network or its activity at the WFMH Lahti (Finland) Congress in1997 succeeded in the sense that consumers/ users/survivors worked toward a public declaration. It was not until a pre-WFMH Congress meeting of selected consumers at Santiago (Chile) in 1999 that a workable rescue plan and restructure proposals were put into place. These were endorsed by the large contingent of consumers, users, and survivors who attended the congress. It was this group who were successful in raising money for the first part-time secretariat of the World Network of Users and Survivors of Psychiatry (WNUSP), located in Odense, Denmark, and for its direction and development from then onwards. The WNUSP obtained some limited secretariat funding in July 2000. They have had a struggle to survive but are now progressing their development. Their first General Assembly was held in Vancouver, Canada in July 2001 where the members endorsed their constitution and it became incorporated. It had an interim committee and two consumer link persons from the board of the World Federation for Mental Health, contributing to the process that we now see as an independent international organization linking consumers of mental health services, users, and survivors on a worldwide level (Meagher 2003).

This story of the development of an international voice for consumers/users/survivors serves as a 'case history' for agencies to consider. A simplification of the history allows one to see that the original welcoming and facilitation of the consumer voice by the World Federation for Mental Health way back in 1983 has led to the routine recruitment and retention of consumer board members for that organization for about the last two decades, and also to the development of the independent international consumer organization, the WNUSP, which has played a strong role in the negotiations for the development of the Convention on the rights of persons with disabilities. Both organizations have played different but valuable roles in the raising of rights awareness.

There is an important case for engaging people with lived experience of mental health problems and disorders.

In 1986 the WHO Initiative of Support to People Disabled by Mental Illness, which continued through 1999 should be mentioned. This programme, running in partnership with the decisive involvement of service users and family organizations, produced a series of WHO technical documents still widely used up to now (e.g. on quality assurance, guidelines on human rights, essential treatments, housing, psychosocial rehabilitation, and more).

◆ Consumers, as a proportion of the population, are, statistically, a very significant group. The real surprise is that there is not more consumer engagement or more impactful consumer influences internationally when mere numbers are taken into account. Many reasons can be cited to explain or excuse this anomaly; perhaps we are now on the cusp of agencies realizing the significant growth and potential of this group.

◆ Whether organizations utilize the opportunity to reach this full potential or dissipate it is a matter for serious consideration. It is important to note that at this time consumers ought to have unprecedented hope and real potential for an effective say in matters that affect their rights and their lives. In some places this is already happening.

◆ The growth of consumer activity and influence locally and internationally is an unprecedented social change movement with impact and potential for rights protection yet to be fully realized. Most agree on the statistical predictions of the incidence of mental health problems and disorders, yet express surprise at the growth of consumer influence!

- Worldwide, consumers are active and contribute significantly to every aspect of mental health: action, promotion, prevention, policy, support, service delivery, and research agendas. However, it must be said that the documentation of these activities and input is very poor, with few exceptions. It has been suggested that this reflects the overall socio-economic status of consumers and their consequent lack of access to the support and expertise that would facilitate the reporting and recording of activity and the history of achievement. The inevitable result is a failure to truly grasp the input, impact and outcome value, mutual support, expertise, and credibility or otherwise of the majority of consumer groups, projects, and initiatives, internationally or locally. They exist, their numbers are growing, they are an influence that can no longer be ignored. Somehow, the collation of experiences, influences, sub-cultures, innovations, and the role of significant individuals in the consumer movement and the documentation of this will need to be addressed. By whom, and how it will be done, remains a mystery and an activity that is yet to be begun.

What needs to be done to enhance the voice of consumers/users/survivors' participation?

As discussed above, elements of human rights protection mechanisms for persons with mental health problems or disorders already exist; however, they need further sculpturing and refinement. Those protection elements and the processes for their refinement may be regarded as a commitment to both further and develop the following potentials:

- Facilitating and enabling empowerment of consumers, service users, and survivors of mental health services in order for them to participate at all levels of organizations, in services, policy formulation, evaluation, promotion, and prevention programmes. This inevitably requires a move beyond blind adherence to the dominant 'medical model' (currently in vogue in most parts of the world) and a step into 'the brave new world' 'with an explicit social development dimension . . . The medical and welfare approaches to disability were the direct result of society's views that people with disabilities were sick, unable to take care of themselves and in need of charity' (United Nations 2006) .

- Awareness and utilization of human rights protection mechanisms by consumers, service users, survivors of mental health services and service providers, policy makers, organizations, governments, and international agencies to enhance service improvement, quality assurance, and promote best practice models, e.g. by meaningful participation in formulating a United Nations Convention. This is expressed by the World Network of Users and Survivors of Psychiatry (WNUSP) in the following statement:

> An international team of users and survivors of psychiatry…participated actively in the negotiations at the United Nations (UN) in New York from the first session of the Ad Hoc Committee in August 2002 through the adoption of the completed text on December 13, 2006. The Ad Hoc Committee was a unique process for all of us. We seized a historic opportunity and accomplished something basic and fundamental that has changed the human rights landscape for us and for all people with disabilities… Users and survivors of psychiatry finally had a seat at the table and spoke with a passion and clarity that was heard around the world (WNUSP 2007).

- Promotion and education of the public in awareness of the relevant United Nations statements, articles, declarations, conventions, etc., in order for ordinary people to develop a sense of ownership and begin to understand the powers and protections contained within those international instruments.

- Engagement of national and representative mental health organizations in international non-government associations and alliances.

- Communication between international mental health organizations and mutual cooperation in such issues as those which enhance the common good and promote rights protection, e.g. World Federation for Mental Health participation and contribution to the programme of the Conference of World Association for Psychosocial Rehabilitation (WAPR) in Kobe, Japan, October 2004.

- Engagement of international non-government associations and alliances in activities that link them into United Nations agencies and alliances, e.g. World Federation for Mental Health leadership and continuing participation in the United Nations NGO Committee on Mental Health at the UN building in New York as well as having a representative attached to UNESCO and other Geneva based agencies.

- Critical to all the above is the diversity of influences and engagement of a full range of stakeholders at every level from local to international in the relations between mental health and human rights protection, e.g. the World Federation for Mental Health's Strategic Objective: 'Strengthen and enhance WFMH's global advocacy network and its recognition as the only international networking organization for mental health professional, consumer/ carer, and advocacy organizations and interested individuals' (WFMH 2005 official documentation).

- Formal representation. Currently it appears only three of the world associations are publicly committed to formal consumer/user/survivor representation on boards (WFMH, WAPR, and Alzheimer's Disease International) and none of the UN agencies or professional associations have yet expressed a commitment or desire to do so. Admittedly, some do make an effort to engage from time to time but that is insufficient for the purpose of mutual respect and rights awareness issues to ever be addressed from within the organizations concerned.

- The United Nations and its agencies must commit at some point to seeking positions within their ranks for formal consumer/user/survivor representation with a specific task of coordination of reports of rights infringement and facilitation of action/reaction in the international arena. Liaison with UN NGO Committees and world associations as well as national state representatives would be essential duties of such a role.

Consumer/user/survivor representation and involvement in international agencies is a relatively new phenomenon. The case of the development and growth of a consumer voice can be well illustrated as we have mentioned by the World Federation for Mental Health as the first international association to commit to welcoming the consumer/user/survivor voice to its ranks.

A statement such as 'mental health and human rights have long been so closely aligned that they are inextricably linked by both circumstance and need' was used to commence this part of the discussion on the 'role of world associations and the UN'. We trust that as a result of this there are now some new dimensions that involve the consideration by both world associations and the UN of deeper and more committed engagement with people with lived experience of mental health problems and disorders in order to personalize and strengthen their universal commitment to protect human rights and prevent abuse in this sector.

'This is not the end, nor the beginning of the end: but it is, perhaps, the end of the beginning.' (Winston Churchill).

The important voice of the family in shaping policy: what needs to be done

Many consumers of mental health services rely on families for support and in some instances for protection. Governments tend to encourage this for obvious reasons.

The 1991 United Nations Principles for the Protection of Persons with Mental Illness and for the Improvement of Mental Health Care (United Nations 1991) include:

◆ The right to the best available mental health care which shall be part of the health and social care system (Principle 1.1).

◆ Every person with a mental illness shall have the right to live and work, as far as possible, in the community (Principle 3).

In order to achieve the above, families which are an integral part of the community have an important role to play. The concept of the family, however it is defined, is important to the general well-being of the world population. It is, however, a rapidly changing concept and the nuclear family (mother, father, and the children) is rapidly disappearing. The 'family' relationships that now exist are myriad, and can range from the single parent family to the extended family which to some extent still exists in low- and some middle-income countries. Friends and even pets can now be regarded as part of the family. In the high-income parts of the world with all the technology that is readily available families can, however, become isolated even in the urban environment and this urbanization can lead to many social problems including mental illness. People often do not know their neighbours, who in years gone past would have been part of what could be called the community family and willingly available to offer help and support. No matter how 'families' are defined, they can still offer support, nurture, and encouragement.

Such support is particularly important in caring for people with mental illness. Often the responsibility for caring falls upon the family of the person that has the mental illness and yet this important role is commonly overlooked. In the determination of what is the 'family', allowance should be given for the person who has a mental illness to define their family. This caring role can be taken on for different reasons including a lack of services, but often the family will regard it as their responsibility although sometimes it is forced upon them because there is nothing else available. This can have a 'knock on' effect, with the family carers becoming physically and mentally unwell because of the lack of support they receive in this caring role. In addition, they can become socially isolated and experience the stigma that mental illness attracts, and in some cultures the mental illness within the family can remain hidden because of shame. It must be acknowledged that each family will face a different set of circumstances and that not all families require the same level of support. Some may not even recognize the need for support because it is accepted as the family's responsibility to provide the required care.

The family caring role is in itself diversified. The overwhelming majority of families care for one person but those caring for someone with a mental illness or learning disability are more likely to be caring for more than one. This often places a particular burden on the mother, who accepts the primary responsibility as part of her role when it is a child that needs care.

In addition to the caring role families have an important role in the assessment and treatment of their family member. Mental health clinicians working alongside families can help support and empower families to assist in the treatment, care, and recovery process for their family member as well as dealing with their own trauma and distress. The losses, grief, and adaptations that families usually face are different to those arising where there is a congenital or birth-related condition, or one which is evidenced in early childhood. They are different again from the losses associated with care of an ageing parent or partner. Due to this different age of onset and the unpredictable course of mental illness, roles and relationships need to be changed and re-formed on an ongoing basis. A profound sense of grief is experienced, which can be compounded by the professional attitudes encountered and the long search for help.

> To develop a partnership with mental health care providers is vital to the success of families in caring for their loved ones—to their providing crisis intervention, case management, counselling, basic needs support, socialization, advocacy and insight into their loved one's illness. (National Alliance on Mental Illness 2006).

Families have clearly been involved in health care for centuries but their involvement in mental health care in the way envisaged by this quote is a fairly recent development and one that is progressing slowly. It is at varying stages of implementation throughout the world and will not always be possible because of family conflict and disengagement from the family.

Family involvement at all levels is a global issue that the World Federation for Mental Health is concerned about in its endeavours to improve the well-being of all peoples throughout the world and to make mental health a global priority for everyone.

It should be noted that in its Resolution 52/81 of 12 December 1997 the UN General Assembly recognized that the basic objective of the follow up on the International Year of the Family (1994) should be to strengthen and support families in performing their societal and developmental functions and build upon their strengths, in particular at the national and local levels.

Whilst there is a need to support families globally, it is particularly important for there to be a strong focus on the least developed and developing countries to reinforce family related concerns in respect of mental illness and the promotion of mental health.

What needs to be done is the development of:

◆ Increased awareness of family issues around mental health among governments as well as the private sector;

◆ Strengthened capacity of local organizations to formulate, implement, and monitor mental health policies particularly as they relate to or affect families;

◆ Efforts to respond to problems affecting and affected by mental health issues in families;

◆ Reviews at all levels of the situation and needs of families; and

◆ Improved collaboration among national and international non-government organizations for the support of families and identifying specific mental health issues and problems.

A long way still to go

In the end, it has to be said that NGOs on the whole, the United Nations, and the WHO have failed collectively to achieve the four important human rights goals which we identified in the introduction. They have not been able to persuade governments that mental health is as fundamental to well-being as physical health, in fact more so: the preference is usually for a sound mind in a sound body or failing that at least for of a sound mind in an unsound body, not the reverse. They have failed to speak out consistently against the continual abuse of the mentally ill or to find ways of tackling this problem with governments. It would seem that no country, whatever its economic status, is without evidence of abuse, some of which might be described as torture. They have not instituted proper training, especially in nursing homes for the elderly mentally disordered or infirm and in the many mental hospitals, both public and private, which continue to exist in many countries, nor have they succeeded in monitoring adequately the infringements of human rights which are frequently exposed by the media using concealed cameras and other surveillance, nor tackled the excesses of some native healers. Although the WHO has pointed out the lack of mental health legislation in many member countries of the United Nations, it has only partially succeeded in insisting that such legislation be put in place. However, some of those countries which have responded are those which had the worst mental health legislation. Nevertheless, it is not for lack of examples which could easily be adapted in most cases, but lack of national motivation or a failure of governments to take human rights seriously. It has, nevertheless, set out standards and repeatedly pressed governments to act. The most exciting development is the user/consumer and family movements which we have documented here and which form such an important focus of the WFMH. It may, in the end, be the grass roots organizations which finally rebel against governments' inaction and lack of resource allocation. It is sometimes suggested that the mental health world is divided in its attitude to essential issues, and that excuse is used to delay action by the appropriate authorities. That is why the World Federation for Mental Health has mounted a Global Consensus programme in the expectation of demonstrating that the mental health world is very clear what is important and what should be enacted by governments and does agree on fundamental issues which should guide the policy of the United Nations and its Agencies. In the first round there was agreement of over 95 per cent on the 'Principles' of the World Federation, see <http://www.wfmh.org/>.

There have been a number of world reports detailing the evidence for the importance of mental health and the importance of mental illness. Governments have shown little movement. WFMH has recently put forward a global campaign 'The Great Push for Mental Health' in strategic alliance with the Movement for Global Mental Health to raise mental health up the agenda of governments. It concentrates on the four elements 'Unity', 'Visibility', 'Rights', and 'Recovery'; now is the time to act—this campaign should soon be coming to a locality near you.

Unless the mental health community can unite around these fundamental issues, and stand firm against complacency and stigma while achieving greater visibility, the progress of advance, the recognition of the importance of mental health to the world, and the humanitarian need to relieve mental illness wherever it is found will be slow, but by working together and with determination it will eventually succeed. Having written such, as this book went to press the WHO Executive Board (130th session) passed a recommendation to the 65th World Health Assembly for the adoption of a resolution with the intention to include a 'comprehensive mental health action plan'; the move forward has begun!

References

Beers, CW (1908, 1937) *A Mind that Found Itself*. New York: Doubleday, Draw & Co.

Bertolote, J (ed.) (1993) *Guidelines for the Primary Prevention of Mental, Neurological and Psychosocial Disorders: Suicide*. Geneva: World Health Organization.

Brody, E (1993) *Biomedical Technology and Human Rights*. France: UNESCO and England: Dartmouth Publishing Co.

Brody, E (1998) *The Search for Mental Health. A History and Memoir of WFMH 1948–1997*. Baltimore: Williams & Wilkins.

Jacob, KS, Sharan, P, Mirza, I, et al. (2007) 'Mental health systems in countries: where are we now?', Global Mental Health, *The Lancet*, 370, 59–75.

Meagher, J (2003) *Partnership or Pretence*. Australia: Strawberry Hills.

National Alliance on Mental Illness (2006) *Grading the States*. Available at <http://www.nami.org/Content/NavigationMenu/Grading_the_States/Full_Report/GTS06_final.pdf>, accessed 8 November 2011.

United Nations (2006) *Convention on the Rights of Persons with Disabilities. United Nations Development, Economic and Social Affairs. Division of social policy and development*. GA Doc A/61.611.

United Nations General Assembly (1971) *declaration on Rights of Mentally Retarded Persons*, GA Resolution 2856 (XXVI), UN Doc. A/8429.

United Nations General Assembly (1991) *Principles for the Protection of Persons with Mental Illness and for the Improvement of Mental Health Care*. GA UN Doc A/RES/46/119.

WHO, (2005a) *Mental Health Atlas: revised* . Geneva: WHO.

WHO, (2005b) *Resource Book on Mental Health, Human Rights and Legislation*. Geneva: WHO.

The World Network of Users and Survivors of Psychiatry, (2007) *Implementation Manual for the United Nations Convention on the Rights of Persons with Disabilities*. Odense C, Denmark: WNUSP.

Chapter 33

Whose Voices Should Be Heard?

The Role of Mental Health Consumers, Psychiatric Survivors, and Families

David W. Oaks

My recruitment room

I found my own voice to speak out about human rights in the mental health system in what I now call my 'recruitment room' for what would become my career in human rights. I found my voice inside a solitary confinement cell in a psychiatric institution after once more being held down and forcibly injected with a powerful psychiatric drug.

For the more than three decades since then I've been a human rights activist in the field of mental health. I've talked to countless individuals who have experienced human rights violations that could be called far more serious than mine, including various friends who had had involuntary psychosurgery, days tied down in four-point restraints, dozens of forced electroshock, beatings, illegal experimentation, months of unnecessary confinement, years of homelessness, and so much more.

For me, however, my several forced psychiatric druggings along with a few days alone in a bare psychiatric facility cell were enough to motivate me to speak out. My story feels to me like it happened yesterday. Some of my worst nightmares to this day are that I am back there, getting forcibly drugged, and no one will listen.

I was raised by a supportive working class family on the south side of Chicago. All of my grandparents immigrated from Lithuania, and both of my grandfathers were coal miners. For whatever reason, I was not prepared culturally or emotionally when I received scholarships to attend Harvard. At times in my sophomore, junior, and senior years I entered into extreme and overwhelming mental states that led to being locked up in psychiatric institutions five times. There were times I thought the CIA was making my teeth grow, rapidly. I thought the voice of God was on my radio. I believed technology, including the television, was a living force on Earth that communicated with me. I swore I saw a spaceship hovering in my bedroom. Some psychiatrists labeled me *schizophrenic*. Other psychiatrists felt I was *manic depressive,* now known as *bipolar.* Psychiatry's Diagnostic and Statistical Manual gave me a frightening label: psychotic.

More than once in these psychiatric institutions, guards brought me into what was euphemistically called a 'quiet room' or 'seclusion' which was empty except for a bare mattress on the floor. Several attendants held me down to administer an injection. I felt violated, and the unwanted drugs felt highly intrusive to my innermost thoughts and feelings. At a time when I most needed for some form of empathetic human contact, I was left alone for days in this isolation.

Covering a window in one solitary confinement cell was an impenetrable steel mesh screen which I recall pounding with my fist as I vowed, 'When I get out of here I am going to help change this mental health system.'

Thankfully, between my fourth and final institutionalization, I visited Harvard's student-run organization Phillips Brooks House that places community volunteers. I explained I wanted to do mental health advocacy, saying, 'It's medieval in there!' PBH cautiously referred me to a grassroots organization of people diagnosed with psychiatric disabilities where I found advocacy and a mutually-supportive community among other psychiatric survivors. Emerging from the social change turmoil of the early 1970s, the group had a radical name: 'Mental Patients Liberation Front'. I wrote my senior paper on MPLF's unique organizational structure, and somehow graduated with honors in 1977.

Severe human rights violations continue to this day

When I recount my story of forced psychiatric drugging in the 1970s, I am sometimes told that the state of human rights for people in mental health care has vastly improved, and that my story is no longer relevant. However, I have an easy reply. Since then I have had the privilege of working with thousands of fascinating human beings all over the world who have been given a psychiatric label, or who are allies, for more than three decades. I like to say I have had a front seat watching the human spirit come back over and over and over again.

In our advocacy office, we receive letters, phone calls, e-mails, and visits from people all over the world who continue to receive involuntary psychiatric drugging, and even involuntary electroshock. Certainly, there have been some improvements over these decades. There are some marvellous support and advocacy programmes run by caring mental health consumer peers, for example, many of whom are on countless advisory boards. However, in my opinion, the state of human rights violations in mental health care is worse than ever, and harms far more people than ever before. While I respect an individual's choice to take prescription psychiatric drug, a veritable avalanche of psychiatric drugs is being pushed upon the general population as never before, from infancy to old age. In most situations I examine, the individual has not been offered adequate information, alternatives, and advocacy. In fact, the biggest potential increase in human rights violations in mental health lies in front of us, especially in poor and developing countries.

The main improvement in these decades is that our social change movement exists, and we finally have the potential to directly name and challenge these violations. Educated by our social change movement's efforts, journalist Robert Whitaker, in his book *Anatomy of an Epidemic: Magic Bullets, Psychiatric Drugs, and the Astonishing Rise of Mental Illness in America* (2010), pulls together hundreds of research studies to argue that in many ways, during the past few decades, while any one particular individual may certainly find help in mental health care, the overall results of the mental health system's over-reliance on powerful psychiatric drugs have been profoundly and disturbingly negative.

We are, together, sometimes known as the *mad movement*. There's little agreement about the best language for us. *Psychiatric survivors* for me means we are individuals who experienced human rights violations in the mental health system and lived to tell about it. We are not passive victims, we are now citizen activists for human rights and alternatives in mental health. *Mental health consumers* or *users* for me means selecting mental health care in an empowered way, like choosy customers. There are no perfect words, but I ask not to be called *mentally ill*. Individuals may call themselves that, but calling me by that phrase lends too much power to an already-dominant medical model.

Not all of us in the mad movement have a psychiatric diagnosis. Among us are dissident mental health workers, curious researchers, human rights advocates, compassionate family, and concerned members of the general public. When we unite I glimpse democracy beginning to shape the future of the mental health system.

It is time to hear about mental and emotional well being from the perspective of those labelled crazy. We folks on the sharp end of the needle have a voice.

A voice for mad pride

Today a few experts might mistakenly call me *normal*. I have not used the psychiatric system for more than thirty years. I'm married to a loving woman, Debra. We are tax-paying homeowners with a nice big garden. For more than two decades, I've directed a respected nonprofit human rights group in this field, MindFreedom International, that unites 100 sponsor and affiliate groups.

I suspect, though, that some mental health professionals would describe many of my beliefs as *delusional.* As an activist sounding an alarm, I tend to announce these beliefs far more bluntly than my friends in academia. Here are a few:

- *I believe* thousands of us so-called mad citizens and allies are making history by transforming how we as a society approach the subject of the mind.

- *I believe* the psychiatric industry would like to screen everyone for mental and emotional problems, and place millions of new customers onto their powerful drugs.

Please, allow me to say more than once that I am pro-choice about your personal health care decisions. If an individual knows the risks, has access to a range of alternatives, and willingly chooses prescribed pharmaceuticals, that is his or her business and no one else's. I have been there. I know what it's like to beg for a psychiatric drug. I also know what it's like to quit psychiatric drugs, and care must be taken to do this well.

- *I believe* many of these psychiatric drugs can be addictive, brain damaging, and deadly, but much of this information is covered up from patients and their families.

- **I believe** many psychiatric drug corporations act like bullies by lying and choking out non-drug, humane options for mental health care.

- *I believe* there is no scientific evidence for claims by some in the psychiatric industry that a 'chemical imbalance' is the basis for mental disorders.

- *I believe* much of the mental health industry is traumatizing, damaging, and even killing mental health clients who are, by some measures, among the most powerless in our society.

- *I believe* these human rights violations amount to a hurricane of unscientific psychiatric labels. . . psychiatric drugging without informed consent or non-drug options. . . torture in institutions using restraints, aversive therapy, electroshock. . . isolation in the community with segregation, impoverishment, and discrimination. . . a criminal lack of options for good housing, for decent jobs, and for humane alternatives to the traditional mental health system.

- *I believe* developing countries ought to be warned that this psychiatric hurricane is invading poor nations, and that this *globalization* of corporate psychiatry's human rights violations could impact hundreds of millions of people.

- *I believe* those of us who society perceives as having gone over the edge of sanity, and who have since returned, have something valuable to offer to citizens who are commonly considered *normal*.

- *I believe* our society is in extreme, global catastrophe such as the climate crisis, yet humanity seems transfixed in a hypnotic trance of passive conformity.

- *I believe* we so-called mad citizens may help humanity wake up from this so-called normality and reach some of its highest goals of social and ecological justice.

- **I believe** this is Mad Pride!

For centuries there has been a war between citizens called *normal* and citizens called *mad*. It is time to say to both, 'Let's talk.' When people are unfairly divided by skin colour, *racism* is traumatizing. When people are unfairly treated because of gender, *sexism* causes suffering. But humans often define ourselves as *the thinking* or *rational animal*. The minority of us perceived as irrational is considered inferior in our most basic essence, our chemistry, our genes. There is a name for this prejudice. I do not hear this word much. It is *sanism*. Sanism has a long history.

That story of the quivering line between normal and mad goes back millennia. Psychiatric institutions have existed only for centuries. It is revealing that it was mainly in the fairly-recent 1800s that the first huge psychiatric institutions were built. Europeans wanted to leave behind their centuries of religious infighting. For better or worse, the Western world was eager to urbanize, colonize, and industrialize.

What to do about us eccentric citizens who do not fit in the Great Modernization? Country folk who spout bizarre beliefs? Joan of Arcs when they have no army? Witches? Head injured? Fools? Developmentally disabled? Shamans? In the 1800s we strange others on the margins were seen as impediments in the transition to a rational citizen (Goldberg 1999).

The extreme of this oppressive approach can be seen in how we citizens with psychiatric labels were eventually treated in Europe. In the 1930s, Nazi Germany targeted children diagnosed with mental disabilities as the very first group for mass murder. Psychiatrists helped develop the theory, methods, and even the paperwork used in Nazi genocide. Never forget. Never again.

Unjust deaths continue to this day in the mental health system. I've seen too many autopsy reports. A major 2006 report by the US National Association of State Mental Health Program Directors shows that the life spans of those in the public mental health system are 25 years shorter than the average American. Some researchers suspect psychiatric drugs play direct and indirect roles in this tragedy (Parks 2006).

Mad movement emerges from activism of many movements

The ferment of the 1960s civil rights, women's rights, anti-war movement, and others encouraged citizen activism. This churning change made community organizing seem to be a natural and obvious choice, even for those of us with psychiatric labels. A spirit of liberation was expressed by Reverend Martin Luther King, Jr. Many times in his speeches, sermons, and essays, MLK sounded a theme that seemed to anticipate our movement. He said, 'psychologists today have a favorite word and that word is "maladjusted." And I say I am proud to be maladjusted. We ought to be maladjusted. . . Human salvation lies in the hands of the creatively maladjusted.' In a speech on the First of September 1967, in front of the American Psychological Association, MLK said, 'Thus, it may well be that our world is in dire need of a new organization, The International Association for the Advancement of Creative Maladjustment' (Roysircar 2009). MLK asked us for this IAACM repeatedly, for more than a decade.

By coincidence, only a few years after MLK's speech the first psychiatric survivor groups in this era emerged, such as We Shall Overcome in Oslo, Norway, the tiny Insane Liberation Front in Portland, Oregon, and Project Release in NYC.

I've known several of the organizers of these early groups who we now consider movement heroes. Howie the Harp organized on both coasts and composed a ballad for the new movement, called *Crazy and Proud*. Judi Chamberlin wrote a book called *On Our Own* (1978), comparing her experiences in a state psychiatric institution with a more empowering alternative. Ted Chabasinski experienced forced electroshock at the age of six in New York State. Ted spent his entire youth in a psychiatric institution. Leonard Roy Frank was an early dropout from the business world who turned to mysticism; he was given multiple forced electroshocks. I was able to attend several of the annual gatherings back then called the International Conference for Human Rights and Against Psychiatric Oppression. I wrote for Madness Network News. The movement spread in Europe, Canada, New Zealand, and Australia (Crossley and Crossley 2001).

Allied mental health professionals played a role. At about the time I was in a psychiatric cell, psychiatrist Loren Mosher was head of the US National Institute of Mental Health's schizophrenia division. Loren created a model known as Soteria House where people could find mental and emotional support without the usual bullying and over-drugging so many experienced in the mental health system. In 1998 Loren famously resigned from the American Psychiatric Association, denouncing it as the American Psychopharmaceutical Association. Loren died in 2004 and is missed (Bernstein 2004).

In the 1980s government and mental health system funding helped start a few drop-in centres, support groups, and advocacy centres. Given how poor our constituency is, funding from the mental health system is necessary. But, on the other hand, this money threatened to co-opt or 'cool out' the fire of activism and protest.

This is not a criticism of advocacy groups that accept funding from the mental health system and the government. System funding is crucial to accomplish the goals of a social change movement composed mainly of low-income citizens. However, those groups that receive government and mental health funds ought to pause and take care to acknowledge, appreciate, and nurture an independent mad movement. After all, what would the environmental movement be if all of its activity was funded by the government and the oil industry, if there was no Greenpeace?

What has changed for psychiatric survivors?

I'm often asked what changes I've seen in more than three decades of mad movement work.

As I've noted, there is some change for the better. Today our movement encompasses thousands of citizens, and hundreds of diverse groups working for a voice for people in the mental health system. There are nowhere near enough of us, but psychiatric survivors and mental health consumers are running housing programmes, peer support groups, and advocacy systems. There are non-drug alternative clinics, networks of mental health professionals, and authors criticizing the psychiatric system (Lehman & Stastny, 2010). There are newsletters, conferences, websites, and e-mail lists. There are universities that have academics working with us, including on research guided by psychiatric survivors.

When I meet with local mental health officials in our small city of Eugene, Oregon, USA, or with leaders of the World Psychiatric Association, I witness some positive effects of our movement. I hear new words from mental health leaders such as *empowerment, peer support, advocacy, trauma, alternatives, recovery,* and *self-determination*. Today, in a policy meeting about us, it is not unusual to see one of us, such as an individual with a psychiatric diagnosis, at the table.

We've had a global impact. For years, MindFreedom and World Network of Users and Survivors of Psychiatry have had teams of psychiatric survivors in meetings inside the United Nations headquarters in New York City. MindFreedom is the only group of its kind accredited by the United Nations as a Non Governmental Organization. We have Consultative Roster Status, which gives our members the ability to attend UN meetings. Led by Celia Brown, an African American psychiatric survivor from New York City, our MindFreedom team of psychiatric survivors participated in UN meetings resulting in an international treaty on disability rights—called a convention—that became legally binding internationally on 3 May 2008.

The UN's health agency is the World Health Organization (WHO) based in Geneva, Switzerland. Benedetto Saraceno, MD, from Italy, was WHO's mental health director. We met with him and he agreed to declare a 'global emergency' of human rights violations in the mental health system.

Dr Saraceno said, 'I think that, indeed, there is a global emergency for the human rights of people suffering from mental health problems. I insist on the word "global" as people tend to believe that these kinds of violations always occur somewhere else when, in fact, they occur everywhere' (personal communication 2005).

I enjoy hearing about some of the creative protests and cultural events that educate the public that are sprouting up all over the world. For more than a decade a Mad Pride movement has grown, similar to Gay Pride (Campbell and Roberts 2009). Mad Pride celebrates all of humanity's uniqueness and freedom with events in about a dozen countries.

For example, a Mad Pride Bed Push has been held for several years in England, and that has spread to the US and Canada. In a Bed Push, activists dressed as mental patients in hospital gowns push a hospital bed on wheels that has a mannequin strapped in four-point restraints. The mad activists push the bed through the streets to escape the psychiatric system educating thousands with humour.

One of the largest Mad Pride events is by MindFreedom Ghana Africa. From 2008 to 2010, Mad Pride Ireland has held several Mad Pride events with thousands of participants in each gathering (personal communication 2010).

Mild mental health reform is not enough

However, reflecting back on what I've learned as a grassroots activist in the mental health advocacy field, I've become fond of saying lately to friends and colleagues: 'Oppression in mental health is far, far deeper than I ever imagined when I started this work, and every day I'm discovering it is deeper still.' What I mean, is that the power imbalance between those considered to have a psychiatric disability and the rest of our society is more enormous than I originally suspected.

We want more than new slogans, tokenism, and a few model programmes. Mild reform can at times be a trap. We want a nonviolent revolution. Just like so many other social change movements, I feel we must turn to activism and peaceful protest.

The warnings from our social change movement have come true. When I started this work the psychiatric oppression mainly terrorized the back wards of psychiatric institutions. Now, as we warned, that oppression has gone over the institutional walls. Today it is found in our communities, in our neighborhoods, our homes, our schools.

Our home ought to be our castle, however varieties of 'outpatient commitment' are now widespread in North America, Canada, and Australasia, where we find citizens court-ordered to take powerful psychiatric drugs against their will while living in their own homes out in the community (Kisely and Campbell 2007). There are even mental health delivery services that increase coercion in mental health care by visiting n individual's front door every day to increase 'medication compliance,' such as the Program of Assertive Community Treatment (Gomory 2002).

The psychiatric system is increasingly prescribing psychiatric drugs for children, and marketing them in our schools. There are mental health screening programmes in a number of US schools. It may seem like a good idea to find a troubled youth. But these programmes threaten to march thousands of young citizens to the front door of the mental health system without advocacy, information, or alternatives. Behind that door young citizens often end up in the embrace of the psychiatric industry, putting more young citizens at risk of a lifetime of psychiatric drugs and discrimination. The US President's New Freedom Commission on Mental Health stated that such screenings ought to become 'common practice.'

When I entered the mental health system in the 1970s as a teen, I was almost broken by the experience. The forced drug injections in solitary confinement wore me down. The most powerful blow, though, was when a psychiatrist sat down with me, looked me in the eyes, and claimed I had a chemical imbalance, and I must take psychiatric drugs the rest of my life. That psychiatrist was wrong.

In the 1970s, our movement mainly focused on the human rights violations of force and fraud in the mental health system. What has changed today is that now I feel the mental health system harms the human rights of most citizens through a special brand of fear, a fear that there is no alternative to the conventional mental health system. Psychiatry has largely choked out choice in mental health. Families with a member in crisis deserve more than just a bag of pill bottles and a court order.

The book, *A Way Out of Madness: Dealing with Your Family After You've Been Diagnosed* (Mackler and Morrissey 2010), which also features a chapter by me about my own family's involvement with my mental health system experiences, points out that families with psychiatric survivors need enough self-determination to demand a full range of humane alternatives for their loved ones. Families and family members in crisis can, of course, be in conflict; however, these families and their psychiatric survivors are also ideally on the same voyage, from passive recipients of services, to empowered actors who demand a full range of services.

There ought to be a full range of voluntary, humane, and safe options and alternatives offered to all who choose to use them, including mutual support, jobs, housing, peer run programmes, nutrition, advocacy, quality counselling, and other holistic approaches. A range of choices to achieve mental well-being is not just a good idea. I believe it is guaranteed by the United Nations Universal Declaration of Human Rights.

In other words, why does a young person who has major mental and emotional problems have to live in Finland to find a government-supported alternative such as the 'Open Dialogue' system, which tends to use less or even no psychiatric drugs?

The usual excuse is two words: 'more money.' But the problem is deeper than 'more money.' Poor nations have something to teach the richer nations. In two major studies, WHO researchers visited citizens who had been diagnosed with serious mental health problems in a selection of both rich and poor countries. WHO found that those in less developed nations were far more likely to fully recover and reintegrate back into society (Leff et al. 1992). In other words, nations with less money, fewer psychiatrists and fewer psychiatric drugs appear to have a far better chance. More money is not enough.

Globalization of mental health industry human rights violations

Back in the 1970's, movement activists in richer nations predicted that the labelling and over-drugging we saw in the back wards would some day target the general public. More money was spent. Our prediction came true.

Today I have another prediction. The crisis of globalization of psychiatric human rights violations is going global. For example, I had the opportunity to give a workshop in Istanbul, Turkey, to a room full of psychiatric survivors in a psychiatric community center. I was moved as I heard several psychiatric survivors tell a similar story one after another. As documented by Mental Disability Rights International (now Disability Rights International), a number of these Turkish psychiatric survivors had experienced involuntary electroshock in horrible psychiatric institutions (MDRI 2005). Against their will and without anesthesia, they were held down fully conscious as electricity caused their brains to have convulsions. Although anesthesia would not have protected their brains from the blast of electricity, this 'direct shock' meant they were held down with their eyes wide open and totally aware.

The developing world has been told they must be like the West, that they must be modern and scientific. In mental health that tends to mean the medical model. Drugs are expensive. But electricity is everywhere. So if a poor developing country wants to be like the richer nations, that can mean more electroshock. That is what we are seeing.

This modern approach to mental health is not as much a medical model as it is a *domination model* with a mantra of *label, label, drug, drug, shock, shock*. This domination model is globalizing rapidly. The World Bank and World Health Organization and other large agencies, by their own admission, are promoting multi-billion dollar campaigns to bring western mental health to millions of citizens in poor developing countries. This newest Western export is missing something. This export package has labels, drugs, and shock. But hardly ever does the package include the advocates, alternatives, and activists that exist in the West.

The WHO estimates that 450 million people in the world have a mental disability, and 400 million are not in 'treatment' (WHO 2001). Unchecked and unchallenged, this goal could mean, in my opinion, that over the next few decades hundreds of millions of more people—many of them stressed by war, economic imbalance, and ecological crisis—could be put on psychiatric drugs or electroshocked without adequate advocacy, information, and alternatives.

Today, a child on Ritalin or Prozac is typically North American or European. If the psychiatric drug industry has its way, the face of a child on psychiatric drugs may increasingly be from Asia, from Africa, and from South America.

I am inspired by leaders in poor countries. One of the main organizations in this field is the Center for Advocacy in Mental Health in Pune, India, led by Bhargavi Davar, with a staff of more than a dozen. They educate, they advocate, they help more than 1,000 clients a year. Their leadership for a global nonviolent revolution is essential.

What has changed? When our movement began we warned that psychiatric drugs could cause persistent structural brain changes, including shrinkage of the brain. Science has proven us right. I'll touch on just one particular family of drugs that is typically given during forced psychiatric procedures, the type given to me: *neuroleptics,* also known as *antipsychotics.* They include dozens of drugs with trade names such as chlorpromazine [Thorazine or Largactil], haloperidol [Haldol], thioridazine [Mellaril], and thiothixene [Navane]—all of which I was given—to newer neuroleptics such as clozapine [Clozaril or Zaponex], risperidone [Risperdal], olanzapine [Zyprexa], quetiapine [Seroquel], and aripiprazole [Abilify] (Stip 2001). Neuroleptics, which 50 years ago used to be primarily given to adults inside psychiatric institutions, are now so common they have routinely been advertised on television for years in some countries (Maturo 2010), and are now given to children as young as 18 months (Wilson 2010).

Well-respected mainstream scientists have used modern research, MRI scans, CT scans, animal studies, and autopsies to link high-dose long-term neuroleptics to structural brain change. Let me emphasize one kind. Many studies indicate that long-term, high-dosage, neuroleptics can actually shrink the front of the brain—our lobes linked to higher level functions (Moncrieff and Leo 2010).

Just like with the climate crisis, some corporate defenders sow doubt about this brain crisis. But studies cut through those smokescreens. Some defenders say the shrinkage is from underlying 'mental illness.' But many of these brain changes have also been produced in non-human animal studies. Some defenders even wonder if brain shrinkage may be good for us. But such changes are often linked to worse mental and emotional problems, and can make it difficult to quit the neuroleptics (MindFreedom 2010)

I read about neuroleptic brain changes in the medical literature. But I do not hear about neuroleptic brain damage in the media, mental health conferences, legislative assemblies, or courtrooms. No informed consent sheets I have seen adequately warn anyone of this hazard. Patients and their families may be the last to know.

I know neuroleptics are also associated with other physical problems, such as diabetes. But damage to the higher-level brain system is what places neuroleptics in the same ballpark as psychosurgery, as a lobotomy.

We can easily be pigeon-holed as simply anti-drug. But we are not in a civil war between choosing to take or not take a prescribed drug. There are MindFreedom members who willingly take prescribed psychiatric drugs. But we are united in overthrowing domination by any one model in the mental health system, and two centuries ago the emerging dominant paradigm was the narrow medical model (Scull et al. 1996). This history has shown that minor reform tends to reinforce domination by the medical model, and increase its funding.

If someone personally believes spirituality helps his or her well being, I personally agree. But if the government and mental health system pushed one form of prayer as the only answer for mental problems, if it suppressed non-prayer options, if it claimed science had proven its prayer was the only true way to healing, we would ask, 'By what right? What special evidence can justify the bullying by this one model?' Asking these questions would not make us anti-spirituality. Asking makes us pro-freedom.

Similarly, when I dare to question the wisdom of massive and overwhelming psychiatric drugging of so many people in our society, without adequate advocacy and alternatives, I am sometimes accused of blanket condemnation of all psychiatric drugging. However, I am in fact pro-choice about an individual's personal health care choice to take prescribed psychiatric drugs. In fact, I've found that my colleagues who choose to take prescribed psychiatric drugs have the most at stake about the domination of the medical model. Their very lives are on the line.

A united global campaign for human rights in mental health

There ought to be an enormous united campaign throughout the health, human rights, and disability fields to provide support and technical assistance so that the voices of psychiatric survivors can be heard, especially in poor and developing countries. We also need to hear from advocates, attorneys, dissident mental health workers, and concerned family members who question the mental health system.

In the 20th century, many citizens tended to be intimidated by topics such as energy, urban sprawl, international trade, and gender preference. The public back then was far more likely than now to defer to 'experts' on these topics and to stay silent. We have a long way to go. But today it is more common for a citizen to explore these topics. We are in the beginning stages of citizens becoming confident enough to address mental and emotional well-being.

As I've noted, author Robert Whitaker has applied his skills as a mainstream medical journalist to the question of the efficacy of long-term psychiatric drugging, and has found many of the widely-accepted claims of the psychiatric drug industry to be faulty (Whitaker 2010). I am personally seeing how the data he provides in his book are raising questions among the general public, and among leading professionals within today's mental health system. Whitaker also provides data for the efficacy of alternatives that minimize psychiatric drugging, such as Loren Mosher's Soteria House model, and Finland's Open Dialogue approach.

Our mad movement began by connecting to other movements. We must do so again. One of the most rewarding connections for me is the environmental movement. The numbers are back. What is called *normality* is shredding the very fabric of the whole planet's ecology.

Neuroscientists on the cutting edge of brain research admit they know very little about the mind. Based on the little they suspect, they hypothesize that the mind cannot be understood as a machine. The mind appears to emerge from dynamic feedback loops on a complex edge between chaos and order far from equilibrium.

Today there are revolutions throughout science. Complex emergence displaces *mechanistic reductionism*. Quantum theory posits we cannot absolutely 'grip' reality. Physicists plumbing the depths of subatomic particles say that what we call 'reality' is weirder than they ever imagined. Mathematicians studying what they call 'string theory' hypothesize hidden dimensions.

What has been called *madness* may be at the core of human experience. If any one of us is mad, all of us are in the same mad boat. We all need each other, every one of us. Eliminating the Amazon rainforest may destroy a rare plant that is tomorrow's cancer cure. Eliminating all extreme mental states may destroy tomorrow's prophet.

Citizens cannot dominate complex systems. But one can have influence in what is known as the butterfly effect. The late scientist Edward Lorenz asked, 'Does the flap of a butterfly's wings in Brazil set off a tornado in Texas?' (Hilborn 2004). Simple small actions have long-term unpredictable immense effects.

We can teach citizens about the power of mutual support in un-muting their mute button and reviving morale. We can teach citizens that all strange thoughts are not necessarily good, but all change for the good has begun with one strange thought such as, 'Let us outlaw slavery.' In his best seller *Collapse: How Societies Choose to Fail or Succeed* (2005), physician Jared Diamond finds that some cultures self-destruct, while others learn to think well enough as a group to survive.

When I speak about the movement for nonviolent revolution, I am not speaking only about mental health. I am speaking about a global nonviolent revolution for social and ecological justice for all (Levine 2010).

I ask you those who support us, 'What is your creative maladjustment? What is your role as a leader in a great global nonviolent revolution?' Despite all arguments and grudges, despite all anger and difference, unite and lead MLK's International Association for the Advancement of Creative Maladjustment.

Mad citizens experienced labels and drugs and restraints and shock, and never gave up. Mad citizens experienced discrimination and homelessness and poverty, and never gave up. Mad citizens took the worst hit the mental health system could give, and never gave up. Who is the mad movement? The mad movement is composed of human beings for justice who cannot be stopped, who will not be stopped.

One of our nonviolent weapons is the mind itself. Our peaceful ammunition is inexhaustible. Historians know that more than 500 years ago, German peasant rebellions used this song as an anthem (Bray 1960). This song is a tribute to the free mind. The Nazis would one day ban it. The title is *Die Gedanken Sind Frei*, which in German means, 'Thoughts are free.'

> Die Gedanken Sind Frei [Thoughts Are Free]
> Die gedanken sind frei
> My thoughts freely flower
> Die gedanken sind frei
> My thoughts give me power
> No scholar can map them
> No hunter can trap them
> No one can deny
> Die gedanken sind frei
> I think as I please
> And this gives me pleasure
> My conscience decrees
> This right I must treasure

My thoughts do not cater
To duke or dictator
No one can deny
Die gedanken sind frei
And if tyrants take me
And throw me in prison
My thoughts will burst free
Like blossoms in season
Foundations will crumble
The structures they tumble
And freely we cry
Die gedanken sind frei
Free people will cry
Die gedanken sind frei!

References

Bernstein, A (2004) 'Contrarian Psychiatrist Loren Mosher, 70', *The Washington Post*, 20 July 2004, B06.

Bray, K (1960) *Songs of work and freedom*. Chicago: Roosevelt University.

Campbell, P and Roberts, A (2009) 'Survivors' history', *Journal: A Life in the Day*, 13(3), August 2009, 33–36.

Chamberlin, J (1978) *On Our Own: Patient Controlled Alternatives to the Mental Health System*. New York: Hawthorn Books.

Crossley, M and Crossley, N (2001) 'Patient' voices, social movements and the habitus; how psychiatric survivors "speak out"', *Social Science & Medicine*, 52(10), May 2001, 1477–89.

Diamond, J (2005) *Collapse: How Societies Choose to Fail or Succeed*. New York: Penguin.

Goldberg, A (1999) *Sex, Religion, and the Making of Modern Madness: The Eberbach Asylum and German Society, 1815–1849*. New York: Oxford University Press.

Gomory, T (2002) 'Effectiveness of assertive community treatment', *Psychiatric Services*, 53, 103.

Hilborn, R (2004) 'Sea gulls, butterflies, and grasshoppers: A brief history of the butterfly effect in nonlinear dynamics', *American Journal of Physics*, 72(4), April 2004, 425–27.

Kisely, S and Campbell, L (2007) 'Methodological Issues in Assessing the Evidence for Compulsory Community Treatment', *Current Psychiatry Reviews*, 3(1), 51–56.

Leff, J, Sartorius, N, Jablensky, A, Korten, A, and Ernberg, G (1992) 'The International Pilot Study of Schizophrenia: five-year follow-up findings', *Psychological Medicine*, 22(1), 131–45. Original Article, World Health Organization, Geneva, Switzerland.

Lehman, P and Stastny, P (eds) (2007) *Alternatives Beyond Psychiatry*. Berlin: Peter Lehman Publishing.

Levine, B (2010) *Get Up, Stand Up: Uniting Populists, Energizing the Defeated, and Battling the Corporate Elite*. White River Junction, VT: Chelsea Green Publishing Company.

Mackler, D and Morrissey, M (2010) *A Way Out of Madness: Dealing with Your Family After You've Been Diagnosed*. Bloomington: AuthorHouse.

Maturo, A (2010) 'Bipolar disorder and the medicalization of mood: an epidemics of diagnosis?', in Professor Barbara Katz Rothman (ed) *Understanding Emerging Epidemics: Social and Political Approaches. Advances in Medical Sociology, Volume 11*. Bingley, UK: Emerald Group Publishing Limited, 225–42.

Mental Disability Rights International (2005) *Behind Closed Doors: Human Rights Abuses in the Psychiatric Facilities, Orphanages and Rehabilitation Centers of Turkey*. Washington, DC: MDRI.

MindFreedom International (2010) *Brain Damage Caused by Neuroleptic Psychiatric Drugs*. Available at <http://www.mindfreedom.org/kb/psychiatric-drugs/antipsychotics/neuroleptic-brain-damage>, accessed 8 November 2011.

Moncrieff, J and Leo, J (2010) 'A systematic review of the effects of antipsychotic drugs on brain volume', *Psychological Medicine*, 40, 1409–1422.

Parks, J, Svendsen, D, Singer, P, and Foti, M (2006) *Morbidity and Mortality in People with Serious Mental Illness*. Alexandria: National Association of State Mental Health Program Directors (NASMHPD) Medical Directors Council.

Roysircar, G (2009) 'The Big Picture of Advocacy: Counselor, Heal Society and Thyself', *Journal of Counseling & Development*, 87(3), Summer 2009, 288–94.

Scull, A, MacKenzie, C, and Hervey, N (1996) *Masters of Bedlam*. Princeton: Princeton University Press.

Stip, E (2001) 'Happy birthday neuroleptics! 50 years later: la folie du doute', *European Psychiatry*, 17(3), May 2002, 115–119.

Whitaker, R (2010) *Anatomy of an Epidemic: Magic Bullets, Psychiatric Drugs, and the Astonishing Rise of Mental Illness in America*. New York: Crown.

Wilson, D (2010) 'Child's Ordeal Shows Risks of Psychosis Drugs for Young', *The New York Times*, 2 September 2010, A1.

World Health Report (2001) *Mental Health: New Understanding, New Hope*. Geneva: World Health Organization.

Commentary 7

The Right to Health

Gunilla Backman and Judith Bueno de Mesquita

Introduction

Until recently, the health and human rights communities worked in parallel, rarely engaging with one another. Mental health care was one of the first health issues to attract the attention of the human rights community, back in the 1970s and 1980s. Initially, human rights organizations and experts were primarily concerned with civil and political rights abuses, such as torture and unlawful deprivation of liberty, occurring in some psychiatric institutions around the world (Hunt 2005a). Over the past decade, however, increasing attention has been paid to the right of everyone to the enjoyment of the highest attainable standard of physical and mental health (the 'right to the highest attainable standard of health' or the 'right to health'). This development has occurred as a result of greater attention being paid by the international human rights community to economic, social, and cultural rights, such as the rights to health, education, housing, food, and water. Also important has been the increasing engagement of health organizations and experts, including those working in the field of mental health care, with the right to health.

In 2002, the then Commission on Human Rights decided to appoint a UN Special Rapporteur on the right to the highest attainable standard of health. A Special Rapporteur is an independent expert mandated to monitor and report to the United Nations on a particular human rights issue, including conceptual dimensions and implementation around the world.[1] Mental health care was a central theme in the work of the first Special Rapporteur on the right to the highest attainable standard of health, Paul Hunt (2002–2008). In particular, the Special Rapporteur's annual report submitted to the Commission on Human Rights in 2005 included a chapter on the right to health of persons with mental disabilities (Hunt 2005a).

It is becoming clear that the right to health has a distinctive and practical role to play in improving access to, and the quality of mental health care. In this chapter, drawing on the work of the Special Rapporteur and others, we briefly highlight some aspects of the relationship of the right to health to mental health care in theory and practice.

The legal sources of the right to health

The right to the highest attainable standard of health was first recognized in the Constitution of the World Health Organization (1946). Since then, it has been protected in the majority of international human rights treaties, including the International Covenant on Economic, Social and Cultural Rights (ICESCR 1966), the Convention on the Elimination of All Forms of Discrimination Against Women (1979), the Convention on the Rights of the Child (1989) and the Convention on

---

[1] Special Rapporteurs formerly reported to the Commission on Human Rights, and now report to the Human Rights Council which replaced it in 2006.

the Rights of Persons with Disabilities (2006). Regional human rights treaties in Africa, the Americas, and Europe also include protections of the right to health. Around two-thirds of constitutions worldwide recognise a duty of the state to guarantee health or health care (Kinney and Clark 2004).

In 2000, the Committee on Economic, Social and Cultural Rights (CESCR), a body of independent experts appointed to monitor the implementation of ICESCR, adopted General Comment 14 on the right to health. This document sets out the Committee's interpretation of this human right. CESCR's analysis makes the right to health more accessible and practical. Actors, including the Special Rapporteur on the right to health, have begun to apply and refine CESCR's interpretation to particular issues, such as mental health care (Hunt, 2005a; World Health Organization, 2005; Asociación Pro Derechos Humanos and Mental Disability Rights International, 2004).

As the following paragraphs illustrate, the right to health includes norms which are highly relevant to a range of shortcomings in mental health care around the world. The majority of these norms have long been recognized in the health sector, and have been highlighted in various documents, e.g. the Declaration of Alma-Ata (1978), as being critical to the improvement of health and well-being in the population. However, the added value of human rights is that they convert these norms from permissive standards into legally-binding obligations.

Key right to health norms for mental health care

Today, around 450 million people around the world suffer from mental or neurological disorders, and behavioural health conditions or from psychosocial problems. Mental disabilities disproportionately affect people living in poverty and other vulnerable groups, including women and children (Gable and Gostin 2009). Very few people with mental disabilities receive treatment and care, and where they do, it is often inappropriate. Paul Hunt described mental health as among 'the most grossly neglected elements of the right to health' (Hunt 2005a). People with mental disabilities are often vulnerable and exposed to human rights abuses and frequently face obstacles in claiming their rights or reporting the discrimination which they have encountered.

Around 40 per cent of countries have no mental health policy and around 30 per cent have no mental health plan. The global median percentage of government health budget expenditure devoted to mental health is 2.8 per cent (World Health Organization 2011). In many countries, there is poor coordination between mental health care and other health services, as well as between services provided in health and other sectors (Hunt 2007:43). Further, donor countries rarely support mental health care in developing countries (Hunt 2005a). With increased focus and commitment to reach the Millennium Development Goals, which do not include mental health commitments, mental health is further marginalized or overlooked in discussions among bilateral and multilateral actors in the field of international development.

The right to health contains norms, including the following, which are highly relevant to the mental health care context:

A right to mental health care: The right to health is not a right to be healthy: it is a right to facilities, goods, services, and conditions that are conducive to the realization of the highest attainable standard of physical and mental health. At the heart of the right to health is a functioning health system accessible to all, without discrimination. With this in mind, the right to health makes a number of demands on a health system, including in respect of mental health care. Mental health care must have, at its heart, the well-being and human rights of individuals. General Comment 14 explains that health care, including mental health care, must be widely available within a jurisdiction; accessible geographically, financially, and on a non-discriminatory basis;

gender sensitive, respectful of medical ethics and culturally acceptable; and good quality in respect, among others, of having skilled medical personnel and scientifically approved drugs and medical equipment. There must be an appropriate mix of services and continuum of care with effective referrals, and coordination with other related services and sectors, such as social services and education (Hunt 2008:15). Information on health, including mental health, must also be accessible, which means, *inter alia*, that it must be understandable.

The adoption and implementation of a national health plan including mental health is a requirement for ensuring these mental health care objectives. The plan should be based on recent assessment, e.g. a situation analysis or a rapid assessment; relate to the whole population, including women, men, boys, and girls; be costed, have a timeframe; have health and right to health indicators and benchmarks (Backman et al. 2008); be transparent, available, and accessible to the public; and be periodically reviewed, on the basis of a participatory approach and transparent process. The inclusion of mental health care in a national plan also serves to prevent its marginalization in the broader health care context.

Non-discrimination and equality: Non-discrimination and equality are fundamental rights to health principles. People with psychosocial disabilities frequently encounter stigma and discrimination. Mental health care which unnecessarily isolates or segregates users is inherently discriminatory.

Progressive realization and resource constraints: The right to health does not demand that states develop a comprehensive, integrated health system overnight. In view of resource constraints on states, it requires that they progressively take effective measures to work towards this objective, including in the field of mental health care. While the right to health recognizes that states face resource constraints, it requires that they devote the maximum available resources to health, including mental health care. This includes resources available from the international community.

While many aspects of the right to health are subject to progressive realization, states have some immediate obligations. This includes non-discrimination, and the development of a costed national health plan. It should be noted that the development of a national health plan also has immediate practical purpose, namely in facilitating strategic resource planning. Any attempt at the progressive improvement of the mental health of the population requires the state to identify goals, indicators, and plan resources, including any request for additional resources from the international community. A costed national health plan is a critical first step in achieving this.

Participation: The right to health is not only concerned with outcomes—such as what mental health care is provided and what policies are in place; it is also concerned with processes. Participation is a key process. Under international human rights law, persons with psychosocial disabilities are entitled and must be supported to participate in policy-making processes, including those on mental health care. Involving persons, including children, with psychosocial disabilities, and their families and representative organizations, and reflecting their perspectives and experiences in the design and implementation of relevant initiatives, helps to ensure that their needs are met and their rights are respected. The right to health can be used by persons with mental disabilities and their advocates to insist that governments provide them with, or work towards, the standards they are entitled to, such as community based mental health services, treatment, and rehabilitation (Gostin and Gable 2009).

Accountability: The right to health demands that the state and other responsible actors are held to account, i.e. that those responsible show, explain, and justify how they have realized their obligations in respect of the right to health. Because persons with psychosocial disabilities are often vulnerable to human rights violations in the health care sector and beyond, it is vital that independent, effective, transparent, and accessible monitoring and accountability mechanisms are available to them. There are various types of accountability mechanisms: judicial, e.g. constitutional redress; quasi-judicial, e.g. UN treaty bodies; administrative, e.g. human rights impact assessment; political, e.g. budgetary reviews by Parliamentary committees; and social, e.g. civil society organizations (Potts 2008). It is important to underline the importance of not relying exclusively on legal accountability for a number of reasons, including that approximately 40 per cent of countries lack dedicated mental health legislation (WHO 2011); other countries have outdated mental health legislation which does not incorporate human rights (Gable and Gostin 2009); legal processes are frequently expensive and difficult to access for marginalized groups, including people with mental disabilities; and legal judgments sometimes go unenforced in some countries. The issue of accountability is further explored on p. 583.

International assistance and cooperation: Human rights treaties, such as ICESCR, give rise to responsibilities to respect the right to health in other countries; where possible, prevent third parties interfering with this human right in other countries; and, depending on available resources, facilitate access to health services, goods, and facilities in other countries, including through providing aid. This is particularly relevant in the context of mental health, since donors have rarely prioritized mental health care. This is also why it is critical that the international community respects the Paris Declaration on Aid Effectiveness (2005) and the Accra Agenda for Action (2008), which incorporate the principle of national ownership of development. These global commitments will reinforce assistance to countries to realize their human rights obligations, including to improve the mental health and well-being of the population. Where donors do support mental health care, it is vital that they support the development of appropriate services (Mental Disability Rights International 2002).

The practical contribution of the right to the highest attainable standard of health

The conceptual relevance of the right to health provides opportunities for promoting accessible and good quality mental health care. While we do not describe in detail models for applying the right to health to mental health care, the following paragraphs suggest a number of ways in which the right to health makes a positive contribution in this field.

The policy approach: The importance of integrating human rights, including the right to health, into mental health legislation is well-documented (WHO 2005). Bringing the right to health to bear explicitly upon local, national, and international health policy-making processes, including a national health plan, is another strategy for guaranteeing the right to health.

Worldwide, there are increasing numbers of initiatives to integrate human rights into health care policies and programmes, including in the field of mental health care. Often these initiatives pay particular attention to human rights such as participation, empowerment, equality and non-discrimination, accountability, and civil and political rights (Department of Health (UK) 2008; Scottish Human Rights Commission 2009).

Rosie Winterton, the former Minister of State for Health Services, UK, supported a fundamental reform of health and social care in England, with the aim of creating services which are patient and service user led. The Department of Health decided to apply a human rights-based approach in five National Health Service Mental Health Trusts, with the aim of demonstrating that using a human rights-based approach in the design and delivery of services can make a difference in people's lives. This project was an attempt to show that human rights are not only for other countries, a relic from the past or a legal issue that belongs to the domain of the lawyers. It aimed to demonstrate the practical value of human rights for the whole organization and how human rights can be operationalized, not only in terms of protecting rights but also in terms of promoting them. After six months, the Trusts' work was evaluated, and some of the outcomes indicated that the initiative had:

◆ Increased patient-centred care, with a process involving to a greater extent minority and vulnerable groups;

◆ Meant that service providers were more often given the opportunity to take part in influencing and developing their care programmes;

◆ Empowered staff to challenge decisions, as their arguments were grounded in human rights law and not only good practice;

◆ Created a sense of empowering arising from the awareness that the organization can be held to account;

◆ Resulted in service users being aware of their rights and able to question their treatment.

In 2009, the Scottish Commission on Human Rights published an evaluation of a human rights-based approach adopted at the State Hospital, the high security forensic mental health hospital for Scotland and Northern Ireland. The approach focused on human rights principles such as accountability, non-discrimination, participation, and the empowerment of rights holders, and aimed for public authorities to apply the Human Rights Act, which primarily focuses on civil and political rights, and link to international and regional standards. The evaluation of the Scottish Human Rights Commission founds that the approach had a range of benefits, including:

◆ A more positive and constructive atmosphere with mutual respect between patients and staff, leading to increased engagement between the two groups, increased work satisfaction by staff, and increased satisfaction among patients as regards to their care and treatment;

◆ A reduction in blanket policies and an increased focus on the risks of each patient, as well as on the rights of every member of staff, patient, and carer (Scottish Human Rights Commission 2009).

The right to health is sometimes marginalized in policy approaches. This is disappointing since the normative content of the right to health can provide a useful conceptual and practical framework for mental health policies, leading to more equitable, appropriate, and sustainable policies. It can help focus attention on issues such as whether a policy successfully addresses the availability, accessibility, acceptability, and quality of mental health care; is non-discriminatory and promotes equality; has been developed through a participatory process; aims to enhance participation; and includes appropriate independent monitoring and accountability structures and procedures.

Seeking more resources: Health care is often grossly underfunded and mental health care is often marginalized in the health budget. While the right to health recognizes that states often have limited resources at their disposal, it demands that they devote as much to health as possible, and that they distribute these resources within the health sector in a way which enables an appropriate balance of services.

Ministers of health can use the right to health as a tool to legally underpin requests for greater resources for health. A national health plan is an important framework for demanding greater resources. Mental health policy makers and advocates can also use the right to health to demand greater resources when mental health care is neglected within a health budget. States that have inadequate domestic resources can seek resources from the international community, using the human rights obligation of international assistance and cooperation in health to legally strengthen their requests.

Monitoring and accountability: The right to health is increasingly used to enhance the accountability of the state for the provision of mental health care. The following paragraphs provide examples of international right to health accountability mechanisms which have been used by civil society for improving mental health care.

International human rights courts and commissions have long been used to hold states accountable in relation to human rights abuses occurring in the context of mental health care. While cases have traditionally focused on civil and political rights, recently there has been more attention to the right to health. For example, in *Purohit and Moore v Gambia* (African Commission on Human and Peoples Rights 2003), the African Commission on Human and Peoples' Rights held that Gambia's mental health law, the *Lunatics Detention Act* (1917), was lacking in terms of therapeutic objectives, and that it was inadequate to treat only those persons with mental disabilities for whom there were matching resources and programmes. The Commission, which found the state in violation of a number of human rights including the right to health, ordered the state to replace the Act.

In March 2004, a number of civil society organizations contacted the UN Special Rapporteurs on health, food, and torture concerning the conditions at the Poiana Mare psychiatric hospital in Romania. It was alleged that 17 patients had died as a result of malnutrition and hypothermia since the beginning of that year. The Special Rapporteurs sent a communication to the government of Romania drawing attention to these allegations. The government replied to the Special Rapporteurs, drawing attention to investigations which it was undertaking into the incidents and improvements that it was making to the living conditions at the facility (Hunt 2005b). In 2005, the Special Rapporteur on the right to health undertook a country mission to Romania to learn about how the country implements the right to health. During this visit, he had the opportunity to visit Poiana Mare. In the report on his mission, the Special Rapporteur recommended that the government support further improvements at the facility such as: making appropriate medication available, providing adequate rehabilitation for patients, ensuring that patients are able to access effective complaint mechanisms, and the provision of human rights training for hospital staff (Hunt 2005c).

Civil society has also engaged with treaty monitoring bodies, including CESCR, with a view to improving mental health care. For example, in 2002, when this Committee reviewed Ireland's second periodic report under ICESCR, civil society organizations drew its attention to the situation of many persons with mental disabilities who were unnecessarily living in psychiatric hospitals in Ireland. The Committee's Concluding Observations recommended that 'the State party speed up the process of transferring persons with mental disabilities who are not suffering from serious psychiatric illness and who are still living in psychiatric hospitals, to more appropriate care settings' (CESCR 2002:34). The adoption and entry into force of the Convention on the Rights of Persons with Disabilities has created new opportunities for the protection and enforcement of this human right in the context of mental health care.

Conclusion

The right to the highest attainable standard of health is a key human right in the context of mental health care. Not only are its norms highly relevant, but it brings practical tools and new avenues to improve protection of users of mental health care. The right to health has been increasingly used by the health sector, civil society, and national human rights institutions as a framework for structuring analysis and to demand action to improve mental health care.

While many international human rights mechanisms do not have powers to force a state to comply with their jurisprudence, in the experience of the authors, where cases are taken up and where shortcomings in relation to mental health care are highlighted, governments can be willing to act to improve the situation. Further, where human rights, including the right to health, have been applied and evaluated in health services, health workers have highlighted that this has been a positive and practical experience.

References

African Commission on Human and Peoples' Rights (2003) *Purohit and Moore v The Gambia, African Commission on Human and Peoples' Rights, Communication No. 241/2001, Sixteenth Activity report 2002–2003, Annex VII.*

Asociación Pro Derechos Humanos and Mental Disability Rights International (2004) *Human Rights and Mental Health in Peru.* Lima: Asociación Pro Derechos Humanos and Mental Disability Rights International.

Backman, G. et al. (2008) 'Health Systems and the Right to Health: An Assessment of 194 Countries', *The Lancet,* **372**, 2047–85.

Committee on Economic, Social and Cultural Rights (2002) *Concluding Observations: Ireland, UN doc. E/C.12/1/Add.77.*

Department of Health (UK) (2008) *Human Rights in Healthcare Evaluation: Final Evaluation Report.* London: Department of Health (UK). Available at <http://www.dh.gov.uk>, accessed 16 December 2009.

Gable, L and Gostin, LO (2009) 'Mental Health as a Human Right', in A Clapham and M Robinson (eds) *Realizing the right to health. Swiss Human rights Book. Vol. 3.* Berne: Ruffer & Rub, 249–261.

Hunt, P (2005a) *Report of the UN Special Rapporteur on the right of everyone to the enjoyment of the highest attainable standard of physical and mental health, UN doc. E/CN.4/2005/51.*

Hunt, P (2005b) *Report of the Special Rapporteur on the right of everyone to the enjoyment of the highest attainable standard of physical and mental health: Addendum—Summary of cases transmitted to Governments and replies received, UN doc. E/CN.4/2005/51/Add.1.*

Hunt, P (2005c) *Report of the Special Rapporteur on the right of everyone to the enjoyment of the highest attainable standard of physical and mental health: Addendum—mission to Romania, E/CN.4/2005/51/Add.4.*

Hunt, P (2007) *Report of the Special Rapporteur on the right of everyone to the enjoyment of the highest attainable standard of physical and mental health: Addendum—mission to Sweden, UN doc. A/HRC/4/28/Add.2.*

Hunt, P (2008) *Report of the Special Rapporteur on the right of everyone to the enjoyment of the highest attainable standard of physical and mental health, UN doc. A/HRC/7/11.*

Kinney, E and Clark, B (2004) 'Provisions for Health and Health Care in the Constitutions of the Countries of the World', *Cornell International Law Journal,* **37**, 285–355.

Mental Disability Rights International (2002) *Not on the Agenda: Human Rights of People with Mental Disabilities in Kosovo.* Washington: Mental Disability Rights International.

Potts, H (2008) *Accountability and the Right to the Highest Attainable Standard of Health.* Essex University: Human Rights Centre.

Scottish Human Rights Commission (2009) *Human Rights in a Healthcare Setting: Making it Work.* Available at <http://www.scottishhumanrights.com>, accessed 16 December 2009.

World Health Organization (2005) *World Health Organization Resource Book on Mental Health, Human Rights and Legislation.* Geneva: World Health Organization.

World Health Organization (2011) *Mental Health Atlas 2011.* Geneva: World Health Organization.

Chapter 34

The Right to Participation of People with Mental Disabilities in Legal and Policy Reforms

Oliver Lewis and Nell Munro

'[T]he idea of citizen participation is a little like eating spinach: no one is against it in principle because it is good for you.'

Arnstein 1969:216

Introduction

International policy documents related to improving the lives of people with mental disabilities and securing their human rights often emphasize the importance of involvement. However, involvement in this context is typically defined as involvement in personal health care related decisions[1] and sometimes as involvement in planning services.[2] The UN Convention on the Rights of Persons with Disabilities is the first binding human rights treaty to articulate the importance of involvement and participation in relation to people with disabilities, including those with mental disabilities. It enjoins states to secure the right of people with disabilities—including those with mental disabilities—to 'effectively and fully participate in political and public life on an equal basis with others'.[3]

In this chapter we will argue that ensuring the participation of people with mental disabilities in the legal and policy reforms relating to their lives is a vital dimension to the realization of the full range of human rights. Promoting participation can improve the relevance, credibility, and qualitative outcome of reforms. It can also serve to empower people with mental disabilities and send

---

[1] For example Principle 11(9) of the Principles for the Protection of Persons with Mental Illness and the Improvement of Mental Health Care (1991) states that 'Where any treatment is authorized without the patient's informed consent, every effort shall nevertheless be made to inform the patient about the nature of the treatment and any possible alternatives and to involve the patient as far as practicable in the development of the treatment plan.'

[2] For example Recommendation 5 of World Health Organization (2001) *The World Health Report 2001: Mental Health: New Understanding, New Hope* states that 'Communities, families and consumers should be included in the development and decision- making of policies, programmes and services. This should lead to services being better tailored to people's needs and better used. In addition, interventions should take account of age, sex, culture and social conditions, so as to meet the needs of people with mental disorders and their families.'

[3] United Nations Convention on the Rights of Persons with Disabilities (2006) Art. 29(a).

a message to the wider community that people with mental disabilities are stakeholders in society with a right to have a voice in the legal and policy decisions which affect their lives. No one would expect regulations affecting industry, for example, to be reformed without close consultation with the stakeholders involved. The involvement of people with mental disabilities is just as central to the process as it is to any resultant law and policy reform.

There are, of course, many stakeholders whose participation in policy-making is necessary. The 'direct users' of mental health policy, including mental health service users, as well as carers, relatives, and mental health care professionals, are the primary stakeholders whom governments often involve in law and policy reform. The wider public, each of whom is a potential future mental health service user (including those who are taxpayers and voters) can also claim an entitlement to be heard,[4] and to have a role in ensuring that policy reforms are both relevant and effective. The arguments we will make below about the advantages of securing the participation of people with mental disabilities apply equally to the wider public. However, in this chapter we will focus primarily on the participation of people who use mental health services, since it is their human rights which, we argue, can only truly be achieved through placing their needs, concerns, and aspirations at the front and centre of any reform process.

What is participation?

The terms *participation* and *involvement*, which we use interchangeably, frequently appear in the literature in this field. Because both terms are inherently vague, multiple values have been attached to them. For the purpose of this chapter and the sake of clarity we refer to service user involvement as occurring when the participation of people who use or have used mental health services in any capacity is treated as integral to the processes of legal and policy reform. Practices which can help to secure involvement are explored throughout this chapter, and include actively responding to calls for policy reform initiated by people with mental disabilities, facilitating their participation in policy planning, consulting with people with mental disabilities on policy documents, and employing people with mental disabilities to evaluate and monitor the implementation and effectiveness of new laws and policies.

Participation is necessary when the objective of legislators and policy-makers is to achieve change which reflects the values and concerns of service users. Consultation can be carried out purely for the politically correct but ultimately vacuous purpose of legitimizing policies which may nevertheless be criticized for allowing for underfunded, discriminatory, or excessively coercive practices (Harrison and Mort 1998). The motives of those who claim that they are promoting involvement should, therefore, always be closely scrutinized.

Promoting participation may make policy implementation more efficient

The argument advanced by the World Health Organization is that including service users in decision-making relating to service planning 'should lead to services being better tailored to people's needs and better used' (WHO 2001:xii). We would argue that this is also true at the level of law and policy-making. Using a wide range of participation methods can help to achieve a wide range of better outcomes for policy reforms.

The logic of this argument is that policy reforms which have been designed in consultation with all stakeholders are more likely to be effective in practice. However, to be confident of the validity of this assertion it is necessary to unpack it a little. Historically, societies have not viewed people

---

[4] See, for example, Pollitt, C (2003) *The Essential Public Manager*. Open University Press.

who have mental disabilities as relevant stakeholders when it comes to designing the laws and policies which affect their lives. Other stakeholders have been consulted: governments around the world have long recognized the need to secure the support of the psychiatric profession for legal reforms which will affect their practice and the lives of their patients. But service users have been excluded. This phenomenon is common to other branches of health care. However, over the last twenty years across a number of countries there has been a shift towards the promotion of user involvement in personal health care planning and service planning. These changes have been attributed to, amongst other things, neo-liberal economic policies which link consumer choice to the efficient allocation of resources (Barnes and Prior 1995), a loss of public confidence in medicine, a desire on the part of service users to challenge paternalism (Rowe and Shepherd 2002), and a belief on the part of policy-makers that user involvement may be the best way to drive up quality and improve health outcomes (Rutter et al. 2004).

This final argument of improving health outcomes has encountered some criticism. One systematic review of the research on health care involvement conducted in 2002 found that there was as yet no evidence base to support claims that user involvement promoted improvements in care quality or patient satisfaction (Crawford et al. 2002). In addition, several studies have demonstrated that the adoption of policies to promote involvement do not automatically lead to service users describing themselves as experiencing participation in practice.[5] However, it is significant that these difficulties and the absence of an evidence base for some claims have not been interpreted as a justification for giving up. It is important to emphasize that, behind disputes about the function and object of involvement, there appears to be a growing normative consensus that involving service users, including service users with mental disabilities, in the decisions which affect them, is unarguably the right thing to do.

Participation as a human right

Steiner identifies two ways in which participation has been expressed as a human right: 'the relatively vague and abstract right to take part in the conduct of public affairs or government and the relatively specific right to vote in elections' (Steiner 1988). The right to vote which is enshrined in various legal texts,[6] as well as the parallel right to stand for election, although people with mental disabilities are often denied the benefit of these rights. It is indicative of the invisibility of people with disabilities within public life that in many countries they are not legally entitled to exercise their right to vote because they have been deprived of their legal capacity.[7]

The abstract right 'to take part' tends to prove more contentious, simply because states have competing conceptions of when, why, and how to facilitate citizen participation. The United Nations Convention on the Rights of Persons with Disabilities (CRPD) does, however, define this

[5] Hodge, S (2005) 'Participation, Discourse and Power: A Case Study of Service User Involvement', *Critical social policy*, 25(2), 164–179; Lester, H, Tait, L, et al. (2006) 'Patient Involvement in Primary Mental Health Care: A Focus Group Study', *British Journal of General Practice*, 56(527), 415–422; Peck, E, Gulliver, P, et al. (2002) 'Information, Consultation or Control: User Involvement in Mental Health Services in England at the Turn of the Century', *Journal of Mental Health*, 11(4), 441–451; Rutter, D, Manley, C, et al. (2004) 'Patients or Partners? Case Studies of User Involvement in the Planning and Delivery of Adult Mental Health Services in London', *Social Science and Medicine* 58, 1973–1984.

[6] Art. 25 of the International Covenant on Civil and Political Rights, Art. 29 of the Convention on the Rights of Persons with Disabilities.

[7] See, for example, the series of reports on guardianship and human rights produced by the Mental Disability Advocacy Center, available from <http://mdac.info/> and Bartlett, P, Lewis, O, and Thorold, O (2007) *Mental Disability and the European Convention on Human Rights*. Martinus Nijhof Publishing, 149–175.

concept for the purposes of international human rights law. The CRPD was adopted because it was felt that the pre-existing human rights mechanisms had failed to provide for the rights of persons with disabilities. The convention specifies that term *persons with disabilities* 'include those who have long-term physical, mental, intellectual or sensory impairments which in interaction with various barriers may hinder their full and effective participation in society on an equal basis with others'.[8] The disability-specific convention represents a paradigm shift from viewing persons with disabilities as objects of management, treatment, pity, and fear, towards persons with disabilities as subjects of the full range of human rights on an equal basis with others.

The CRPD establishes a committee at the United Nations level whose members are experts responsible for periodically monitoring state compliance with the CRPD for those states which have ratified the convention and for interpreting the convention generally. The committee also adjudicates upon individual cases brought by individuals against states which have ratified the Optional Protocol to the CRPD.

The CRPD recognizes participation rights in several places. It requires states to 'closely consult with and actively involve persons with disabilities' in the development and implementation of legislation and policies to implement the convention and other decision making processes that concern them.[9] Because much depends on local context, the convention provides no definitions of consultation or involvement nor does it provide any guidance as to how states are supposed to consult and involve.

The CPRD further obliges states to create a society where people with disabilities can 'effectively and fully participate in the conduct of public affairs without discrimination and on an equal basis with others, and encourage their participation in public affairs'.[10] Specifically, states are expected to encourage the participation of people with mental disabilities in non-governmental organizations and associations,[11] including organizations and associations which represent people with disabilities at international, regional, national, and local levels.[12] The CRPD explicitly provides that such organizations should be involved with and participate fully in the national independent bodies responsible for promoting, protecting, and monitoring the implementation of the convention,[13] giving people with disabilities an explicit role in assessing the performance of state bodies in implementing the convention.

Participation in health policies at the local, national, and international levels had already been a principle under international human rights law well before the entry into force of the CRPD in May 2008.[14] The right to health is located in Article 12 of the International Covenant on Economic, Social and Cultural Rights, a 1966 treaty which many states worldwide have ratified, legally

---

[8] CRPD, Art. 1.

[9] CRPD, Art. 4(3).

[10] CRPD, Art. 29(b).

[11] CRPD, Art. 29(b)(i).

[12] CRPD, Art. 29(b)(ii).

[13] CRPD, Art. 33(3).

[14] As well as the United Nations examples below, see for example the opinion of the European Committee on Social Rights, which interpreted Art. 15(3) of the Revised European Social Charter, to include the provision that, 'persons with disabilities and their representative organizations should be consulted in the design, and ongoing review of such positive action measures [seeking to improve the integration of people persons with disabilities in the life of the community] and that an appropriate forum should exist for this to happen' (Conclusion on Slovenia, 2003–1, 507), as cited in de Schutter, O (2005) 'Reasonable Accommodations and Positive Obligations in the European Convention on Human Rights', in A Lawson, and C Gooding (eds) *Disability Rights in Europe*. Hart Publishing.

binding themselves to the provisions therein.[15] This provision has been authoritatively interpreted to include 'the participation of the population in all health-related decision-making at the community, national and international levels'.[16] In 2005 the UN Special Rapporteur on the Right to the Highest Attainable Standard of Physical and Mental Health (hereinafter 'Special Rapporteur') stated that 'the right of persons with mental disabilities to participate in decision-making processes that affect their health and development, as well as in every aspect of service delivery, is an integral part of the right to health',[17] thus emphasizing that the obligation on states to respect, protect and fulfil the right to health includes the obligation to involve the citizenry in development of health and related policies. Commenting specifically on participation in public policy-making, the Special Rapporteur says in the strongest terms:

> It is essential that persons with mental disabilities, and their representative organizations, are involved at all stages of the development, implementation and monitoring of legislation, policies, programmes and services relating to mental health and social support, as well as broader policies and programmes, including poverty reduction strategies, that affect them. States should affirmatively solicit their input. As providers of care and support, family members also have an important contribution to make in legislative and policy processes, as well as decisions concerning care. Involving mental health-care users, their families and representative organizations, and encompassing their perspectives in the design and implementation of all relevant initiatives, helps to ensure that the needs of persons with mental disabilities are met.[18]

The Special Rapporteur additionally expressed that states should support people with disabilities who may have problems in making or communicating decisions. The CRPD solidifies this by placing a legal obligation upon states to ensure that people have the support that they need in order to exercise their legal capacity.[19]

If participation in policy-making is a right, how can it be enforced by those who claim they are victims? In some jurisdictions it may be argued that the right to participate is inherent in the right to respect for private life. The European Court of Human Rights has in at least two cases indicated that process is important in determining whether there has been a breach of the right to private life. In *Hatton v UK*, a case brought by applicants who advocated against night flights at London's Heathrow airport, the European Court of Human Rights said that in connection with the procedural element of its review of cases involving environmental issues it 'is required to consider all the procedural aspects, including the type of policy or decision involved, the extent to which the views of individuals (including the applicants) were taken into account throughout the decision-making procedure, and the procedural safeguards available'.[20] As Olivier de Schutter has suggested, such an analysis could be applied to policy measures which affect people with disabilities. This would 'require public authorities, before adopting such measures, to seek information about the extent of such an impact, the available alternatives, and the means by which the impact could be reduced and kept to a minimum' (de Schutter 2005).

---

[15] 160 states had ratified the UN Covenant on Economic, Social and Cultural Rights at the time this chapter was finalized (1 January 2009).

[16] UN Committee on Economic, Social and Cultural Rights, General Comment No. 14 (2000), para. 11.

[17] 2005 Annual Report to the Human Rights Commission, by the UN Special Rapporteur on the right of everyone to the enjoyment of the highest attainable standard of physical and mental health, Paul Hunt, Reference number E/CN. 4/2005/51, 11 February 2005.

[18] See Hunt above, n. 17, para. 60.

[19] Art. 12(3). See also Chapter 10: 'Universal legal capacity as a universal human right'.

[20] *Hatton and others v UK*, European Court of Human Rights, Application No. 36022/97, Grand Chamber judgment 8 July 2003, para. 104.

User involvement may secure broader human rights compliance

To date, little research has assessed the level, or considered the significance, of involving service users with mental disabilities at the level of national policy-making and legislative reform. However, in other regulatory contexts it is often argued that key stakeholders must be included at the earliest stage of law and policy reform in order to improve their effectiveness. This early participation can help to ensure that reforms will not have an unnecessarily detrimental impact upon the operations of the sector to be regulated. In many cases the cooperation of regulated businesses or public sector agencies is necessitated by the fact that this will be the only way to ensure their compliance with the proposed regulation. Detecting breaches of the law and promoting compliance through enforcement mechanisms may all be complicated in situations where regulators have little actual knowledge of the operations of the regulated sector and where traditional punitive enforcement mechanisms have only a minimal impact (Baldwin and Black 2008).

This argument applies equally well in the case of laws relating to mental disability. Regulatory oversight of mental health service provision in the UK and North America has traditionally taken the form of specialist inspections and audits. In mental health and social care institutions inspectors may have the opportunity to observe and report on human rights abuses. However, independent inspectorate systems simply do not exist in many countries[21] and there are serious concerns about efficacy in those where they do exist.[22] In addition, focusing only on settings where people are detained means that the use and abuse of coercive practices in the community are ignored.[23] In both contexts it is service-users who are present in the setting all the time who should be seen as offering the first line of defence against abusive practice and excessive uses of coercion. In reforming mental health law and policy to promote human rights, service users should be considered key stakeholders, whose participation in monitoring and evaluation may determine the likely effectiveness of the policy in question.

Participation contributes to securing equality and dignity

Ultimately, promoting the participation of people with mental disabilities in law and policy-making sends out powerful messages to the wider society about what it means for all people to be 'born free and equal in dignity and rights'.[24] In defining dignity, Nordenfelt distinguishes between the broad concept of human dignity which typically underpins human rights and which is held equally by all individuals by dint of their common humanity, and a dignity of identity which is grounded in individual integrity and autonomy (Nordenfelt 2004). Violations of the dignity of

---

[21] An indicator of this is that at the time of writing this chapter only forty states had ratified the Optional Protocol to the UN Convention against Torture, a legal instrument which obliges states to establish independent prevention mechanism to monitor the human rights of people in places of detention which includes mental health and social care institutions.

[22] Mental Disability Advocacy Center (2006) *Inspect! Inspectorates of mental health and social care institutions in the European Union* available online at: <http://mdac.info/sites/mdac.info/files/English_Inspect%21%20Inspectorates%20of%20Mental%20Health%20and%20Social%20Care%20Institutions%20in%20the%20European%20Union.pdf >, accessed 12 May 2010.

[23] The scope for coercion in the community extends beyond the use of explicit Community Treatment Orders, strategies such as withholding a proportion of welfare benefits or attaching conditions to the availability of social housing have also been employed to promote treatment compliance, see: Monahan, J, Redlich AD, et al. (2005) 'Use of Leverage to Improve Adherence to Psychiatric Treatment in the Community', *Psychiatric Services*, 56(1), 37–44.

[24] Art. 1, Universal Declaration of Human Rights, 1948.

identity may leave an individual with a permanent sense of injury to his or her self-respect, which cannot readily be restored or reversed.

Experiencing mental disability places individuals at a great risk of experiencing violations of their dignity of identity. Individuals with mental disabilities experience not only the possibly distressing effects of their condition, but also of legal coercion, stigma, and resultant social exclusion. Indeed, the fragility of personal identity has been cited as a considerable limitation upon efforts to promote mental health service user involvement.[25] The problem of how to secure meaningful and effective participation in legal and policy reform is therefore a dimension of the wider problem of ensuring that the human rights of people with mental health disabilities are protected. A government-led programme which validates people with mental health disabilities as experts in relation to their own lives, takes heed of their wishes when initiating reform, and proactively seeks out their counsel when defining its own agenda for reform could go a long way towards challenging the ways in which the opinions of people with mental disabilities are systematically discredited.

Actively promoting participation strengthens democratic societies

Theorists of democracy often claim that recognizing social difference and attempting to accommodate the diverse needs of social groups who experience cultural or structural inequalities can help to promote dynamic and robust democratic societies. Critics of such an approach argue that according special status to identity-based political movements can serve to reify social difference, or simply displace exclusion from the margins of society to the margins of a plethora of different special interest groups (Young 2000).

Within these debates attention is typically focused upon social movements such as the civil rights movement in the US, or upon second wave feminism, where the establishment of a robust political identity for the excluded community was central to the achievement of their aims. It is not clear that an equivalent social movement constructed around a positive assertion of shared interests by people with mental disabilities either has or could emerge (Barnes 1999; Crossley 1999). Whilst there are associations of users their profile both nationally and internationally is often low and most national and local mental health policy reforms processes are neither initiated nor led by users affected by these policies. Some consequences of this are discussed on p. 595.

As Young points out, however, social difference is not identity (Young 2000:87). Political groupings which are defined as identity-based tend to emerge when they share a positive desire to challenge structural inequalities and not out of a negative or exclusionary desire to promote only the interests of those who share their attributes. Democratic societies benefit from the inclusion of different perspectives within debates about law and policy reform because airing conflicting views, and allowing the expression of diverse and sometimes uncomfortable opinions enables conflicts to be defined, refined and ultimately resolved: 'A democratic plurality ought to be fully inclusive because the plurality of perspectives they offer helps to disclose the reality and objectivity of the world in which they dwell together' (Young 2000:112).

---

[25] Barnes, M and Shardlow, P (1996) 'Identity Crisis: Mental Health User Groups and the "Problem" of Identity', in C Barnes and G Mercer, *Exploring the Divide: Illness and Disability*. Leeds: The Disability Press; Hodge, S (2005) 'Competence, Identity and Intersubjectivity: Applying Habermas's Theory of Communicative Action to Service User Involvement in Mental Health Policy Making', *Social Theory and Health*, 3(3), 165–182; Speed, E (2007) 'Discourses of Consumption or Consumed by Discourse? A Consideration of what "Consumer" means to the Service User', *Journal of Mental Health* 16(3), 307–318.

Techniques for promoting participation

Arnstein's seminal critique of so-called participation practices argued that in many cases citizens were being called upon to legitimize otherwise unpopular policies or to act as window-dressing for processes that were ultimately undemocratic. She argued that citizen participation should be modelled as a ladder: the higher up the ladder of participation a practice is, the greater the degree of power citizens have over the outcome. This is depicted in Figure 34.1. In her words, 'citizen participation is a categorical term for citizen power. It is the redistribution of power that enables the have-not citizens, presently excluded from the political and economic process, to be included in the future' (Arnstein 1969).

Criticism has been levied against the ladder model because by focusing on power, being linear, and posing a dichotomy of included/excluded, it 'fails to capture the dynamic and evolutionary nature of user involvement' (Tritter and McCallum 2006). However, the ladder model provides a useful reminder of the relationship between power and participation. Participation typically needs to be facilitated by policy-makers who can determine the degree of control other stakeholders have over the process. Stakeholders whose cooperation may be central to the success of a policy in practice will typically be granted an audience. People with mental disabilities, on the other hand, who can be managed, leveraged, or compelled to adhere to the policies which affect them may not be so fortunate.

With this in mind, the first consideration for policy-makers when attempting to promote participation needs to be 'How serious are we about ensuring participation?' Policy-making is likely to become more fraught and challenging if the values and concerns of people with mental disabilities are heard, listened to, officially recognized, and acted upon. Other stakeholders may complain that their views are not being accorded proper attention and the wider community may be sceptical about the decisions which are reached through this process. Involving more stakeholders creates a greater potential for disagreements (perhaps previously unarticulated), and a greater likelihood that fundamental conflicts will emerge which cannot readily be resolved. These tensions within the policy-making process create powerful incentives for policy-makers to ignore, discredit, and exclude people with mental disabilities. In considering how to promote participation, we have asked what are the possible pitfalls of the various techniques available rather than downplay the significance of this tension.

When and where to seek participation

It is sometimes the case that socially marginalized 'groups' are able to identify and lobby effectively for the policy changes they desire. In other words, they initiate the reform process. However,

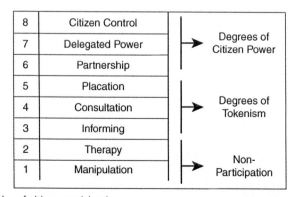

Figure 34.1 A ladder of citizen participation
Arnstein, SR, 'A Ladder of Citizen Participation', *Journal of the American Institute of Planners* 35 (4), p.216 © 1969, Taylor and Francis.

Box 34.1: Public meetings

Before any decision is reached as to whether or not policy reform will be carried out, stakeholders can be consulted on whether or not such reform is needed.

Features: There are a variety of ways that this can happen: roundtable discussions where short presentations are followed up with time for discussion, open public forums which are advertised locally and open to attendance by anyone. Or invitee-only meetings. The difficulty with invitee-only meetings is that they will inevitably be open to criticism as non transparent. Alternatively, a standing citizens' panel—perhaps elected by civil society groups to give them legitimacy, or focus groups—whereby a facilitator picks out people with pre-defined experiences or attributes—could be established, to whom government could turn to for consultation.

Benefits: Face to face meetings allow stakeholders to develop a deeper understanding of other positions that are held. Bilateral follow-up meetings can be scheduled for further discussion, as necessary.

Limitations: Unless the meeting is spread over several days, there may be little time to discuss issues in depth. Prior information needs to be provided so that participants can ponder their responses and interventions. Some users of mental health services may need assistance by way of capacity-building so that their advocacy and participation skills are equalized upwards so that they can contribute on an equal basis with others. Travel and other expenses may need to be paid for users of mental health services who may not have a job, unlike other stakeholders (mental health professionals, for example). Without tight facilitation, participants may move from topic to topic and the discussion could remain at a superficial level. If there are set presentations or panels, participants may adhere to what they have prepared at the expense of involving themselves in a constructive dialogue.

Expert committee

Features: Government can appoint an expert committee to provide recommendations and/or make decisions on its behalf. To be effective everyone serving on the committee needs to be committed to ensuring that people with mental disabilities are included in all discussions and that this is perceived by others.

Benefits: Groups of experts are likely to be better informed than government officials. Committee may be able to use other methods, e.g. consultation. Being part of a committee gives a direct seat at the decision-making table.

Limitations: Experts do not have power in the same way as government does. Neither do they usually have the breadth of knowledge or savvy political skills to deliver policies which will stand a chance of being adopted. Appointment to a committee set up by government is inevitably political, and there will have been some initial screening. It may, therefore, be likely that the members are all 'on-side' already, and thus the experts are unlikely to be representative of the range of views in society. There is a risk of tokenism if there are only be one or two users of mental health services on a committee comprised of several more psychiatrists, nurses, policy-makers, and other professionals. Policy-makers may be lured into recruiting '[t]he "tame" consumer on a committee because we have to have one' (Connor 1999). Another issue is of representativeness, namely to what extent do the users on the committee represent a range of views of others? Finally, financial issues need to be addressed to make sure that the person with mental disabilities is paid for her or his time and expenses on an equal basis with the others on the committee.

Box 34.1: Public meetings *(continued)*

Public consultation

Perhaps the most widely employed participation technique is the use of public consultation after a draft policy document has been published.

<u>Features</u>: Consultation is carried out on the premise citizens have a role in telling what decisions they would like their elected decision-makers to take. Often in governmental structures there is no direct seat for citizens, so consultation is a way of soliciting input from a variety or a segment of the population.

<u>Benefits</u>: Open to any group or individual to provide their feedback. Users can mobilize and snowball information. Consultation can be carried out using web-based technology, but not all citizens have access to the internet so this risks excluding people experiencing poverty.

<u>Limitations</u>: Often the questions have already been set and sometimes the answers are implied in the questions themselves. The questions may not be the questions most relevant to users. Consultation is uni-directional: often a citizen sends her opinion in response to a call for consultation and receives no acknowledgement or feedback on ideas. It may be difficult for citizens to believe that their opinion is being taken into account, and indeed difficult for governments to prove the contrary. A good way to do this is to publish a list of contributors and a summary of the suggestions. Further limitations are that government can legitimize 'bad' policy outcomes by relying on 'good' consultation processes.

Consultation may create the false expectations that citizens actually have authority to make policy; in democratic societies it is elected politicians who have the responsibility to weigh 'public' opinion against other factors such as policy imperatives, financial constraints, and political acceptability. Consultation also needs time, and depending on policy priorities time may be scarce. As well as time, more money may be required, for example, to hire someone to read through and analyse the responses which come in as a result of a consultation process.

A further limitation is that citizens may get consultation fatigue, but the authors have never come across consultation fatigue in mental health sphere, as consultation is unfortunately still rare.

---

it is typical that because of the social exclusion faced by people with mental disabilities, their participation is usually sought only after policy-makers have identified the need for policy reform. We identify three key points in the policy-making process when participation can be actively facilitated, and consider the potential shortcomings of involvement at each stage. This chapter is not intended to offer guidance as to how the problems we identify could be overcome, as this will be dependent on the local context, the financial and time resources available and the dynamism and skills set of the individuals involved. What we do suggest is that those wanting to ensure participation discuss the pros and cons of each methodology as well as adopting a strategy to overcome potential problems (this process itself would benefit from the participation of affected groups).

Who should be involved, and who is responsible for facilitating their participation?

The CRPD makes clear that states need to take proactive measures to facilitate the political participation of people with disabilities, including people with mental disabilities. However, in order to achieve this, states first have to identify whose participation they are aiming to encourage. The effects of stigma and social exclusion may mean that people with mental disabilities are reluctant to own this as a part of their social identity and may be reluctant to participate in policy-making. In turn, the stakeholders who do participate may be subject to criticism for being unrepresentative and not capable of legitimately reflecting the interests of people with mental disabilities. Furthermore, a diagnosis of mental disability is not always static over time. Individuals who are the centre of mental disability policy at one time may not be at another time. Others, who have may not have seen its direct relevance on their lives may nonetheless come to rely on mental disability policy in time.

The problem of identity has already been raised in much of the research in service user participation in service planning and delivery.[26] People with mental disabilities report feeling ambivalent about being accorded a status as 'service users' or consumers. They may avoid efforts made to foster their participation either because they wish to obscure this dimension of their identity from public view, or because they resent having an identity as 'mentally disabled' placed upon them when it does not reflect their own self perception. In addition, people with mental disabilities express heterogeneous views about services (Lammers and Happell 2003), and may not identify with the non-governmental organizations and other activist bodies which claim to act in their name. This is sometimes used to reinforce the claim that the minority of people with mental disabilities who work as activists are outliers pursuing purely personal agendas. This serves to delegitimize the voices of people with mental disabilities. Importantly, there is some evidence that the fact that only a minority of service users actively express a particular view does not automatically mean that this view is not representative of the majority (Crawford and Rutter 2004). However, the problem of identifying whose views should be treated as relevant remains difficult to resolve.

One approach is to adopt a broad definition of relevant stakeholders. Pollitt argues that all of us have the potential to become future users of mental health services, and all citizens are affected by policy to the extent that they are current tax payers (Pollitt 2003). This is a sound argument for making sure that as wide a cross-section of the community is consulted upon proposed policy reforms as possible. But it creates problems for policy-makers trying to identify who to proactively seek to engage in policy-making at earlier stages of the process. It also does not address the question of how much credit should be accorded to the views of those have a mental disability in the present, as opposed to those who may acquire that status in the future.

A concrete answer to the question of whose participation should be encouraged creates a danger of perpetuating the very injustice we are seeking to redress. States have ignored the wishes and feelings of people with mental disabilities for so long because they have viewed them as incapable of forming valid opinions upon the decisions which most affect them. If we attempt to redress this by defining a specific subset of this population as being relevant stakeholders whilst excluding others as not healthy enough, educated enough, or affected enough to be worthy of attention then we simply relocate this problem without resolving it. It is not the case that there is a definable population who should always be included within policy-making, and a larger population whose participation may or may not be relevant. Rather, each policy question requires policy-makers to engage with this issue anew.

Who bears the responsibility of ensuring participation?

International human rights law places the responsibility for ensuring the enjoyment of human rights clearly upon the shoulders of the **government**. The ministries, departments, and individuals

---

[26] See n. 25.

which bear these responsibilities vary across states and across regions within states in federal systems. We emphasize here the need for buy-in from the highest levels of government for participation to have any impact. This means government ministers, heads of department, directors of quasi-governmental agencies, and so on.

The responsibility extends beyond a duty to ensure that users are involved, because involvement needs to be effective and appropriate. Extra resources may be required to pay service users for their time and cover expenses. Coupled with the duty to involve is that states also have a duty to build the capacity of disabled people's organizations. The Special Rapporteur on the Right to Health has said that 'States should support the development and strengthening of advocacy groups of persons with mental disabilities',[27] and the CRPD obliges states to 'promote actively an environment in which persons with disabilities can effectively and fully participate in the conduct of public affairs' by way inter alia of participation in nongovernmental organizations (NGOs) and political parties.[28]

Given the power imbalances within mental health systems, there is a special duty placed upon **mental health professionals** to ensure that people with mental disabilities are involved in law and policy reform. Observing this duty does not necessarily give rise to a conflict of interests. As we have pointed out, the World Health Organization considers participation to generate health benefits both for individuals and community. Professionals sometimes express sceptical attitudes to participation and involvement and professional bodies may therefore also play a particularly important role in ensuring that participation is nonetheless promoted (Soffe et al. 2004; Summers 2003).

Lastly, people with mental disabilities and their representative organizations can demand participation. If they do not get it, they should contact local and domestic bodies which may be able to help: parliamentary committees, national human rights structures such as an ombudsperson or a commission. If this fails, NGOs are advised to seek the input from international actors such as the UN Special Rapporteur on the Right to Health, UN Special Rapporteur on Disability, and UN Committee for the Rights of Persons with Disabilities (where the state has ratified that Convention). There may be regional mechanisms or positions which NGOs can turn to, such as the Commissioner for Human Rights of the Council of Europe.

Conclusions

Participation in political and public life is as important for people with mental disabilities as it is for any other person. We have argued that beyond its importance for them, participation of people with mental disabilities in the policy cycle is useful for policy makers, as the policy and legislative outcomes will be more responsive to needs, and will more likely be effectively implemented.

The participation of people with disabilities has often been overlooked in favour of measures of protection, treatment, and exclusion.[29] The CRPD changes this by placing the rights of people with mental disabilities on an equal footing with the disability rights movement more generally and placing an emphasis on the state's active responsibility to secure participation on an equal basis with others, rather than merely requiring the state not to exclude.

We recommend that policy makers bear in mind three key principles as they ensure the participation of people with mental disabilities. First, the values and concerns of people with

---

[27] See Hunt above, n. 17, para. 61.

[28] CRPD, Art. 29(b).

[29] Declaration on the Rights of Mentally Retarded Persons (1971), Principles for the Protection of Persons with Mental Illness and the Improvement of Mental Health Care (1991).

mental disabilities, as well as those without, should be central to the decisions which affect their lives. Second, participation in law and policy-making is a matter of human rights: national legislatures should put structures in place to ensure participation. Third, policy-makers should think in terms of maximizing participation by using a variety of methodologies, rather than thinking of doing the minimum necessary to legitimize their actions.

The UN Convention on the Rights of Persons with Disabilities provides a right to policy participation and has come into force at a time when states worldwide are beginning to recognize the importance of the views of consumers of health and welfare services in determining their delivery. However, as this chapter has sought to demonstrate, the limits of meaningful participation are not easy to define, and there is no simple recipe to overcome the challenges which proper participation creates.

Acknowledgements

The authors would like to thank Joyce Chamberlain and two anonymous reviewers for their helpful comments on a previous draft.

References

Arnstein, SR (1969) 'A Ladder of Citizen Participation.' *Journal of the American Institute of Planners*, 35(4), 216–24, accessed 26/1/12.

Baldwin, R and Black, J (2008) 'Really Responsive Regulation', *The Modern Law Review*, 71(1), 59–94.

Barnes, M and Prior, D (1995) 'Spoilt for Choice? How Consumerism can Disempower Public Service Users', *Public Money and Management*, 15(July–September), 53–58.

Barnes, M and Shardlow, P (1996) 'Identity Crisis: Mental Health User Groups and the "Problem" of Identity', in C Barnes and G Mercer (eds) *Exploring the Divide: Illness and Disability*. Leeds:The Disability Press, 114–34.

Barnes, M (1999) 'Users as Citizens: Collective Action and the Local Governance of Welfare', *Social Policy and Administration*, 33(1), 73–90.

Bartlett, P, Lewis, O, and Thorold, O (2007) *Mental Disability and the European Convention on Human Rights*. Leiden: Martinus Nijhof Publishing, 149–75.

Beazley, M, Griggs, S, and Smith, M (2004) 'Rethinking Approaches to Community Capacity Building', discussion paper. School of Public Policy, Birmingham: University of Birmingham, as cited in Block 2, *Doing Public Policy*. Open University.

Beresford, P (2006) 'Service Users, Social Policy and the Future of Welfare', in L Budd, J Charlesworth, and R Paton (eds) *Making Policy Happen*. London: Routledge and Milton Keynes: The Open University, 141–152.

Connor, H (1999) 'Collaboration or Chaos: A Consumer Perspective', *Australian and New Zealand Journal of Mental Health Nursing*, 8, 79–85.

Crawford M, Rutter D, Manley C, et al. (2002) 'Systematic Review of Involving Patients in the Planning and Development of Health Care', *British Medical Journal*, 325, 1263–67.

Crawford, M and Rutter, D (2004) 'Are the Views of Mental Health User Groups Representative of those of "Ordinary" Patients? A Cross-sectional Survey of Service Users and Providers', *Journal of Mental Health*, 13(6), 561–8.

Crossley, N (1999) 'Fish, Field, Habitus and Madness: The First Wave Mental Health Users Movement in Great Britain', *British Journal of Sociology*, 50(4), 647–70.

Harrison, S and Mort, M (1998) 'Which Champions, Which People? Public and User Involvement in Health Care as a Technology of Legitimation', *Social Policy and Administration*, 32(1), 60–70.

Hodge, S (2005) 'Participation, Discourse and Power: A Case Study of Service User Involvement', *Critical Social Policy*, 25(2), 164–79.

Hodge, S (2005) 'Competence, Identity and Intersubjectivity: Applying Habermas's Theory of Communicative Action to Service User Involvement in Mental Health Policy Making', *Social Theory and Health*, 3(3), 165–82.

Lammers, J and Happell, B (2003) 'Consumer Participation in Mental Health Services: Looking from a Consumer Perspective', *Journal of Psychiatric and Mental Health Nursing*, 10(4), 385–92.

Lester, H, Tait, L, England E, and Tritter J. (2006) 'Patient Involvement in Primary Mental Health Care: A Focus Group Study', *British Journal of General Practice*, 56(527), 415–22.

Monahan, J, Redlich, AD, Swanson J, et al. (2005) 'Use of leverage to improve adherence to psychiatric treatment in the community', *Psychiatric Services*, 56(1), 37–44.

Nordenfelt, L (2004) 'The varieties of dignity', *Health Care Analysis*, 12(2), 69–81.

Peck, E, Gulliver P, and Towel D. (2002) 'Information, Consultation or Control: User Involvement in Mental Health Services in England at the Turn of the Century', *Journal of Mental Health*, 11(4), 441–51.

Pollitt, C (2003) *The Essential Public Manager*. Maidenhead: Open University Press.

Rowe, R and Shepherd, M (2002) 'Public Participation in the NHS: No Closer to Citizen Control?', *Social Policy and Administration*, 36(3), 275–90.

Rutter, D, Manley, C, Weaver T, Crawford, MJ, and Fulop, N, (2004) 'Patients or Partners? Case Studies of User Involvement in the Planning and Delivery of Adult Mental Health Services in London', *Social Science and Medicine* 58, 1973–84.

de Schutter, O (2005) 'Reasonable Accommodations and Positive Obligations in the European Convention on Human Rights', in A Lawson and C Gooding (eds) *Disability Rights in Europe*. Oxford: Hart Publishing, 35–63.

Soffe, J, Read, J, and Frude, N (2004) 'A Survey of Clinical Psychologists' Views regarding Service User Involvement in Mental Health Services', *Journal of Mental Health*, 13(6), 583–92.

Speed, E (2007) 'Discourses of Consumption or Consumed by Discourse? A Consideration of what "Consumer" means to the Service User', *Journal of Mental Health*, 16(3), 307–318.

Steiner, HJ (1988) 'Political Participation as a Human Right', *Harvard Human Rights Yearbook*, 1(1), 77–134.

Summers, A (2003) 'Involving Users in the Development of Mental Health Services: A Study of Psychiatrists' Views', *Journal of Mental Health*, 12(2), 161–74.

Tritter, JQ and McCallum, A (2006) 'The Snakes and Ladders of User involvement: Moving beyond Arnstein', *Health Policy*, 76, 156–68.

World Health Organization (2001) *The World Health Report : 2001 : Mental Health : New Understanding, New Hope*. Geneva: World Health Organization.

Young, IM (2000) *Inclusion and Democracy*. New York: Oxford University Press, 83–120.

Chapter 35

Human Rights in the Real World

Exploring Best Practice Research in a Mental Health Context

Susan Rees and Derrick Silove

'You cannot be independent in researching oppression: you are either on the side of the oppressed or the oppressor'

Barnes 1996

Introduction

Interest in the link between human rights and mental health has grown in recent decades, yet consensus has not yet been achieved in establishing a core research paradigm for examining their interaction. The present chapter considers the emerging research models that have been used in recent inquiries with the aim of forging greater convergence in methodologies across the field.

The relationship between human rights and mental health is complex. Human rights concepts are derived primarily from philosophical, moral, and legal principles, now codified in international covenants and conventions. Legal remedies potentially allow transgressions to be addressed at a national or international level (Robertson 1999). Nevertheless, the legal forum represents only one component of the overall human rights endeavour. The full realization of a comprehensive human rights regime depends on the adoption of universal standards that protect citizens from a wide range of abuses and deprivations and that prescribe conditions of life that promote optimal well-being and personal development.

In that broad context, it is evident that there is a synergistic relationship between mental health and human rights. Promoting mental health requires close attention to protecting human rights, and conversely, the fulfilment of human rights principles is a *sine qua non* for ensuring the attainment of optimal mental health (Mann 1999). In that respect, many of the risk factors predicting poor mental health (poverty, disruption of families, social disintegration, exposure to violence, and abuse) represent breaches or neglect of fundamental rights, although it is unusual when referring to these risk factors for explicit reference to be made to human rights in mental health research.

The Convention on the Rights of Persons with Disabilities and its Optional Protocol (adopted on 13 December 2006) has taken an important step in forging close links between human rights and mental health. In the convention, persons with disabilities, including those with mental disorders, are regarded as being capable of asserting their rights, making decisions relevant to their lives and participating as active members of society. The convention specifically emphasizes the role of research as a path towards establishing, claiming, and protecting the rights of persons with disabilities (UNEnable 2010). Nevertheless, as indicated, there is no established single method or guiding framework for conducting research that explicitly explores the relationship between human rights and mental health. In this chapter, we consider the methods that have been used, focusing specifically on research with communities exposed to mass conflict, gross human rights violations, and displacement. We attempt to identify a typology of emerging human rights research methods by considering examples from the field, giving consideration to the advantages and limitations of each approach.

Translation of research into practice

Central to any research endeavour linking human rights to mental health is the degree to which the process encourages translation of data into practice. We divide this translation process conceptually into *intra-research* or processual factors (that is, the direct and immediate impact of the ongoing research process on participants and their communities), and *extra-research* outcomes, or the extent to which the data transforms (or has the capacity to do so) the conditions leading to abuses or their consequences. A translation focus matches the express priorities of funding organizations that universally require that research applications outline the concrete benefits of the proposed investigation to the community. Translational research in a mental health and human rights framework might take several forms, including evaluating whether the principles of conventions are applied in policy and practice; whether the rights of communities are promoted in a manner that advances their mental health; and whether persons with mental disorders have access to best practice treatments and/or are treated in a manner that protects their human rights. A more challenging notion of translational research would involve the identification of fundamental structural factors that act as impediments to the realization of both rights and mental health. For example, research may focus specifically on the foundations of political oppression and discrimination, thereby revealing the root causes of human rights abuses and consequent mental health problems. In that sense, research can be challenging to the status quo, and the process itself may be directly emancipatory in relation to participating communities. Inquiries of this nature can put researchers and participants at risk, however, raising complex ethical issues which we consider hereunder.

A provisional typology of human rights and mental health research methods

Based on existing studies drawn from the field of refugee and post-conflict mental health, we offer a provisional overarching typology of research methods which we refer to as: 'Translational Human Rights Research in Practice' (THRRIP). As will be seen, the THRRIP typology includes a heterogeneous range of methodologies and approaches.

Although there is substantial overlap in methods, there are also key differences amongst them including in the informing epistemic traditions, in the extent to which the process is participatory, the explicit priority given to human rights, and the extent to which the focus is on immediate translation or social change. To highlight the distinctions in objectives, methods, outcomes, and benefits of each type, we present models in a somewhat stereotypic manner, acknowledging that in practice, research projects commonly draw on elements of more than one model, as is illustrated by the examples we provide.

Research with a primary human rights focus

Documentary research (Type 1)

Although we do not deal with this typology in detail in this chapter, we note that the case study approach to documenting human rights standards and violations, most often at the country level, is the most direct and explicit human rights focused research type. Amnesty International,

Human Rights Watch, and Physicians for Human Rights are at the forefront of recording and documenting human rights cases so they can be used as evidence to advocate for change in societies experiencing violations of rights and to challenge current illicit practices such as the use of torture (Physicians for Human Rights 2008). Published documents of this type can also be used as a secondary source, or reference, for related empirical research. When included, mental health indices are often treated as corroborating evidence, rather than as the primary focus. For example, the presence of post-traumatic stress disorder (PTSD) supports other evidence that the person is likely to have been tortured. This form of documentary research is a powerful mechanism for challenging breaches of human rights by providing evidence of actual cases of abuse, often recording the names of victims, dates, place where the abuse occurred, witness accounts, and identification of perpetrators. Guidelines are now available for recording and collecting human rights data of this kind (Andrews and Hines 1987; Tobin 1994). Some relevant organizations have an explicit health focus, for example, the International Federation of Health and Human Rights Organisations (IFHHRO 2008).

Research with a primary mental disorder focus

The trauma or implicit human rights model (Type 2)

The introduction of the construct of post-traumatic stress disorder (PTSD) into the Diagnostic and Statistical Manual of the American Psychiatric Association edition III (DSM-III) in 1980, has led to an exponential increase in epidemiological research in the field of traumatic stress. The operationalization of the criteria for PTSD has allowed the field to apply standardized measures to studying diverse population samples in order to assess the impact of trauma exposure on psychiatric outcomes. Definitions have varied, but according to the contemporary consensus, reflected in Criterion A of DSM-IV, trauma represents a threat to life involving the self or close others. As such, the construct of PTSD does not derive from human rights principles, but is based on principles of the psychological and physiological response to life threat, whatever the cause. In many instances, however, life threat is integrally related to human rights violations, for example, the traumas suffered by persons exposed to torture, mass violence, and politically motivated sexual cause. In some settings, trauma and human rights violations may not be directly connected, for instance amongst populations exposed to ecological disasters or civilian accidents.

An important question is why researchers in the refugee and post-conflict mental health field have adopted this trauma-defined model when the outcome, PTSD, does not necessarily imply a response to human rights abuses. In general, reference to human rights issues tends to be subordinated to concepts of trauma, even though the risk factors identified, such as torture, mass rape, and political murder, represent fundamental contraventions of human rights. The evident advantage of adopting the trauma model is that it allows scientists to standardize their measurements for the purposes of comparison within the field and more generally across diverse fields focusing on other forms of trauma. The less overt reason may be that the trauma model confers respectability on the post-conflict field which has a relatively low scientific status in both Psychiatry and Medicine. Employing the constructs and lexicon of the trauma model, as opposed to a human rights framework, therefore offers an entry point into the scientific-medical arena and increases the likelihood that findings will be publishable in leading psychiatric and medical journals. There are some exceptions to this general rule, where investigators have incorporated explicit human rights concepts within the trauma model of research (Basoglu et al. 2005; Silove et al. 2009). As a consequence, the results will reach a wide audience of health professionals and commonly, attention from the media. It can also be assumed that the implicit human rights message will be conveyed to or inferred by the reader, even if this intent is somewhat muted by the language of the trauma model. The disadvantage, however, is that researchers are limited to the constructs and measures used in the trauma field. For example, the focus on PTSD has overshadowed consideration of other psycho-social responses such as anger that may be more relevant to experiences of injustice (Silove 1999; Silove et al. 2009).

Hence, one of the unforeseen risks of adopting the trauma model as the key research framework for the field of refugee and post-conflict mental health is that it inadvertently may attenuate the human rights focus. With the drive to standardization of diagnostic measures, a development that facilitates comparison of findings at an international level, there is a risk that studies will become somewhat de-contextualized, that is, there will be less focus on the unique history, culture, and human rights conditions in each setting. Determinants of mental disorder such as unemployment, poverty, and exposure to trauma are treated as 'risk factors', again obscuring the fundamental human rights issues underpinning these forms of deprivation and abuse, or considering, even implicitly, the potential structural underpinnings and socio-political remedies for these problems.

An added consideration is that unless researchers take a strong human rights stance, they may comply too readily with restrictions placed on their research by autocratic governments—or inadvertently impose such constraints on themselves to avoid difficulties. A study based firmly on human rights principles will ensure that if any compromises need to be made, then they are fully acknowledged, highlighting the contextual and structural obstacles to revealing abuses within the inquiry.

It would be erroneous, however, to assert that all these risks render research founded on the trauma model of little value to human rights. The data may be of benefit in addressing the unmet need for mental health services, for example, in developing countries affected by conflict. The involvement of local academics and field workers in large-scale epidemiological studies may help to build the research capacity of emerging institutions, a process which, in itself, can be empowering. Researchers often engage with NGOs and health services, providing opportunities for the cross-fertilization of skills and ideas related to research practices and procedures. Professionally isolated indigenous practitioners working with conflict-affected communities benefit from the expertise and knowledge of expatriate researchers. 'Behind the scenes' and in the grey literature, the findings are often transduced into human rights language and discussed explicitly in those terms.

Research with both a mental health and human rights focus

An empiricist model of rights research (EMORR) (Type 3)

The designated Type 3 model is related to Type 2 in that it applies standard research methods that are consistent with the orthodox scientific framework (and hence publishable in leading scientific journals), but the focus is explicitly on a core human rights concern as reflected in the stated aims and hypotheses of studies. There is an avowed or implicit commitment to making the data available for those who guide policy and/or practice. The method does not mandate active researcher or community involvement in the application of the data to practice or policy change, however, and in that sense, the research process itself is not necessarily directly empowering in relation to participants. The research team's responsibility is to adhere to accepted ethical standards and to produce data of the highest scientific value. Consultations informing the research design invariably include the community itself, but may extend to policy makers or human rights advocates. Hereunder, we will describe projects focusing on the mental health of detained asylum seekers to illustrate this model.

Research with a psycho-social focus

Social science research amongst disaster and conflict-affected communities (Type 4).

The social science research literature investigating the effects of humanitarian disasters and conflict-affected communities represents a fourth type of human rights oriented research. This broad approach commonly distinguishes itself from the empiricist or quantitative method by claiming a focus on the community as a whole, rather than on individuals. The orientation is towards the strengths of the community, reflected in terminology such as psycho-social recovery and resiliency rather than mental disorder or disability. Research frameworks commonly draw on the precepts of academic disciplines such as anthropology, social work, community psychology, and sociology. Although most studies apply qualitative approaches, methodologies may vary, including elements of ethnography, in-depth semi-structured interviews, focus groups, and participant observation techniques.

Social science research is distinguished from participatory action methods (see hereunder) in that it does not necessarily mandate active participation in directing the research process by community members or stakeholders and there is no explicit requirement that the research process itself will bring about direct social transformation for the target community. Explicit reference to human rights varies according to the study, with some mentioning rights without elaboration, and others giving an explicit focus to documenting abuses as a mechanism for addressing psycho-social problems related to structural disadvantage.

The social science approach based on qualitative methods often is depicted as a preferred alternative to the clinical focus of mental health research. A review (Batniji et al. 2005) of qualitative research in the disaster and conflict field noted that there was an overweening preoccupation across studies with a critique of the category of post-traumatic stress disorder (PTSD), with many studies garnering evidence to demonstrate that this psychiatric disorder represents a Western construct of little relevance across cultures and contexts. In contrast, the social science approach purports to concentrate on communal issues such as poverty, unemployment, and political injustice, argued to be of greater relevance to psycho-social well-being. Individual-level clinical interventions are often depicted as impractical and unnecessary, potentially obscuring human rights issues, considerations of cultural resiliency, practical needs for economic advancement, and strategies to enhance the community's inherent 'capacit(ies) to carry on materially and emotionally' (Zarowsky 2004:202).

The controversy concerning individual and collective responses to mass conflict has exerted a strong influence on the field, the division often reflecting professional allegiances (medical versus social science) and expressed in debates about the value of qualitative versus quantitative methods, and psycho-social versus psychiatric conceptualizations. In our view, the distinction between mental illness and psycho-social well-being tends to be overdrawn with insufficient acknowledgement that there is substantial overlap in these two domains. For example, it remains difficult to define clear-cut boundaries between normative and pathological forms of depression, grief, and anxiety. Equally, there is a paucity of data concerning which forms of distress and/or disability respond to psycho-social as opposed to clinical interventions, and how the two approaches may achieve synergistic outcomes. These desiderata in knowledge should be the substance of scientific inquiry rather than that of ideologically-driven debate. A step forward would be to design and implement multidisciplinary, mixed method research inquiries that include both qualitative and quantitative methods, and that focus both on severe forms of mental disorder as well as the spectrum of psycho-social problems generated by conditions of mass conflict.

Participatory action human rights research (PAHRR) (Type 5)

The fifth subtype of research that we identify is referred to here as Participatory Action Human Rights Research (PAHRR). The approach is consistent with a broad range of participatory research methodologies, both qualitative and quantitative. Unlike other forms of social science research (Type 4), PAHRR has an explicit human rights orientation. Although, within that tradition, there is substantial variation in methods, researchers share a core philosophy of inclusivity and active participation by users, stakeholders, and beneficiaries throughout the process (intra-research outcomes) and in the use of the products of the research (extra-research outcomes). Hence processual or intra-research issues are as important as end point outcomes. PAHRR tends to be applied in settings involving oppressed and marginalized groups, the aim being to empower participants in a manner that fosters their mental well-being and human rights. Critical theory commonly is the informing philosophy that guides the research endeavour (see Cargo and Mercer 2008; Reason and Bradbury 2001). That model focuses primarily on the structural inequalities impacting on health, as well as on the collective actions that may advance social transformations that will address injustices.

PAHHR recognizes that research is inevitably influenced and potentially constrained by political forces. As such, the approach challenges the notion of epistemological neutrality. Political choices inevitably influence micro-level decisions including the framing of hypotheses and the selection of research methods. Context is regarded as crucial in locating the study within a theoretical framework and understanding how the methodology unfolds to match the issues that require investigation. Intrinsic to PAHRR is the notion that engagement and active involvement of grassroots communities in partnership with researchers, at all levels in the exercise, is fundamental to achieving the intended transformations. Together, the coalition of researchers and community members engages with the process and the products of the research to challenge oppressive authority structures that often benefit from and support the status quo, conditions that frequently involve the denial of human rights. The focus may be more complex in Western societies, where authorities may profess a progressive approach to ameliorating social problems but in reality avoid confronting the fundamental structural inequalities that impinge on both human rights and mental health, particularly amongst marginalized sectors of society. PAHRR therefore is a model of research in which the process itself aims to be intrinsically emancipatory, that is, it has an explicit mission to realize in action key tenets of the human rights project.

As described, this emancipatory or critical approach to research positions the researcher as a politically strategic actor in supporting change. Yet such a position may create a dilemma for university-based researchers who need to harmonize the intended goal of advancing community transformations with the demands for scientific rigour and credibility. As indicated, in principle, the two goals should be compatible. As noted, research funding bodies, governments, and society as a whole increasingly demand that research findings should be translatable, that is, contribute directly to policy development, social change, and/or practical outcomes. An implicit but rarely voiced qualification, however, is that the changes brought about by research should not disrupt the status quo or the existing power relationships within the society. Our case studies highlight these inherent dilemmas.

Case studies

We offer some examples from our own research to illustrate aspects of the aforementioned research subtypes, particularly emphasizing categories 3 and 5. We aim to illustrate the benefits as well as the disadvantages of undertaking research using these differing approaches.

Empirical model of human rights research (EMOHHR)

This case study illustrates research that has an explicit human rights focus in assessing policies that may impact on the mental health of a vulnerable group, namely asylum seekers (Steel et al. 2004), in a setting where there is political resistance to the topic under study.

Australia was the first Western country to introduce a policy of indefinite, non-reviewable, mandated detention for certain categories of asylum seekers, particularly those who arrived by boat or who did not have valid entry documents at the port of arrival in the country. From the introduction of the policy and for almost two decades thereafter, mental health workers and human rights groups raised concerns about the mental health consequences of detaining asylum seekers, periods that could extend for several years in immigration detention centres. Yet government officials and detention centre authorities steadfastly refused to allow the conduct of systematic research to assess the mental health and well-being of detainees.

As a consequence, the research unit led by the second author initiated a study that involved phone interviews with the families from one ethnic group held in a remote detention centre. Legal representatives and support groups provided information and obtained consent from detainees during visits to the centre. Independent ethical advice indicated that detention did not remove detainees' rights to choose to participate in research. The process involved psychologists from the same ethnic and linguistic background interviewing adults and (older) children by phone.

The study, published in a public health journal (Steel et al. 2004), reported that all adults and children in the sample met diagnostic criteria for at least one current psychiatric disorder, many having several co-morbid conditions. In the majority of cases, the onset of the disorder had occurred since being detained. Respondents reported high levels of exposure to trauma within the centre, consistent with reports from a succession of commissions of inquiry and other sources (Silove et al. 2007).

The project illustrates the complexities of undertaking rights-based research of this kind in a mental health framework. Debate ensued about the ethics of undertaking such a study without government consent (Minas 2004; Zion, Briskman, and Loff 2010). The rejoinder (Kirmayer, Rousseau, and Krepeau 2004; Rousseau and Kirmayer 2010) was that in extreme situations, where access to vulnerable groups is prevented, the moral and scientific imperative to reveal data concerning their mental health plight can take precedence over the principle, generally preferred, to obtain endorsement of a study by all relevant stakeholders. The documentary work of international human rights agencies such as Amnesty International and Human Rights Watch provides obvious examples where data obtained about conditions of oppression would never be revealed if the research was dependent on the consent of the authorities. A further concern raised was that the participants in the project might be put at risk by revealing information about their suffering in detention. Investigating and revealing human rights violations invariably incurs risks; an absolute prohibition against such research because of the risk involved would curtail most human rights inquiries worldwide. It would be paradoxical indeed if, in the low risk environment of a democratic country such as Australia, human rights research were stifled because of this concern. In each instance of research of this type, it is necessary to undertake a risk-benefit analysis, always a difficult calculation given that prediction of outcomes is far from easy in these fraught contexts. In the Australian context of the time, there was evidence of a shift in communal and political views, with growing concerns about the mental health impact of detention, making the timing of the research particularly important. The reality was that soon after the research was completed and published, all participating families were released from detention, although we cannot be sure to what extent the data contributed to that outcome. The study results were used extensively, however, by asylum advocates in Australia and the data proved central to the deliberations of an inquiry into the impact of detention on children undertaken by the Australian Human Rights and Equal Opportunities Commission (HREOC). In concert, these developments, together with a range of social and political factors at the time, ultimately resulted in major changes being made to the detention policy in Australia. With a change of government, the detention policy initially was modified to address many of the concerns raised but there have been reversals in recent times with the arrival of larger numbers of asylum seekers by boat. In general terms, however, this example of research highlights the challenges of studying controversial society-wide issues that are located at the intersection point of human rights and mental health. The aim, however, was to illustrate how the use of standard scientific methods to record the mental health consequences of these violations provided the credibility that allowed the data to be used in multiple ways to help shape policy on this issue.

Research Type 5—participatory action human rights research

We illustrate some elements of the PAHHR model of research by describing two studies that involved East Timorese asylum seekers residing in Australia in the 1990s. This marginalized group lived under the constant threat of being forcibly returned to their homeland prior to and just following its independence in 1999. Both studies explicitly focused on the stresses associated with statelessness and asylum seeking amongst a community displaced by mass violence and gross human rights violations.

East Timor was a Portuguese colony for over 400 years before being invaded and occupied by Indonesia in 1974–5 with the tacit approval of the major powers including Australia (Taudevin 1999). Extensive human rights abuses were documented in East Timor after the invasion, with a quarter of the population dying or being killed between 1975 and 1999 (Taylor 1999). Deaths occurred as a consequence of starvation, forced displacement, and war, with the Indonesian military being accused of arbitrary arrests, extra-judicial detentions, disappearances, systematic rape, and torture (Amnesty International 1995). These atrocities occurred in the context of an ongoing guerrilla war waged by the East Timorese independence army, Falintil.

In 1999, following the fall of the longstanding Suharto regime, the interim Indonesian government bowed to international pressure to hold a referendum in East Timor to test popular support for independence. Leading up to and following the plebiscite (that strongly supported a move to independence), Indonesian-backed militia perpetrated widespread atrocities (Taudevin 1999) with an estimated 10,000 people being killed and 300,000 being forcibly displaced, many to neighbouring West Timor. Almost all infrastructure including buildings and services were damaged or destroyed (Rees and Silove 2006).

One of the asylum seeker studies reported is referred to as the M-D project (based in Melbourne and Darwin, Australia) (Rees 2003) and the other, the Sydney project (Silove et al. 2002). In spite of disciplinary differences across the two studies (one being based in the social sciences and the other in psychiatry), both projects embraced a human rights-oriented approach. The rationale, planning, and trajectory of both studies made explicit the researchers' focus on structural inequalities and political challenges (both in the homeland and in the country of refuge) that impacted on the target groups. In effect, the projects included elements of EMORR (Type 3) and PAHHR (Type 5), demonstrating how research methods overlap.

The M-D project aimed to identify and analyze intersecting psychological, political, social, and cultural factors impacting on the well-being of East Timorese women asylum seekers. Timorese women faced long periods living with uncertainty and fear of repatriation, with the Australian government asserting that they had the right to protection in Portugal, given the colonial history. The qualitative inquiry comprised in-depth semi-structured interviews, questionnaires administered to professionals working with the community, and an analysis of secondary source material.

The research was intended to be transformative (Truman et al. 2000:24), providing knowledge that asylum seekers could use as a tool for achieving changes to the specific post-migration challenges they faced. The M-D study aimed to be inclusive, in that it engaged non-academic researchers (community workers, asylum seekers, and East Timorese community representatives) in most aspects of the research process. The findings were used by Timorese community leaders in lobbying for asylum seekers to remain in Australia, a campaign that ultimately was successful.

The M-D study demonstrated how cooperation between academic and non-academic partners can assist existing systems to promote individual empowerment and advance social policy. Community workers, particularly those who share the same ethnic background as the target population, are 'natural researchers' in that they can observe and relay community realities to academic researchers and also assist in translating findings into policies and health practice (Perez and Martinez 2008) including in mental health. From a policy perspective, the East Timorese community health worker involved in the M-D study used the research findings to support the ultimately successful lobbying initiative to achieve permanent residency for this displaced group.

The Sydney project (Silove et al. 2002) piloted a researcher-advocacy model highlighting aspects of the Type 5 approach in that it: 1. involved an explicit analysis of social, political and cultural factors impacting on the well-being of the target group; 2. aimed to address human rights issues; 3. involved an interdisciplinary group of researchers and research staff with representatives from the Timorese community, a trauma agency working with the Timorese community, and academics with a long history of support for the Timorese; and 4. explicitly aimed to overcome obstacles to service access in a group known not to be utilizing the wide range of agencies available, including mental and general health, government and non-government agencies, social support, and legal services. The empirical data gathered included core mental health as well as broader psycho-social indices, assessing for the impact of trauma and ongoing living difficulties, with the aim being to develop strategies to assist the East Timorese community in all these interrelated areas. The priority was to provide immediate assistance (clinical and practical) to participants in the study, based on the information obtained. The results of the social, mental, and general health data were communicated directly to participants in a form they could understand, leading to joint decision-making about what further action was needed. Outcomes included further medical assessments followed by emergency and long-term treatment; engagement in counselling, psychiatric assessment, and treatment; referral and/or advocacy for social, financial, or work-related problems; family interventions; and report-writing to assist with legal proceedings. At a wider level, the data collected was made available to the community for its own advocacy needs (Rees and Silove 2006).

Participatory action studies of this type are arduous and time consuming. A systematic review found that only four of 60 studies identified as participatory actually documented community involvement across all research phases (Viswanathan et al. 2004), indicating the challenges in achieving that goal. Differences in priorities may become evident within teams, with service providers and community members understandably being focused on advocacy and the action components, whilst academic team members have the added concern about the quality of data collected. These potentially divergent priorities can lead to some tensions in relation to the time and effort apportioned to each element of the project.

Conclusions

This chapter offers a framework for considering the range of methodologies that have emerged in researching the link between human rights and mental health, with special reference to the refugee and post-conflict field. Given the diversity of professional and theoretical frameworks that contribute to the field, it is not surprising that disparate approaches and methods have been applied. We have deliberately highlighted the differences across the five models identified in order to illustrate their distinctive features. In practice, many studies appropriately draw on elements from several models.

One purpose of the chapter is to emphasize the need for researchers to match methods to hypotheses rather than vice versa. In other words, the key research issue should be identified first and then consideration should be given to which, of an array of possible methods, would best be applied in the context to yield the most informative data. In many instances, an eclectic or mixed methods approach may suit the subject matter being investigated. Sequencing of research methods may provide a powerful approach to gathering data in an iterative manner, with each step offering a test of earlier hypotheses in a cybernetic manner. For example, in the postconflict mental health field, there is a growing consensus that indigenous constructs of distress need to be identified when first studying a population, both for scientific reasons and as an expression of respect for the cultural rights of participating communities. The initial documenting of these constructs and their phenomenology generally requires qualitative approaches. Quantitative methods may become more central in the subsequent psychometric testing of derived instruments and in the application of measures in epidemiological surveys. Our unit has applied this sequence of inquiries to several populations including the Vietnamese (Steel et al. 2009), East Timorese (Silove et al. 2008; Silove et al. 2009) and, in an ongoing research programme, amongst West Papuans (Rees, Silove, and Kareth 2009). These examples illustrate the principle that no single method is adequate to studying the complex interplay of culture, human rights, and mental health.

We have not focused substantially on gender in this chapter but this issue is central to considering both research methods and the content of inquiries. The experience of being a refugee differs substantially according to gender (Rees and Pease 2007; Ward 2005) and gender-neutral research is at risk of obscuring the specific realities and therefore the rights of women. Considerations in studying key concerns such as gender-based violence have led to the development of special methodologies and approaches to address these issues (WHO 2007).

We have tried to emphasize that there is substantial room for an expansion of the scope of research to extend beyond (but at the same time include) the approach of the dominant trauma model (Type 2) in order to ensure that the eco-social context which is directly salient to human rights issues becomes central to the research endeavour. We do not advocate removing standard measures of mental health but instead suggest that the value of a broader approach to data gathering is that the results of the core mental health inquiry can be better understood within the context, culture and human rights concerns of the particular community. Conversely, studies based solely on ethnographic or participatory approaches to research (Types 4 and 5) may be enhanced by including mental health indices that can help in linking the findings to the wider international literature.

The post-conflict mental health field is only emerging from its pioneering period. Experienced researchers in the field commonly were groomed in research methods applicable to other areas of mental health or psycho-social inquiry. As the post-conflict field matures, researchers will benefit from developing or adapting methodologies to suit the subject matter rather than relying entirely on approaches 'imported' from other fields. Interdisciplinary differences in epistemological perspectives could become a growing strength rather than a point of divergence. The task also involves educating the gatekeepers of research (granting bodies, journal editors) about the value of innovative approaches to research. Within the field, however, the first step in achieving a comprehensive, multidisciplinary approach is to recognize how little we know, and how difficult it is for any single method to provide a comprehensive account of the complexities involved in studying the interface of human rights, context, and culture in assessing mental health and psycho-social outcomes.

References

Amnesty International (1995) *East Timor Violations of Human Rights*. Melbourne: Amnesty International.

Andrews, JA and Hines, WD (1987) *Key guide to information sources on the international protection of human rights*. New York, NY: Facts on File Publications.

Barnes, C (1996) 'Disability and the myth of the independent researcher', *Disability and Society*, 11, 107–112.

Basoglu, M, Livanou, M, Crnobaric, C, Franciskovic, T, Suljic, E, Duric, D, et al. (2005) 'Psychiatric and cognitive effects of war in the former Yugoslavia: Association of lack of redress for trauma and posttraumatic stress reactions', *JAMA*, 294, 580–90.

Batniji, R, Van Ommeren, M, and Saraceno, B (2005) 'Mental and social health in disasters: Relating qualitative social science research and the Sphere standard', *Social Science and Medicine*, 62, 1853–64.

Cargo, M and Mercer, S (2008) 'The value and challenges of participatory research: Strengthening its practice', *Annual Review of Public Health*, 29, 325–50.

International Federation of Health and Human Rights Organisations (IFHHRO) (2008) Available at <http://www.ifhhro.org>, accessed 11 September 2008.

Kirmayer, LJ, Rousseau, C, and Crepeau, F (2004) 'Research ethics and the plight of refugees in detention', *Monash Bioethics Review*, 23(4), 85–92.

Mann, JM (1999) 'Introduction', in JM Mann, S Gruskin, M Grodin, and G Annas (eds) *Health and human rights*. New York: Routledge, 3–7.

Minas, IH (2004) 'Detention and deception: Limits of ethical acceptability in detention research', *Monash Bioethics Review*, 23(4), 69–77.

Perez, L and Martinez, J (2008) 'Community health workers: Social justice and policy advocates for community health and well-being', *American Journal of Public Health*, 98, 11–16.

Physicians for Human Rights (2008) *Broken laws, broken lives. Medical evidence of torture by US personnel and its impact*. Cambridge, MA: Physicians for Human Rights.

Reason, P and Bradbury, H (2001) *Handbook of action research: Participative enquiry and practice*. Thousand Oaks, CA: Sage.

Rees, S (2003) 'Refuge or Retrauma? The impact of prolonged asylum seeker status on the well being of East Timorese women asylum seekers residing in the Australian community', *Australasian Journal of Psychiatry*, 11(Supplement), S96–S101.

Rees, S and Pease, B (2007) 'Domestic Violence in Refugee Families in Australia: Rethinking Settlement Policy and Practice', *International* Journal of Immigrant and Refugee Studies, 5, 1–19.

Rees, S and Silove, D (2006) 'Rights and advocacy in research with East Timorese asylum seekers in Australia. A comparative analysis of two studies', *Journal of Immigrant and Refugee Studies*, 4, 49–68.

Rees, S and Silove, D (2007) 'Speaking out about health and human rights in West Papua', *The Lancet*, 370, 637–39.

Rees, S, Silove, D, and Kareth, M (2009) 'Dua sakit (double sick): trauma and the settlement experiences of West Papuan refugees living in North Queensland', *Australasian Psychiatry*, 17(S1), August 2009, S128–S132.

Robertson, G (1999) *Crimes against humanity: The struggle for global justice*. London: Penguin.

Rousseau, C and Kirmayer, L (2010) 'From complicity to advocacy: The necessity of refugee research', *American Journal of Bioethics*, 10(2), 65–67.

Silove, D (1999) 'The Psychosocial Effects of Torture, Mass Human Rights Violations, and Refugee Trauma: Toward an Integrated Conceptual Framework', *Journal of Nervous & Mental Disease*, 187(4), 200–207.

Silove, D, Austin, P, and Steel, Z (2007) 'No Refuge from Terror: The Impact of Detention on the Mental Health of Trauma-affected Refugees', *Transcultural Psychiatry*, 44(3), 359–93.

Silove, D, Bateman, C, Brooks, R, Fonseca, M, Steel, Z, Roger, J, Soosay, I, Fox, G, Patel, V, and Bauman, A (2008) 'Estimating Clinically Relevant Mental Disorders in a Rural and an Urban Setting in Postconflict Timor Leste', *Archives of Gen Psychiatry*, 65(10), 1205–1212.

Silove, D, Brooks, R, Bateman Steel, C, Steel, Z, Hewage, K, Roger, J, and Soosay, I (2009) 'Explosive anger as a response to human rights violations in post-conflict Timor-Leste', *Social Science & Medicine*, 69(5), 670–77.

Silove, D, Coello, M, Tang, K, et al. (2002) 'Towards a researcher-advocacy model for asylum seekers: A pilot study amongst East Timorese living in Australia', *Transcultural Psychiatry*, 39, 4, 452–468.

Steel, Z and Silove, D (2004) 'Science and the common good: indefinite, non-reviewable mandatory detention of asylum seekers and the research imperative', *Monash Bioethics Review*, 23(4), 93–103.

Steel, Z, Momartin, S, Bateman, C, Hafshejani, A, and Silove, DM (2004) 'Psychiatric status of asylum seeker families held for a protracted period in a remote detention centre in Australia', *Australian and New Zealand Journal of Public Health*, 28, 527–36.

Steel, Z, Silove, D, and Nguyen, MG (2009) 'International and indigenous diagnoses of mental disorder among Vietnamese living in Vietnam and Australia', *The British Journal of Psychiatry*, 194, 326–33.

Taudevin, L (1999) *East Timor, too little, too late*. Sydney: Duffy and Snellgrove.

Taylor, JG (1999) *East Timor: The price of freedom*. Annandale, Australia: Pluto Press.

Tobin, J (1994) *Guide to human rights research*. Cambridge, MA: Harvard Law School Human Rights Program.

Truman, C, Mertens, D and Humphries, B (2000) *Research and Inequality*. London: University College Press.

UN Enable (2010) *Convention on the Rights of Persons with Disabilities*. Available at <http://www.un.org/disabilities/default.asp?id=150> Accessed 3 May 2010.

Viswanathan, M et al. (2004) *Community-Based participatory research: Assessing the evidence*. Evidence Report/Technology Assessment No. 99 (Prepared by RTI—University of North Carolina Evidence-based Practice Center under Contract No. 290–02-0016). AHRQ Publication 04-E022–2. Rockville, MD: Agency for Healthcare Research and Quality. July 2004.

Ward, J (2005) *Conducting population based research on gender-based violence in conflict affected settings: An overview of a multi-country research project*. Expert paper prepared from the Expert Group Meeting of UN Division for Advancement of Women, Economic Commission for Europe and World Health Organization, April 2005.

WHO (2007) *Ethical and safety recommendations for researching, documenting and monitoring sexual violence in emergencies*. Geneva: World Health Organization.

Zarowsky, C (2004) 'Trauma stories: Violence, emotion and politics in Somali Ethiopia', *Transcultural Psychiatry*, 27, 383–40.

Zion, L, Briskman, L, and Loff, B (2010) 'Returning to History: The Ethics of Researching Asylum Seeker Health in Australia', *The American Journal of Bioethics*, 10(2), 48–56.

Chapter 36

Reflections from a Mother–Infant Intervention

A Human Rights-Based Approach to Research Collaboration

Mark Tomlinson, Peter J. Cooper, Leslie Swartz, and Mireille Landman

Introduction

The human rights component of collaborations in health research between institutions in rich[1] countries and those in low- and middle-income (LAMI) countries may not be initially apparent. The subtle exploitation of research participants when power is not appropriately acknowledged and interrogated constitutes a breach of human rights and is an issue which has been receiving considerable more attention in recent years (Benatar 2003). Benatar (1998) has stated that even well planned and ethical research has the potential to be exploitative, as all research is conducted in a relationship and in any relationship one has to give due consideration to the question of power.

In this chapter we reflect on the nature of research collaborations and argue that using a human rights-based approach adds a nuanced but significant dimension to the analysis. This will be done with a focus on the ethics of research and the nature of the relationships between collaborators, as well as on the complex interplay between researchers and their participants. In addition, we will argue that while an analysis of the relationship between researchers in rich countries and those in LAMI countries is important, an exploration of the power differentials within countries and between researchers in the same country is also crucial.

We use a South African mother–infant intervention project to illustrate the principles of an ethical approach to such research (Costello and Zumla 2000), and include analysis of within-country dynamics. We show how simply focusing on the rich-poor country level, simplifies the complexity of other levels of interaction that may be operative.

Human rights, ethics, and power

The Nuremburg Trials that followed the end of the Second World War and the adoption of the Universal Declaration of Human Rights by the United Nations General Assembly in 1948 firmly

---

[1] A number of terms have been used to describe the wealthier (often formerly colonizing) countries and the poorer (often formerly colonized), including 'developed'/'undeveloped', 'first world'/'third world', 'Western'/'non-Western', and 'north'/'south'. None of these terms is wholly accurate, and in this chapter we also use another contemporary nomenclature, rich/low- and middle-income (LAMI) countries.

entrenched in the legal apparatus of countries the notions of human rights and human dignity. The Declaration of Helsinki of 1964 (World Medical Association 2004) provided 12 principles for conducting research using human participants, but as Bhutta (2002) correctly points out, the declaration was physician focused, and did not directly address the issue of research in LAMI countries. The Council for International Organizations of Medical Sciences (CIOMS) together with the World Health Organization has developed International Ethical Guidelines for Biomedical Research Involving Human Subjects (CIOMS-WHO 1993). Macklin (1999) argues that both the Helsinki Declaration and the CIOMS guidelines are open to different interpretations; indeed, they may in fact be internally inconsistent and there are occasions when elements in the different codes or declarations conflict. Zion et al. (2000) argue that the Declaration of Helsinki does not address the type of exploitation present in many poor countries where research subjects are often rendered passive because they are dependent on the goods and services that accompany the research. They argue that the CIOMS guidelines go some way to addressing this but they argue that the guidelines do not provide a sufficiently comprehensive understanding of exploitation (Zion et al. 2000).

Benatar (2002) argues that the ethical merit of a piece of research (which is as important as its scientific merit) must embrace respect for the dignity of research subjects, such as their privacy, safety (no harm should accrue to them in the course of conducting the research) and integrity (their opinions and viewpoints are to be respected). These are fundamental issues about respect for individuals and thus of human rights. The core components of a rights-based approach involves the systematic integration of human rights principles such as participation, non-discrimination, transparency, and accountability into policy and programme responses; and a focus on key elements of the right to health—availability, accessibility, acceptability, and quality when defining standards for provision of services (Gruskin et al. 2007).

Benatar (2003), as noted above, argues that research is about relationships and that all relationships involve (at some level) considerations of power. In his view there is an intimate link between ethics and power. He distinguishes between what he calls 'hard power' (largely comprising military power) and that of 'soft power', one aspect of which is the power of knowledge. Benatar (2003) argues that hard power will be used less and less, and be replaced by the use of soft power such as financial power and that of the power of knowledge. The intimate access to knowledge about people characteristic of health care, and certainly of much research, can easily be used to expose and exploit vulnerability (Benatar 2003).

Research collaboration

If we accept Benatar's (2003) notion that knowledge is power, and that in the future 'soft power' is likely to replace 'hard (military) power', then the present bias in research publication between rich and LAMICs is instructive. For example, while 90 per cent of the 135 million infants born in the world each year live in low-income or developing countries (Population Reference Bureau 2002), in a recent survey only 4 per cent of the articles in 12 major international infancy and developmental journals were found to address the experience of infants living in the developing world (Tomlinson and Swartz 2003). The term 'the 10/90 gap' has also been coined to describe the discrepancy between disease burden and research funding, with only 10 per cent of the world's annual health research budget being spent on diseases which contribute 90 per cent of the global burden of disease (Edejer 1999).

Together with acknowledging the nature of such discrepancies and ensuing efforts to reduce this gap (e.g. Global Forum for Health Research (Global Forum for Health Research 2009), there has been an examination of the nature of existing research collaborations and the extent to which they have adequately negotiated issues of power and exploitation. Increasingly, researchers are asking how collaborations between rich and LAMI countries are formulated in practice, and what is the nature of the relationships that characterize these collaborations when they happen.

Types of collaboration

Various forms of research partnerships have come to characterize the interaction between researchers in rich countries and those in LAMI countries. An example in the medical field has been characterized by what has become known as 'postal research', where researchers from rich countries receive biological samples collected and sent by colleagues in LAMI countries (Costello and Zumla 2000). 'Postal research' is the most extreme example of research that adds very little value to the LAMI country, and where the research does not inform practice in the host country. Similarly, researchers sometimes 'parachute' into communities, collect data, and leave.

Another model has been that of the more sophisticated 'annexed site' field research, where the research in LAMI countries is led and managed by expatriate staff (Costello and Zumla 2000). Annexed site research has been very productive in terms of the innovative research and findings that have emerged. Supporters have argued that this approval permits, in difficult circumstances, tight control over research quality, while at the same time avoids falling prey to the shortcomings of postal research. The annexe site model has been described as semi-colonial in nature; the research agenda is dominated by outsiders; line management is the preserve of foreigners; dissemination is focused on international journals and conferences; and the research agenda has the effect of attracting staff away from local institutions.

These models are often exploitative in that it is unlikely that the intervention/drug being tested will be implemented in the host country following the completion of the research. The issue of whether research in a LAMI country should be conducted at all (ethical or otherwise) if the intervention being tested is not intended for implementation in that country, or if the health systems of that country does not have the capacity to implement the intervention if made available, is an increasingly pertinent one (Declaration of Helsinki 2008), but not within the scope of this chapter.

Partnership model of collaboration

In an attempt to prevent the limitations of postal and annexed site research, Costello and Zumla (2000) posit a 'partnership model' of research collaboration. They argue that this is a more equal form of research, characterized by a research agenda that is negotiated with researchers from the host country and where line management is the preserve of locals. In addition, in a partnership model, international dissemination is balanced by outputs in national and local journals, and implicit to the research agenda is the attempt to build local research and academic infrastructure. The notion of the partnership model is useful, and increasingly research collaborations between rich countries and LAMI countries (certainly in the social sciences) are being characterized by this approach. Many authors point to the importance of considering how best to conduct non-exploitative, capacity-building research in developing countries (Costello and Zumla 2000; Eastwood et al. 2001; Edejer 1999). Butler (2000) has outlined an initiative by the Institut de Recherche pour le Developpement (French national agency for scientific research for development) that attempts to redress the balance of power between researchers in rich countries and those in LAMI countries by adopting an International Code of Ethics for Research Collaboration (see Box 36.1). Pang (2002) has also argued (in line with this) that because of the imbalance in power consideration should be given to adopting an international code of ethics for collaborations between rich countries and LAMI countries, and that the notion of 'research ethics' should be expanded to include an emphasis on 'development ethics'.

Box 36.1: Draft Declaration of French National Agency for Scientific Research for Development (Butler 2000)

1. No research in a developing country can be done without the participation of teams from that country.

2. The scientific quality of research conducted in cooperation with developing countries must be the same as that in industrialized countries.

3. Northern partners must help train scientific and technical staff in developing countries, and limit the risk of a 'brain drain'.

4. Industrialized countries' rules relating to the planning and management of research programmes must be strictly respected in any joint projects.

5. Each project must undergo systematic ethical examination, taking into account the developing country's culture.

6. Health and safety conditions must be the same for everyone involved.

7. All participants must be informed about every part of the programme, particularly of any risks and any possible economic or social implications.

8. Everyone involved must have right of access to the various methods of publication and be given the chance to maximize the benefit of their results.

9. Partners must make a systematic effort to maximize the benefits for the populations and countries involved, without necessarily waiting for official completion.

10. No cooperation-based research should be undertaken which, in the present state of knowledge, could be considered potentially harmful to populations, individuals or their environment.

11. Intellectual property rights on data and results obtained must be shared fairly among the participants, in accordance with their overall contributions.

Reprinted by permission from Macmillan Publishers Ltd: *Nature*, 406 (6794), Butler, 'Call for North/ South code of research ethics', copyright, 2000.

Within country relationships

One aspect of research collaborations that has received very little consideration in the literature, however, is the nature of relationships within the host country itself. Many LAMI countries are characterized by enormous differentials in terms of wealth and living conditions, and LAMI country researchers are commonly very different from their compatriots, and even research assistants, in terms of education, status, and financial position. These researchers often do not come from the impoverished communities which are commonly the focus of research and intervention enterprises. In fact, these researchers may share more in terms of their social position, lifestyle, and interests with researchers from wealthier countries, than they do with their fellow citizens who are the objects of research. We examine a South African mother–infant intervention project in light of the principles of the partnership model as outlined by Costello and Zumla (2000), and add to the analysis the key issue of within-country dynamics. We show that simply focusing on the rich-poor country level, simplifies the complexity of other levels of interaction that may be operative.

Thula Sana mother–infant project

In 1995, discussions began between the Winnicott Research Unit (then at Cambridge University, UK), the Child Guidance Clinic at the University of Cape Town, South Africa, and the Parent Centre, a Cape Town-based non-governmental organization, about setting up a randomized controlled trial of a mother–infant intervention in Khayelitsha, a peri-urban settlement of around 500,000 people on the outskirts of Cape Town. By early 2004, after appropriate preparatory work (Cooper et al. 1999, 2002), the randomized controlled trial had been completed. We named our project 'Thula sana' which in the local Xhosa language means 'hush baby'.

Khayelitsha is a predominantly informally organized settlement, made up of serviced and unserviced shacks. There is considerable overcrowding and the population is highly unstable, partly because of steady migration from the rural areas, and partly because of sustained movement within Khayelitsha itself from unserviced to serviced shacks, from violent to less turbulent areas, and from flooded to drier areas. The study was carried out in two adjoining areas of Khayelitsha: SST and Town II. The former is an informal settlement characterized by particularly high levels of unemployment (two-thirds of the population are estimated to be unemployed) and poverty (predominantly shacks with no electricity or running water); the latter is characterized by a somewhat better standard of living (many of the houses are made of brick and receive basic services). The setting for this study bears all the hallmarks of those discussed by Costello and Zumla (2000). As we will show, the conceptualization, planning, and implementation of the Thula Sana study fundamentally followed the tenets of the partnership model of collaboration. This study demonstrates that consideration of within-country dynamics (some specific to South Africa but others that apply more generally to other contexts) can add significantly to a rich description and understanding of the complexities of collaborative research.

Levels of collaboration

An essential feature of the type of analysis proposed by Costello and Zumla (2000) is that it is concerned with the relationships between 'insiders'—people living in the country being studied—and 'outsiders'—researchers from wealthier countries. In describing different levels of collaboration in this study we suggest that there are in fact many layers of insiders and outsiders, and that a simple binary distinction based on country of residence may obscure more complex relationships.

Level 1: British university—South African university

The UK partner (based at the University of Reading) secured the funding from a British trust, and the principal grant holder was at the University of Reading (United Kingdom). With regard to the partnership model (Costello and Zumla 2000) however, two of the grant holders were South African, and the research team in South Africa consisted entirely of South Africans. No expatriates were used in the day to day management of the study, although they had significant input at the level of planning, overall supervision, and quality control. The South African partners were involved in planning at all stages and were solely responsible for implementation on the ground. The project therefore was neither a semi-colonial, nor an annexed site model of research but a project fundamentally characterized by a partnership model of interaction.

Level 2: South African university—South African non-governmental organization

The Parent Centre is a non-governmental organization (NGO) with extensive experience in communities in Cape Town as well as having some experience in the implementation of an early mother–infant intervention on a small scale. In the randomized controlled trial (RCT) that we implemented, their focus was on the clinical intervention, while the academic partners from the University of Cape Town (to which we were attached at the time) and University of Reading had both the clinical intervention as well as the randomized controlled trial (research component) in mind. Colleagues from the Parent Centre spoke at times about feeling that they were playing 'second fiddle' to the research agenda, particularly in terms of what was seen to be the favoured product (i.e. publications and conference presentations). For the Parent Centre, the power, to some extent, lay in the perceived primacy given to peer reviewed publications. While they were never excluded from authorship, the subtle hierarchy between research output (publication) and clinical supervision (task of implementation) was apparent.

Level 3: South African university—university research base in the community

There is a small industry in South Africa and other (mostly developing) countries organized to set up satellite research bases in communities. In this study, we erected a prefabricated structure with interview and observation rooms that was necessary for us to run an intervention and collect data in the community. The set-up was appropriate to the project needs but was in its nature rudimentary in comparison to facilities on the university campus. It was also a substantial distance from the university campus and relatively isolated, for example having no email link or internet access. The logistics of organizing something as simple as petty cash from the university were complex, and there was also some physical danger in cash having to be carried from the university to the site.

Level 4: South African-based university—project assessment team

For the data to be gathered it was necessary to employ a Xhosa-speaking assessment team who spent most of their time in the community collecting data. The skills required of assessors were complex, and most assessors had some tertiary qualifications. Largely for historical reasons associated with racial policy in South Africa, none of the assessors had had access to postgraduate research training. Therefore assessors had specialist knowledge and skills (largely through their understanding of the language and cultural issues in the community) but had been excluded from the opportunity to become researchers in their own right. The differential in privilege between the white university-based researchers and the black assessors, without whom the work could not have been possible, was a source of discomfort, especially as difference between these two groups could be attributed to social factors rather than to differences in research ability. The particular stressors faced by the most senior assessor in this project are discussed elsewhere (Nama and Swartz 2002).

Level 5: Project assessment team—community-based intervention team

In order to preserve blindness to the intervention, the assessors who were hired and trained did not come from the community itself, while the intervention team did. This served a crucial methodological research purpose in a randomized controlled trial with blind assessment. In addition, it was felt that hiring women as counsellors from the community in which the intervention was to take place would assist in trust building and ensuring counsellors were seen as credible by the mothers who received the intervention. In both these aims we believe the study was successful. Our mother–infant counsellors were readily accepted by the community and the relationships between the project and the community remained good for the duration of the study. We also believe that hiring assessors from another community in Cape Town achieved our stated aim of blindness. The manner in which the project was set up however created an additional level of insider-outsider dynamics, with the assessment team having to negotiate carefully around issues of 'community belonging' and 'who could speak' on behalf of the community.

The research context

In a context where racial discrimination was institutionalized for decades, and where gender disparities remain extreme, both race and gender demand immediate consideration. Race and gender have particular resonance in a society for so long stratified on discriminatory lines. Henderson (1999) outlines how race and gender became dominant in defining how she was perceived as a white woman who entered another part of Cape Town during the turbulent run up to South Africa's first democratic elections in 1994. Could predominantly white academics and researchers say anything about the experience of black South Africans? This was highlighted by the institutional silencing of the voices of black South Africans during South Africa's apartheid past, and the patronizing way in which white people often spoke about and for black people. In relation to gender, it is necessary to ask whether it is possible for a male to think meaningfully about the experiences of motherhood, postpartum depression, and the mother–infant relationship?

An additional factor was the notion of motherhood in South Africa. An enduring image throughout the apartheid years which persists, was that of the African mother single-handedly holding the family together despite cruel privations, including endemic poverty, discrimination, the migrant labour system,[2] and ongoing harassment from the security forces. For South African white men to begin planning a study into the prevalence of postpartum depression and its effects on the mother–infant relationship amongst black South Africans was immediately ideologically sensitive. The mere suggestion, in the political climate of that time, that African mothers might in fact be distressed (regardless of the reason), was seen by many people to be highly provocative or contentious. As the idea for the project was being formulated, and prior to any funding having been secured, a prominent black female academic opposed our project aimed at assessing mothers and their infants, arguing that there was nothing to be studied and that the idea of depressed mothers was a Western construct which had no relevance in South Africa (personal communication). In line with this, on another occasion when the project was being presented at a departmental seminar, a colleague was criticized for the perceived Western bias of the intervention. This issue speaks both to the reality that depression is a DSM (Diagnostic and Statistical Manual of Mental Disorders) diagnosis and as such is located within a particular Western discourse, but also to South Africa's apartheid history and discourses regarding who has the right to speak for whom.

In designing the intervention we made significant attempts to ensure that any bias was minimized. One example was the fact that one of the grant holders was a leading expert in the field of culture and mental health, and while the support of the World Health Organization had been enlisted, the person responsible for the training and development of the intervention material had experience in the implementation of such projects in diverse communities within South Africa. In addition (and of crucial importance) was the fact that no assumption was made that postpartum depression existed or that it was related to impaired mother–infant interaction

---

[2] One of the more infamous apartheid laws was the system whereby wives and children were refused permission to live in the areas where their husbands had secured employment—usually on the mines. This ensured a cheap labour force—the belief being that salaries could be limited to providing for one person. Families were assumed (in one of the classic self deluding ideologies produced by the apartheid regime) to be self sufficient, while being banished (on the basis of tribal affiliation) to remote areas designated as 'homelands'.

within Khayelitsha. Instead, as groundwork to the randomized controlled trial, and in order to assess community needs and conditions, an epidemiological study investigating prevalence rates and the possibility of such disturbed interactions was conducted (Cooper et al. 1999). Collaboration with the health system, with non-governmental organizations working in the field of family well-being and with community leaders, was also given priority. Some critics were not convinced and continued to identify a 'Western bias' that did not take into account the South African reality.

In this regard, we were also very clear from the start about not imposing our ideas about what constituted 'good parenting' on the women in our study. It can be argued that in a mother–infant intervention (perhaps more so than in other forms of interventions) notions of expert/non-expert are particularly prevalent, and what constitutes 'good enough parenting' cannot be assumed. Many parents are understandably cautious about 'an expert' giving advice about how to 'parent' their infant. In the South African context this was only partly about culture, but also about power, status, and those who are 'assumed to know'. This was exacerbated by decades of white supremacy and the assumption of white knowledge dominance. Can a 'cultural' or 'racial' outsider' speak with any authority in a context such as this and determine as researchers or as parenting 'experts' the best way to care for infants?

In the Thula Sana project and in work with infants in general, a crucial aim is to create a space in which the unspeaking baby can be thought about and responded to. Some of the dilemmas related to knowledge are foregrounded by the fundamental need in this kind of work to accept a condition of 'not knowing' (about the correct way to parent in this case) while at the same time continuing to try to think about and make sense of the baby's needs. For the community worker this involves taking a quiet, but active and thoughtful role in relation to the needs of the mothers and their babies. It also involves encouraging the mothers themselves to adopt a reflective stance. The methodology of a RCT requires that the intervention is clearly specified. Our intervention was a manualized one specifying content to be covered at each visit. We would argue that a 'manualized' focus on the early abilities of infants and creating a space in which the mother can problem solve and think about her infant, falls within the strict demands of a rigorous RCT methodology, and more importantly was a crucial aspect of any possible intervention in the socio-political context within which we were working.

The brutalizing effects of the trauma as a consequence of apartheid has implications for the ways in which a nation thinks about infancy. Children's pain may have become too unbearable for words or thoughts. Those responsible politically and socially for children may have found it impossible to think about children's pain. The facilitation of these reflective capacities in Thula Sana was done hand in hand with a didactic programme. Often community projects run into difficulty or fail because of a perceived sense by members of the community that they have not 'been given' anything. The idea of a silent listener is not always prized. On the other hand, where input is given (as in our case), we run the ongoing risk of being accused of 'telling mothers what to do', and of a naïve cultural imperialism in assuming things about infancy, motherhood, and the nature of gender relationships in Khayelitsha. Not surprisingly, perhaps, there have been criticisms that the project claimed knowledge in what is ideologically constructed as the 'sacred' sphere of mothers and babies in a different cultural and class context.

It would in many ways be easier to limit the researchers' role purely to a facilitative one which allows for the development of a thinking space. However there are occasions on which our knowledge gleaned through training and research suggests a fundamentally different approach to that commonly held by community members. For example, in the Thula Sana project we were working in a deprived and embattled community, and found ourselves offering as part of our expertise a view of infancy which was at odds with the emphasis on infants' strength and capacity to withstand harm held by many community members. We have often been told that young Xhosa children need not be pampered or picked up each time they cry. Growing up strong and 'getting on with it' are seen as important developmental milestones. In a recent interview, a mother said that during the apartheid years this was particularly the case with a boy child, because one never knew if he might have to leave the country and join the armed struggle. Independence was not so much a developmental task as a survival necessity.

As well as recognizing the importance of these ideas for the emotional protection they provided for the community, it was also felt necessary to offer alternative ways of thinking which might facilitate shifts in understanding. In taking up a position on the need of infants for more active care-giving a strong and potentially painful challenge was issued to the community. The potential benefits outweigh the obvious risks in taking up this kind of position in relation to the community.

Entry into the community and informed consent

In any partnership model a core element is the negotiation of entry into the host country as well as the community that is to be researched. In South Africa in the mid-1990s this involved a significant political as well as social and research element. The question of how or whether it is possible, in an intervention such as this, to negotiate entry in a democratic and culturally respect-ful manner has implications for the work. The intervention described above depends heavily for its design on research in Europe and the US, though there has been considerable care taken to adapt this to the local context. Before the intervention was implemented, extensive negotiations were undertaken with community leaders and people experienced in working with mothers and infants in the area in which the shack settlement is located. The political climate necessitates sensitive and careful negotiations around entry, particularly for white professionals. The issue of cultural sensitivity and the dangers of cultural imperialism are well known in this community, and there was no possibility of our working in the area had community members felt imposed upon inappropriately.

The gaining of true informed consent is a complex issue. Annas and Grodin (1998) question whether in an impoverished setting, where the offer of anything is seen as 'better than nothing', the consent that is gained truly informed and truly consensual. In the process of entering the Khayelitsha community all efforts were made to ensure that all community leaders and stakehold-ers were involved in the consultation process in a transparent and inclusive manner. There are questions though about the extent to which it was possible to receive informed consent from community representatives as many of the specialized research driven concerns may not have been fully understood.

In the face of extensive community 'buy in' to the project, there is also the question whether any individual woman felt in a position to decline the offer of participation. Every attempt was made to ensure that participants knew that they could decline participation (at any point) but it is possible that (unspoken) community pressure may have undermined this. Although they may voice their willingness to participate it remains unclear whether individual mothers felt able to refuse participation given expressed support by community leaders. Informed consent should also aspire to moral and not simply legal requirements (Benatar 1998).

Levels within levels

At different times in the research process, and for different reasons, relationships between differ-ent levels in the partnership were highlighted and at times difficult. An interesting phenomenon was the manner in which elements of the dynamics between the NGO and university staff and those between the assessment and counselling teams in the research base were replicated in terms of what was seen to be 'more valuable': the clinical intervention or the research output. To the counselling team, it was clear that the intervention itself was of crucial concern; to the university staff however, for the sustainability of the project, there had also to be a focus on research output. In reality, of course, each element was as important as the other, but investments differed and shifted, and were valued differently.

There were interesting anomalies in the relationships in the project. For example, at times it appeared that the research team based in Britain were viewed with less suspicion by people from the Khayelitsha community than were the white South African researchers. Furthermore, relationships between the British team and community members sometimes appeared less strained than those between the South African researchers and the community. This is understandable given South Africa's racial history, but represents a phenomenon which may be obscured by looking only at inter-country relationships in research partnerships.

Culture and power

One of the justifications for the partnership model is that insiders understand the culture of the group being studied. It is important to note, as we have suggested, that just as there are complex layers of being inside and outside, there are gradations of cultural knowledge. Who, within any group, can be seen to stand for, represent, and advocate on behalf of the cultural norms of that group (assuming, incorrectly, that cultural norms are static and uncontested, or that communities are homogeneous)? In this study, the assessment team were black, Xhosa-speaking women, but in certain important ways even they were not seen as belonging to the community we were studying. It is quite possible to gloss over these complexities and to give the illusion that the 'cultural problem' has been overcome by a racially or culturally heterogeneous research team. There will always be tensions about what is and what is not culturally acceptable, about who may and may not speak on whose behalf. It entrenches the power and credibility of those writing up research, to argue that cultural issues can be entirely resolved. Cultural tensions inevitably remain within the work, tensions which need to be considered and reconsidered through the research process.

Sharing in the fruits

One aspect of the partnership model as discussed by Costello and Zumla (2000) concerns the issue of authorship and dissemination. We argue that if research and academic infrastructure is to be developed in the host country this has to move beyond words and be reflected in deeds. For instance, when the relationship between the rich/LAMI countries is discussed in the literature it commonly takes the form of authors from rich countries interrogating different models, or outlining the fact that the relationship between them is skewed in one way or another. A good example of this is a paper on collaboration entitled 'Research relationships between the South and the North: Cinderella and the ugly sisters' (Jentsch and Pilley 2003). They make suggestions about how to address difficulties and imbalances in this research relationship. The article makes a number of important points, but interestingly, both authors are from rich countries. In our view, a large part of the role of collaborative research must be in terms of the development of publication expertise amongst collaborators in LAMI countries. In our collaboration there have been a number of publications emanating from the more traditional source (University of Reading together with University of Cape Town researchers and academics; Cooper et al. 1999). In addition, there has also been an article whose lead author was one of the research assistants in Khayelitsha and where both authors were from South Africa (Nama and Swartz 2002).

With regard to the issue of how the findings might be of benefit locally, we have recently published the first results from our RCT (Cooper et al. 2009) and we are at present in negotiations with government authorities about employing this intervention in a planned roll out of early child development services in the context of the Integrated Management of Childhood Illness.

Discussion

With increasing knowledge about the limitations of postal and annexe site models of research there has been a move towards more partnership oriented models of research collaboration between researchers in developed and developing countries. This move is welcome and will undoubtedly serve as a more equitable blue-print in future research. One difficulty with the partnership model is that much of its emphasis is on the country divide. There is little interrogation of the crucial issue of within country, or within research group dynamics. In South Africa, within-country divides are marked and we suspect that the dynamics of class, culture, and differential access to resources are common themes in most countries. It is entirely feasible that as a result of in-country divides, the relationship between research assistants on the ground in the host country may be easier with the principal investigator from the rich country than with in-country researchers. Failure to understand this can have important implications in how a research project is managed and the data that are produced.

A cautionary note is in order. True collaboration must be, and continue to be, the ideal towards which any research endeavour must strive. There is a reality, however, of power differentials, differing agendas, and the fact that different participants within a collaboration may have different resources and investments in the success of any project. This implies that it can never be assumed that simply because most elements of a partnership model have been fulfilled, the resulting collaboration is one of true equality. In a research context with inevitable differentials in terms of power, knowledge, investment, and expertise, such an equal collaboration is something of a Platonic ideal.

Acknowledgements

We would like to thank the two reviewers for their useful comments.

References

Annas, GJ and Grodin, MA (1998) 'Human rights and maternal-fetal HIV transmission prevention trials in Africa', *American Journal of Public Health*, 88, 560–63.

Benatar, SR (1998) 'Imperialism, research ethics and global health', *Journal of Medical Ethics*, 24, 221–22.

Benatar, SR (2002) 'Reflections and recommendations on research ethics in developing countries', *Social Science and Medicine*, 54, 1131–41.

Benatar, SR (2003) 'Bioethics: Power and Injustice: IAB Presidential Address', *Bioethics*, 17, 387–98.

Bhutta, Z (2002) 'Ethics in international health research: a perspective from the developing world', *Bulletin of the World Health Organization*, 80, 114–20.

Butler, D (2000) 'Call for North/South code of research ethics'. *Nature*, 406, 337.

Cooper, PJ, Tomlinson, M, Swartz, L, Woolgar, M, Murray, L, and Molteno, C (1999) 'Postpartum depression and the mother-infant relationship in a South African peri-urban settlement', *British Journal of Psychiatry*, 175, 554–58.

Cooper, P, Landman, M, Tomlinson, M, Molteno, C, Swartz, L, and Murray, L (2002) 'The impact of a mother-infant intervention in an indigent peri-urban South African context: pilot study', *British Journal of Psychiatry*, 180, 76–81.

Cooper, PJ, Tomlinson, M, Swartz, L, et al. (2009) 'Improving the quality of the mother-infant relationship and infant attachment in a socio-economically deprived community in a South African context: a randomised controlled trial', *British Medical Journal*, 338: b974.

Costello, A and Zumla, A (2000) 'Moving to research partnerships in developing countries', *British Medical Journal*, 311, 827–29.

CIOMS–WHO (1993) *Council for International Organizations of Medical Sciences and World Health Organization: International Ethical Guidelines for Biomedical Research Involving Human Subjects.* Geneva: CIOMS.

Declaration of Helsinki (2008) Available at <http://www.wma.net/en/30publications/10policies/b3/>, accessed 27 March 2011.

Eastwood, JB, Plange-Rhule, J, Parry, V, and Tomlinson, S (2001) 'Medical collaborations between developed and developing countries', *Quarterly Journal of Medicine*, 94, 637–41.

Edejer, TT (1999) 'North-south research partnerships: the ethics of carrying out research in developing countries', *British Medical Journal*, 319, 438–41.

Global Forum for Health Research (2009) Available at <http://www.globalforumhealth.org/>, accessed 7 November 2011.

Gruskin, S Mills, EJ, and Tarantola, D (2007) 'History, principles, and practice of health and human rights', *The Lancet*, 370, 449–55.

Henderson, PC (1999) *Living with fragility: Children in New crossroads.* Unpublished PhD thesis, Rondebosch, SA: University of Cape Town.

Jentsch, B and Pilley, C (2003) 'Research relationships between the South and the North: Cinderella and the ugly sisters?', *Social Science and Medicine*, 57, 1957–67.

Macklin, R (1999) 'International research: Ethical imperialism or ethical pluralism', *Accountability in Research*, 7, 59–83.

Nama, N and Swartz, L (2002) 'Ethical and social dilemmas in community-based controlled trials in situations of poverty: A view from a South African project', *Journal of Community and Applied Social Psychology*, 12, 286–97

Pang, T (2002) 'Commentary on "reflections and recommendations on research ethics in developing countries" by SR Benatar', *Social Science and Medicine*, 54, 1145–46.

Population Reference Bureau (2002) Population trends, June 2001. Available at <http://www.prb.org/Publications/PolicyBriefs/PopulationTrendsandChallengesintheMiddleEastandNorthAfrica.aspx>, accessed 7 November 2011.

Tomlinson, M and Swartz, L (2003) 'Imbalances in the knowledge about infancy: the divide between rich and poor countries', *Infant Mental Health Journal*, 24, 547–56.

World Medical Association. (2004) *World Medical Association Declaration of Helsinki: Ethical Principles for Medical Research Involving Human Subjects.* Note of clarification of paragraph 30 added by the WMA General Assembly, Tokyo, 2004. Available at <http://www.wma.net/en/30publications/10policies/b3/>, accessed 7 November 2011.

Zion, D, Gillam, L, and Loff, B (2000) 'The Declaration of Helsinki, CIOMS and the ethics of research on vulnerable populations', *Nature Medicine*, 6, 615–617.

Chapter 37

Can Cognitive Behaviour Therapy Act as a Human Rights Intervention for Consumers Experiencing Severe Mental Disorder?

Peter Walker, Zachary Steel, and Julia Shearsby

The last two decades have seen the rapid expansion of cognitive behavioural models and treatments for psychosis, following a long period of little development in this regard. This has occurred contemporaneously with a re-invigorated social movement advocated by mental health consumers as active participants in the management of their illness. This chapter will examine the historical origins of this particular social movement, consider human rights issues that arise for those experiencing psychosis, and discuss why a relatively standard model of care, Cognitive Behavioural Therapy (CBT), is being utilized as an important human rights based intervention in psychosis. It will illustrate the nature in which CBT with a human rights focus has been used in clinical practice with a case description.

Cognitive Behavioural Therapy

Cognitive Behavioural Therapy is a widely used psychological therapy that was developed in the late 1960s and 70s (Beck 1967). It is theoretically related to learning models of behaviour (Barlow and Durand 1995). It is an active and directive treatment that targets symptoms that are experienced as distressing or impair functioning. For this reason CBT interventions tend to be highly pragmatic, drawing on a range of techniques which are hypothesized to directly target a constellation of symptoms that are identified as constituting a target problem. CBT interventions generally commence with developing a shared explanatory model for the target problem that identifies areas for intervention. Cognitive strategies will aim to help consumers identify the relationship between their behaviour, the content of their thoughts, and associated emotional states. Through a collaborative, therapeutic relationship, thinking and behavioural patterns that maintain distress are explored and challenged. Behavioural strategies, such as relaxation, breathing control, or exposure therapy that target specific symptoms or support the cognitive work will also be taught with regular homework practice recommended.

Despite considerable success in many other areas of mental health work including treatment of anxiety and mood disorders and somatic and physical disorders, until recently cognitive behavioural psychological models and interventions have made little contribution to understanding or supporting people affected by psychosis (Bellack 1986). In the last two decades this has changed both in the development of cognitive models of psychosis, providing a rationale for intervention, and the adaptation of CBT as an intervention for drug resistant psychotic symptoms. The effectiveness of CBT in treating psychotic symptoms is supported by an increasing body of outcome trials and meta-analytic reviews (Rector and Beck 2001; Tarrier and Wykes 2004; Gould et al. 2001). CBT as an adjunct intervention for psychotic conditions such as schizophrenia and bipolar affective disorder is now widely recognized and is increasingly being incorporated into best practice guidelines (NICE 2002). Of particular note, and underpinning why CBT has emerged as an unlikely human rights intervention, is that psychological models of psychosis have challenged many long held assumptions about psychosis in emphasizing the continuity between normal and psychotic experiences and through the study of cognitive processes in the context of psychotic symptoms. These approaches contrast with the more traditional approaches that have dominated mental health services, which emphasized the discontinuity of psychosis, discouraging clinicians from actively engaging with the subjective experience and content of psychotic symptoms.

The consumer movement and auditory hallucinations

The *consumer movement*, also referred to variously as the *user movement*, *psychiatric survivor movement*, or the *patients' rights movement*, is organized internationally in a range of different organizations, engaging in a diversity of political action to promote the rights, welfare, and respectful treatment of people with mental disorders (Cohen 1998; Shera et al. 2002). One arm of this movement developed in the Netherlands around Marius Romme, a social psychiatrist who developed an approach to the experience of voices and visions that emphasized acceptance and saw the voice hearer as an expert in the experience (Romme and Escher 1989). This model was broadened into the development of self-help groups for individuals who hear voices, organized by networks of volunteer consumers, carers, and mental health professionals. Hearing Voices Networks now exist in 20 countries including Australia and are considered an important resource for those experiencing distressing voices or visions. From the outset there was a clear alliance between the interests of consumers seeking to validate their experience of hearing voices and the emerging psychological models of psychosis (Kingdon and Turkington 2004; Bentall et al. 2007; Kuipers et al. 2006). Of particular significance in this process was a clinical encounter between Marius Romme and Patsy Haagen, a voice hearer. Patsy's experience of voice hearing showed little response to a variety of treatments and she refused to understand the voices as merely psychotic symptoms. Drawing on the work of psychologist Julian Jaynes (1976), who placed psychotic symptoms within the context of a broader bio-evolutionary model, Patsy 'normalized' her experience as adaptive for her. Romme was particularly interested in the positive psychological consequences that resulted from Patsy's understanding of her psychotic symptoms. In response to Patsy's case, Romme appeared on Dutch television and conducted an interview about her experience of hearing voices. Around 450 people identifying as voice hearers rang in after the programme and, contrary to the common sense assumption, approximately one third of callers had not utilized psychiatric services and a significant number viewed their experience of hearing voices as positive. This stimulated Romme and colleagues to initiate research into the factors that predict effective coping strategies when hearing voices (Romme et al. 1992).

In October 1987, Romme helped to organize a peer support network which became known as 'Foundation Resonance'. This group organized consumer-led workshops, provided lectures, and ran discussion groups for mental health workers. It aimed to break down the social taboo associated with the experience of hearing voices. The movement gained momentum when Paul Baker, a community development worker from Manchester, attended a conference in north-eastern Italy (a region that had implemented a radical approach to community care for mental health problems) and met with Romme who encouraged him to establish a Hearing Voices Group in the United Kingdom. Baker stated 'my goal is not to change psychiatry, not to change the patients, but to offer the hearers of voices an organization through which they can emancipate themselves' (Baker 1990). In 1988, the Hearing Voices Network was established in the UK. While the UK and continental Europe have well established consumer led networks, the formation of such groups in Australia is a recent phenomenon with the Hearing Voices Network of NSW being established in 2007.

The following section draws on the authors' experience of working with voice hearers in Australia using cognitive behavioural approaches. It became apparent to all of us that many of the consumers we had the opportunity to work with responded to CBT in a qualitatively different way to consumers we had worked with who had other problems such as anxiety, depression, or physical symptoms. CBT provided a framework that was seen by consumers as promoting consumer empowerment and the advancement of consumer rights.

CBT for psychosis from a human rights perspective

As in other settings, the background to our clinical work in Australia is that Mental Health Services have been consistently criticized on the basis of the neglect of human rights of those experiencing mental illness (Richmond 1983; Burdekin et al. 1993; Mental Health Council of Australia 2005; Senate Select Committee on Mental Health 2006). It is an unsettling context with problems of limited resources, stigma, and social and economic exclusion making it difficult to negotiate for clinician and consumer alike. This in turn may contribute to a general pessimism about the potential for consumer recovery (Hugo 2001). In this environment it is impossible to ignore issues of human rights, yet clinicians are not offered frameworks through which to resolve human rights dilemmas. Professional codes of conduct primarily focus on individual professional and consumer interactions and fail to address the broad social and institutional complexities leading to loss of effective citizenship and exclusion.

The experience of consumers, as outlined in various reports (Richmond 1983; Burdekin 1993; Mental Health Council of Australia 2005; Senate Select Committee on Mental Health 2006) and in the author's experience from working with those traversing the mental health systems is described as 'coercive', with limited opportunity to collaborate in determining the course of treatment. Consumers use prison terminology, referring to 'release' instead of discharge and the 'lock-up' rather than 'seclusion'.

The internalization of stigma by consumers is often inevitable in such contexts. They come to accept worker and society stereotypes, and view themselves as an 'outsider', as being out-of-control, as dangerous, and with limited prospects for a future (Ridgeway 2001). There is often a complete absence of recovery narratives within the workplace, of living successfully with symptoms, of valuing the struggles and victories in consumers' lives.

A number of factors intrinsic to CBT have placed it in a unique position as a promoter of human rights for consumers experiencing psychosis. The authors do not consider that CBT is the only psychological treatment that is able to promote human rights in those affected by psychosis. Rather, aspects of the approach that will be elaborated on make it impossible for the consumer and clinician working effectively together to avoid the discussion and promotion of human rights issues. Further, CBT is ubiquitous, with the vast majority of mental health workers having at least some knowledge of it if not considerable expertise in its delivery. Although the authors would consider that in the Australian context cognitive behavioural treatments for psychosis are not as easily accessible as they should be, they are far more influential and available than other potentially useful psychological approaches.

It will be argued that CBT for psychosis works to uphold many specific human rights principles including freedom of expression, the right to self-determination, and independence. Elements of treatment reinforce the inherent dignity of the consumer. Further, we argue for clinicians to expand interventions to include advocacy for the adherence to other rights such as adequate housing, the right to work and study, and the right to continuity of care. The clinician advocates limiting coercive or punitive treatments regardless of service limitations and for treatment to occur in the least restrictive environment possible.

Psychologists and other allied health professionals, who are primarily (although not exclusively) associated with the provision of CBT in this context, are perhaps in an advantageous position within the mental health system, having little influence on questions of involuntary detention or medical management. Pressure to admit and discharge is placed firmly in the hands of Psychiatric Consultants and Registrars who are left with little opportunity to explore psychosocial interventions in an under-resourced environment. Being removed from this aspect of care allows the psychologist to avoid role confusion associated with the need to make clinical decisions that may be against a consumer's stated wishes. This, in the author's experience, allows for greater collaboration.

CBT: a person focused intervention

The collaborative therapeutic alliance

Intrinsic to the CBT approach is collaborative empiricism. This requires the consumer and clinician, as far as possible, to meet as equals in order to consider the nature of a person's beliefs and experiences, to discuss their interpretation, and to design experiments to test those interpretations. Utilizing a non-judgemental empirical framework to understand the experience of symptoms creates an environment that validates the meaning of experiences and sends a message that they are being taken seriously. CBT approaches to psychosis encourage clinicians to maintain a lack of investment in any particular interpretation, letting the data inform conclusions (Nelson 2005). It was our experience that for many of the consumers the resulting working relationship with a health professional was an entirely new experience that broke through the dominant coercive model of care.

The therapist as witness

In order to engage with, collect evidence, and if appropriate challenge a delusion or the meaning of voices, the clinician has to attend to all of the interconnecting elements. Treatment protocols suggest that clinical assessment is considerably longer than the CBT based assessments for non-psychotic disorders (Chadwick et al. 1996). Through this process the clinician is doing the very opposite of 'silencing', the more traditional strategy for managing the discussion of psychotic experiences. For many consumers this was the first time that they had been able to fully describe their experiences and associated feelings. These encounters make it clear that the experience of psychosis is associated with a great deal of trauma and distress (Jackson et al. 2004). As clinicians it becomes clear that an important component of our role is to stand as witnesses to this experience and know the person's story.

There are clear parallels to the role that documentation plays in other contexts, particularly as a tool to support survivors of human instigated trauma recover from their experiences and tell their stories (Steel et al. 2009). Lira and Weinstein (who published at the time under the pseudonyms of Cienfuegos and Monelli 1983) developed testimony therapy amongst victims of the Pinochet regime in Chile. In this approach the clinician works with the survivor to create a life narration integrating the traumatic experiences into a self, social, and political narrative. The resulting testimonies not only served the purpose of telling a story but are used to advance the work of human rights organizations such as Amnesty International. Recently, Neuner et al. (2004) have combined testimony therapy with exposure therapy (a commonly used treatment within the cognitive behavioural tradition) amongst Sudanese refugees living in a Ugandan refugee settlement, demonstrating improved clinical outcomes over other models of care. Hence, CBT for psychosis and testimony therapy share a commitment to witnessing and documenting rather than silencing and denying.

Amongst consumers with psychosis the importance of understanding psychosis within a person's life story emerged as a major area of clinical gain. Clinicians also provide a role in witnessing the experience of distress associated with the mandated infringement of their rights. In their formulations, clinicians encounter both the horror of the experience of psychotic symptoms as well as the distress and feelings of injustice associated with an involuntary psychiatric admission.

Shared formulation

An important and often challenging component of CBT treatments for all psychological presentations is the development of a shared psychological formulation. With respect to psychotic disorders, after a relatively long process of assessment (Chadwick et al. 1996), a psychological formulation that hypothesises factors maintaining distress and impaired functioning is developed (An example of a problem formulation has been published previously by the authors Shearsby et al. 2007). It is reasoned that, if a consumer is to engage in the process of therapy earnestly, the clinician and consumer need to agree on the problem areas and the consumer must understand the process by which change is expected to occur. This component of CBT offers dignity to the person by valuing their perspective, acknowledging experiences of distress while offering hope of the alleviation of that distress.

Consumers as participatory agents

CBT is an active approach. It works against the passivity that is common in mental health settings. Within many Australian acute hospital inpatient settings, consumers are largely required to wait passively for their medication to take effect. They are not routinely encouraged to engage in other therapeutic activities and even when ward programmes are in place they are optional and not always prioritized by staff. In contrast, CBT requires clinician and consumer to collaboratively formulate the nature of a problem, discuss the evidence for beliefs about voices, engage in behavioural experiments, and practice non-pharmacological methods for managing mood or anxiety symptoms. All these components require active engagement by both the consumer and the therapist.

Psychological models of the negative symptoms of psychosis have emphasized the role of low expectancy beliefs. These low expectancies are often reinforced by mental health services (Rector et al. 2005) which, in combination with the illness symptoms, lead to the increasing exclusion of the consumer from participatory engagement. CBT treatments for psychosis encourage consumers to determine their own limitations through experimentation. Through goal setting and the implementation of behavioural experiments, consumers are encouraged to learn their real limits, such as the intensity with which they are able to study, the type and hours of employment, or the amount of time they are able to socialize before feeling overwhelmed. The capacity of CBT approaches in this regard is illustrated by the substantial evidence base that CBT interventions can reduce functional disability across a wide range of chronic somatic disorders (Sumathipala 2007). In this respect CBT appears to assist the individual consumer in the progressive realization of a range of second generation rights that they are effectively excluded from due to the debilitating nature of their illness and the associated paternalism of contemporary mental health care models.

The boundaries of disability are discovered through challenging and confronting disability. While there is substantial evidence that psychotic illness can lead to significant impairment, the CBT model begins with no assumptions in this regard. It stands in opposition to any approach that encourages pessimism about the likelihood of recovery. Goal setting, treatment planning, and exposure treatments all help a consumer to identify their strengths and limitations. Once disability has been more clearly delineated through this process, active strategies for adaptation are applied.

CBT and the biopsycho-social context

As noted previously there has been a strong confluence between consumer advocacy groups such as the Hearing Voices Network and leading researchers in developing cognitive behavioural formulations of psychosis. Despite this, there has been little discussion in the literature of the role of CBT in addressing issues of social justice for consumers with psychosis. As a manualized treatment approach, CBT runs the risk of being viewed solely as a therapeutic technology that can be delivered irrespective of the clinical context. There is a tendency in standard treatment manuals to downplay the broader context of care. Little discussion is given, for example, to the suffocating effect of stigma, and the barriers to employment, accommodation, and relationships in current manualized CBT programmes (Corrigan 1998). The focus tends to be on individual symptom management without recognition of the impact of the illness and the associated removal of autonomy and human rights within a mental health facility or in interaction with mental health services in the community (Bracken and Thomas 2001). Clinicians are often asked to provide CBT when other interventions have failed and CBT is often conceptualized as another treatment approach which can be 'rolled out' (Birchwood and Trower 2006). This is in contrast to the avowed commitment of this approach to a full biopsycho-social formulation requiring CBT practitioners to consider all levels of disease from the molecular to the social, including the human rights context (Engel 1977).

Practitioners are encouraged in treatment manuals to ensure that CBT formulations and interventions are personalized, attending to the rich interaction between an individual's set of symptoms, their context, and their history. Although rarely specified, this includes the broader social and institutional context of their illness experience.

The CBT practitioner as human rights advocate

The failure to recognize the role that CBT has in the broader human rights for people with psychosis is an important oversight in the existing literature. It is our experience that CBT is enhanced when promoting human rights outcomes. It may be that CBT approaches can be of most value when they directly address the very real difficulties associated with negotiating the mental health system as well as an individual's distressing symptoms. Therefore it is critical to provide the space for consumers to have their experiences recognized. With this view in mind, the clinician's role expands out from individual face-to-face work to include issues of social justice. This may take multiple forms, from supporting consumer led 'community meetings' for the discussion of problems in the ward environment and the running of groups for the education on consumer rights in mental health, tempering the expansion of 'risk assessment', or confronting the use of derogatory and stigmatizing language.

The following section presents a case study of CBT for psychosis from a human rights framework. The following description has been written and presented with the full permission of

Steve who declined to be a co-author but agreed to review it. Steve's story has been modified to avoid identification.

Case illustration

Steve is a 42-year -old man who lives in government subsidized housing in an inner city suburb of Sydney. He had received a diagnosis of schizophrenia after being misdiagnosed with depression and was taking an atypical antipsychotic medication.

He was born in an industrial town several hours west of Sydney. He described himself as the 'runt of the litter', stating that he was 'awkward' as a child, and performed poorly at school and at sport. This theme, 'the runt of the litter' was hypothesized to shape the nature of his psychotic symptoms.

In early high school he started smoking marijuana and this became an important part of his life. He left high school early and started working in a factory. He described this workplace as 'hard' and 'intimidating'. This is where he first experienced psychotic symptoms. He described a sense that his workmates were 'getting inside my head'.

In reaction to this perceived threat, Steve joined a local martial arts academy. He noticed soon after this that his martial arts trainer had started to communicate to him 'as a voice'. Although initially encouraging, the voice soon became threatening. It generalized to others in the community such that when he was in public he was convinced that passersby were communicating with him telepathically. He reasoned that he lacked the ability to get inside others heads due to his 'runt' status. He believed he was ostracized because he wasn't conforming to the status quo, that is, people getting inside each other's mind for personal gain. He reported being 'against the cut and thrust of social climbing'.

He had several previous admissions in busy inner city psychiatric units. He described a sense of humiliation around his most recent admission after being detained by police when leaving a fast food outlet on a suburban street. He had to be physically restrained as he was reluctant to go to hospital as previous admissions had been experienced as traumatic. He had his clothes torn in the process of being restrained. He was tormented by psychotic symptoms, was intimidated by the distress displayed by other consumers, and felt unsupported by staff. He was given a hospital gown to wear and was unable to have clothes or other possessions brought in for several days. He said that this just confirmed his fears.

The therapist engaged Steve during the early part of a month-long admission. It was agreed that, when discharged, his outpatient appointments would be conducted in his home as he had developed a traumatic association with the hospital.

Witnessing the experience

An important component early in the intervention was the witnessing of Steve's experience of psychosis. He described horrific details and appreciated that it was being documented. Steve experienced voices as uniformly derogatory and malevolent. He heard that he would be caught and tortured and this included being burned, having his lips cut with razor blades, and impaled.

During the early period of treatment Steve considered that his treating psychologist was 'in on it' but was a 'nice guy' who felt sorry for him. Regardless, he believed it important to establish a 'paper trail' in the event he was harmed. Later in the intervention, as he developed a different understanding of what was happening to him, the necessity of documentation became less relevant.

With the establishment of a solid trusting relationship the details of Steve's beliefs, his experience of voices, and how these influence one another was explored in great detail. He remarked that he had never been asked about these details before and that in fact he had been encouraged by family and mental health workers alike not to discuss them. He said that previously those working with him had acted to remove his freedom to express his concerns. He reflected on the equality of the relationship, and the fact that the psychologist prioritized his goals and seriously considered his beliefs. Gradually a shared formulation was established and links to formative early life experiences were made. Steve described details of his early life that led him to believe he was intrinsically weaker than others, that he was a 'runt'. This belief remained in adulthood and maintained his distress.

Steve's experience of being detained and subsequently having medical treatment mandated with a Community Treatment Order was a further aspect of his experience that required recognition. He said that there was no discussion of his choices of treatment and that he was not provided with information on the treatments provided. His experience of feeling powerless, humiliated, and treated with hostility became a focus for intervention. They formed part of the psychological formulation and were referred to as violations of his dignity, his self-determination, freedom to make choices, and decisions regarding treatment.

Collaboration

Steve was introduced to the concepts of cognitive therapy and commenced monitoring his thoughts when distressed and was encouraged to develop a series of alternative explanations to thoughts associated with distress. Importantly, beliefs about the difficulties associated with traversing the mental health system were accepted and validated.

Consistent with recommendations for use of CBT with psychotic symptoms (Nelson 2005) the therapist was not invested in confirming or disconfirming particular beliefs. Rather, it was emphasized that the aim was to assist Steve to be rigorous in collecting evidence that would allow for the most likely conclusions to emerge. The approach was collaborative, with Steve determining the topics for discussion during each session.

Steve designed and implemented a number of experiments to test the idea that others could hear his thoughts. One experiment involved Steve walking into a quiet home-wares store in his local area, standing close to the shop assistant so that he could observe their facial expression, and 'shouting' expletives his head. He observed the shop assistant for any signs of reaction. Evidence for and against his beliefs was tested and documented and gradually Steve's understanding of his experience changed. Over the course of treatment he considered a variety of developmental, neuro-psychological, and biological explanations for his symptoms. For example, he describes a neuro-psychological 'self-monitoring deficit hypothesis' that explains voices and a schema based developmental explanation that incorporates his belief that he was a 'runt of the litter' accounting for his belief in his persecution.

Steve was active in the process of developing dynamic psychological formulations, performed his own research into newer developments within CBT for psychosis (such as Meta Cognitive Therapy—see Moritz and Woodward 2007), and encouraged the therapist to assist in their implementation.

Normalization and stigma

A key component of treatment involved education about the dimensional nature of psychotic phenomena and the development of a normalizing rationale (Kingdon and Turkington 2004). This approach built on the work of Marius Romme, emphasizing that each of us has the potential to develop psychotic symptoms if put into certain, often stressful, situations. Further, it identifies key creative, scientific, and philosophical figures who were thought to suffer from psychosis. This approach does not romanticize psychosis and in no way down-plays the suffering and distress associated with the experience. Rather, it attempts to address the stigma associated with psychosis. By demonstrating that these are extensions of thinking and behaviour that occur in the general population, it reduces the distinction between the 'mentally ill' and the 'well' that is reinforced by the media and also often by mental health services.

Steve had internalized the stigma that exists within Australia regarding the disability of those experiencing psychosis. Despite there being no history of aggression or hostility in Steve's behavior, he had initially believed in an inherent violent potential and unpredictability associated with psychosis. He had a view that, as a 'schizophrenic', he should maintain low expectations of what he would be able to achieve in his life. He let go of any ambition to work or study.

The implementation of the normalization rationale reduced the distinction Steve felt between himself and the rest of society. It offered a strategy for living a life less constrained by stigma. It encouraged him to challenge some of his expectations by conducting behavioural experiments and engaging with consumer advocates who encouraged him to test out his personal limits. Examples included taking a course in horticulture at a local college and working on a voluntary basis in a nursery.

The value Steve derived from the normalizing rationale encouraged him to become involved in the newly-formed Self Help Group for voice hearers in his local area. This group, affiliated internationally with the organization originally established by Marius Romme, Foundation Resonance, offered a unique contribution to Steve's recovery. He said that the group offered support and encouragement. His self-esteem improved as he assisted and encouraged others and he became inspired by others who had successfully rejected the limitations that can be associated with a diagnosis of schizophrenia.

He became less socially isolated despite the fact that he was still bombarded by voices and the sensation that people were invading his mental life when in public.

The steady achievement of goals, renewed social engagement, and meaningful activity afforded an improvement of Steve's sense of self-efficacy. He challenged himself physically, interpersonally, and intellectually (reading complex neuro-psychological literature in order to formulate explanations for his experiences). His self-esteem improved dramatically and this allowed him to encourage others.

Self-determination

Goal setting identified that Steve wanted to eventually study at a tertiary level, that he wanted to establish a high degree of fitness, and he would one day like to work in the field of landscaping. He is working toward these goals and has completed a TAFE course and established a physical training regimen. These initiatives provided further information on his true limits.

Treatment became less frequent over time with Steve and the therapist meeting mostly once a month. There are occasions where Steve organizes a period of more regular appointments to manage a set-back or to address some stressful situation. Almost exclusively, he sets the agenda and keeps up to date with his goals.

Advocacy

Issues of advocacy arise regularly when working with those who access mental health services. We consider that it is highly problematic to ignore or avoid their discussion. Firstly, clinicians have an obligation to protect and uphold standards of human rights in the areas in which they work, regardless of perceived lack of resources or other constraints. Further, to be taken seriously by consumers, clinicians must be able to attend to those things that matter to consumers most and be able to assist in their resolution. Most importantly, being aware of and advocating for consumers' human rights offers a clear framework for intervention in an environment whose intrinsic complexity can lead to therapeutic nihilism.

Advocacy was a vital part of the intervention for Steve. He was provided with information about his rights with respect to his interaction with health services. This included information on the Mental Health Act, the role of Official Visitors in inpatient facilities, and information about support services such as the Mental Health Advocacy Service. He read the various reports on the status of human rights in Australian mental health services.

The CBT oriented approach was extended to include open discussion of human rights and the development of strategies to advocate for these. Steve expressed considerable anger about his experiences with mental health services. Initially this was difficult to overcome as, in reality, the treating psychologist was a part of this system. Steve and the therapist carefully reviewed and documented the injustices that he experienced and, through instruction in the use of structured problem solving, developed strategies to deal with these events if they were repeated. Steve was encouraged to assert himself during discussion with his treating team about possible pharmacological treatments. He was able to find a team with whom he felt able to collaborate and where he felt his preferences and concerns were heard.

On several occasions, when there was a change in his case-worker or psychiatrist, Steve was offered a psychiatric admission in order to alter his medication in a controlled environment or as a threat to motivate him to abstain completely from marijuana. He was terrified by this possibility and expressed this clearly. His psychiatrist advocated strongly and often effectively against any unreasonable restriction in his care.

Concluding comments

There remains considerable concern about the human rights inadequacies of contemporary models of service delivery for people experiencing psychotic disorders across most Western countries. A cursory review of the international literature (Hazelton 2005) suggests a discernable trend towards a proportionate reduction in investment in community models of care with a commensurate increase in investment in acute inpatient care. The emergence of an associated narrative of risk mitigation and management appears to have, at least in part, reinforced stereotypes of people with psychosis as being the dangerous 'other', displacing alternative clinical narratives of treatment or rehabilitation. The lived experience of mental health consumers with psychosis, as recorded in numerous reports and testimonials, is one of disempowerment and loss of self-directed autonomy (Richmond 1983; Burdekin et al. 1993; Mental Health Council of Australia 2005; Senate Select Committee on Mental Health 2006).

The factors contributing to such outcomes represent a complex mix of disability associated with psychosis, under-resourced services, and coercive management practices; stigma; and social disenfranchisement. Both consumer and clinician can be rendered powerless in the face of such formidable structural barriers to the full realization of their human rights. In implementing CBT treatments for psychosis we have discovered how a model of collaborative formulation and treatment helps to redress key areas where consumers experienced restriction in autonomy and been rendered passive recipients of care. At the same time, the CBT interventions can be made considerably more important and meaningful to consumers by expressly incorporating human rights based analysis and understanding.

References

Baker, P (1990) 'I Hear Voices and I'm Glad To!', *Critical Public Health*, 4, 21–27.

Barlow, DH and Durand, VM (1995) *Abnormal Psychology: An Integrative Approach.* Pacific Grove: Brooks Cole Publishing Company.

Beck, AT (1967) *Depression: clinical, experimental, and theoretical aspects.* New York: Harper & Row.

Bellack, AS (1986) 'Schizophrenia: Behavior therapy's forgotten child', *Behavior Therapy*, 17, 199–214.

Bentall, RP, Fernyhough, C, Morrison, AP, Lewis, S, and Corcoran, R. (2007) 'Prospects for a cognitive-developmental account of psychotic experiences', *British Journal of Clinical Psychology*, 46, 155–73.

Birchwood, M and Trower, P (2006) 'The future of cognitive behavioural therapy for psychosis: not a quasi neuroleptic', *The British Journal of Psychiatry*, 188, 107–108.

Bracken, P and Thomas, P (2001) 'Postpsychiatry: a new direction for mental health', *British Journal of Psychiatry*, 322, 724–27.

Burdekin, B, Guilfoyle, M, and Hall, D (1993) *Human Rights and Mental Illness.* Report of the National Inquiry into the Human Rights of People with Mental Illness. Canberra: Australian Government Publishing Service.

Chadwick, PD, Birchwood, MJ, and Trower, P (1996) *Cognitive Therapy for Delusions, Voices and Paranoia.* Oxford, UK: John Wiley & Sons.

Cienfuegos, AJ and Monelli, C (1983) 'The testimony of political repression as a therapeutic instrument', *American Journal of Orthopsychiatry*, 53, 43–51.

Cohen, M (1998) 'Users'movement and the challenge to psychiatrists', *Psychiatric Bulletin*, 22, 155–57.

Corrigan, PW (1998) 'The impact of stigma on severe mental illness', *Cognitive and Behavioural Practice*, 5, 201–22.

Engel, GL (1977) 'The need for a new medical model: A challenge for biomedicine', *Science*, 196, 129–36.

Gould, RA, Mueser, KT, Bolton, E, Mays, V, and Goff, D (2001) 'Cognitive therapy for psychosis in schizophrenia: an effect size analysis', *Schizophrenia Research*, 48, 335–42.

Hazelton, M (2005) 'Mental health reform, citizenship and human rights in four countries', *Health Sociology Review*, 14, 230–41.

Hugo, M (2001) 'Mental Health Professionals' Attitudes Towards People who have experienced a Mental Health Disorder', *Journal of Psychiatric and Mental Health Nursing*, 8, 419–25.

Jaynes, J (1976) *The Origin of Consciousness in the Breakdown of the Bicameral Mind.* Boston: Houghton Mifflin.

Jackson, C, Knott, C, Skeate, A, and Birchwood, M (2004) 'The trauma of first episode psychosis: the role of cognitive mediation', *Australian and New Zealand Journal of Psychiatry*, 38, 327–33.

Kingdon, DG and Turkington, D (2004) *Cognitive Therapy of Schizophrenia.* New York: Guilford Press.

Kuipers, E, Garety, P, Fowler, D, Freeman, D, Dunn, G, and Bebbington, P (2006) 'Cognitive, Emotional, and Social Processes in Psychosis: Refining Cognitive Behavioural Therapy for Persistent Positive Symptoms', *Schizophrenia Bulletin*, 32, S24–31.

Mental Health Council of Australia (2005) *Not for Service: Experiences of injustice and despair in mental health care in Australia.* Deakin, ACT: Mental Health Council of Australia.

Moritz, S and Woodward, TS (2007) 'Metacognitive training in schizophrenia: from basic research to knowledge translation and intervention', *Current Opinion in Psychiatry*, 20, 619–25.

National Institute for Health and Clinical Excellence (2002) *Schizophrenia: core interventions in the treatment and management of schizophrenia in primary and secondary care.* London: NICE Clinical Guideline 1.

Nelson, H (2005) *Cognitive Behavioural Therapy with Delusions and Hallucinations.* Cheltenham, UK: Nelson Thornes.

Neuner, F, Schauer, M, Klaschik, C, Karunakara, U, and Elbert, T (2004) 'A comparison of narrative exposure therapy, supportive counseling, and psycho-education for treating posttraumatic stress disorder in an African refugee settlement', *Journal of Consulting & Clinical Psychology,* 72, 579–87.

Rector, NA and Beck, AT (2001) 'Cognitive behavioral therapy for schizophrenia: an empirical review', *Journal of Nervous and Mental Disease,* 189, 278–87.

Rector, NA, Beck, AT, and Stolar, N (2005) 'The Negative Symptoms of Schizophrenia: A Cognitive Perspective', *The Canadian Journal of Psychiatry,* 50, 247–57.

Richmond, D (1983) *Inquiry into health services for the psychiatrically ill and developmentally disabled.* Sydney: NSW Department of Health.

Ridgeway, P (2001) 'Re-storying Psychiatric Disability: Learning from First Person Recovery Narratives', *Psychiatric Rehabilitation Journal,* 24, 335–43.

Romme, MAJ and Escher, AD (1989) 'Hearing voices', *Schizophrenia Bulletin,* 15, 209–216.

Romme, MA, Honig, A, Noorthoorn, EO, and Escher, AD (1992) 'Coping with hearing voices: An emancipatory approach', *British Journal of Psychiatry,* 161, 99–103.

Senate Select Committee on Mental Health (2006) A national approach to mental health- from crisis to community. Commonwealth of Australia: Senate Select Committee on Mental Health.

Shearsby, J, Walker, P, and Steel, Z (2007) 'From passive acceptance to active engagement: The path of CBT for psychosis', in DA Einstein (ed) *Innovations and Advances in Cognitive Behaviour Therapy.* Bowen Hills, QLD, Australia: Australian Academic Press, 123–41.

Shera, W, Aviram, U, Healey, B, and Ramon, S (2002) 'The Mental Health System Reform: A Multi Country Comparison', *Social Work and Mental Health,* 35, 547–75.

Steel, Z, Bateman-Steel, CR, and Silove, D (2009) 'Human rights and the trauma model: Genuine partners or uneasy allies?', *Journal of Traumatic Stress Studies,* 22(5), 358–65.

Sumathipala, A (2007) 'What is the evidence for the efficacy of treatments for somatoform disorders? A critical review of previous intervention studies', *Psychosomatic Medicine,* 69(9), 889–900.

Tarrier, N and Wykes, T (2004) 'Is there evidence that cognitive behaviour therapy is an effective treatment of schizophrenia? A cautious or cautionary tale?', *Behaviour Research and Therapy,* 42, 1377–1401.

Chapter 38

Promoting a Just Society and Preventing Human Rights Violations

A Post-Nuremberg Inheritance for the Helping Professions

Fran Gale and Michael Dudley

The post-Nazi reckoning saw justice linked with the development of human rights standards. The lessons from this time and the inheritance of international human rights have had far-reaching implications for the helping professions and for civil society.

This chapter focuses on responses that helping professionals are making or may make, as they reconfigure their practice in response to these developments. It follows these responses through a series of themes.

After considering the relationship of science and technology to instrumental rationality and utility, particular attention is given to the burgeoning area of post-conflict interventions, including justice, forgiveness, and reconciliation processes. We examine professionals' role in programmes that promote a just society and prevent genocide, such as Holocaust education, anti-racism and discrimination programmes, and the cultivation of communities that care. The chapter begins and finishes with reflections on codes of ethics in medicine, psychiatry, and helping professions, and how professionals might deploy their skills and authority, adopt forms of practice that respect service users' rights, and realize social justice.

Helping professionals and social justice: opportunities, challenges, and pitfalls

How may the duties and aspirations of the helping (and specifically, mental health and psychiatric) professions to defend and promote human rights, be best understood? What powers and resources must be harnessed, and what barriers must be overcome?

Professions may be defined as possessing specialized skills and knowledge that they apply for the collective good (ABIM Foundation, ACP-ASIM Foundation, and EFIM 2002; Pellegrino and Relman 1999; Robertson 2007; Coady 2009). They mirror cultural and communal norms, which for health professionals may influence diagnosis and treatment through laws, ethical codes, and cultural practices. However norms may be problematic: the language of consensus, 'partnerships', and 'community capacity' in many contemporary government documents addressing health and social problems, may conceal unequal power arrangements and does not guarantee ethical solutions (Dudley and Gale 2002).

Justice comes down to being treated according to what is fair, due, or owed (Beauchamp 2009); while 'distributive justice' refers to the fair, equitable apportioning of social goods and burdens according to justified norms of distribution (Robertson 2007; Kymlicka 2002). Acting justly is one of the four planks of medical and psychiatric ethics, along with respect for patient autonomy and dignity, not harming, and acting beneficently (Beauchamp 2009). Social-justice criteria underpin international conventions, charters, and codes, from the Universal Declaration of Human Rights (UDHR) to the recent Convention on the Rights of Persons with Disabilities (CRPD). The advent of mental health epidemiology and universal, evidence-based preventive strategies, together with consumer movements, media attention, state regulation, and the internet, highlight questions of social justice within mental health.

Professions as communities of practice are not immune to the seductions of power and wealth. Some see the latter, in an era where self-interest is often regarded as primary, as dominant motivations expressed through elitism, restrictive knowledge, price-fixing, and other collusive practices disempowering users (Coady 2009). Professional bodies and institutions may also generate roles and obligations that can lead to unethical acts (Luban 1988), especially in certain cultural contexts. The situation of psychiatry under Nazism (Dudley and Gale 2002 and Chapter 11, this volume) and in the Soviet Union and China (van Voren, this volume) exemplify the outcomes when professionals' opportunism goes unchecked. Health programmes, whether corporate or state-sponsored, may marginalize and exclude disadvantaged groups, as the Nazi ones did. Arguably many US Managed Care programmes do much the same thing (Sabin and Daniels 2009). Managerialism, fiscal rationing, and other *forces majeures* can also thwart professional and ethical standards.

Through their knowledge and intimate involvement in their patients' lives and deaths, doctors bear a unique responsibility and influence. This is especially so in the case of psychiatrists in whom sweeping powers are vested when illness undermines their patients' autonomy.

Psychiatrists are trained to diagnose and treat mental illness. Their classifications do not include racism and genocide, nor do they generally tackle the social problems that affect people's well-being. Yet, as noted, questions about normality arise when epidemiological surveys find so many people suffer from diagnosable mental illnesses, for instance, in the US (Kessler et al. 2005) and Australia (Slade et al. 2009). Health demands more than absence of disease, as UN conventions attest, and mental health is inseparable from well-being and the satisfaction of basic needs such as love, justice, and meaning (Fromm 1965). The 'right' to health care implies that access to health care belongs with other civil rights, such that health care itself constitutes one of the essential social goods (Daniels 1995). As the mental health of individuals and populations meshes inextricably with socio-economic and cultural factors, so the right to health and health care are to be understood broadly: they encompass individual medical services, preventative interventions, public health initiatives, employment, workplace safety, and social resources (such as housing and welfare) for chronically ill and disabled people. For those with severe and persistent mental illness, they also entail reducing stigma, and changing policies that cause social stress (Prilleltensky et al. 2008).

Responses by the helping professions to these challenges, related to self-regulation and equity, are further elaborated in this chapter.

Science, value, human limits, and eugenics revisited

The Nazi psychiatrists illustrate the temptation to side with the forces of instrumental rationality, treating the environment and people as objects whose utility is to be exploited, rather than as human subjects or moral agents imbued with inviolable dignity and rights (Higgins and Ramia 2000). Those who contrast Nazi psychiatry with contemporary ethical debates about science and medicine should not be beguiled by the latter's innocence of explicit racial hygiene theories (Caplan 2007:71). Instrumental rationality can still raise its ugly head, for instance, in the 'new eugenics', which raises serious concerns about treating humans as means to policy ends rather than as ends in themselves.

Despite sometimes adverse effects, Western culture has compelling reasons for highly prizing science and technology. Equating scientific and technological progress with human progress, however, translates into valiant commitments to prolong life through 'conquering' human diseases, with the hope of new 'wonder' drugs, vaccines, stem cell research, and gene therapies. Excessive fervour, underestimation of risk, and harms have sometimes accompanied these advances. Though some have celebrated a human capacity to re-design the world and transform themselves into something 'other', belief in the progressive advancement of medical science needs to be tempered with recognizing the limitations of human life and of medical interventions, including unintended harms that may arise from unreflective initiatives (Fox 2007:157). For example, the stem cell research debate has been shaped by ethical concerns about human embryo 'farming', but has been somewhat re-configured since it became possible to use non-embryonic stem cells with clear therapeutic advantages. However, fears of losing out in international competition may goad countries to undertake such research, even if they cannot afford the innovations in question (La Fleur 2007; Komatsu 2007; Shimazono 2007:212–5).

Similarly, 'cultural and spiritual concerns, so basic to formulations of personhood and social reality to persons across the globe, fall outside the strict confines of (a European) international psychiatry' (Fabrega 2000), which often has a biomedical focus. Unacknowledged values surrounding medical science require clarification. The methods of natural science do not consider power relations between people and groups, nor value an historical perspective: science lives in the present (Müller-Hill 2007). From a 'natural-science' viewpoint, bringing human rights commitments into research practice compromises 'objectivity'. This assumes that objectivity exists, that facts can be quarantined from values. Affirming a linear narrative of progress may foster violence, for example, against 'backward' indigenous peoples (Rose 2004). Research funding oftentimes depends on political influence, and funding bodies do not welcome challenges to conventional Western social norms and conceits (Rees and Silove, this volume).

The eugenic implications of new technologies raise particular concerns. For example, pre-implantation genetic diagnosis (PGD) of human embryos, which can detect inherited diseases like Huntingdon's disease, Duchenne muscular dystrophy, and cystic fibrosis, was recently extended to managing mutations that confer increased breast cancer risk. This initiative is controversial, since other factors may affect the risk (Pray 2008). The further possibility of improving inherited traits to make 'designer babies' raises many ethical issues. For example, safety concerns include the multiple effects of genes, other factors determining whether embryos with altered genes develop desired traits, and unintended negative effects of genetic manipulations. Insufficient regulatory control and commercial marketing may spark a techno-eugenic race among prospective parents. Children cannot consent to their parents' manipulating their genes. Also, access to such technology is inequitable, which violates principles of distributive justice (Simmons 2008).

Where can we draw the line between clinical genetics on the one hand, and eugenics on the other? Various nations have enforced sterilizations and abortions for those with presumed genetic disorders, and the Nazis extended this principle to the systematic killing or 'euthanasia' of 'lives unworthy of life' (*lebensunwertes Leben*). Despite this history, arguments are sometimes advanced against knowingly giving birth to a child with a genetic disease or physical or cognitive disability. Insurance companies—and sometimes new technology proponents—may suggest that pre-natal genetic screening should be standard practice, and if a serious condition is diagnosed, abortion is the right choice. What message does that give to children who are born with genetic conditions, and to those who should meet their needs? For whom are physical or mental disabilities painful, the people who have them, or those who take care of them? (Annas and Grodin 2007; Shimazono

2007:202–203; Ogino 2007). The World Health Organization (WHO) stated such practices cannot be called 'new eugenics' because there is no coercion to have tests, and a woman's right to choose to continue a pregnancy is guaranteed (Wertz et al. 1993). However, feminist activists with a disability assert that selective abortion after PGD or pre-natal screening should not be considered a 'woman's reproductive right', rather that it is a woman's right not to select her children. The social model of disability, which informs the CRPD, places the obligation for inclusion squarely back on society. Disability is part of the human experience (Belfer and Samarasan, this volume). Information and support around the bearing and rearing of a child with a disability should be provided (Ogino 2007).

Similarly, the principle of self-determination manifested in the 'right to die', for example, obscures the fact that death is not a matter for the individual alone, any more than it is solely a matter for the state. Death generally occurs in the context of (and is influenced by) networks of relationships, and its effects reverberate throughout a family and community (Komatsu 2007:194–196).

Thus, better public education and awareness would extend to the history of medicine, and the risks entailed in research, including uncritical trust in potential therapeutic benefits (Schmidt 2006:17). In its zeal for tackling disability, medicine needs to better understand disability's social foundations. How this may be accomplished is addressed in the final sections of this chapter.

Helping professionals and recovery after mass human rights violations: an overview of justice, forgiveness, and reconciliation

When genocide or other large-scale human rights violations occur, professionals may become involved in various roles: as perpetrators, bystanders, victims, survivors, rescuers, or facilitators of recovery. The contested histories of professions—as well as of nations, communities, and families—reflect the struggle for collective memory and understanding in the face of collective denial and amnesia (Dudley and Gale 2002). Forgetting and repressing a past incur costs for everyone involved (Schlink 2009:52). Truth-telling is vital for combating denial. Societal and cultural remembrance discourages repeated transgression and bolsters civil society, while strengthening individual and collective identity. However, remembrance can be harrowing, as victims who testify at truth commissions face those who have harmed them, and as nations re-examine inglorious moments in their histories. Individual and collective memories will differ, and victims disrupt the amnesia and denialist narratives of perpetrators in particular. Remembrance evokes questions and strong emotions, including between affected descendants. Commemorations run the risk of provoking resistance, expressed as ennui, or denial and historical revisionism.

In Germany, the historical disgrace of the Holocaust has unleashed a 'cultural civil war' to determine the meaning of German history, identity, citizenship, and belonging. Compelled to exonerate or disassociate families from Nazi contamination, or to escape it by inventing new identities, generations of Germans have wrangled over collective guilt, 'inherited sin', and national pride. For some, German nationalism cannot be trusted, and national belonging can only be expressed through civic patriotism, consumerism, and economic progress. The traumatized national self has affected the 'emotional economy' and well-being of many, resulting in efforts to either defend or renovate the culture (Moses 2007; Schlink 2009; Miller-Idriss 2009). Australia has seen similar over its foundational colonial violence—invasion, dispossession, mass slaughter of the original inhabitants, and 'the stolen generations' (Manne 2003) (see further below).

Moreover, recovery from individual and collective trauma may require a great deal of time, even extending over generations. It may be postponed, blocked, aborted, or indefinitely suspended. Resolution means not being chained to, or fixated on, a traumatic past—being able to both forget and remember (Schlink 2009). Traumatic affects and themes include powerlessness, fear of annihilation, loss, torture, psychological isolation, and stigma. Survivors react to normative life stresses and post-Holocaust trauma with more extreme responses, and can experience negative affect and adaptive functioning years later, although instrumental adaptation may disguise this pattern (Greene and Graham 2009; Kahana et al. 2007; Sadavoy 1997). These survivors often exemplify ambivalence in emotional expression. For victims suffering post-traumatic stress disorder (PTSD), apparently neutral events (dealing with a policeman, crossing a border) may awaken incapacitating memories of repression, insecurities, or homelessness (Staub 2003:462).

Understandably, victims resent the impunity extended to perpetrators and demand justice, which may be retributive (punishing perpetrators) or restorative (benefiting victims). Justice encompasses accountability through apology, public acknowledgement of wrongdoing, truth-telling through dialogue, listening, and story-telling, reparations, and/or improved national economic well-being (Staub 2003:441–442). The requirements of retribution on the one hand, and restoration (entailing forgiveness and reconciliation) on the other, diverge, and both approaches pose challenges.

In cases of wholesale transgression, the punishment of principal offenders becomes paramount. One objective may be to ensure that rights violators never again hold public office (Smith 2010). However, spontaneous summary justice may overtake both the innocent and the guilty, when formal judicial processes cannot deal with all those implicated. De-nazification identified higher and lower level decision-makers, direct perpetrators, and facilitators, and limited punishment to those directly responsible (Schlink 2009). Children of perpetrators and bystanders, and even ensuing generations, may be caught in the web of guilt, collective amnesia, and sometimes communal hostility to those who recall the horrors (Staub 2003:432–450; Schlink 2009).

Forgiveness and reconciliation

Forgiveness undergirds many religions, and has recently been extensively examined in philosophy, mental health, social science, and neurobiology. Griswold (2007) offers an extended treatment, which we touch on here. Forgiveness may encompass economic forgiveness (of debts), political pardon, judicial pardon, metaphysical forgiveness, and significantly, political apology (considered below). Scenarios may include forgiving wrongs done to others, to the dead, forgiving the unrepentant, oneself, God, or being forgiven by God. But paradigmatically, forgiveness is a moral relation between two individuals, one of whom has wronged the other; the individuals concerned ideally can communicate with each other; and forgiveness entails reciprocal duties. The wrongdoer must acknowledge responsibility, repudiate the deeds, express regret to the injured party, commit to personal amendment, acknowledge the damage done (from the injured person's perspective), and offer an intelligible narrative of the wrongdoing. If the wrongdoer fulfils these conditions, the injured party, while not condoning or excusing the wrongdoer's deeds, relinquishes revenge and commits to moderating resentment, re-envisions the wrongdoer, and communicates to the wrongdoer that he is forgiven.

Reconciliation takes place in civic contexts, especially in recent truth commissions. The process acknowledges past suffering in order to achieve sustainable peace, national integration, and an ongoing interdependent future (Hamber 2007; Brouneus 2008). Reconciliation seeks to transform broken relationships, institutional structures, and social practices. It unites mourning and restoration, justice and mercy, vision and pragmatism. The closely related question of political apology invokes complex questions, such as contested public histories, reparations, and who has a mandate to speak for whom. Like forgiveness, political apology is costly, voluntary, entails vulnerability, and involves bargaining, compromise, and deal-making (Long and Brecke 2003). The parties need not be those originally concerned, or even individuals except as members of a social or political body (Griswold 2007:135–146). As public performance, symbolism, and memory, it signifies a renewed willingness to cooperate and collaborate (Griswold 2007:179).

The relationship between forgiveness and reconciliation is complex. As we have indicated they have been understood as operating at different levels, though civic forgiveness as conceived in South Africa elevated it to a virtue for political as well as individual life. Some commentators hold that reconciliation, though often involving forgiveness, need not do so: its motivation may be primarily instrumental (e.g. financial, familial, restoring working relationships), akin to negotiation (Glas 2006). Others (for instance Enright 2001) argue that true reconciliation entails changing the victim's inner feelings and attitudes towards the wrongdoer. Conversely, true forgiveness—without forgetting (see below)—may occur without reconciliation.

Forgiveness is lauded for various reasons, including its capacity to heal victims and wrongdoers, and to harmonize personal and public relationships. It can be taught, and its practice can improve physical and mental health, as well as reduce anxiety and depression (Verhagen 2006). It can overcome avoidance and speechlessness by grappling with pain and traumatic memories. It opposes ferocity and hardness (Glas 2006:198–200; Griswold, 2007). Understanding and potential empathy for perpetrators, sometimes as equals, also facilitates reconciliation, as may perpetrators' acknowledging responsibility, apologizing, and asking forgiveness (Staub 2003: 444). Forgiveness as a mode of cooperation also receives experimental support from the classic Prisoner's Dilemma experiment which illuminates problems with recurring 'defection' and retribution and advantages for reciprocal altruism, since the reward of each is greater if each cooperates (Axelrod 1984; Ridley 1996).

Thus forgiveness appears to 'pay', and maintaining rage may endanger health. If forgiveness is psychologically healthy as well as morally desirable, and if it can be taught, ought it to be prescribed as part of therapy or cultural reconciliation? Several problems arise here. A civic culture of forgiveness and apology may confer on victims an expectation which amounts to duress, or may be used to humiliate, or it may become staged, or trite (Griswold 2007:180–183). What of heinous crimes? Where social exclusion or oppression prevails, is prescribing forgiveness possible or even desirable?

One conceptual objection holds that forgiveness may be regarded as a free gift. Exceptional, extraordinary as it is, it 'arrives', overturning common patterns in history, politics, and the law (Derrida 2001). Neither earned nor compelled, forgiveness can arise independent of apology, unconditional, potentially limitless (Macaskill 2005). Offering and accepting it involves risk: a lack of calculation, vulnerability, even faith (see Griswold 2007:117–119). Likewise, apology may be independent of forgiveness: both involve vulnerability, and are voluntary (Griswold 2007: 175–176). Although forgiveness may be learnt, and even taught in non-coercive situations, prescribing forgiveness is impossible.

Secondly, forgiveness after genocide or mass violence may be inconceivable, incomprehensible, or regarded as subverting justice (Staub 2003:433). Although unconditional love and forgiveness are celebrated in various religious traditions, Griswold (2007:59–72) argues that unconditional forgiveness erodes the offender's accountability. In abuse and in marriages, women may be expected or prevailed on to forgive, thus suppressing violence and betrayal and derailing personal growth (Lamb 2006). Where perpetrator behaviours persist and are sanctioned, 'forgiveness' may resemble capitulation. A reading of Judeo-Christian, Buddhist, and other religious sources suggests that forgiveness is not (ideally) unconditional, that repentance is important in restoring broken relationships, but also that releasing resentment has value regardless of the offender's response (e.g. Meninger 2008; Sacks 2003; Blumenthal 1998).

Pragmatically, however, distress caused by human rights violations, or anger replacing passive acceptance of abuse, may complicate or curtail the emotional work of forgiveness. Individual healing and collective healing may not coincide. Some wrongs are accessible to truth-telling, dia-logue, listening, story-telling, and forgiveness. Other, more radical wrongs, such as those experienced by Nazi death-camp survivors, are more intractable, because victimization that decimates groups is often random, frustrates basic needs, and potentially creates negative outlooks on the world, the self and the future, such that members of victim groups often suffer from a diminished capacity to lead satisfying lives (Staub 1989). Many have noted the affective impact, the toxicity of working close to such terrible events (e.g. Levi 1987; Higgins 2003). Thus the nature of the offender, the offence, or situation will sometimes render forgiveness possible, sometimes not (Griswold 2007:90–98). It is not a panacea.

Descendants of victims may request apologies from descendants of perpetrators for their forebears' crimes, and descendants of perpetrators may apologize or seek forgiveness. Can such parties meaningfully undertake these actions? People other than victims themselves cannot offer forgiveness, unless the victims accord them the standing to do so. Schlink (2009:71–73) notes strategic considerations, such as descendants of victims obtaining (quasi-)legal title, and sees hollowness in politicians participating in such rituals. Yet if colonizers still benefit from dispossession (see Hunter, in this volume), official apologies may enjoy a profound psychological impact, paving the way to further structural reform (Grace 2002).

Similarly, reconciliation processes may have mixed intentions and effects. Apologies to and reparations for victims, through providing accountability and restoring the moral and social standing of victims and perpetrators, have assisted conflict resolution and communal restoration (Griswold 2007:180)). For some post-conflict societies, economic justice is essential. Rwandan women identified this prerequisite to their country's Unity and Reconciliation Commission (Staub 2003:442). However, Truth and Reconciliation Commission (TRC) proceedings generally entail risks of insecurity and retraumatization for witnesses. Reconciliation may be limited or precluded if important social structures or institutions are rigid or hostile (Schlink 2009; Spitz 2006). In some settings, being a victim and residing in locations that have witnessed high levels of violence, decreases the propensity for forgiveness (Ferguson et al. 2007). Justice and politics, national and individual needs may conflict, and criminal trials may cause further division and fear in former enemy groups (Brouneus 2008, Mullet et al. 2008). For indigenous people in Australia, reconciliation programmes have sometimes had elements of coercion that contradict well-being (Altman and Hinkson 2007).

For warring groups, reconciliation requires that victims forgive, if not individual perpetrators, at least members of the group which perpetrated violence, and that the latter assume responsibility. Where both groups are victims and perpetrators, both need to forgive and assume responsibility (Staub 2003:468). Acknowledging mutual victimization may help perpetrators heal and open themselves to their victims (Staub 2003:440). For therapists, finding the victim in the perpetrator is an important tool in building empathy; while for victims, seeing perpetrators as weak and flawed may strengthen and sustain them (Zachar 2006).

The prominent South African TRC promoted forgiveness and relied on the idea of a continuous relationship to resolve conflict (Zachar 2006; Kruger 2006). Criticisms levelled against it included the perpetrators' escape from judgment (even for those who refused to cooperate), amnesties for serious crimes, limited or no financial restitution for victims, and with the futility of 'prescribed' forgiveness.

Truth, reconciliation, and mental health: recent research

Is public TRC testimony transformative and cathartic? Still-scarce South African empirical research has considered this question (Minow 1998) and the results have been mixed. Many victims who appeared before the South African TRC spoke about their witnessing as an experience that gave them a degree of control over their trauma. One study (admittedly retrospective and not randomly sampled) noted no significant association between TRC participation and current psychiatric status or forgiveness attitudes, with low forgiveness associated with poorer psychiatric health (Kaminer et al. 2001). TRC data transcripts and participant focus groups showed perpetrators were obdurate, and victims and families disinclined to forgive. Among white, Asian, and coloured South Africans, but not black South Africans, knowledge of and exposure to the TRC's work and accepting TRC-elicited truths about apartheid appeared to correlate with people being more racially reconciled, with reconciliation depending on levels of contact (Gibson 2004). The difference for black South Africans may have been attributable to reduced levels of contact (Gibson 2004), or their having been more targeted for violence (Brouneus 2010). In a representative South African population survey, having a TRC-relevant experience to share, increased distress, anger, and negative perceptions of the TRC's view of survivors' testimony: some survivors contradicted the perceived helpfulness of bearing testimony. At a community level, however, the survey showed that perceptions of the TRC were moderately positive, irrespective of various demographic variables (Stein et al. 2008).

Other TRC research broadly confirms these findings. A multistage, stratified cluster random survey of 1,200 Rwandans found that witnesses at the *gacaca*, the Rwandan village tribunals utilized for truth and reconciliation after the 1994 genocide, suffered from higher levels of depression and PTSD than did non-witnesses, including when controlling for important predictors of psychological ill health. This may be because gacaca testimony is like short-term intensive trauma exposure that re-traumatizes, although those involved in pilot gacaca courts for longer periods were no better off psychologically. Such an outcome may also mean that willingness to witness affects mental symptomatology, because those with more mental illness are more willing to witness, or that gacaca witnesses are not secure, psychologically or physically (Brouneus 2010). The gacaca courts' partisanship (ignoring crimes by the Rwandan Patriotic Front) and their failed adherence to international standards for due process and for protecting children's identities in particular, would confirm this (Smith 2010).

This research suggests that truth-telling, while essential for nations and potentially valuable for individuals, is not a cure-all, and that TRCs offer no substitute for comprehensive psychological interventions. While therapeutic exposure to traumatic memories has been used successfully for PTSD in traumatized civilians, refugees, and civil war survivors, TRC participants should be properly protected, and followed up to clarify risks for adverse emotional reactions and to ensure timely interventions (Silove et al. 2006).

Thus the South African and other TRC research has been informative for new situations where TRCs are operating or contemplated. A related question is how well witnesses understand the purposes, operation, and limitations of truth commissions. In one study, 344 educated East Timorese citizens who had been particularly exposed to their country's trauma and were familiar with truth commissions, nominated the goals of truth commissions as knowledge of atrocities and historical recording, overcoming denial, strengthening global respect for human rights, and restoring collective dignity, including perpetrators, whom they favoured healing rather than condemning. Most participants were aware of the limited scope of the truth commissions and did not have unrealistic expectations regarding the outcomes (Mullet et al. 2008).

The South African TRC neglected intergroup forgiveness (as compared with interpersonal forgiveness) (Chapman 2007). Post-conflict survivors have conceived of intergroup forgiveness as a democratic, public process with special deference to the offended group, aiming at reconciliation between two conflicting groups (Kadiangandu and Mullet 2007). This insight is relevant to (and has been taken into account in) Northern Ireland, the Democratic Republic of Congo, and Australia (Mellor et al. 2007).

Staub et al. (2005) have undertaken important, culturally sensitive work in Rwanda on group-based forgiveness. In Rwanda, Tutsi and Hutu staff of NGOs working with community groups underwent an experiential and psycho-educational intervention that aimed to foster psychological healing from trauma. The skills acquired promoted healing among Tutsi survivors and returning exiles and Hutus touched by their group's violent actions, and effected reconciliation and more positive orientation to members of the other group. The participants listened together to materials about genocide, impacts of trauma, basic human needs, and avenues to healing, and with empathic support, told their stories and listened to the stories of others. The intervention's effectiveness was evaluated for the community groups that the participants served, rather than for the participants themselves. The intervention was associated with reduced trauma symptoms and a more positive orientation towards members of the other group, both over time (from before to two months afterwards) and in comparison to two control groups: one with untrained facilitators using their traditional procedures, and a no-treatment control group (Staub, 2003:432–450; Staub et al. 2005).

The healing of children affected by mass human rights violations

The effects of human rights violations on children can prove transgenerational through loss, direct exposure to or witnessing of violence, and can also arise indirectly through the impact of the actions and emotions of exposed others on children. Perpetrators' offspring can be profoundly affected by the silence around their parents' actions, vexed relationships with them, other intimate relationships, isolation and damaged personal identity, and cultural amnesia. Denial is central to genocidal perpetrators and bystanders, cultures and nations. Many strategies must be used to address children's needs, but school education, witnessing parents who are committing to personal healing and reconciliation, and work with individual perpetrator groups, can all ameliorate the harm suffered by children (Staub 2003:446).

In wars, combatants have long forced children into terrorism, violence, and social destruction. Such violations have been increasingly outlawed by the near-universal ratification of the Convention on the Rights of the Child (CRC); Graça Machel's 1996 landmark study, *Impact of Armed Conflict on Children*; the adoption in 2000 of the Optional Protocol to the CRC on the involvement of children in armed conflict; and the 2002 establishment of the International Criminal Court (ICC) that criminalizes serious crimes, including those targeting children. The 2005 United Nations Basic Principles and Guidelines on the Right to a Remedy and Reparation for Victims of Gross Violations of International Human Rights Law and Serious Violations of International Humanitarian Law also provides that victims of such abuses, including children, have a right to prompt, adequate, and effective reparation (Smith 2010).

The involvement of children in transitional justice is thus relatively recent, and newly researched (UNICEF Innocenti Research Centre 2011; Parmer et al. 2010). TRCs in Sierra Leone and Liberia in particular have explicitly involved children through formalizing relationships with child protection organizations. Framed by the CRC and the African Charter on the Rights and Welfare of the Child, their procedures emphasize respect for children, confidentiality, and informed and voluntary participation (with parental consent as appropriate), and their roles as victims and witnesses. Different challenges are faced by girls and boys, adolescents and younger children, refugee and internally displaced children, those orphaned by war, children from different religious and ethnic backgrounds, children with disabilities, and children recruited into armed forces and groups. To date, children accused of crimes have not been held legally accountable for perpetration. Where children not under direct adult supervision have killed people, this omission is problematic: an appropriate forum for achieving accountability under international law has yet to be set up (Smith 2010).

In Sierra Leone, for example, children were especially targeted. For the TRC, partnerships between children's networks, experts on child protection and children's rights, and TRC members enhanced child participation and protection. Allowing young people to shape and adapt the process promoted healing and citizenship. Confidential testimony informed a child-friendly TRC report which was widely disseminated. However, miscommunication sometimes occurred: in exchange for participation, children (often from impoverished situations) expected financial or other practical support in education or health care, which was not forthcoming. The TRC also arguably lacked sufficient dedicated resources and capacity to deliver on its goals (Smith 2010). The TRC experience showed that children making statements needed adequate orientation to— and support during—the process, and ongoing support afterwards within their environment. Despite the crucial importance of active child and youth engagement, human rights had to be linked with development for TRC truth-telling and reintegration to achieve healing and reconciliation. Thus children and young people's basic economic, educational, and protection needs had to addressed, and post-conflict social policy reforms needed to be undertaken in education, health care, social welfare, protection, and justice. For future action, the authors of one report on this TRC commended the role of family and community engagement; of extending knowledge of child development in war, and the implications for social reconstruction and children's citizenship; and potential connections of transitional justice to traditional and collective practices of trust, accountability, forgiveness, and reconciliation (Cook and Heykoop 2010).

To this detailed analysis we would add the inclusion of mental health intervention in planning similar future responses. The mental health challenge is especially great for those with existing mental disorders and intellectual disabilities, as well as victims of sexual abuse, former child soldiers, and others with persistent war-related trauma. Former child soldiers in particular share common characteristics: for example, more PTSD and clinical depression than non-conscripts (Kohrt et al. 2008), with these symptoms and related experiences appearing associated with less openness to reconciliation and more revengeful feelings (Bayer et al. 2007). Torture, conflict-related bereavement and poverty, and physical abuse at home all predict poor outcomes in Nepalese former child soldiers, whilst education improves this outlook (Kohrt et al. 2010). Among 23 Ugandan youth returning from the Lord's Resistance Army (LRA), fears about being accused, joblessness, learning new norms, and conflict resolution collided with the community's fear of recurring violence, overstretched resources, and concern for children still in captivity: hence interventions need to encompass both returning youth and their communities (Annan et al. 2009). Noting that returned child soldiers frequently face community rejection, and that psychosocial reintegration initiatives generally neglect issues of impunity, Veale and Stavrou (2007) suggest that traditional justice and reconciliation approaches, complemented by international child rights and protection safeguards, could further reconciliation and identity resolution. Trauma-focused and psycho-social approaches are both necessary in post-conflict interventions (Miller and Rasmussen 2010), as is cultural specificity and respect.

In Australia, the removal of indigenous children from their families for placement with white families and in orphanages from the 19th century to the 1970s, was the subject of an official inquiry in 1997. Yet the practice only attracted a delayed, long-awaited official apology when the newly-elected Labor government issued one in 2008 (Smith 2010). Various initiatives have ensued, including community and school educational programmes, and oral history and story collections, but financial compensation has been refused.

Promoting a just society

In the shadow of the Holocaust, Alexander assessed whether nations were likely to engage in such behaviour in future; he cited indicators such as a country's success in dealing with social problems (and whether authorities advocated destruction of life), the extent to which fear governed decision-making processes for most people, the existence of civil rights and their exercise by individuals, and freedom of information (Schmidt 2006:270).

Genocide prevention

Despite various arguments and proposals that individuals, groups, states, and the community of nations must influence governments to prevent genocide (Charny 1991; Staub 2003), early warning systems are still under development. The international campaign Genocide Watch—which exists to predict, prevent, stop, and punish genocide and other forms of mass murder—describes early warning signs in eight different stages (<http://www.genocidewatch.org/>). Similarly the 'Minorities at Risk' project (<http://www.cidcm.umd.edu/mar/>) uses computer-modelling systems to monitor and analyze conflicts in politically-active communal groups (Baum 2008:32). The ICC, operating since 2002, covers genocide, war crimes, crimes against humanity, and crimes against peace, but its influence is yet to be evaluated. However, it only has complementary jurisdiction: that is, it does not operate unless a state in question is unable or unwilling to investigate, and if warranted, prosecute these crimes. Genocides have continued, presenting major international challenges over intervention.

Conventions and legislation

In recent decades, the development and monitoring of human rights conventions and the work of international human rights NGOs have more effectively addressed human rights neglects and abuses. Changes in international human rights law and institutions have facilitated prosecution of those accused of crimes against humanity (Robertson 2006). Legislation against hate speech and bullying, for example, has also protected minorities and enabled nations and communities to restrain and correct racism and negative discrimination through legal action. Many strategies have been employed to hold governments accountable for rights abuses, such as diplomacy, boycotts, and ostracism. The introduction to this book and several other chapters address the role of conventions and legislation more comprehensively.

Education against social exclusion

Educational attainments did not prevent the Holocaust, and misinformation facilitated it. For schoolchildren in Nazi Germany, the taboo against mass killing was broken down by asking them to make calculations of resources required to support people with disabilities, using inflated figures (Weindling 2006:256).

Can anti-racist education reduce or eliminate prejudice or racist behaviour? There is a contrast between individualistic and conservative views that hold that human nature is relatively immutable, and critical theories of society that suggest that criteria of a good society provide a yardstick for genocide-proof societal development.

Racism takes many forms, and empirically evaluated anti-racism interventions are sparse, usually brief, and have other methodological limitations, such as ill-defined or poorly-measured outcomes. Though no one approach suffices, reviews (for instance Pedersen et al. 2003) nevertheless propose certain conclusions. Combining grassroots and top-down approaches in local settings works best. Crucially, 'education' is more than rational discussion or provision of information alone. Successful programmes promote behavioural change, particularly concrete skills, irrespective of attitudinal change which may prove hard to achieve. Individual strategies include challenging false beliefs about target groups, allowing participants to feel dissonance (psychological discomfort arising from incompatibility between their beliefs); and teaching empathy, perspective-taking, and skills for challenging racism. Interpersonal strategies are more likely to work if they are longitudinal, re-define in-groups as tolerant, diverse, and inclusive; and while emphasizing sameness and diversity, they generalize this learning to other marginal groups. Contact between groups works if institutional authorities sanction it, and if the parties are equal, non-competitive, and have a superordinate goal (Allport 1954). The issue of safety may mediate outcomes. Also effective is providing consensus information challenging prejudiced people's beliefs that their views are the norm; and dialogue (which is more effective than being lectured at). Clear unambiguous political leadership and coalitions are also vital (Pedersen et al. 2003).

Recounting the Holocaust, its related histories, and antecedents, illuminates crimes of obedience and moral choices confronting individuals, cultures, and societies. This may be of value to a wider audience than those directly affected, also enabling understanding of the plight of victims and the long-term medical and psycho-social consequences. After the genocide in Rwanda, understanding the social and situational determinants of evil helped survivors and members of perpetrator groups who were not themselves perpetrators to feel 'more human' (Staub 2003:6, 47–51).

Thus, Holocaust and related education against social exclusion aims to stimulate action against discrimination, devaluation, and violence. Contact with victims and survivors and exposure to their testimony forms a vital part of this strategy. The latter will often require (and result in) revision of national, cultural, and/or group narratives. Where antagonism and hostility persist, dialogue groups and problem-solving workshops may promote community-rebuilding. There are numerous examples of this happening in (post-)conflict zones, such as Israel-Palestine and Northern Ireland. The role and responsibility of the media also requires consideration (Thornicroft 2006; Staub 2003:456). Other measures include developing caring schools (see below), and governments preventing human rights violations (Zimbardo 2007; Staub 2003).

Promoting critical thinking, mutual acknowledgement, and accommodation of plural identities, and disobedience where necessary, is essential to cultivating a just society (Baum 2008:223). Teaching empathy and targeting perpetrators, for example bullies, is also critical. Many anti-discrimination programmes in schools and communities counter racism. For example, the Anne Frank travelling exhibition contains historical and contemporary information about persecution, and employs youth guides (<http://www.annefrank.org/en/Worldwide/Travelling-exhibition/>). The Courage to Care programme is a travelling exhibition that aims to inform and educate Australian students about the dangers of prejudice and discrimination (<http://www.couragetocare.com.au/index.aspx>). Other fine examples could be noted. In the wake of conflict and terror, Staub (2007) highlights the resources available for preventing violence and promoting positive group relations, including humanizing out-groups, dialogue, psychological healing, promoting pluralism, contact between groups, and exploring shared history. This includes changing school practices.

In this vein, Zimbardo (2007) celebrates and re-invents heroism. Exemplifying the virtues of courage, justice, and transcendence, heroism is voluntary, sacrificial, and undertaken in service of others without expectation of gain. Rather than being an individual characteristic of extraordinary people, he sees heroism as socially constructed, and as banal. In speaking of 'the banality of heroism', Zimbardo signals its ordinariness, its (potential) ubiquity. Paradoxically, while heroism re-imagined is a socially owned rather than an individual characteristic, holding the democratic possibility of anyone being a hero, it also promotes resistance to (unwanted) social influences. Zimbardo discusses cultivating an heroic imagination, including the need for children and adults to re-engage with epic myths and stories of our own and other cultures; and being instructed or shown how to manifest civil and moral courage (Zimbardo 2007; Schlink 2009). This may include pro-social models that represent desired actions, admitting mistakes, and learning not to fear personal conflict or social ostracism. Charny (2006) also explores the contrasts and choices between fascist and democratic mindsets for individuals, families, and societies.

For helping professionals, a broad-based curriculum will reflect on cultural values and ideologies that influence their world view. Possible examples include stigma, the history and philosophy of science, applied ethics, and cultivation of a 'moral-historical imagination' (Glover 1999). Utilitarian scientific (or 'instrumental') rationality in modern societies and organizations frequently delimits human life-goals to action, material well-being, and pleasure. It de-legitimizes accounts of humans as free moral agents, open through contemplative reason to ultimate reality and meaning (Moreno-Riaño 2001) and demotes human beings to mere objects, means to ends. Thus any strategy to prevent victimization must challenge instrumental rationality's trumping of ethical, intersubjective motivations. This requirement extends to challenging the belief that self-interest is humanity's sole ruling principle, and that kindness is weakness (Phillips and Taylor 2009). After conflict or actual genocide, some victims heal by devoting themselves to creating a world where self-interest is not sovereign (Oliner and Oliner 1988), as noted above.

However, is learning moral courage sufficient (Schlink 2009)? Individual morality may be insufficient if institutions that recognize inclusive and equal citizenship are absent. Given the fragile foundations of culturally advanced civilization that the Holocaust revealed, how safe are we today?

Although mass human rights violations occur in all manner of polities, a flourishing democracy may be the best safeguard to prevent their recurrence. Universal rationalistic, liberal, and/or cosmopolitan approaches promote Holocaust education, anti-denialism, international conventions that define and criminalize genocide and uphold universal human rights, and atrocity-exposing work by international NGOs. Yet these may not suffice. Personal choices are not simply part of individual psychological dispositions or universal values or principles. Higgins (2003) distinguishes ethnic and civic nationalisms, arguing that they differ in their propensities to provide the preconditions for genocide. Early modern states pursued ethnic homogeneity and ethnocide against external and internal 'others' as the basis of national belonging. Ethnic nationalism, with traditional elites resisting the incursions of the representative state and democracy, is exemplified in the early 20th century histories of Germany, Australia, and South Africa. By contrast, the modern civil society which developed, for example, in Britain from the late 17th century and in France a century later, illustrated an evolving vital interdependence between the rule of law, the constitutional, representative state, and the state's subjects (later 'citizens') organizing and bargaining to influence state policy. This civic nationalism tended to promote diversity and inclusivity in citizenship, in contrast to the older ethnic nationalism's exclusivity and ethnic homogeneity.

Nazism represented an extreme ethnic nationalism which murderously resisted ethnic diversity. Thus Higgins suggests that preventing genocide requires a civic-nationalist inclusivity that encompasses ethnic diversity, and that the health of national institutions also requires assessment. National belonging and citizenship provide a crucial focus for collective moral responsibility and agency, as well as personal identity.

Since socio-structural and personal factors operate interdependently in the perpetration of inhumanities, civilized life requires not only humane personal codes that are modelled and inculcated from early in life, but effective safeguards against the abuse of power. Arguably, authoritarian systems with limited public access to media and internet offer greater scope for moral disengagement than do pluralistic systems that support critically socially engaged citizens. Pluralism encourages diverse perspectives and interests, public debate and dissent (Bandura 1999), and promotes shared goals and connections using education and experiential methods. None of this, of course, obviates the need for positive leadership (Staub 2003:368).

Child-rearing practices as formative for social responsibility

Child rearing that promotes caring, helping, and non-aggression is also essential: fostering the positive evaluation of human beings, concern about others' welfare, and feelings of personal responsibility for it (Staub 2003:117, 161). Significant building blocks and practices here include parental warmth, affection, reasoning with the child (especially about consequences of their behaviour for others), firm control, and guiding and modelling prosocial behaviour. Such practices contrast with formerly entrenched views that emphasized obedience and forcefully break children's will (De Mause 1974). A humanistic rather than conventional orientation will promote the good and responds to others' needs even if this means breaking conventions or disturbing social order (Hoffman 1970) and 'just world' assumptions (Staub 2003:121–122). Providing opportunities for children to 'stand in another's shoes' can enhance this effect. Cultivating capacities for managing stress and exercising independent judgment, confidence and competence in making decisions, and preparedness (for instance, in having existing plans and the ability to generate them in the future) as well as awareness of one's actions' impacts, are vital to standing apart if required, and to taking action. Children may learn responsibilities for others by being assigned specific duties related to others' welfare, for example contributing to family maintenance or the care of others (Whiting and Whiting 1975, cited in Staub 2003:174; Staub 2003:173–198).

Individual identities founded on excessive dependence on (or independence from) the group, obstruct genocide prevention, while connected but autonomous identities are best equipped for resistance. Similarly, those who are constructively rather than blindly patriotic (that is, who express love for the nation as well as a willingness to question and criticize its policies and practices that are contrary to human welfare) will embody this capacity for resistance against genocide (Staub 2003:351–359).

Prevention of human rights violations also includes halting or preventing violence as such. The cultural and societal roots of violence among young people and families include harsh living conditions, poverty, individualism, reduced community cohesion, discrimination, unreconstructed male roles, violence on television (e.g. 'reality' TV shows), and cyberbullying. Strategies for identifying and responding to these factors lie outside the scope of this chapter, but are nevertheless also vital.

Other desiderata include creating caring schools through warmth and sensitivity, reasoned standards and discipline, training in helpfulness, expanding understanding of others and respect for difference, community-building, and specifically dealing with aggression and trauma. At the school and community levels, moral engagement can be enhanced by discussing the impacts of bullying with students, training and peer modelling of non-bystander behaviour, conflict-resolution training, and learning to fulfil needs in constructive ways (Staub 2003:173–198, 212–226, 267–286). In this context, programmes like 'Courage to Care' enjoy considerable relevance. Effective anti-bullying policies and programmes exemplify one kind of response that can mobilise children, parents, schools and teachers around this issue (see the Method of Shared Concern as one example (Pikas 1989)).

Responses by the helping professions

Prevention also demands the cultivation and training of a socially aware workforce. A survey of US health-ethics policy documents found that they seldom address resource allocation, advocacy, and care for the most vulnerable (Berkman et al. 2004). Applied ethics training has come to inform the education of mental health and helping professionals, but traditionally focuses on clinical encounters and environments rather than social issues impinging on professionals and their clients. During the drafting of the RANZCP code of ethics, the inclusion of a principle concerning the role of psychiatrists in society was hotly debated. Those against inclusion of this aspect saw it as a matter for personal choice, preferring that the code confine itself to professional–patient and intercollegial relationships. Others affirmed the profession's vital role of advocating for clients and raising awareness of mental health. The latter group won out (Bloch and Pargiter 2009:167).

Under the social influences mentioned above, paternalism has yielded to a contractual relationship, for example between the psychiatrist and patient. Yet as conceived in liberal discourse, contracts present problems for furthering human rights. Firstly, they emphasize original autonomy rather than connection. Although contracts (implicit or explicit) exist between medicine or psychiatry and society, the liberal contractual position is primarily self-interested (Gauthier 1994; Midgley 1994). In his famous thought experiment in *A Theory of Justice*, John Rawls suggested that this would be true even of a model of distributive justice negotiated by rational agents, none of whom knows their own position in a hypothetical new society, so that the least advantaged person is protected through a process of 'constrained maximization' that allocates resources accordingly (Rawls 1972).

Secondly, contractarianism marginalizes groups who cannot negotiate and enter into contract, since their capacity for rational choice is compromised, as is the case, for example, with those with mental disorders, intellectual disabilities, and prisoners, but also animals and the environment (Nussbaum 2006; Midgley 1994). In these circumstances, the helping professions have a duty of advocacy.

The social contract also fails when the state fails morally, through oppressing its citizens or when the social order collapses in warfare or natural disaster (Robertson 2007). Totalitarian states present particular dilemmas for Western beliefs, law, and practices concerning individual autonomy. The mental stability of individuals may be judged on the basis of whether they adhere to correct political thought and action or advance the well-being of society as a whole. In these circumstances, helping professionals confront fundamental dilemmas over compliance with government policy. In the Nazi and Soviet cases, there were a range of responses within psychiatry to its political abuse as a means to enforce obedience (Chodoff 2009; see van Voren, this volume).

If contracts are unpromising, and community-based initiatives are dependent on what notion of community is being invoked, other promising approaches for furthering the human rights agenda in mental health may involve adopting and promoting organizational codes and international charters, including virtue-based approaches; and initiating emancipatory or empowering practices (Prilleltensky et al. 2008; Zion et al. 2012).

For example, efforts to codify and regulate the powers of the medical profession date from Hippocrates. Codes and charters may range from minimal legal rules (perhaps forestalling external interventions) or with deterrent intent (e.g. the Nuremberg code) to principles and attendant duties, to virtue-based oaths and conventions. Such standards may serve multiple purposes, including promoting professional status and self-regulation on the one hand, and moral sensitizing and educational functions on the other (Bloch and Pargiter 2009). The RANZCP Code of Ethics recognizes that (mental) health professionals have a responsibility to society, through improving quality of and access to mental health services, the just allocation of health resources and community awareness of mental health and illness (Code of Ethics, Principle 11). The Code also admonishes psychiatrists to refrain from 'misuse their professional knowledge and skills': to not participate in torture, or other forms of cruel, inhumane or degrading punishment and executions, to declare their purpose when interventions are not inherently therapeutic, and to follow accepted ethical guidelines in situations of conflict or war. US evidence suggests, however, that compared with doctor–patient relationships, socio-political aspects of practice have been relatively neglected in the implementation of medical codes of ethics (Berkman et al. 2004;

Bloch and Pargiter 2009). At this stage, little if any research illuminates whether training and continuing education programmes around values and ethics can foster openness and reduce breaches of ethical codes.

As a helping professional, one may accept the status quo, or engage critically with institutions, disciplines, communities, colleagues, and clients for emancipatory purposes. The latter choice implies acknowledging power (the capacity and opportunity to fulfil or obstruct personal, relational, or collective needs) as central to personal well-being, in the helping professions and all helping practice. Acknowledging psychopolitical validity (Prilleltensky et al. 2008; Zion et al. 2012) means challenging ineffective, reactive, disempowering, and merely individualistic approaches. It entails understanding how helping professions may hinder people, engaging with service users' concerns and pain, and promoting citizenship that involves advocacy and genuine partnerships across social divides.

Such re-imagining and reconfiguring of mental health practice means exploring how social processes generate economic inequalities and psychiatric disorders; how oppression, liberation, and well-being operate in psychological, relational, and collective domains. Such an 'emancipatory' approach eschews positivism and the colonizing, divisive Western narrative of progress. Highlighting neglected cultural and interpersonal domains, its context-sensitive interventions contrast with one-size-fits-all Western medical approaches (this problem is discussed in the Introduction and chapters by Steel and by Silove and colleagues). In clinical practice, case formulations and therapies that draw on feminist and narrative insights understand the individual in social context, the personal as political, and identify and support the strengths and flourishing of service users. In research, social-psychiatric inquiry is needed to engage with policies that stress democracy, citizenship, and socio-cultural contexts in health care. Global mental health advocates suggest that mental health policy and service planning require the development of vigorous primary health and community mental health programmes that reinforce and support each other, with basic interventions available at all levels (Saraceno et al. 2007; Patel and Prince 2010). Training programmes may teach advocacy skills and developing partnerships with service users who co-generate strategies for systemic change (Muntaner et al. 2008; Prilleltensky et al. 2008).

While a huge literature exists on promotion and prevention in mental health, empowering approaches harness the expertise of many disciplines, groups, and sufferers in the service of mutual learning about what works in promotion, in services, and in research and evaluation. Agencies may positively discriminate in favour of service users, employing them as consumer helping professionals or peer support workers (Warner 2010). Helping professionals may be trained to act as advocates with service users, publicly questioning prevailing policies and attitudes which disadvantage and stigmatize groups, effecting changes in governance of health organizations to facilitate user representation, and working more closely with users for full citizenship when this is lacking (Dudley and Gale 2002). Partnerships of mental health and helping professionals and service users are needed with all relevant stakeholders (for instance, primary health care workers, medical and health staff, communities, government, and NGOs) to reduce stigma and to identify and advocate for the mental health needs of populations. Culturally informed and sensitive training with communities in what has sometimes been called 'mental health literacy' (Jorm et al. 1997) and 'mental health first aid' (Jorm et al. 2010) is also indicated.

Empirical research reveals the overriding convictions of psychiatrists, including the value of patients, a need for sophisticated, reflexive understanding of their situations, and the importance of advocacy. The need for a jointly constructed narrative of the patient's experience emerges, to consider and, where possible, prevent the potential misuse of the power differential in relationships with third parties, to anticipate and respond to potential abuses of psychiatry (especially through dual roles), and to advocate assertively for better services, including within institutions (Robertson et al. 2009).

Conclusion

This chapter, as a companion to Chapter 11, has considered challenges in promoting a just society and preventing human rights violations, particularly in the light of the Nazi era and the Nuremberg trials, and the social responsibilities of helping professionals in particular. The place of social justice within mental health—issues such as liberty, equity, social inclusion, and advocacy—is evident in a range of social developments. Developments in science and technology pose ethical questions, with the 'new eugenics' in particular introducing serious concerns about failing to treat human beings as ends in themselves. Understanding disability's social foundations requires better public and specialist education, for example about the history of medicine and psychiatry, managing expectations raised by research participation, applied ethics reflection, for instance on the centrality of individual service users' well-being and choice over the advancement of science. Professionals need to reflect on disability rights in particular. Common to all these initiatives has been a rediscovery of the fundamental dignity of persons.

The post-conflict tasks of transitional justice, forgiveness, and reconciliation raise important questions about how mental health and justice can work together to further community reconstruction whilst meeting the needs of those adults and children most at risk. Civil societies must consider how to combat social exclusion and rear children who are emotionally attuned and pro-social. Warning systems that potentially prevent genocide and development programmes that promote a just society and teach conflict resolution and to prevent or halt violence, are also desirable. For this purpose, we addressed the role of conventions and legislation, education that combats social exclusion through Holocaust-focused and related forms of instruction, promoting critical thinking, empathy and respect for difference, and challenging views of humanity bounded by utilitarian scientific rationality. Contact with sufferers, and with those from opposing social or victim groups, is vital. Nor should the necessity for vigilance in renewing democracy be underestimated.

Social engagement by helping professionals is crucial if we want to help shape developments rather than simply reacting to exigencies: we need to bolster human rights through contributing to strengthening civil society. Our mandate for such engagement is embedded in international conventions, charters, and codes from the earlier UN declarations of rights to the recent Convention on the Rights of Persons with Disabilities, in which social justice constitutes a core theme. Being socially engaged, however, is a matter of exercising one's citizenship whatever one's profession might be.

Acknowledgements

We thank Winton Higgins and Alan Rosen for a number of significant scholarly and editorial suggestions.

References

ABIM Foundation, ACP-ASIM Foundation, and EFIM (2002) 'Medical professionalism in the new millennium: a physician charter', *Annals of Internal Medicine*, 136, 243–46.

Allport, GW (1954) *The nature of prejudice*. Reading, MA: Addison-Wesley.

Altman, J and Hinkson, M (2007) *Coercive reconciliation: stabilise, normalise, exit Aboriginal Australia*. North Carlton, Melbourne: Arena Publications.

Annan, J, Brier, M, and Aryemo, F (2009) 'From "Rebel" to "'Returnee": Daily Life and Reintegration for Young Soldiers in Northern Uganda', *Journal of Adolescent Research*, 24, 639.

Annas, G and Grodin, M (2007) *Address* at Medical Malice conference, Boston University, 30 March 2007.

Axelrod, R (1984) *The evolution of cooperation*. New York: Basic Books.

Bandura, A (1999) 'Moral Disengagement in the Perpetration of Inhumanities', *Personality and Social Psychology Review*, 3(3), 193–209.

Baum, SK (2008) *The psychology of genocide: perpetrators, bystanders and rescuers*. New York: Cambridge University Press.

Bayer, CP, Klasen, F, and Adam, H (2007) 'Association of trauma and PTSD symptoms with openness to reconciliation and feelings of revenge among former Ugandan and Congolese child soldiers', *JAMA*, 298(5), 555–59.

Beauchamp, TL (2009) 'The philosophical basis of psychiatric ethics', in S Bloch and S Green (eds) *Psychiatric ethics*. 4th edn. Oxford: Oxford University Press, 25–48.

Berkman, ND, Wynia, MK, and Churchill, LR (2004) 'Gaps, conflicts, and consensus in the ethics statements of professional associations, medical groups, and health plans', *Journal of Medical Ethics*, 30, 395–401.

Bloch, S and Pargiter, R (2009) 'Codes of ethics', in S Bloch and S Green (eds) *Psychiatric ethics*. *Psychiatric ethics*. 4th edn. Oxford: Oxford University Press, 151–73.

Blumenthal, DR (1998) 'Repentance and forgiveness', *Cross Currents*, (Spring). Available at <http://www.crosscurrents.org/blumenthal.htm>, accessed 30 June 2011.

Brounéus, K (2008) 'Analyzing reconciliation: a structured method for measuring national reconciliation initiatives, peace and conflict', *Peace and Conflict: Journal of Peace Psychology*, 14, 3, 291–313.

Brounéus, K (2010) 'The trauma of truth-telling: effects of witnessing in the Rwandan gacaca courts on psychological health', *Journal of Conflict Resolution*, 54(3), 408–37.

Caplan, A (2007) 'The ethics of evil: the challenge and lessons of Nazi medical experiments', in WR Lafleur, G Böhme, and S Shimazono (eds) *Dark Medicine: rationalising unethical medical research*. Bloomington: Indiana University Press, 63–72.

Chapman, A (2007) 'Truth commissions and inter-group forgiveness: the case of the South African Truth and Reconciliation Commission', *Peace and Conflict: Journal of Peace Psychology*, 13(1), 51–69.

Charny, I (1991) 'Genocide intervention and prevention', *Social Education*, 55(2), 124–27.

Charny, IW (2006) *Fascism and democracy in the human mind: a bridge between mind and society*. Lincoln and London: University of Nebraska Press.

Chodoff, P (2009) 'The abuse of psychiatry', in S Bloch and S Green (eds) *Psychiatric ethics*. 4th edn. Oxford: Oxford University Press, 99–110.

Coady, A (2009) 'The nature of professions: implications for psychiatry', in S Bloch and S Green (eds) *Psychiatric ethics*. 4th edn. Oxford: Oxford University Press, 85–98.

Cook, P and Heykoop, C (2010) 'Child Participation in the Sierra Leonean Truth and Reconciliation Commission', in S Parmar, MJ Roseman, S Siegrist, and T Sowa (eds) *Children and Transitional Justice: Truth-Telling, Accountability and Reconciliation*. Human Rights Program, Harvard Law School (United Nations Children's Fund (UNICEF)), 159–91. Available at <http://www.unicef-irc.org/publications/series/17/>, accessed 30 June 2011.

Curtis, I (2010) *Paper: a clinical response*. 21 June 2010. Available at <http://iancurtispsychiatrist.com/a-clinical-response/>, accessed 28 December 2010.

Daniels, N (1995) *Just Health Care*. Cambridge: Cambridge University Press.

DeMause, L (ed) (1974) *The history of childhood*. New York: Harper Torchbook.

Derrida, J (2001) *On cosmopolitanism and forgiveness*. Trans. Mark Dooley and Michael Hughes. London & New York: Routledge.

Dudley, M and Gale, F (2002) 'Psychiatrists as a moral community? Psychiatry under the Nazis and its contemporary relevance', *Australian and New Zealand Journal of Psychiatry*, 36, 585–94.

Enright, R (2001) *Forgiveness is a choice: A step-by-step process for resolving anger and restoring hope.* Washington, DC: American Psychological Association.

Fabrega, H Jr (2000) 'Culture, spirituality and psychiatry'. In Forum—Culture, spirituality and psychiatry, *Current Opinion in Psychiatry*, 13, 531–43.

Ferguson, N, Binks, E, Roe, MD et al. (2007) 'The IRA Apology of 2002 and forgiveness in Northern Ireland's Troubles: A cross-national study of printed media', *Peace and Conflict: Journal of Peace Psychology*, 13, 93–113.

Fox, RC (2007) 'Toward an ethic of iatrogenesis', in WR Lafleur, G Böhme, and S Shimazono (eds) *Dark Medicine: rationalising unethical medical research.* Bloomington: Indiana University Press, 149–64.

Fromm, E (1965) *Escape from freedom.* New York: Avon Books.

Gauthier, D (1994) 'Why contractarianism?', in P Singer (ed) *Ethics.* (Oxford Readers). New York: Oxford University Press, 367–73.

Gibson, JL (2004) 'Does truth lead to reconciliation? Testing the causal assumptions of the South African truth and reconciliation process', *American Journal of Political Science*, 48, 201–217.

Glas, G (2006) 'Elements of a phenomenology of evil and forgiveness', in NN Potter (ed) *Trauma, truth and reconciliation: healing damaged relationships.* New York: Oxford University Press, 171–202.

Glover, J (1999) *Humanity: a moral history of the twentieth century.* London: Jonathan Cape.

Grace, D (2002) 'Apologising for the past: German science and Nazi medicine', *Science and Engineering*, 8, 31–42.

Greene, RR and Graham, SA (2009) 'Role of Resilience Among Nazi Holocaust Survivors: A Strength-based Paradigm for Understanding Survivorship', *Family & Community Health*, 32(1), (January/March), S75–82.

Griswold, CL (2007) *Forgiveness: a philosophical exploration.* New York: Cambridge University Press.

Hamber, B (2007) 'Forgiveness and reconciliation: paradise lost or pragmatism?', *Peace and Conflict: Journal of Peace Psychology*, 13(1), 115–25.

Higgins, W (2003) *Journey into Darkness.* Sydney: Brandl and Schlesinger.

Higgins, Wand Ramia, G (2000) 'Social citizenship', in W Hudson and J Kane (eds) *Rethinking Australian citizenship.* Melbourne: Cambridge University Press, 136–49.

Hoffman, ML (1970) 'Moral development', in PH Mussen (ed) *Carmichael's manual of child psychology.* New York: Wiley, 261–359.

Jorm, AF, Kitchener, BA, Fischer, J, and Cvetkovski, S (2010) 'Mental health first aid training by e-learning: a randomized controlled trial', *Australian and New Zealand Journal of Psychiatry*, 44(12), 1072–81.

Jorm, AF, Korten, AE, Jacomb, PA, Christensen, H, Rodgers, B, and Pollitt, P (1997) '"Mental health literacy": a survey of the public's ability to recognise mental disorders and their beliefs about the effectiveness of treatment', *Medical Journal of Australia*, 166, 182–86.

Kadiangandu, JK and Mullet, E (2007) 'Intergroup forgiveness: A Congolese perspective', *Peace and Conflict: Journal of Peace Psychology*, 13(1), 37–49.

Kahana, B, Harel, Z, and Kahana, E (2007) *Holocaust Survivors and Immigrants: Late Life Adaptations.* US: Springer.

Kaminer, D, Stein, DJ, Mbanga, I, Zungu-Dirwayi, N (2001) 'The Truth and Reconciliation Commission in South Africa: relation to psychiatric status and forgiveness among survivors of human rights abuses', *The British Journal of Psychiatry*, 178, 373–77.

Kessler, RC, Berglund, P, Demler, O, Jin, R, Merikangas, KR, and Walters, EE (2005) 'Lifetime Prevalence and Age-of-Onset Distributions of DSM-IV Disorders in the National Comorbidity Survey Replication', *Archives of General Psychiatry*, 62, 593–602.

Kohrt, BA, Jordans, MJD, Tol, WA, Speckman, RA, Maharjan, SM, Worthman, CM, and Komproe, IH (2008) 'Comparison of mental health between former child soldiers and children never conscripted by armed groups in Nepal', *JAMA*, 300(6), 691–702.

Kohrt, BA, Jordans, MJD, Tol, WA, Perera, E, Karki, R, Koirala, S, and Upadhaya, N (2010) 'Social ecology of child soldiers: Community determinants of mental health, psychosocial well-being and reintegration in Nepal', *Transcultural Psychiatry*, 47(5), 727–53.

Komatsu, Y (2007) 'The age of a '"revolutionised human body" and the right to die', in WR Lafleur, G Böhme, and S Shimazono (eds) *Dark Medicine: rationalising unethical medical research*. Bloomington: Indiana University Press, 180–200.

Kruger, C (2006) Spiral of growth: a social psychiatric perspective on conflict resolution, reconciliation and relationship development', in NN Potter (ed) *Trauma, truth and reconciliation: healing damaged relationships*. New York: Oxford University Press, 29–66.

Kymlicka, W (2002) *Contemporary political philosophy: an introduction*. 2nd edn. Oxford: Oxford University Press.

La Fleur, W (2007) 'Refusing Utopia's bait: research, rationalisations and Hans Jonas', in WR Lafleur, G Böhme, and S Shimazono (eds) *Dark Medicine: rationalising unethical medical research*. Bloomington: Indiana University Press, 233–45.

Lafleur WR, Böhme G, and Shimazono S (eds) (2007) *Dark Medicine: rationalising unethical medical research*. Bloomington: Indiana University Press.

Lamb, S (2006) Forgiveness therapy in gendered contexts: what happens to the truth?', in NN Potter (ed) *Trauma, truth and reconciliation: healing damaged relationships*. New York: Oxford University Press, 229–56.

Levi, P (1987) *The drowned and the saved*. New York: Summit.

Long, W, and Brecke, P (2003) *War and reconciliation: reason and emotion in conflict resolution*. Cambridge: MIT Press.

Luban, D (1988) *Lawyers and justice*. Princeton: Princeton University Press.

Macaskill, A (2005) 'Defining forgiveness: Christian clergy and general population perspectives', *Journal of Personality*, (Oct), 73(5), 1237–65.

Manne, R (ed) (2003) *Whitewash. On Keith Windschuttle's Fabrication of Aboriginal History*. Melbourne: Black Inc. Agenda.

Mellor, D, Bretherton, D, and Firth, L (2007) 'Aboriginal and non-aboriginal Australia: The dilemma of apologies, forgiveness, and reconciliation', *Peace and Conflict: Journal of Peace Psychology*, 13(1), 11–36.

Meninger, W (2008) 'Why forgiveness is needed', *Tikkun*, (March/April), 23(2), 26. Available at <http://www.tikkun.org/article.php/Meninger-Whyunconditionalforgiveness/print>, accessed 30 June 2011.

Midgley, M (1994) 'Duties concerning islands', in P Singer (ed) *Ethics*. (Oxford Readers). New York: Oxford University Press, 367–73.

Miller, KE and Rasmussen, A (2010) 'Mental health and armed conflict: the importance of distinguishing between war exposure and other sources of adversity: a response to Neuner', *Social Science and Medicine*, 71, 1385–89.

Miller-Idriss, C (2009) *Blood and culture: youth, right-wing extremism and national belonging in contemporary Germany*. Durham, NC and London: Duke University Press.

Minow, M (1998) *Between vengeance and forgiveness: Facing history after genocide and mass violence*. Boston: Beacon.

Moreno-Riaño, G (2001) 'The Etiology of Administrative Evil: Eric Voegelin and the Unconsciousness of Modernity', *The American Review of Public Administration*, 31, 296.

Moses, AD (2007) *German intellectuals and the Nazi past*. New York: Cambridge University Press.

Müller-Hill, B (2007) 'The Silence of the Scholars', in WR Lafleur, G Böhme, and S Shimazono (eds) *Dark Medicine: rationalising unethical medical research*. Bloomington: Indiana University Press, 57–62.

Mullet, E, Neto, F, and Pinto, M (2008) 'What can Reasonably be Expected from a Truth Commission: A Preliminary Examination of East Timorese Views', *Peace and Conflict: Journal of Peace Psychology*, 14(4), 369–93.

Muntaner, C, Borrell, C, and Chung, H (2008) 'Class exploitation and psychiatric disorders: from status syndrome to capitalist syndrome', in CI Cohen and S Timimi (eds) *Liberatory Psychiatry: philosophy, politics and mental health*. Cambridge: Cambridge University Press, 131–46.

Nussbaum, M (2006) *Frontiers of justice: disability, nationality, species membership*. Boston and London: Belknap (Harvard University Press).

Ogino, M (2007) 'Eugenics, reproductive technologies, and the feminist dilemma', in WR Lafleur, G Böhme, and S Shimazono (eds) *Dark Medicine: rationalising unethical medical research*. Bloomington: Indiana University Press, 223–32.

Oliner, SP and Oliner, PM (1988) *The altruistic personality: rescuers of Jews in Nazi Europe*. New York: Free Press.

Parmar, S, Roseman, MJ, Siegrist, S, and Sowa, T (eds) *Children and Transitional Justice: Truth-Telling, Accountability and Reconciliation*. Human Rights Program, Harvard Law School (United Nations Children's Fund (UNICEF)). Available at <http://www.unicef-irc.org/publications/series/17/>, accessed 30 June 2011.

Patel, V and Prince, M (2010) 'Global mental health: a new global health field comes of age', *JAMA* 303(19), (May 19), 1976–77.

Pedersen, A, Walker, I, Rapley, M, and Wise, M (2003) *Anti-racism: What works. An evaluation of the effectiveness of anti-racist strategies*. Murdoch University, WA: SSHE Research (Social Change and Equity). Available at <http://www.omi.wa.gov.au/resources/clearinghouse/antiracism_what_works.pdf>, accessed 8 November 2011.

Pellegrino, E and Relman, AS (1999) 'Professional medical associations: ethical and practical guidelines', *Journal of the American Medical Association*, 282, 984–86.

Phillips, A and Taylor, B (2009) *On kindness*. London: Penguin.

Pikas, A (1989) 'The common concern method for the treatment of mobbing', in E Roland and E Munthe (eds) *Bullying, an international perspective*. London: Fulton, 195–202.

Pray, L (2008) 'Embryo screening and the ethics of human genetic engineering', *Nature Education*, 1(1). Available at <http://www.nature.com/scitable/topicpage/Embryo-Screening-and-the-Ethics-of-60561>, accessed 2 April 2010.

Prilleltensky, I, Prilleltensky, O, and Voorhees, C (2008) 'Psychopolitical validity in the helping professions: applications to research interventions, case conceptualisation and therapy', in CI Cohen and S Timimi (eds) *Liberatory Psychiatry: philosophy, politics and mental health*. Cambridge: Cambridge University Press, 105–30.

Rawls, J (1972) *A theory of justice*. Cambridge, MA: Harvard University Press.

Ridley, M (1996) *The origins of virtue*. London: Viking (Penguin), Chapter 3 (51–66).

Robertson, G (2006) *Crimes against Humanity: the struggle for global justice*. 3rd edn. Melbourne: Penguin.

Robertson, M (2007) 'Psychiatrists and social justice: the concept of justice. (Part I)', *Journal of Ethics in Mental Health*, 2(2), 1–4.

Robertson, M, Kerridge, I, and Walter, G (2009) 'Ethnomethodological study of the values of Australian psychiatrists: towards an empirically derived code of ethics', *Australian and New Zealand Journal of Psychiatry*, 43, 409–419.

Rose, DB (2004) *Reports from the wild country: ethics for decolonisation*. Sydney: University of New South Wales Press.

Sabin, JE and Daniels, N (2009) 'Allocation of mental health resources', in S Bloch and S Green (eds) *Psychiatric ethics*. 4th edn. Oxford: Oxford University Press, 111–26.

Sacks, J (2003) *The dignity of difference: how to avoid the clash of civilisations*. Revised edn. London: Continuum.

Sadavoy, J (1997) 'Survivors: A review of the late-life effects of prior psychological trauma', *American Journal of Geriatric Psychiatry*, 5, 287–301.

Saraceno, B, van Ommeren, M, Batniji, R, Cohen, A, Gureje, O, Mahoney, J, Sridhar, D, and Underhill, C (2007) 'Barriers to improvement of mental health services in low-income and middle-income countries', *The Lancet*, 370, 1164–74.

Schlink, B (2009) *Guilt about the past*. St Lucia, Qld: University of Queensland Press.

Schmidt, U (2004, 2nd edn 2006) *Justice at Nuremberg: Leo Alexander and the Nazi Doctors' Trial*. Basingstoke, UK: Palgrave Macmillan.

Segal, SP and Burgess, PM (2008) 'Use of community treatment orders to prevent psychiatric hospitalisation', *Australian and New Zealand Journal of Psychiatry*, 42, 732–39.

Shimazono, S (2007) 'Why we must be prudent in research using human embryos', in WR Lafleur, G Böhme,and S Shimazono (eds) *Dark Medicine: rationalising unethical medical research*. Bloomington: Indiana University Press, 201–22.

Silove, D, Zwi, AB, and Le Touze, D (2006) 'Do truth commissions heal? The East Timor experience', *The Lancet*, 367, 1222–24.

Simmons, D (2008) 'Genetic inequality: Human genetic engineering', *Nature Education*, 1(1). Available at <http://www.nature.com/scitable/topicpage/Genetic-Inequality-Human-Genetic-Engineering-768>, accessed 2 April 2010.

Singh, SP and Fisher, HL (2005) 'Early intervention in psychosis: obstacles and opportunities', *Advances in Psychiatric Treatment*, 11, 71–78.

Slade T, Johnston A, Oakley-Browne MA, Andrews G, Whiteford H (2009) '2007 National Survey of Mental Health and Wellbeing: methods and key findings', *Australian and New Zealand Journal of Psychiatry*, 43(7), 594–605.

Smith, Alison (2010) 'Basic assumptions of transitional justice and children', in S Parmar, MJ Roseman, S Siegrist, and T Sowa (eds) *Children and Transitional Justice: Truth-Telling, Accountability and Reconciliation*. Human Rights Program, Harvard Law School (United Nations Children's Fund (UNICEF)), 31–65. Available at <http://www.unicef-irc.org/publications/series/17/>, accessed 30 June 2011.

Spitz, D (2006) 'How much truth and how much reconciliation? Intrapsychic, interpersonal and social aspects of resolution', in NN Potter (ed) *Trauma, truth and reconciliation: healing damaged relationships*. New York: Oxford University Press, 127–38.

Staub, E (1989) *The roots of evil: the origins of genocide and other group violence*. New York: Cambridge University Press.

Staub, E (2003) *The psychology of good and evil: why children, adults and groups help and harm others*. Cambridge, UK: Cambridge University Press.

Staub, E (2007) 'Preventing violence and terrorism and promoting positive relations between Dutch and Muslim communities in Amsterdam', *Peace and Conflict: Journal of Peace Psychology*, 13(3), 333–60.

Staub, E, Pearlman, LA, Gubin, A, and Hagengimana, A (2005) 'Healing, reconciliation, forgiving and the prevention of violence after genocide or mass killing: an intervention and its experimental evaluation in Rwanda', *Journal of Social and Clinical Psychology*, 24(3), 297–334.

Stein, DJ, Seedat, S, Kaminer, D, Moomal, H, Herman, A, Sonnega, J, and Williams, DR (2008) 'The impact of the Truth and Reconciliation Commission on psychological distress and forgiveness in South Africa', *Social Psychiatry and Psychiatric Epidemiology*, 43(6), 462–8.

Thornicroft, G (2006) *Shunned: Discrimination against People with Mental Illness*. Oxford: Oxford University Press.

UNICEF Innocenti Research Centre (2011) *Children's truth commissions*. UNICEF Innocenti Research Centre. Available at <http://www.unicef-irc.org/publications/series>, accessed 30 June 2011.

Veale, A and Stavrou, A (2007) 'Former Lord's Resistance Army Child Soldier Abductees: Explorations of Identity in Reintegration and Reconciliation', *Peace and Conflict: Journal of Peace Psychology*, 13(3), 273–92.

Verhagen, P (2006) 'Forgiveness: a critical appraisal', in NN Potter (ed) *Trauma, truth and reconciliation: healing damaged relationships*. New York: Oxford University Press, 203–27.

Warner, R (2010) 'Does the scientific evidence support the recovery model?', *The Psychiatrist*, 34, 3–5.

Weindling, PJ (2006) *Nazi medicine and Nuremberg trials: from medical war crimes to informed consent.* Basingstoke, UK: Palgrave Macmillan.

Wertz, DC, Fletcher, JC, and Berg, K (1993) *Guidelines on ethical issues in medical genetics and the provision of genetic services.* Geneva: World Health Organization.

Whiting, B and Whiting, JWM (1975) *Children of six cultures.* Cambridge, MA: Harvard University Press.

World Health Organization (2005) *WHO Resource Book on Mental Health, Human Rights and Legislation.* Geneva: World Health Organization.

World Psychiatric Association (2005) Madrid Declaration on Ethical Standards for Psychiatric Practice. Available at World Psychiatric Association > About WPA > Consensus Statements and Declarations > Declarations on Ethical Standards. Amended September 2005. <http://www.wpanet.org/detail.php?section_id=5&content_id=31>, accessed 5 January 2011.

Yamaori, T (2007) 'Strategies for survival versus accepting impermanence: rationalizing brain death and organ transplantation today', in WR Lafleur, G Böhme, and S Shimazono (eds) *Dark Medicine: rationalising unethical medical research.* Bloomington: Indiana University Press, 165–79.

Zachar, P (2006) 'Reconciliation as compromise and the management of rage', in NN Potter (ed) *Trauma, truth and reconciliation: healing damaged relationships.* New York: Oxford University Press, 67–81.

Zimbardo, P (2007) *The Lucifer effect: how good people turn evil.* London: Rider.

Zion, D, Briskman, L, and Loff, B (2012) 'Psychiatric ethics and a politics of compassion: the case of detained asylum seekers in Australia', *Journal of Bioethical Inquiry*, 9(1), 67–75.

Part 5

Towards the Future

Afterword: Global Mental Health and Human Rights: Barriers and Opportunities

Norman Sartorius

The remarkable group of experts—leaders in the field of psychiatry, behavioural sciences, ethics, philosophy, and legislation—whom Michael Dudley, Derrick Silove, and Fran Gale have brought together produced chapters rich in evidence as well as in experience and hopes about the protection of human rights in relation to illness. Some of the contributions before us are particularly relevant for the care of people with mental illness, others have a wider focus, embracing human rights issues related to other diseases, to research, education, and policy-making.

The wealth of information that has been assembled presents a platform on which it should be possible to fight for the rights of the mentally ill. At present, most planks of that platform are either demonstrations that there is much abuse of the human rights of the people with mental illness (in the process of mental health care, in daily life, in psychiatric research, in the management of co-morbid physical illness, and in many other situations) or exhortations about the need to ensure that rights be respected. The latter arguments are mainly justified by overarching ethical considerations which, while often accepted in principle, do not necessarily have the power of persuasion that would make those involved change their ways. To use the platform well, to make it help in ensuring that the rights of the people with mental illness are protected, it will be necessary to complement the presentation of these studies by a description in concrete terms of the benefits that the protection of human rights of the mentally ill may bring, in addition to satisfying an ethical demand.

These benefits include, at least: (i) the guarantee that people with mental illness will receive the same amount of care as people who suffer from other illnesses which, in turn, will reduce the length of their illness, diminish the probability that they will remain impaired and disabled after the illness, and reduce the chances that they will die from physical illness at present frequently neglected when occurring in a person with a serious mental disorder; (ii) the confirmation—by the provision of appropriate care to the mentally ill who need it—that the society in which we live is on the way to becoming a civic society in which all have the obligation to help others in need and the right to expect the same amount of help if they were to suffer from a similar condition; (iii) the creation of an antidote to the currently growing epidemic of burn-out in personnel working in mental health institutions who feel that their work is of little significance because it helps people who are of so little value that the society did not even recognize that they have the same rights as any other citizen.

There are two additional points that need to be included in the coda to such an excellent collection of essays. The first concerns the need to add to each chapter and each commentary a 'sunset clause', as is the case for many other texts which are valid for a time, and have to be re-examined at regular intervals. The world is changing very fast and many moral prescriptions or needs clearly present today will be replaced by others, tomorrow. The protection of human rights as a permanent objective may well remain relevant for a long time: but which rights, in which situations, or which people should receive priority? We should ensure that these questions are continually reviewed and perhaps urge governments to establish Standing Human Rights Committees that would identify what needs changing. While governments are considering the establishment of such committees, it will be important to assign the role of the standing commit-tees to professional associations, patient and family organizations, and others who might help in keeping the effort well-focused and useful; a second revised edition of this book should already today be on the calendar of Dr Dudley and his colleagues, perhaps for the year 2015.

The second point that the coda should include is that of hope that the difficulties and non-observance of human rights described in this book will move people in power and all others to fight for the protection of human rights and to make this fight central to their activity. Having defined what needs to be done is not enough: we should each look in our own field of action and apply the principles and desiderata described in this book in our daily work, our publications, our education of others, and in the orientation of our research.

Author Index

Note: 'n.' after a page number indicates a footnote on that page.

Subject Index

Note: 'n.' after a page number indicates a footnote on that page.

7382

law and legislation (*cont.*)
   and human rights 297, 299–300
   intellectual disabilities 467–72
   lived experience in Australia 376–7, 380
   older people 490, 493
   participation in reforms 585–97
   poorly resourced settings, protecting
      rights in 528–31, 536
   severe and persistent 309, 313, 314, 315
  and rights, relationship between 15
  rule of law 56
  standards, human rights 541
  stigma and discrimination 121
  substance abuse 513
  suicide 516
  torture 255, 260–1
League of Nations 61, 189, 451
learned helplessness 182, 227
least restrictive environment principle, civil
   commitment 287
legislation *see* law and legislation
lesbians *see* homosexuality
Levit, V.G. 243
Lewis, Teresa 184
liberalism 12–13, 25, 29
  capabilities 14
  citizenship 77
  development of human rights 57
  group rights 18
Liberia 643
libertarianism 13, 288–9, 300
liberty
  negative v positive 73, 74
  right to 468–9
al-Libi, Ibn al-Shaykh 259, 335
life, right to 467–8
life insurance 126
life-support 191
Like Minds Like Mine campaign 121
Lincoln, Abraham 260
literacy issues 170
lithium 348
Lithuania 520
Litvak, Anatole, *The snake pit* 63
lived experience of mental illness 376–81, 566–8,
   571–2
living wills 309, 315
Living with Memory Loss Program 490
Locke, John 25, 57, 62
London Charter, development of human rights 64
Lorenz, Edward 575
'love failure' 519
low and middle-income countries (LAMICs)
  burden of mental disability 5
  consumers', survivors', and families' voices
   572, 573, 574
  global inequity for mental health 29, 31
  human rights 554
  mental health interventions 7
  population mental health 27
  protecting the rights of the mentally ill in 527–36
  research collaboration 611–21
  resources for mental health 6, 7, 38

loyalty, world 189–90
Lunacy Act (New South Wales, 1878) 376, 377,
   379, 380
Lunatics Detention Act (Gambia, 1917) 583
Lunts, Daniil 246
Luther, Martin 57

Machel, Graça 643
mad movement 567–76
Mad Pride movement 571
Madrid Declaration 27, 34, 237 n. 2, 303
Magna Carta 9, 56
Malaysia 35, 509
Malik, Charles 61
Mann, Jonathan 165
manners, and development of human rights 58–9
Maudsley, Henry 283
Mauritius 543
Maximin Theory 153
McIvor, Trevor 432
Médecins Sans Frontières 388
media 284, 333, 335–6, 36–7, 457, 646
Medical Foundation for the Care of Victims
   of Torture 76
Medical Research Council 355
medical professionals *see* health professionals
medical students 351, 378–9
Medicare (Australia) 377, 490
medication
  coercion 32–3
  consumers', survivors', and families' voices 567, 568,
   569, 571–2, 573–4
  economics of mental health 156
  global inequity 30
  HIV 163, 168, 169
  international dissemination of drugs 40
  lived experience 376, 566, 568, 571–2
  older people with mental illnesses 482, 492
  PTSD 258
  race factors 140
  research collaboration 613
  in secure settings 284, 287
  severe and persistent mental illness 302
  substance abuse 508–9
  women's health 418, 421, 423
Medicines Australia 357, 358
Mehta, Hansa 61, 62
Melbourne, University of 354
MENCAP 473
Mengele, Josef 218
menopause 419
menstruation, onset of 419
Mental Capacity Act (UK, 2005) 288
mental disabilities *see* mental illnesses and disabilities
Mental Disability Advocacy Centre (MDAC) 27, 88,
   88 n. 56, 119, 468, 558
Mental Disability Advocacy Centre (MDAC)
   v Bulgaria 543
Mental Disability Rights International (MDRI, later
   Disability Rights International) 572
Mental Disorders Act (Zambia, 1951) 530–1
mental health, definition 3
Mental Health Act (New South Wales, 1958) 376, 380